SIXTH EDITION

EBERSOLE and HESS'
Gerontological Nursing
& Healthy Aging

Theris A. Touhy, DNP, CNS, DPNAP
Emeritus Professor
Christine E. Lynn College of Nursing
Florida Atlantic University
Boca Raton, Florida

Kathleen Jett, PhD, GNP-BC, DPNAP
Gerontological Nurse Practitioner, Board Certified
Memphis, Tennessee

ELSEVIER

ELSEVIER

3251 Riverport Lane
St. Louis, Missouri 63043

Previous editions copyrighted 2018; 2014, 2010, 2005, and 2001.

Library of Congress Control Number 2020949527

Content Strategist: Sandra Clark
Content Development Manager: Lisa Newton
Content Development Specialist: Sara Hardin
Publishing Services Manager: Shereen Jameel
Project Manager: Rukmani Krishnan
Design Direction: Margaret Reid

Printed in the United States of America

Last digit is the print number: 9   8   7   6   5   4   3   2   1

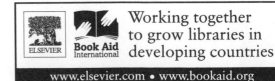

To Danny

You touched our family and so many others in your social work practice with your presence, caring, deep love, and your music. Your gentle spirit lives on.

To all the students who read this book. I hope each of you will improve the journey toward healthy aging through your competence and compassion.

To all of my students who have embraced gerontological nursing as their specialty and are improving the lives of older adults through their practice and teaching.

To the older adults I have been privileged to nurse, and their caregivers, thank you for making the words in this book a reality through your caring and for teaching me how to be a gerontological nurse.

Theris Touhy

To my husband, Steve, and our wonderful children and grandchildren, who never cease to remind me that the best parts of life are in the adventures we share.

To Dr. Michael Johnson, who is a never-ending guide in pathfinding through chaos.

And to the persons around me who teach me both the challenges and opportunities of aging with grace and dignity.

Kathleen Jett

REVIEWERS AND EVOLVE WRITERS

REVIEWERS

Linda Gambill, RN, MSN/Ed
Practical Nursing Program Director
Assistant Professor
Practical Nursing/Health Technologies Division
Southwest Virginia Community College
Cedar Bluff, Virginia

Catherine Graeve, PhD, MPH, BSN
Associate Professor of Nursing
St Catherine University
St Paul, Minnesota

Linda Henningsen, MSN, MS, RN
Assistant Professor of Nursing
Department of Nursing Education
Kansas Wesleyan University
Salina, Kansas

Rebekah Mullins, RN, BSN, MSN
Nursing Instructor
Abilene Christian University
Abilene, Texas

Victoria Alaina Schad, RN, MSN-BC Gerontological Nursing
Professor of Nursing Practice
Utica College
Utica, New York

EVOLVE WRITERS

Charla K. Hollin, RN, BSN
Allied Health Division Chair
University of Arkansas Rich Mountain
Mena, Arkansas

Bethany H. Sykes, EdD MSN, RN
Marco Island, Florida

Linda Turchin, MSN, CNE
Professor Emeritus
Fairmont State University
Fairmont, Wyoming

We are very excited to have been able to offer a timely and completely revised 6th edition of this text guided by the National Council of State Boards of Nursing (NCSBN) new model of clinical judgment. The NCSBN has identified the need to enhance the clinical judgment skills of entry-level nurses and in a few years, the Next Generation NCLEX® Examination for nursing licensure will be based on the new model of clinical judgment. Using the NCSBN Clinical Judgment Measurement and Action Model, our emphasis is on use of the six cognitive skills identified as essential for nurses to make appropriate clinical judgment in care of older adults: Recognize cues; Analyze Cues, Prioritize Hypotheses, Generate Solutions, Take Action; Evaluate Outcomes.

The model is especially relevant to guide the design of nursing actions in care of older adults. Older adults are complex and their responses to illness are often subtle and may not meet standard diagnostic criteria seen in younger individuals. Cues to impending health concerns are often missed or blamed on age, leading to unnecessary disability, complications, and quality of life issues. Nurses are key to recognizing and analyzing cues leading to the prioritization of hypotheses needed to generate solutions, taking action and evaluating outcomes leading to the healthiest aging while dealing with the most common challenges facing an aging population. The text provides the comprehensive information to guide the development of competent clinical judgment in nursing practice with older adults across the continuum of care.

We have held true to our belief that gerontological nursing is a part of the practice of nurses in all fields. In 2020, up to 75% of nurses' time was spent with older adults, and every older person should expect care provided by nurses with competence in gerontological nursing. We continue with our use of a holistic framework to address the needs of the body, mind, and spirit along a continuum of wellness, and grounded in caring and respect for the person as an individual with worth and dignity. The text begins with an introduction to gerontological nursing and provides nurses, faculty, and students with the basic but key information needed to promote heathy outcomes in persons as they age.

We draw on the most current evidence-based information whenever it is available. As in the fifth edition, all content has been updated and is consistent with the *Recommended baccalaureate competencies and curricular guidelines for the nursing care of older adults* developed by the AACN in collaboration with the John A. Hartford Foundation Institute for Geriatric Nursing at New York University. At the time of the writing the 2030 revisions to *Healthy People 2020* were not available, but references to goals relevant to older adults found in the 2020 edition remain.

We have written this to be used in all courses, to provide more expansive coverage than in the brief discussions of aging usually found at the end of many text chapters. In this way it is complementary to any other text and provides more thorough information essential when caring for older adults. It is especially directed to the needs of the undergraduate student in both associate and bachelor's degree programs. For faculty considering a text for use in master's and doctoral programs, we refer you to our sister text, *Toward healthy aging*.

We have divided the chapters into five sections that build on one another. Section 1, **Foundations of Healthy Aging**, presents key elements that provide the background—in other words, context—to all other sections. In Section 2, **Foundations of Gerontological Nursing**, gerontological nursing care across the continuum of settings and economic and common legal issues faced by nurses are addressed. Section 3, **Fundamentals of Caring**, provides in-depth coverage of cues that may indicate and affect functional abilities and presents nursing and interprofessional actions to enhance wellness and prevent unnecessary morbidity and mortality. Many of these topical areas are part of what are referred to as "geriatric syndromes." All have the potential to significantly impact on the quality of life while aging. Section 4, **Promoting Health in Chronic Illness**, presents a number of the most common disease processes. They are so common that they are referred to as "age-related disorders" in some of the geriatric literature and are thought to be explained, in part, by the extant biological theories of aging. Nonetheless, they are still not considered "normal changes with aging." The chapters are brief, and content is pointedly directed at how the normal changes with aging (Chapter 4) influence the cues observed, the priority of the hypotheses, and the nursing actions required to move toward outcomes reflecting healthy aging. The content is designed to enhance that found in physiology texts. Finally, Section 5, **Caring for Older Adults and Their Caregivers**, addresses circumstances of living, loss, dying, and aging within social and cultural spheres and issues that often affect older adults and their families/significant others. Content includes care of older adults with neurocognitive disorders, late life transitions such as retirement, relationships in later life, loss of spouse/life partner, sexuality, caregiving, and promotion of healthy aging when experiencing loss, dying, death, and palliative care.

The text is organized in a way that we hope optimizes student learning. Each chapter begins with the phenomenological consideration of the lived experience of an elder. The chapters end with key concepts, learning activities, and discussion questions to stimulate further educational growth. Selected chapters include Next-Generation NCLEX® Examination-style Questions. Where appropriate, the cues necessary for clinical judgment to address healthy aging are provided. For readers who wish to seek additional information, resources are provided at http://evolve.elsevier.com/Touhy/gerontological.

Gerontological nurses have always assumed a leadership role in improving care for older adults and promoting healthy aging. Since the first edition of this text, there has been an explosion, not only of persons in later life, but also of knowledge, research, interest, and resources in gerontological nursing. Today the expectation is that all nurses will be prepared to provide culturally proficient care for the growing number of diverse older adults all over the globe and have the knowledge and skills to promote healthy aging for people of all ages. We can look forward to the coming years when aging in health will be the norm, and we hope this text will provide the knowledge nurses need to play a key role in making this happen.

ANCILLARIES

Ancillaries are available at http://evolve.elsevier.com/Touhy/gerontological.

For Instructors

- **TEACH for Nurses Lesson Plans:** Detailed listing of resources available to instructors for each book chapter include learning objectives; key terms; student and instructor resources; suggested classroom activities; answers to Critical Thinking Activities in the book; and clinical activities that can be used for classroom discussion, projects, and further study. Also included is an outline of nursing curriculum standards for each chapter that includes QSEN, Concepts, and BSN Essentials, and a unique Case Study for each book chapter.
- **PowerPoint Presentations:** Lecture slides to accompany each chapter (approximately 750 slides total)
- **Answers to Activities and Discussion Questions:** Solutions to the questions that appear at the end of each chapter.
- **Test Bank:** Approximately 500 questions in the latest NCLEX® examination format
- **Next-Generation NCLEX® (NGN)–Style Case Studies for Gerontological Nursing:** Six NGN-style case studies focused on using clinical in care of older adults.
- **Image Collection:** Over 75 illustrations and photos that can be used in a presentation or as visual aids

For Students

- **NCLEX®-Style Review Questions:** Questions organized by chapter for additional help in preparing for the NCLEX® examination
- **Case Studies:** Accompanying select chapters, these provide short case studies with questions to help students see content put into practical use

ACKNOWLEDGMENTS

We would like to thank Priscilla Ebersole and Patricia Hess, the creators of the first edition of this book, for their trust in providing us the opportunity to continue their legacies as we share their beautiful words and passion for gerontological nursing. We hope that our work honors them and the specialty we all love. It has been a real privilege for us to be a part of the work of two gerontological nurses from whom we have learned to care.

We would also like to thank the people at Elsevier who helped produce this book, including Sandy Clark and Sara Hardin.

Theris A. Touhy
Kathleen Jett

CONTENTS

Gerontological Nursing and Promotion of Healthy Aging

Theris A. Touhy

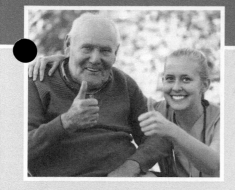

THE LIVED EXPERIENCE

I don't think I will work in gerontological nursing; it seems depressing. I don't know many older adults, but they are all sick without much hope to get better. I'll probably go into labor and delivery or the emergency room where I can really make a difference.

Student Nurse, age 24

Because geriatric nursing especially offers nurses the unique opportunity to dramatically impact people's lives for the better and for the worst, it demands the best that you have to offer. I am very optimistic about the future of geriatric nursing. Increasing numbers of older adults are interested in marching into old age as healthy and involved. Geriatric nursing offers a unique opportunity to help older adults meet these aspirations while at the same time maintaining a commitment to the oldest and frailest in our society.

Mathy Mezey, Professor Emeritus and Retired Founding Director, The Hartford Institute for Geriatric Nursing, New York University College of Nursing (Ebersole & Touhy, 2006, p. 142)

CARE OF OLDER ADULTS: A NURSING IMPERATIVE

Healthy aging is now an achievable goal for many. It is essential that nurses have the knowledge and skills to help people of all ages, races, and cultures to achieve this goal. Older adults today are healthier, better educated, and expect a much higher quality of life as they age than did earlier generations. Enhancing health in aging requires attention to health throughout life, as well as expert care from nurses. Most nurses care for older adults during the course of their careers, and it is estimated that up to 75% of nurses' time is spent with older adults. In addition, the public will look to nurses to have the knowledge and skills to assist people to age in health. Every older adult should expect care provided by nurses with competence in gerontological nursing. Knowledge of aging and gerontological nursing is core knowledge for the profession of nursing.

The terms *geriatric nursing* and *gerontological nursing* are both used in the literature and in practice to describe the specialty of caring for older adults. While both terms are used in the text, we prefer gerontological nursing because this reflects a more holistic approach encompassing both health and illness.

Who Will Care for an Aging Society?

By 2040, the number of older adults in the world will be at least 1.3 billion. It is a critical health and societal concern that gerontological nurses, other health professionals, and direct care workers are prepared to deliver care in all settings across the globe. The aging workforce is in short supply in most of the developed world, and the increased aging population is posing challenges for many countries to meet the expanding need for care services for older adults. The developing countries are experiencing the most rapid growth in numbers of older adults and at the same time lack systems of care and services.

The geriatric workforce shortage also presents a looming crisis for the 43.5 million unpaid family caregivers providing care for someone 55 years or older. Without improvement in the eldercare workforce, even more stress will be placed on family and other informal caregivers. With smaller family sizes, the rising divorce rate, and the increase in geographical relocation, the next generation of older adults may be less able to rely on families for caregiving (Chapter 26). Will there be enough care workers to assist families in the care of loved ones? *Healthy People 2020* (US Department of Health and Human Services, 2012) includes goals related to geriatric education (Box 1.1).

In the United States, care of older adults is projected to be the fastest-growing employment sector in health

care. In spite of demand, the number of health care workers who are interested and prepared to care for older adults remains low (Institute of Medicine [IOM], 2008). Less than 1% of registered nurses and less than 3% of advanced practice nurses (APNs) are certified in geriatrics. "We do not have anywhere close to the number of nurses we need who are prepared in geriatrics, whether in the field of primary care, acute care, nursing home care, or in-home care" (Christine Kovner, RN, PhD, FAAN, as cited in Robert Wood Johnson Foundation, 2012).

Geriatric medicine faces similar challenges, with about 7000 prepared geriatricians, 1 for every 2546 older Americans—and this number is falling, with the trend predicted to be less than 5000 by 2040 (IOM, 2008). Less than 3% of medical students chose to take geriatric electives (Campaign for Action, 2016). Other professions such as social work, physical therapy, and psychiatry have similar shortages. It is estimated that by 2030, nearly 3 million additional health care professionals and direct care workers will be needed to meet the care needs of a growing older adult population.

HISTORY OF GERONTOLOGICAL NURSING

Historically, nurses have always been on the front line of caring for older adults. They have provided hands-on care, supervision, administration, program development, teaching, and research and are, to a great extent, responsible for the rapid advancement of gerontology as a profession. Gerontological nurses have made substantial contributions to the body of knowledge guiding best practice in the care of older adults. Nurses have been, and continue to be, the mainstay of care of older adults (Mezey & Fulmer, 2002).

Gerontological nursing has emerged as a circumscribed area of practice only within the past six decades. Before 1950, gerontological nursing was seen as the application of general principles of nursing to older adults with little recognition of this area of nursing as a specialty similar to obstetric, pediatric, or surgical nursing. Whereas most specialties in nursing developed from those identified in medicine, this was not the case with gerontological nursing because health care of the older adult was traditionally considered within the domain of nursing.

The foundation of gerontological nursing as we know it today was built largely by a small cadre of nurse pioneers, many of whom are now deceased. The specialty was defined and shaped by those innovative nurses who saw, early on, that older adults had special needs and required the most subtle, holistic, and complex nursing care. This history is similar to the development

BOX 1.1 **Healthy People 2020**

Older Adults

- Increase the proportion of the health care workforce with geriatric certification (physicians, geriatric psychiatrists, registered nurses, dentists, physical therapists, dietitians)

From US Department of Health and Human Services, Office of Disease Prevention and Health Promotion. (2012). *Healthy people 2020.* http://www.healthypeople.gov/2020.

of pediatric nursing and the recognition that pediatric nursing is "not med-surg nursing on little people" (Taylor, 2006, p. E128) and that nurses needed special skills to care for children. When examining the history of gerontological nursing, we must marvel at the advocacy and perseverance of nurses who have remained committed to improving the care of older adults despite struggling against great odds over the years. Box 1.2 presents the views of some of the geriatric nursing pioneers, as well as those of current leaders, on the practice of gerontological nursing and the reasons they are attracted to this specialty.

Nursing was the first of the professions to develop standards of gerontological care and the first to provide a certification mechanism to ensure specific professional expertise through credentialing. The most recent edition of *Gerontological Nursing: Scope and Standards of Practice* (American Nurses Association [ANA], 2018) provides a comprehensive overview of the scope of gerontological nursing, the skills and knowledge required to address the full range of needs related to the process of aging, and the specialized care of older adults as a group and as individuals. The document also identifies levels of gerontological nursing practice (basic and advanced) and standards of clinical gerontological nursing care and gerontological nursing performance.

Current Initiatives

The most significant influence in enhancing the specialty of gerontological nursing has been the work of The Hartford Institute for Geriatric Nursing, established in 1996 and funded by the John A. Hartford Foundation. Initiatives in nursing education, nursing practice, nursing research, and nursing policy include enhancement of geriatrics in nursing education programs through curricular reform and faculty development, creation of the National Hartford Centers of Gerontological Nursing Excellence, predoctoral and postdoctoral scholarships for study and research in geriatric nursing, and clinical practice improvement projects to enhance care for older adults (http://www.hartfordign.org).

The National Hartford Center of Gerontological Nursing Excellence offers a Distinguished Educator in Gerontological Nursing Program as well as Leadership Conferences on Aging. Another resource is Sigma Theta Tau's Center for Nursing Excellence in Long-Term Care, which sponsors the Geriatric Nursing Leadership Academy (GNLA) and offers a range of products and services to support the professional development and leadership growth of nurses who provide care to older adults in long-term care (Box 1.3 provides additional resources).

BOX 1.2 Reflections on Gerontological Nursing From Gerontological Nursing Pioneers and Current Leaders in the Field

Mary Opal Wolanin, Gerontological Nursing Pioneer

"I believe that one of the most valuable lessons I have learned from those who are older is that I must start with looking inside at my own thinking. I was very guilty of ageism. I believed every myth in the book, was sure that I would never live past my seventieth birthday, and made no plan for my seventies. Probably the most productive years of my career have been since that dreaded birthday and I now realize that it is very difficult, if not impossible, to think of our own aging." (From interview data collected by Priscilla Ebersole between 1990 and 2001.)

Terry Fulmer, Dean, College of Nursing, New York University, and Co-Director, John A. Hartford Institute for Geriatric Nursing

"I soon realized that in the arena of caring for the aged, I could have an autonomous nursing practice that would make a real difference in medical outcomes. I could practice the full scope of nursing. It gave me a sense of freedom and accomplishment. With older patients, the most important component of care, by far, is nursing care. It's very motivating." (From Ebersole, P., & Touhy, T. (2006). *Geriatric nursing: Growth of a specialty.* New York: Springer, p. 129.)

Jennifer Lingler, PhD, FNP

"When I was in high school, a nurse I knew helped me find a nursing assistant position at the residential care facility where she worked. That experience sparked my interest in older adults that continues today. I realized that caring for frail elders could be incredibly gratifying and I felt privileged to play a role, however small, in people's lives. At the same time, I became increasingly curious about what it means to age successfully. I questioned why some people seemed to age so gracefully, while others succumbed to physical illness, mental decline, or both.

As a Building Academic Geriatric Nursing Capacity (BAGNC) alumnus, I now divide my time serving as a nurse practitioner at a memory disorders clinic, teaching an ethics course in a gerontology program, and conducting research on family caregiving. I am encouraged by the realization that as current students contemplate the array of opportunities before them, seek counsel from trusted mentors, and gain exposure to various clinical populations, the next generation of geriatric nurses will emerge. And, I am confident that in doing so, they will set their own course for affecting change in the lives of society's most vulnerable members." (Jennifer Lingler as cited in Fagin, C., & Franklin, P. (2005). Why choose geriatric nursing? Six nursing scholars tell their stories. *Imprint* [September/October], p. 74.)

American Nurses Credentialing Center: Nursing Case Management Certification (RN-BC): https://www.nursingworld.org/our-certifications/nursing-case-management/

American Association of Managed Care Nurses: Certification, educational resources

APRN Gerontological Specialist-Certified (GS-C) Exam: https://www.gapna.org/certification

Case Management Society of America: Standards of Practice, certification, educational resources: https://www.cmsa.org/

ConsultGeri.org: The evidence-based geriatric clinical nursing website of The Hartford Institute for Geriatric Nursing, at the NYU College of Nursing. There are also two iPad/iPhone apps that give access to evidence-based information and tools to treat common problems encountered in the care of older adults, including one specific to dementia: (https://itunes.apple.com/us/app/consultgeri-dementia/id962437779 and https://itunes.apple.com/us/app/consultgerirn/id578360141)

Core Competencies for Gerontological Nurse Educators: https://www.nhcgne.org/core-competencies-for-gerontological-nursing-excellence

End of Life Nursing Consortium (ELNEC): Education programs for end of life care: https://www.aacnnursing.org/ELNEC

Hospice and Palliative Nurses Association: Education, research, certification examination (Certified Hospice and Palliative Nurse)

National Hartford Center of Gerontological Nursing Excellence: https://www.nhcgne.org/

National Hospice and Palliative Care Organization: https://www.nhpco.org/

GERONTOLOGICAL NURSING EDUCATION

Essential educational competencies and academic standards for care of older adults have been developed by national organizations such as the American Association of Colleges of Nursing (AACN) for both basic and advanced nursing education. *The Essentials of Baccalaureate Education for Professional Nursing Practice* (AACN, 2008) specifically address the importance of geriatric content and structured clinical experiences with older adults across the continuum in the education of students.

In 2010, AACN and The Hartford Institute for Geriatric Nursing, New York University, published the *Recommended Baccalaureate Competencies and Curricular Guidelines for the Nursing Care of Older Adults,* a supplement to the *Essentials* document. In addition, gerontological nursing competencies for advanced practice graduate programs have also been developed. All of these documents can be accessed from the AACN website. There are also competencies for gerontological nursing

educators published by The National Hartford Center of Gerontological Nursing Excellence (Box 1.3). There has been some improvement in the amount of geriatrics-related content in nursing school curricula, but it is still uneven across schools and hampered by lack of faculty expertise in the subject.

The vast majority of schools have no faculty members certified by the American Nurses Credentialing Center in gerontological nursing. There is a critical need for nurses with master's and doctoral preparation and expertise in the care of older adults to assume faculty roles. Most schools still do not have freestanding courses in the specialty similar to courses in maternal/child or psychiatric nursing. This means that a substantial number of graduating nurses have not had the education needed to competently meet the needs of the burgeoning number of older adults for whom they will care. "In the past, nursing education has been dogged about assuring that every student has the opportunity to attend a birth, but has never insisted that every student have the opportunity to manage a death, even though the vast majority of nurses are more likely to practice with clients who are at the end of life" (AACN, 2007, p. 7). Best practice recommendations for nursing education include provision of a stand-alone course, as well as integration of content throughout the curriculum so that care of older adults is valued and considered an integral part of nursing care.

Curriculum and clinical experiences have to be inspirational, and so do faculty and clinical mentors teaching students. Care of older adults now covers a 50-year age span between the ages of 60 and 110 years and older; therefore practice experiences need to be provided in a variety of settings, including community and long-term care (Kydd et al., 2014). Experience with older adults in the community and opportunities to focus on health promotion should be the first priority for students. This will help them develop more positive attitudes, understand the full scope of nursing practice with older adults, and learn nursing responses to enhance health and wellness. Practice in rehabilitation centers, subacute and skilled nursing facilities, and hospice settings is suited for more advanced students and provides opportunities for leadership experience, nursing management of complex problems, interprofessional teamwork, and research application (Sherman & Touhy, 2017).

ORGANIZATIONS DEVOTED TO GERONTOLOGY RESEARCH AND PRACTICE

The Gerontological Society of America (GSA) demonstrates the need for interdisciplinary collaboration in research and practice. The divisions of Biological

Sciences, Health Sciences, Behavioral and Social Sciences, Social Research, Policy and Practice, and Emerging Scholar and Professional Organization include individuals from myriad backgrounds and disciplines who affiliate with a section based on their particular function rather than their educational or professional credentials. Nurses can be found in all sections and occupy important positions as officers and committee chairs in the GSA.

This mingling of the disciplines based on practice interests is also characteristic of the American Society on Aging (ASA). Other interdisciplinary organizations have joined forces to strengthen the field. The Association for Gerontology in Higher Education (AGHE) has partnered with the GSA, and the National Council on Aging (NCOA) is affiliated with the ASA. These organizations and others have encouraged the blending of ideas and functions, furthering the understanding of aging and the interprofessional collaboration necessary for optimal care. International gerontology associations, such as the International Federation on Aging and the International Association of Gerontology and Geriatrics, also have interdisciplinary membership and offer the opportunity to study aging internationally.

Organizations specific to gerontological nursing include the National Gerontological Nursing Association (NGNA), the Gerontological Advanced Practice Nurses Association (GAPNA), the National Association Directors of Nursing Administration/Long Term Care (NADONA/LTC) (also includes assisted-living RNs and LPNs/LVNs as associate members), the American Association of Directors of Nursing Services (AADNS), American Assisted Living Nurses Association (AALNA), and the Canadian Gerontological Nursing Association (CGNA).

RESEARCH ON AGING

Inquiry into and curiosity about aging is as old as curiosity about life and death itself. Gerontology began as an inquiry into the characteristics of long-lived people, and we are still intrigued by them. Anecdotal evidence was used in the past to illustrate issues assumed to be universal. Only in the past 60 years have serious and carefully controlled research studies on aging flourished.

The impact of disease morbidity and impending death on the quality of life and the experience of aging have provided the impetus for much of the study by gerontologists. Much that has been thought about aging has been found to be erroneous, and early research was conducted with older adults who were ill. As a result, aging has inevitably been seen through the distorted lens of disease. However, we are finally recognizing that

aging and disease are separate entities albeit frequent companions.

Aging has been seen as a biomedical problem that must be reversed, eradicated, or controlled for as long as possible. The trend toward the medicalization of aging has also influenced the general public. The biomedical view of the "problem" of aging is reinforced on all sides. A shift in the view of aging to one that centers on the potential for health, wholeness, and quality of life, and the significant contributions of older adults to society, is increasingly the focus in the research, popular literature, the public portrayal of older adults, and the theme of this text.

The National Institute on Aging (NIA), the National Institute of Nursing Research (NINR), the National Institute of Mental Health (NIMH), and the Agency for Healthcare Research and Quality (AHRQ) continue to make significant research contributions to our understanding of older adults. Research and knowledge about aging are strongly influenced by federal bulletins that are distributed nationwide to indicate the type of research most likely to receive federal funding. These are published in requests for proposals (RFPs). Ongoing and projected budget cuts are of concern in the adequate funding of aging research and services in the United States.

Nursing Research

Nursing research draws from its own body of knowledge, as well as from other disciplines, to describe, monitor, protect, and evaluate the quality of life while aging and the services more commonly provided to the aging population, such as hospice care. Nurses have generated significant research on the care of older adults and have established a solid foundation for the practice of gerontological nursing. Research with older adults receives considerable funding from the National Institute of Nursing Research (NINR), and their website (http://www.ninr.nih.gov) provides information about results of studies and funding opportunities. Gerontological nurse researchers publish in many nursing journals and journals devoted to gerontology, such as *The Gerontologist* and *Journal of Gerontology* (GSA), and there are several gerontological nursing journals including *Journal of Gerontological Nursing, Research in Gerontological Nursing, Geriatric Nursing,* and the *International Journal of Older People Nursing.*

Nursing research has significantly affected the quality of life of older adults and gains more prominence each decade. Federal funding for gerontological nursing research is increasing, and more nurse scholars are studying nursing issues related to older adults. Some of the most important nursing studies have investigated methods of caring for individuals with dementia, reducing falls and the use of restraints, pain management, delirium, care transitions, and end-of-life care.

Knowledge about aging and the experience of aging has changed considerably and will continue to change in the future. Past ideas and current practices will not be acceptable to present and current cohorts of older individuals. Nursing research will continue to examine the best practices for care of older adults who are ill and living in institutions, but increasing emphasis will be placed on strategies to maintain and improve health while aging, especially in light of the increasing numbers of older individuals across the globe. Primary and acute care provided to older adults is an important area of focus that needs attention (Kovach, 2018).

Current research priorities include a focus on community and home-care resources for older adults, an emphasis on family caregiving issues, and a shift from the attention on illness and disease to the expectation of wellness, even in the presence of chronic illness and functional impairment. Improving quality of life for individuals with chronic illness and end-of-life and palliative care are two areas of scientific focus in the National Institute for Nursing Research (NINR) Strategic Plan (2016). Translational research and continued attention to interprofessional studies are increasingly important.

GERONTOLOGICAL NURSING ROLES

Gerontological nursing roles encompass every imaginable venue and circumstance. The opportunities are limitless because we are a rapidly aging society. Specialized knowledge in gerontological nursing is essential for nurses to fulfill these emerging roles. The National Council of State Boards of Nursing has identified the need to enhance the clinical judgment skills of entry-level nurses, and the NCLEX® will be modified toward a greater focus on clinical judgment. Increasing client age and acuity, as well as changes in health care, make this especially important for nurses who care for older adults. Nursing education must ensure that students are assisted to develop the clinical judgment skills necessary to care competently for older adults.

The dearth of content and practice experiences, as well as faculty preparation and interest in care of older adults, makes improvement of clinical judgment skills in care of older adults challenging. Older adults are complex and their responses to illness may not meet standard diagnostic criteria and are often missed, leading to unnecessary disability, complications, and quality-of-life issues. Nurses are key to recognizing and analyzing cues and taking action to improve outcomes of care. The text provides comprehensive information to guide the

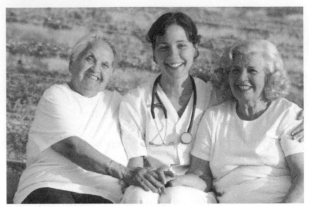

Gerontological nursing is important in this rapidly aging society. (© iStock.com/DianaHirsch.)

development of competent clinical judgment in nursing practice with older adults across the continuum of care.

A gerontological nurse may be a generalist or a specialist. The generalist functions in a variety of settings (primary care, acute care, home care, post-acute and long-term care, and the community) providing nursing care to individuals and their families. National certification as a gerontological nurse is a way of demonstrating special knowledge in care for older adults and should be encouraged (http://www.nursecredentialing .org/GerontologicalNursing).

The gerontological nursing specialist has advanced preparation at the master's level and performs all of the functions of a generalist but has developed advanced clinical expertise, as well as an understanding of health and social policy and proficiency in planning, implementing, and evaluating health programs.

Specialist Roles

Under the Consensus Model for APRN Regulation, advanced practice registered nurses (APRNs) must be educated, certified, and licensed to practice in a role and a population. APRNs are educated in one of four roles, one of which is adult–gerontology. This population focus encompasses individuals from age 13 years (adolescent) to older adults. Titles of APRNs educated and certified across both areas of practice include the following: Adult–Gerontology Acute Care Nurse Practitioner, Adult–Gerontology Primary Care Nurse Practitioner, and Adult–Gerontology Clinical Nurse Specialist. Certification is available for all of these levels of advanced practice; in most states this is a requirement for licensure. The APRN Gerontological Specialist–Certified (GS-C) is also available to APRNs and recognizes expertise at the proficient level in managing complex older adults (Box 1.3).

Advanced practice nurses with certification in adult–gerontology will find a full range of opportunities for collaborative and independent practice both now and in the future. Direct care sites include geriatric and family practice clinics, long-term care, acute care and post-acute care facilities, home health care agencies, hospice agencies, continuing care retirement communities, assisted living facilities, managed care organizations, and specialty care clinics (e.g., Alzheimer's disease, heart failure, diabetes). Gerontological nursing specialists are also involved with community agencies such as local Area Agencies on Aging, public health departments, and national and worldwide organizations such as the Centers for Disease Control and the World Health Organization. They function as care managers, eldercare consultants, educators, and clinicians.

One of the most important advanced practice nursing roles that emerged over the last 40 years is that of the gerontological nurse practitioner (GNP) and the gerontological clinical nurse specialist (GCNS) in skilled nursing facilities. Nurse practitioners have been providing care in nursing homes in the United States since the 1970s, in Canada since 2000, and only recently in the United Kingdom. Recommendations from expert groups in the United States and Canada have called for a nurse practitioner in every nursing home; however, numbers remain small and there is a need for continued attention at the policy and funding level for increased use of nurse practitioners in LTC settings (Harrington et al., 2000; Ploeg et al., 2013). This role is well established, and there is strong research to support the impact of advanced practice nurses working in LTC settings (Campbell et al., 2019, 2020; Dwyer et al., 2017; Mellilo et al., 2015; Oliver et al., 2014; Ploeg et al., 2013) (Box 1.4).

An encouraging trend is that the number of doctors and advanced practitioners in the United States who focus on nursing home care (skilled nursing facility providers: SNFs) rose by more than a third between 2012 and 2015. This suggests the rise of a significant new specialty in medical and nursing practice that will affect patient outcomes. It is very important that these providers have competency in geriatric care, since most do not have educational preparation in the specialty. The Society for Post–Acute and Long-Term Medicine provides educational programs (Morley, 2017).

Generalist Roles

Acute Care

Older adults often enter the health care system with admissions to acute care settings. Older adults comprise 60% of the medical–surgical patients and 46% of the critical care patients. Acutely ill older adults frequently

---

> **BOX 1.4 Outcomes of APNs Working in LTC Settings**
>
> - Improvement in or reduced rate of decline in incontinence, pressure injuries, aggressive behavior, and loss of affect in cognitively impaired residents
> - Lower use of restraints with no increase in staffing, psychoactive drug use, or serious fall-related injuries
> - Improved or slower decline in some health status indicators including depression
> - Improvements in meeting personal goals
> - Lower hospitalization rates and costs
> - Fewer ED visits and costs
> - Improved satisfaction with care

Data from Ploeg J., Kaasalainen S., McAiney C., et al. (2013). Resident and family perceptions of the nurse practitioner role in long term care settings, *BMC Nurs 12*(1):24; Campbell T, Bayly M, Peacock S. (2019). Provision of resident-centered care by nurse practitioners in Saskatchewan long-term care facilities: Qualitative findings from a mixed methods study. *Res in Geron Nurs 6*, 1–9.

---

have multiple chronic conditions and comorbidities and present many challenges. Others appear in the emergency department after falls or suffering from cardiovascular conditions or infection (Cowan-Lincoln, 2015). Hospitals can be dangerous for older adults.

In spite of almost two decades of research to counter harmful iatrogenic problems, iatrogenic complications occur in as many as 29% to 38% of hospitalized older adults, a rate three to five times higher than that seen in younger patients (Inouye et al., 2000; Parke & Hunter, 2014). Older adults may be admitted for heart failure or pneumonia and, during their stay, their condition improves; however, the person who came in walking and able to perform activities of daily living on their own often leaves unable to function (Box 1.5). In most cases, iatrogenic complications could be prevented (Sourdet et al., 2015).

Common iatrogenic complications associated with hospitalization include functional decline, pneumonia, delirium, new-onset incontinence, malnutrition, pressure injuries, medication reactions, and falls. Many of these are geriatric syndromes that require prevention and treatment to prevent untoward consequences for older adults. The geriatric syndromes (also called geriatric giants) are discussed in Chapters 8, 10–15, and 25. Recognizing the impact of iatrogenesis, both on patient outcomes and on the cost of care, the Centers for Medicare and Medicaid Services (CMS) has instituted changes that will reduce payment to hospitals relative to these often preventable outcomes (https://www.cms.gov/medicare/medicare-fee-for-service-payment

BOX 1.5 Example: The Spiral of Iatrogenesis

An 84-year-old man lives alone and has no family. He has osteoarthritis, hypertension, and wears bilateral hearing aids and glasses for reading. He is independent in ADLs and IADLs and takes care of his small home. He avidly reads the newspaper, watches sports, drives, and participates in a water aerobics class at the local YMCA. He is admitted to the hospital following a fall on the sidewalk in front of his home. Neighbors called an ambulance and he was admitted through the emergency department (ED). X-ray examination revealed no fracture but he has pain in the left leg and in his back. Unfortunately, he was not wearing his hearing aids when he was admitted, and communication has therefore been problematic. He often appears distracted and does not always respond readily. He was unable to participate in the brief cognitive assessment and has been labeled confused on the chart.

He has been agitated at night and not sleeping, and a benzodiazepine was therefore ordered. An indwelling catheter was inserted in the ED, and he is being given narcotics for pain. Oral intake is poor, and he has not had a bowel movement in the 3 days post admission. He has been maintained on bedrest and identified as a high fall risk. When the catheter is removed, he is unable to hold his urine and is placed in adult briefs. His mental status has deteriorated further, he is dehydrated, in a negative caloric balance, incontinent, and constipated. He is unable to ambulate and is considered unsafe to return home, and discharge plans are therefore being made for an assisted living facility.

/hospitalacqcond/hospital-acquired_conditions.html). The changes target hospital-acquired conditions (HACs) that are high cost or high volume, result in a higher payment when present as a secondary diagnosis, are not present on admission, and could have reasonably been prevented through the use of evidence-based guidelines. Targeted conditions include several of the common geriatric syndromes such as catheter-associated urinary tract infections, pressure injuries, and falls.

To improve acute care of older adults, it is essential that all health care professionals (hospitalists, primary care providers, members of the interprofessional team, and nurses) are knowledgeable about care of older adults. "Acute care nursing specialty knowledge alone is not enough to ensure quality hospital care for older adults. Important nursing care interventions are overlooked when gerontological expertise is absent from medical and surgical inpatient units. Acute care nursing of older adults must reflect a sense of responsibility for functional outcomes, not just carrying out interventions associated with biomedical concerns. Nursing care of hospitalized older adults requires integration of acute care specialty knowledge with gerontological nursing knowledge and skill" (Parke & Hunter, 2014, pp. 1574, 1579).

Roles for nurses caring for older adults in hospitals include direct care provider, care manager, discharge planner, care coordinator, transitional care, and leadership and management positions. Many acute care hospitals are adopting new models of geriatric and chronic care to meet the needs of older adults and maintain cognitive and physical function when hospitalized. These include geriatric emergency departments and specialized units such as acute care for the elderly (ACE), geriatric evaluation and management units (GEMs), and transitional care programs. These new models of care have been successful in coordinating care, maintaining physical and cognitive function, preventing iatrogenesis, and reducing the risk of delirium (Chapter 25).

ACE units are distinct areas of a hospital specifically designed to reduce the incidence of functional disability of older adults occurring during hospitalization for acute medical illness (Palmer, 2018) by proactively identifying and managing geriatric syndromes to help maintain the patient's function (Box 1.6). Three randomized clinical trials and systematic review of ACE or related interventions demonstrate reduced functional disability, reduced risk of nursing home admission, and lower costs of hospitalizations. ACE principles could improve care of older adults in any acute setting, and future designs of medical units for adults should resemble the ACE unit (Palmer, 2018).

Other initiatives include The Nurses Improving Care for Healthsystem Elders (NICHE), a program

BOX 1.6 Characteristics of ACE units

- Patient-centered as opposed to disease-centered care
- Comprehensive geriatric assessment with emphasis on functional abilities
- Transition planning from beginning of a patient's stay
- Involvement of patient and all caregivers from physicians to family in care planning
- Interdisciplinary teams (geriatrician, nurse coordinator, nurses, physical and occupational therapists, pharmacists, dieticians, social workers) making daily rounds
- Environmental modifications such as handrails in patients' rooms, bathrooms, hallways; contrasting colors to aid people with vision loss and other safety features
- Promotion of self-care activities
- Homelike atmosphere, common rooms where patients can gather to socialize and engage in cognitive stimulation and therapeutic activities

From: Cowan-Lincoln, M. (2015). 10 things geriatricians want hospitalists to know. *The Hospitalist* (10). https://www.the-hospitalist.org/hospitalist/article/122103/10-things-geriatricians-want-hospitalists-know; Palmer, R. (2018). The acute care for elders unit model of care. *Geriatrics 3*(3),59.

developed by the Hartford Geriatric Nursing Institute in 1992 designed to improve outcomes for hospitalized older adults (http://www.nicheprogram.org). NICHE-LTC was recently developed to enhance quality of care delivered to older adults in long-term and residential care facilities and is designed around the Centers for Medicare and Medicaid Services (CMS) Five-Star Quality Measures (Greenberg et al., 2018) (Chapter 6). NICHE offers many opportunities for new roles for acute and long-term care nurses such as the geriatric resource nurse (GRN). The GRN role emphasizes the pivotal role of the bedside nurse in influencing outcomes of care and coordination of interprofessional activities. NICHE-LTC also utilizes Geriatric Certified Nursing Assistant (GCNA) roles to promote geriatric expertise among front-line staff. These types of initiatives will increase the need for well-prepared geriatric professionals working in interprofessional teams to deliver needed services.

Community- and Home-Based Care

Nurses will care for older adults in hospitals and long-term care facilities, but the majority of older adults live in the community. Community-based care occurs through home and hospice care provided in people's homes, independent senior housing complexes, retirement communities, residential care facilities such as assisted living facilities, and adult day health centers. It also takes place in primary care clinics and public health departments. Care will continue to move out of hospitals and long-term care institutions into the community because of rapidly escalating health care costs and the person's preference to "age in place" (see Chapters 6 and 16). Gerontological nurses will find opportunities to create practices in community-based settings with a focus not only on care for those who are ill but also on health promotion and community wellness.

Nurses in the home setting provide comprehensive assessments including physical, functional, psychosocial, family, home, environmental, and community. Care management and working with interprofessional teams are integral components of the home health nursing role. Nurses may provide and supervise care for older adults with a variety of care needs (including chronic wounds, intravenous therapy, tube feedings, unstable medical conditions, and complex medication regimens) and for those receiving rehabilitation and palliative and hospice services. Hospice care is provided in residential hospices, long-term and skilled facilities, and acute in-patient hospice units. However, the majority of hospice care is provided in the individual's home.

The ability to form caring relationships with patients and families, similar to nursing in long-term care settings, is a rewarding component of hospice nursing practice. Nurses described "working with the dying as an honour, as life affirming, and as encouraging them to appreciate their own lives more fully" (Ingebretsen & Sagbakken, 2016). However, nursing education in palliative care is limited, and this lack of education can be a source of moral distress for nurses working with individuals who are dying (Wolf et al., 2019). Schools of nursing must increase education and practice experiences for nursing students in home- and community-based as well as hospice and palliative care. Chapter 28 discusses hospice and palliative care in greater depth.

Case and Care Management Roles

Nurses are especially well suited for roles as case managers and care managers in acute, long-term, and community-based care. Insurance companies, Medicaid managed care, and Medicare Advantage plans also utilize nurses in roles of case/care managers. Nonprofit community agencies, such as Catholic Senior Services and Area Agencies on Aging, also utilize nurses in these roles. There are increasing opportunities for these roles both in care of individuals with chronic illnesses and in transitional care (see Chapter 6). Many nurses enter private practice as case/care managers. Although the terms *case manager* and *care manager* have slightly different connotations, in practice the roles are seldom that clear and there is much overlap. Both of these roles include that of advocate, broker, leader, manager, counselor, negotiator, administrator, and communicator. Ideally the care manager follows the individual through the entire continuum of care.

Care managers must be experts regarding community resources and understand how these can best be used to meet the person's needs. They are expected to make appropriate referrals within the person's expectations and abilities and to monitor the quality of arranged services. The care or case manager is a resource person whom the older adult or caregiver can consult for advice and counsel and for brokering (negotiating, arranging) the flow of services. The care manager works to optimize the resources and outcome for the client and the agency or community in which the individual resides. There are Standards of Practice and certifications available for care/case manager roles (Box 1.3).

Certified Nursing Facilities (Nursing Homes)

Certified nursing facilities, commonly called nursing homes, have evolved into a significant location where health care is provided across the continuum, part of long-term post-acute care services (LTPAC). Over a quarter of Medicare patient admitted to hospital are discharged to post-acute (PAC) facilities, many with acute health conditions (Horney et al., 2017). The old image

BOX 1.7 Caring Nurse and Resident Relationships in Long-Term Care

"The residents become our friends and surrogate family. Nowhere else in healthcare are relationships formed the way they are in LTC. I would say that we have more value for our residents as people and patients than they are given elsewhere in healthcare."

From Sherman R, Touhy T. (2017). An exploratory descriptive study to evaluate Florida nurse leader challenges and opportunities in nursing home settings, *SAGE Open Nurs 3*, 1–7.

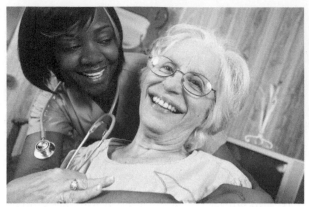

Gerontological nurses have a significant role in the healthy aging of older adults. (© iStock.com/Pamela Moore.)

of nursing homes caring for older adults in a custodial manner is no longer valid. Today, most facilities have post-acute care units that more closely resemble the general medical-surgical hospital units of the past. Most people enter nursing homes for short stays that last no more than 1 week to 3 months (Toles et al., 2014). Post-acute care in nursing facilities will continue to grow with health care reform, and there are many new roles and opportunities for professional nursing in this setting.

Roles for professional nursing include nursing administrator, manager, supervisor, charge nurse, educator, infection control nurse, Minimum Data Set (MDS) coordinator (see Chapter 8), case manager, transitional care nurse, quality improvement coordinator, and direct care provider. Professional nurses in nursing facilities must be highly skilled in the complex care concerns of older adults, ranging from post-acute care, to rehabilitation, to end-of-life care. Excellent assessment skills; ability to work with interprofessional teams in partnership with residents and families; skills in acute, rehabilitative, and palliative care; and leadership, management, supervision, and delegation skills are essential.

Practice in this setting requires independent decision-making and is guided by a nursing model of care because there are fewer physicians and other professionals on-site at all times. In addition, stringent federal regulations governing care practices and greater use of licensed practical nurses and nursing assistants influence the role of professional nursing in this setting. Chapter 6 provides more information on long-term care. The opportunity to form long-term relationships with individuals and families is valued by nurses and cited as one of the most rewarding aspects of practice in LTC facilities (Box 1.7).

❖ USING CLINICAL JUDGMENT TO PROMOTE HEALTHY AGING

With the promise of a healthier old age, health care professionals, particularly nurses, will play a significant role in creating systems of care and services that enhance the possibility of healthy aging for an increasingly diverse population. In times of health, illness, rehabilitation, and end-of-life care, outcomes for older adults most often depend on the nursing care received. Expert clinical judgment skills, developed through education in gerontological nursing, are needed to create and evaluate nursing actions that improve outcomes in health and illness for older adults. Continued attention must be paid to the recruitment and education of health professionals and direct care staff to meet the critical shortages that threaten the health and safety of older adults.

Exciting roles for nurses with preparation in gerontological nursing are increasing across the continuum of care and eldercare is projected to be the fastest growing employment sector in health care. Nursing education is required to prepare graduates to assume positions across the continuum of care, with increasing emphasis on community-based and post–acute care settings. Dare we say that gerontological nursing will be the most needed specialty in nursing as the number of older adults continues to increase and the need for our specialized knowledge becomes even more critical in every specialty and every health care setting?

▌ KEY CONCEPTS

- Older adults are complex, and their responses to illness may not meet standard diagnostic criteria and are often missed, leading to unnecessary disability, complications, and quality-of-life issues. Nurses are key to recognizing and analyzing cues and taking action to improve outcomes of care through competent clinical judgment.
- The major changes in health care delivery and the increasing numbers of older adults have resulted in

numerous revised, refined, and emergent roles for nurses in the field of gerontological nursing. There is a critical shortage of nurses trained in the care of older adults.

- Nursing has led the field in gerontology, and nurses were the first professionals in the nation to be certified as geriatric specialists.
- Certification assures the public of nurses' commitment to specialized education and qualification for the care of older adults.
- Advanced practice role opportunities for nurses are numerous and are seen as potentially cost-effective in health care delivery while facilitating more holistic health care.
- All students graduating from nursing programs and all practicing nurses working with older adults should have competency in gerontological nursing.

ACTIVITIES AND DISCUSSION QUESTIONS

1. Consider and discuss with classmates the various gerontological nursing roles that you find most interesting and stimulating.
2. Discuss the gerontological organizations of today and their significance to the practicing nurse.
3. Why do you think more students do not choose gerontological nursing as a specialty? What would increase interest in this area of nursing?
4. What do you think are the most important issues in gerontological nursing education at this time?
5. Discuss your clinical education experiences and reflect on how they have influenced your views about care of older adults and gerontological nursing.

REFERENCES

American Association of Colleges of Nursing (AACN). *The essentials of baccalaureate education for professional nursing practice* 2008. http://www.aacnnursing.org/portals/42/publications /baccessentials08.pdf.

American Association of Colleges of Nursing (AACN). *White paper on the education and role of the clinical nurse leader* Feb 2007. https://nursing.uiowa.edu/sites/default/files/documents /academic-programs/graduate/msn-cnl/CNL_White_Paper .pdf.

American Nurses Association (2018). *Gerontological nursing: Scope and standards of practice* (ed. 2). Silver Springs, MD: Nursesbooks .org.

Campaign for Action 2016. *Not enough nurses prepared to care for those older than 65.* https://campaignforaction.org /not-enough-nurses-prepared-to-care-for-americas-65/.

Campbell, T., Bayly, M., & Peacock, S. (2019). Provision of resident-centered care by nurse practitioners in Saskatchewan long-term care facilities: Qualitative findings from a mixed methods study. *Res Geron Nurs, 6,* 1–9.

Campbell, T., Bayly, M., & Peacock, S. (2020). Provision of resident-centered care by nurse practitioners in Saskatchewan long-term care facilities. *Res Gerontol Nurs, 13*(2), 73.

Cowan-Lincoln, M. (2015). 10 things geriatricians want hospitalists to know. *The Hospitalist, 10.* https://www.the-hospitalist.org /hospitalist/article/122103/10-things-geriatricians-want -hospitalists-know.

Dwyer, T., Craswell, A., Rossi, D., & Holzberger, D. (2017). Evaluation of an aged care nurse practitioner service: Quality of care within a residential aged care facility hospital avoidance service. *BMC Health Serv Res, 17,* 33.

Ebersole, P., & Touhy, T. (2006). *Geriatric nursing: Growth of a specialty.* New York: Springer.

Greenberg, S., Gilmartin, M., D'Amico, C., & Sullivan-Marx, E. (2018). NICHE (Nurses Improving Care for Healthsystem Elders) Program: Long-term care. *Jour of Post-Acute and Long-Term Care Medicine, 19*(3), B12–B13.

Harrington, C., Kovner, C., Mezey, M., et al. (2000). Experts recommend minimum nurse staffing for nursing facilities in the United States. *Gerontologist, 40*(1), 5–16.

Horney, C., Capp, R., Boxer, R., & Burke, R. E. (2017). Factors associated with early readmission among patients discharged to post-acute care facilities. *J Am Geriatr Soc, 65*(6), 1199–1205.

Ingebretsen, L., & Sagbakken, M. (2016). Hospice nurses' emotional challenges in their encounters with the dying. *Int J Qual Stud Health Well-being.*

Inouye S., Bogardus S., Baker D., et al. (2000). The Hospital Elder Life Program: A model of care to prevent cognitive and functional decline in older hospitalized patients. *J Am Geriatr Soc, 48,* 1657–1706.

Institute of Medicine (IOM): *Retooling for an aging America: Building the healthcare workforce,* 2008. https://www.nap.edu/catalog /12089/retooling-for-an-aging-america-building-the-health-care -workforce.

Kovach, C. (2018). Research in gerontological nursing: How are we doing. *Research in Gerontol Nurs, 11*(5), 227–229.

Kydd, A., Engstrom, G., Touhy, T., et al. (2014). Attitudes of nurses and student nurses towards working with older people and to gerontological nursing as a career in Germany, Scotland, Slovenia, Sweden, Japan and the United States. *Int J Nurs Educ, 6*(2), 33–40.

Mellilo, K. D., Remington, R., Abdullah, I., et al. (2015). Comparison of nurse practitioner and physician practice models in nursing facilities. *Ann Long-Term Care, 23*(12), 19–24.

Mezey, M., & Fulmer, T. (2002). The future history of gerontological nursing. *J Gerontol A Biol Sci Med Sci, 57,* M438–M441.

Morley, J. (2017). The future of long-term care. *J Am Med Dir Assoc, 18,* 1–7.

National Institute of Nursing Research: *The NINR strategic plan: advancing science: improving lives,* 2016. NIH Publication #16-NR-7783. https://www.ninr.nih.gov/sites/files/docs/ninr _stratplan2016_reduced.pdf. Accessed October 6, 2020.

Oliver, G., Pennington, L., & Revelle, S., et al. (2014). Impact of nurse practitioners on health outcomes of Medicare and Medicaid patients. *Nurs Outlook, 62*(6), 440–447.

Palmer, R. (2018). The acute care for elders unit model of care. *Geriatrics, 3*(3), 59.

Parke, B., & Hunter, K. (2014). The care of older adults in hospital: if it's common sense why isn't it common practice. *Jour Clin Nurs, 23,* 1573–1582.

Ploeg, J., Kaasalainen, S., McAiney, C., et al. (2013). Resident and family perceptions of the nurse practitioner role in long term care settings: A qualitative descriptive study. *BMC Nurs, 12*(1), 24.

Available at http://www.biomedcentral.com/content/pdf/1472
-6955-12-24.pdf.

Robert Wood Johnson Foundation: *United States in search of nurses with geriatrics training*, 2012. https://www.rwjf.org/en/library/articles-and-news/2012/02/united-states-in-search-of-nurses-with-geriatrics-training.html.

Sherman, R., & Touhy, T. (2017). An exploratory descriptive study to evaluate Florida nurse leader challenges and opportunities in nursing home settings. *SAGE Open Nurs, 3*, 1–7.

Sourdet, S., LaFont, C., Rolland, Y., et al. (2015). Preventable iagrogenic disability in elderly patients during hospitalization. *JAMDA*. http://dx.doi.org/10.1016/jamda.2015.03.011.

Taylor, M. (2006). Mapping the literature of pediatric nursing. *J Med Libr Assoc, 92*(2 Suppl), E128–E136.

Toles, M., Anderson, R., Massing, M., et al. (2014). Restarting the cycle: Incidence and predictors of first acute care use after nursing home discharge. *J Am Geriatr Soc, 62*(1), 79–85.

U.S. Department of Health and Human Services (2012). *Office of Disease Prevention and Health Promotion: Healthy People 2020.* http://www.healthypeople.gov/2020.

Wolf, A. T., White, K. R., Epstein, E. G., & Enfield, K. B. (2019). Palliative care and moral distress: an institutional survey of critical care nurses. *Critical Care Nurse, 39*(5), 38–50.

2

Introduction to Healthy Aging

Kathleen Jett

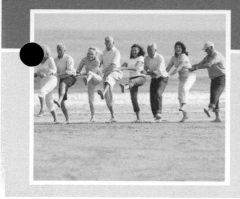

http://evolve.elsevier.com/Touhy/gerontological/

LEARNING OBJECTIVES

Upon completion of this chapter, the reader will be able to:
- Identify at least three factors that influence the aging experience.
- Define health and wellness within the context of aging and chronic illness.
- Describe the trends seen in global aging today.
- Utilize specialized clinical judgment when working with a wide range of older adults.

THE LIVED EXPERIENCE

I believe a human life is like a river, meandering through its course, rushing through rapids, flowing placidly over the plains, twisting and turning through countless bends until it spends itself. It is the same river; yet it looks very different from one place to another. So it is with our lives; circumstances vary from one time to another in the course of a life but there is also value to living.

Georgia, age 80

Caring for older adults gives us a unique opportunity to influence their quality of life in so many ways.

Nursing student, age 19

Aging is part of the life course. Caring for persons who are aging is a practice that touches nurses in all settings: from pediatrics involving grandparents and great-grandparents; to the residents of skilled nursing facilities and their spouses, partners, and children; to nurses providing relief support in countries outside of their own. Core gerontological knowledge and clinical judgment affects all of the nursing profession and is not limited to any one subgroup of nurses.

Gerontological nurses can help shape a world in which persons can thrive and grow old, not merely survive. They have unique opportunities to facilitate wellness in those who are recipients of care. As we move forward in the 21st century, the way nurses respond to our aging society will determine our character because we are no greater than the health of the country and the world in which we live. This chapter provides an introduction to how the nurse can help facilitate some level of health for persons in later life regardless of where they are on the continuum between complete well-being and the final moments of life.

THE YEARS AHEAD

As we look to the future, the world's population will soon include more persons older than 60 years than ever before (Fig. 2.1). In the United States, the number of persons at least 65 years old is expected to almost double between 2018 and 2060 (Fig. 2.2). The older population is also becoming more diverse; by 2060, those who identify as non-Hispanic white is expected to drop from 77% to 55% of the total (PRB [Population Reference Bureau],

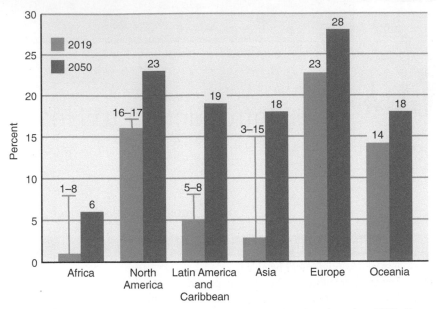

FIG. 2.1 Percent of population aged 65 and over by continent, 2018 and projected to 2050. (Data extracted from PBR: World Population Data Sheet (2018; 2019). www.worldpopdata.org/chart).

2019). In 2020, the number of persons at least 60 years of age outnumbered those under 5 for the first time. It is expected that between 2015 and 2050, the population of older persons worldwide will double to more than 1.2 billion. The majority of those in this exploding population are women (World Health Organization, [WHO], 2020).

This population growth will change the face of aging as we know it and present many new challenges today and in our future. Although healthy aging is now an achievable goal for many in developed and developing regions, it is still only a distant vision for many living in less developed areas of the world, where lives are shortened by persistent communicable

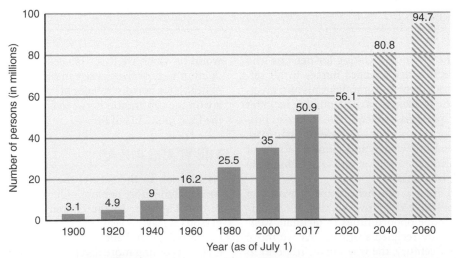

FIG. 2.2 Number of persons 65+, 1900-2060. (From AOA: *2018 Profile of older Americans* (2019). Available at https://acl.gov/aging-and-disability-in-america/data-and-research/profile-older-americans).

diseases, inadequate sanitation, and lack of both nutritious food and health care. It is essential that nurses across the globe have the knowledge and skills to help people of all ages achieve the highest level of wellness possible. Some questions must be asked. How can global conditions change for those who are struggling? How can the years of elderhood be maximized and enriched to the extent possible, regardless of the conditions in which one lives?

HOW OLD IS OLD?

Each culture has its own definition of when one is recognized as "old." A range of terms is used to refer to those considered old, including senior citizens, elders, granny, older adult, tribal elder, or "na" among the !Kung San of Botswana (Rosenberg, 1990). Elderhood may be defined in functional terms—when one is no longer able to perform one's usual activities (Jett, 2003). Social aging is often determined by changes in roles, such as retirement from one's usual occupation, appointment as a wise woman/ man of the community, or at the birth of a grandchild. *Biological aging* is a complex and continuous process involving every cell in the body (Chapter 4). The physical and biological traits by which we identify one as "older" (e.g., gray hair, wrinkled skin) are referred to as the aging phenotype and are the external expression of one's individual genetic makeup and internal changes. *Chronological aging* may be used alone or combined with either social or biological aging. In most developed and developing areas of the world, chronological late life is recognized as beginning sometime between 50 and 65 years of age. These arbitrary numbers had been set with the expectation that persons are in the last decade or two of their lives. Yet this is no longer applicable to men and women in many developed countries where life expectancies are rising.

The transition between mid-life and late life may be marked by special rituals, such as birthday and retirement parties, invitations to join groups such as the American Association of Retired Persons, the qualification for "senior discounts" (Box 2.1), or recognition of special honor.

Chronological Aging

In most developed and developing areas of the world, chronological late life is recognized as beginning sometime between the ages of 50 and 65. In 1935, with the establishment of a national retirement system (Social Security), the time when one became "old" was set at 65 in the United States. In the 2000s, the age when one becomes eligible for age-dependent benefits (and therefore old?) is creeping upward.

BOX 2.1 The Aging Phenotype

A few years ago I stopped coloring my hair, which is almost completely silver now. It was quite a surprise to me the first time the very young clerk in the booth at the movie theater assumed I was 65 and automatically gave me the "senior discount." My husband's hair is only fading to a dull brown. When he goes to the theater alone, they tentatively ask, "Do you have any discounts?"

Kathleen, at age 60

Arbitrary numbers used to describe "old" have been defined with the expectation that persons are in the last decade or two of their lives; however, in many countries the median age of the population is such that few will ever reach 60. According to the World Population Review (2018), the median age (half of the population older and half younger) in Mali was 15.8 years of age with only 3% of the population 65 or older. In contrast, the median age was 47.3 years of age in Japan and older adults make up 27% of the population. In the United States, the median age is 38.1 years of age (World Population Review, 2018). In the United States, life expectancy at birth increased steadily, with a slight drop in 2018 (one-tenth of a year) attributed to the "opioid crisis."

Life expectancy at the age of 65 varied greatly as well (Fig. 2.3) (PBR, 2018). Although racial/ethnic disparities continue to exist, Black females overtook White males in about the year 2000, and Hispanic men and women have the longest life expectancy at birth of all ethnicities. At the age of 65, the life expectancy of White men is lower than other men (Fig. 2.4) (CDC, 2018).

In the countries where the average life expectancies have expanded most rapidly, the following four generational subgroups have emerged: the super-centenarians, the centenarians, the baby boomers, and those in-between. Elderhood has the potential to span 40 years or more, attributable in a large part to increased access to quality health services and emphasis on improving the health of the public.

The Super-Centenarians

The super-centenarians are those who live until at least 110 years of age (Box 2.2). This elite group emerged in the 1960s as those first documented to have lived so long. The Gerontology Research Group has an ongoing study to verify and record at least the top 30–40 validated super-centenarians. Although Jeanne Louise Calment has long been considered the person to have lived the longest, her age has not been completely verified (Gerontology Research Group, 2019). All the oldest living persons have been women, the majority Japanese.

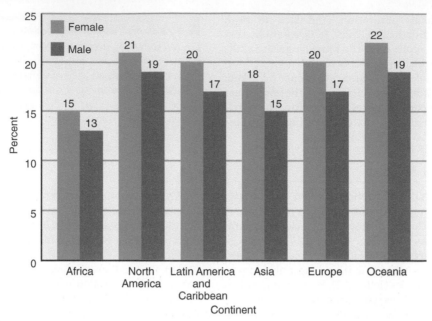

FIG. 2.3 Life expectancy at 65 years of age by continent. (Data extracted from PBR: *Worldpopdata* (2018). www.worldpopdata.org/chart).

Based on the number of living centenarians, 300–450 supercentenarians should be alive at any point in time. In January 2020 it was reported in *USA TODAY* that the oldest person in the world was thought to be Kane Tanaka of Japan (117) (Bode, 2020). While the number of countries with validated information is limited, the countries with the known number of centenarians (in decreasing order) are Japan, the United States, and France (Aging Analytics Agency, with Gerontology Research Group, 2020).

We now know that longevity is influenced by genetics, the environment, and lifestyle. Environmental improvement, at least in developed countries, began in the 1900s with the availability of clean water and adequate food supplies. Current research finds that many long-lived persons do not smoke, are not obese, and handle stress

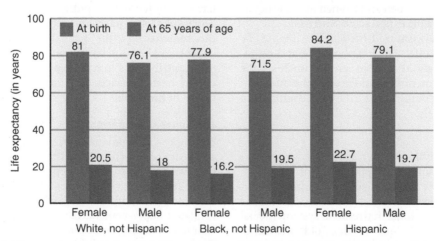

FIG. 2.4 Life expectancy at birth and at 65 years of age, by gender and race/ethnicity, in the United States. (Data extracted from CDC. (2017). *Health, United States, 2017 – Data finder*. https://www.cdc.gov/nchs/data/hus/2017/015.pdf).

BOX 2.2   Super-Centenarian Extraordinaire: Jeanne Louise Calment

It has been reported that Jeanne Louise Calment died in France at age 122. At that time she was believed to be the longest-lived person in the world. She outlived her husband, her daughter, her only grandson, and her lawyer. Her husband died in 1942, just 4 years before their 50th anniversary. Her daughter died in 1936 and her grandson in 1963. She was 4 years old when the Eiffel tower was built and reportedly once sold art supplies to Vincent Van Gogh. She not only lived a long life but also approached life with vigor. Madame Calment took up fencing at 85 and was still riding a bike at 107. She smoked until she was 117 and ate a lifelong diet rich in olive oil. Her longevity remains a mystery to experts and researchers.

From Dollemore D. (2006). *Aging under the microscope: A biological quest,* Bethesda, MD, National Institute of Aging, National Institutes of Health, Publication #02-2756.

well. They are less likely than others to develop a number of chronic diseases such as hypertension, heart disease, cancer, or diabetes (NIII, 2020; Sebastiani et al., 2013). A study of 32 super-centenarians in the United States found that "A surprisingly substantial portion of these individuals were still functionally independent or required minimal assistance" (Schoenhofen et al., 2006, p. 1237). Most functioned independently until after age 100, with no signs of frailty until about the age of 105. They were found to be remarkably homogeneous. None had Parkinson's disease, only 25% had ever had cancer, and stroke and cardiovascular disease were rare if they occurred at all. Few had been diagnosed with dementia. A study of super-centenarians in Japan corroborated these findings. It is theorized that these unusual persons have survived this long for "rare and unpredictable" reasons (Willcox et al., 2008). Although the number of super-centenarians alive today is small, it is predicted to grow as upcoming centenarians live longer because of healthier lifestyle (Robine & Vaupel, 2001).

The Centenarians

Centenarians are those between 100 and 109 years of age, the majority of whom are between 100 and 104 years old. Many centenarians had all or most of the "childhood" diseases, such as measles, mumps, chickenpox, and whooping cough; some lived through polio as children.

In 2016 there were about 82,000 persons at least 100 in the United States. In 2020, this number was expected to have grown to about 92,000 and is expected to reach over half a million by 2060 (Duffin, 2020). The increase has been attributed to improvement in vaccines, antibiotics, hygiene, and sanitation. Genetics has also played

a large role (Fessenden, 2020). Based on the US Census report of 2010, centenarians were overwhelmingly White women living in urban areas of the Southern states. Men most often lived with family members (43.5%) whereas women most often lived in nursing homes. The state with the largest population of those over 100 was North Dakota, at 3.29 per 10,000 persons (U.S. Census, 2019).

Those In-Between

There is also a unique cohort born in the years between 1920 and 1945, that is, between those referred to as the baby boomers and the centenarians. This age group includes some of the last survivors of the Holocaust. Some fought in World War II, the Korean War, and the youngest also fought in Vietnam.

Polio infection was a major fear for this cohort; either they or their friends were affected. A vaccine was not available in the United States until 1954, providing the most benefits to the youngest of the "in-betweeners." It was eradicated in the Western Hemisphere in 2007 but continues to be found in other parts of the world (College of Physicians of Philadelphia, 2020). Many had friends and loved ones who died of the AIDS epidemic before treatment was available.

The number of persons in this age group is growing at an exponential rate, especially those 85+ years of age. There is also a growing racial and ethnic heterogeneity among older adults. The number of persons from racial and ethnic statistical minority groups is projected to increase from 7.2 million in 2007 (19% of older population) to 27.7 million in 2040 (34% of older adults) (ACL/AOA, 2019).

The "Baby Boomers"

The youngest of the "older generation" are referred to as "baby boomers" or "boomers." They were born sometime between 1946 and 1964 (26% of those over 65). In the United States, the first to become baby boomers turned 64 in 2010; the last will do so 18 years later in 2028. More babies were born in the United States in 1946, the year after the end of WWII, than any other year—3.4 million or 20% more than in 1945. These numbers increased every year until they tapered off in 1964. In just 18 years, about 76 million babies had been born (History, 2020). Each day another 10,000 "boomers" turn 65 years old (multiple sources).

Although the super-centenarians and centenarians may not have received the immunizations as they became available, they became a standard of care from 1960 on, when the eldest boomer was 13 years of age. The ability to produce the potent antibiotic penicillin and those that followed has been significantly influential in the survival of this cohort. The baby boomers of today have better access to medication and other treatment regimens than previous cohorts in many parts of the world. Although they have high rates of chronic conditions, especially obesity, diabetes, arthritis, heart disease, and dementia, today's baby boomers will, nevertheless, live longer with these chronic diseases than any of their predecessors. It is hoped that today's social emphasis on healthier lifestyles will go far to help persons reach higher levels of wellness, but for this group, the challenges are many.

MOVING TOWARD HEALTHY AGING

From a perspective of Western medicine, health was long considered the absence of physical or psychiatric illness. It was measured in terms of the presence of accepted "norms," such as a specific range of blood pressure readings and results of laboratory testing, and the absence of established signs and symptoms of illness. When any of the parameters negatively affected the ability of the individual to function independently, debility was assumed. The measurement of a population's health status was usually inferred almost entirely from morbidity and mortality statistics: how long we live, what illness we have, and how many people die from a specific illness. The numbers provided information about illness and death, but the quality of life and wellness of the population could not be inferred. Neither did the data reflect the lives of persons with functional limitations, their ability to contribute to the community, or their self-esteem.

Although there had been efforts for many years to recognize that health meant more than the absence of disease, a national effort was not organized in the United States until 1979. At that time initial national goals were set and described in the document *The Surgeon General's Report on Health and Disease Prevention*. This has been updated every 10 years with the most current document referred to as *Healthy People 2020* and *Healthy People 2030* in development. Many new topical areas that are especially important to the promotion of health while aging were added to the 2020 version. Among these are goals related to quality of life and wellness while aging and the preparation of health care professionals to provide the highest-quality care to adults as they age (ODPHP, 2020).

The strong emphasis on holistic health has resulted in ever-broadening definitions of health and wellness. Wellness now involves one's whole being—physical, emotional, mental, and spiritual (Fig. 2.5). Wellness involves achieving a balance between one's internal and external environment and one's emotional, spiritual, social, cultural, and physical processes. It is a state of being and

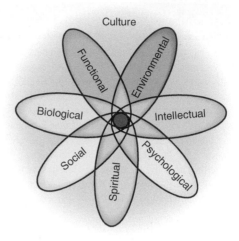

FIG. 2.5 Flower model.

feeling that one strives to achieve wellness through effective health practices. Instead of snapshots in time during a person's illness, a state of wellness can be uniquely defined anywhere along the continuum of health. Age and illness influence the ease at which one moves along the continuum but do not define the individual.

An individual must work hard to achieve wellness. In working toward wellness, an individual may reach plateaus in their ascension to higher-level wellness. Even for those with chronic illnesses, regression from an illness or acute event or crisis can be a potential stimulus for growth and a return to moving along the wellness continuum (see Chapter 17).

Health in later life is often thought of in terms of functional ability (i.e., the ability to do what is important to a given person) rather than the absence of disease. This may mean the person's ability to live independently or the ability to enjoy great-grandchildren when they visit at the nursing home, but it is always individually determined. Although functional status is an important factor, wellness is affected also by socioeconomic factors, degree of social interaction, marital status, and aspects of one's living situation and environment.

Approaching aging from a holistic viewpoint of health emphasizes strengths, resilience, resources, and capabilities rather than searching for cues only related to potential pathological conditions. A wellness perspective is based on the belief that every person has an optimal level of health independent of his or her situation or functional ability. Even in the presence of chronic illness or multiple disabilities or while dying, movement toward higher wellness is possible if the emphasis of care is placed on the promotion of well-being in the

From U.S. Department of Health and Human Services. *Healthy People 2020. Topics and objectives: older adults.* http://www.healthypeople.gov/2020/topicsobjectives2020/overview.aspx?topicid=31.

BOX 2.3 Healthy People 2020
Emerging Issues in the Health of Older Adults

- Coordinate care.
- Help older adults manage their own care.
- Establish quality measures.
- Identify minimum levels of training for people who care for older adults.
- Research and analyze appropriate training to equip providers with the tools they need to meet the needs of older adults.

least restrictive environment, with support and encouragement for the person to find meaning in the situation, whatever it is (Box 2.3).

❖ USING CLINICAL JUDGMENT TO PROMOTE HEALTHY AGING

As life expectancy increases, how will we define aging? How will these definitions, as well as the meaning and the perception of aging, change as the health and wellness of individuals, communities, and nations improve? How will nursing roles and responsibilities change? How can we promote wellness in those who have a much greater chance of living into their 100s?

It is the responsibility of the nurse to assist older adults to achieve the highest level of wellness in relation to whatever situation exists. The nurse can, through knowledge and affirmation, empower, enhance, and support the person's movement toward the highest level of wellness possible. The nurse assesses and helps explore the underlying situation that may be interfering with the achievement of wellness, and works with the person and significant others to develop affirming and appropriate plans of care. The nurse can utilize the resources available, such as *Healthy People 2020/2030* and the *Clinical Preventive Services Guidelines,* to maximize the potential for health (Table 2.1). The nurse and the older adult collaboratively implement strategies to achieve individual goals and evaluate their outcomes. Throughout this text there are multiple suggestions of how this can be done. The goals of the nurse are to care and comfort always, to cure sometimes, and to prevent that which can be prevented.

TABLE 2.1 Example of Interventions to Promote Wellness

Preventive Service	Wellness and Person-Oriented Intervention
Promoting influenza and pneumococcal immunizations Yearly	Consider new approaches to community outreach, such as home visits, neighbor-to-neighbor campaigns. Develop effective reminder systems.
Breast cancer screening Yearly	Develop effective reminder systems. Provide one-to-one education and counseling. Reduce structural barriers, such as transportation difficulties.
Colorectal screening Every 10 years or as directed	Develop effective reminder systems. Reduce structural barriers, such as transportation difficulties.
Vaginal and cervical cancer screening Stops at 65 under certain circumstances	Help women determine eligibility and appropriateness.
Diabetes self-management training Annual	Encourage participation to help the person achieve glycemic goals.
Hearing and balance exams Annual	Offer exams for those with identified problems. For those with impairments, work with them to obtain care.
Shingles vaccination Two doses of Shingrix at age 60	Promote public education regarding the importance of this. Engage in policy activism to promote insurance coverage.
HIV screening Anytime at increased risk	Encourage open conversations to include discussions of "safe sex" and the importance of screening.
Prostate screening (PSA and DRE) Individually determined	Stay informed about current status and recommendations about these screening exams.

KEY CONCEPTS

- Gerontological nursing is an opportunity to make a significant difference in the lives of older adults.
- The meaning of aging is influenced by many factors.
- Nurses have a responsibility to contribute to the nation's goals of increasing the quality of life lived.
- Individuals become more unique the longer they live. Thus, one must be cautious in attributing any specific characteristics of older adults to "old age."
- All persons, regardless of age or life and/or health situation, can be helped to achieve a higher level of wellness, which is uniquely and personally defined.
- Gerontological nurses have key roles in the provision of the highest quality of care to older adults in a wide range of settings and situations.

ACTIVITIES AND DISCUSSION QUESTIONS

1. Discuss the ways in which older adults contribute to society today.
2. Interview an older person and ask how they have changed since they were 25 years of age.
3. Discuss health and wellness with your peers. Develop a definition of aging.
4. Explain wellness in the context of chronic illness.
5. Discuss how you seek wellness in your own life.
6. Discuss what you can do to enhance the quality of life for the persons to whom you provide care.
7. Draw a picture of yourself at 80 years of age. Compare your drawing to those of others who have done the same and discuss the implications of the representation.
8. Discuss how older adults are portrayed in popular TV shows, commercials, and movies.
9. What was the effect of the coronavirus pandemic on each segment of the older population?

REFERENCES

ACL/AOA [Administration on Aging]: *2018 Profile of older Americans,* 2019. https://acl.gov/news-and-events /announcements/now-available-2018-profile-older-americans.

Aging Analytics Agency (with the Gerontology Research Group): *Supercentenarians Landscape Overview: Top-100 Living, top-100 longest lived, top-25 socially and professional active,* 2020. https:// www.aginganalytics.com/supercentenarians.

CDC: *Health, United States,* 2018. www.cdc.gov/nchs/hus/.

College of Physicians of Philadelphia: *All timeline overview,* 2020. https://www.historyofvaccines.org/timeline/all.

Duffin E: *Number of centenarians in the U.S. 2016-2060.* March 6, 2020. https://www.statista.com/statistics/996619 /number-centenarians-us/.

Fessenden, M. There are now more Americans over age 100 and they're living longer than ever 2020. Smithsonian January 22, 2016. https://www.smithsonianmag.com/smart-news/there-are -more-americans-over-age-100-now-and-they-are-living-longer -180957914/.

History: *Baby boomers,* 2020. http://www.history.com/topics/baby -boomers.

Jett, K. F. (2003). The meaning of aging and the celebration of years. *Geriatr Nurse, 24*(4), 209–293.

NIH [National Institute of Health]. (2020). *Is longevity determined by genetics?* https://ghr.nlm.nih.gov/primer/traits/longevity.

Office of Disease Prevention and Health Promotion [ODPHP]. (2020). *Older adults.* https://www.healthypeople.gov/2020 /topics-objectives/topic/older-adults.

PRB [Population Reference Bureau]. (2019). *Fact sheets: aging in the United States.* https://www.prb.org/aging-unitedstates-fact -sheet/.

Robine, J., & Vaupel, J. W. (2001). Supercentenarians: slower aging individuals or senile elderly? *Experimental Gerontology, 36*(4–6), 915–930.

Rosenberg, H. (1990). Complaint discourse, aging, and caregiving among the !Kung Sun of Botswana editor. In J. Sokolovsky (Ed.), *The cultural context of aging: A worldwide perspective* (pp. 19–42). New York: Bergin and Garvey.

Sebastiani, P., Fangui, X. S., Andersen, S., et al. (2013). Families enriched for exceptional longevity also have increased health-span: Findings from the Long Life Family Study. *Front Public Health, 1,* 38.

Schoenhofen, E. A., Wyszynski, D. F., Andersen S., et al. (2006). Characteristics of 32 supercentenarians. *JAGS, 54,* 1237–1240.

U.S. Census Bureau. (2019). *Facts for features: Older Americans month: May 2019.* https://www.census.gov/newsroom/stories /2019/older-americans.html.

Willcox, B. J., Willcox, D. C., & Ferrucci, L. (2008). Secrets of healthy aging and longevity from exceptional survivors around the globe: Lessons from octogenarians to supercentenarians. *J Gerontol A Biol Sci Med Sci, 63*(11), 1201–1208.

WHO. (2020). *Ageing and health.* https://www.who.int/news-room /fact-sheets/detail/ageing-and-health.

World Population Review: (2018). *Countries by median age 2018.* http://worldpopulationreview.com/countries/median-age/.

3

Making Clinical Judgments in the Cross-Cultural Setting With Older Adults

Kathleen Jett

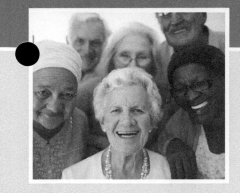

LEARNING OBJECTIVES

Upon completion of this chapter, the reader will be able to:
- Compare and contrast factors influencing health outcomes for vulnerable populations.
- Identify nursing actions appropriate for the increasingly diverse population of older adults.
- Develop strategies that incorporate culturally sensitive actions to facilitate improved outcomes for diverse populations of older adults.

THE LIVED EXPERIENCE

I feel so out of place here. If my children weren't so busy, I suppose I could live with them, but they seemed relieved when this retirement home accepted me. I wonder if they knew I was the only Chinese person in this place. A sweet young Chinese student tried to talk with me, but she only spoke Mandarin and I speak Cantonese. She had never lived in China. I want so much to talk to someone my age that lived in China and speaks my language.

Shin, a 75-year-old woman

I thought all old people were the same. I am very surprised that they are not!

Helen, an 18-year-old nursing student

As the number and diversity of persons of all ages grows, it has become mandatory for nurses to provide culturally proficient care to persons with different life experiences and perspectives, values and beliefs, styles of communication, and ages.

Providing skillful cross-cultural care is especially important in gerontological nursing because of the numbers of older adults immigrating to the United States and other countries. Some have spent their lives in self-contained, homogeneous communities and have not become accustomed to the outside culture of their adopted countries. They are now faced with confronting unfamiliar health care actions when they receive the specialized care needed for the treatment of acute and chronic conditions that are more prevalent with aging. This situation is likely to result in cultural conflict in the health care setting and a high risk for poor outcomes.

This chapter provides an overview of culture and aging, as well as strategies that gerontological nurses can use to best respond to the changing face of aging (see Chapter 2). In doing so, the nurse promotes healthy aging and helps reduce health inequities. These strategies include the skills needed to work with a person who is different from the nurse to find a way to achieve goals for healthy aging. It is moving from cultural destructiveness to culturally proficient care of older adults.

CULTURE

Culture is most often referred to in terms of the shared and learned values, beliefs, expectations, and behaviors of a group of people. Culture guides thinking and decision-making, as well as beliefs about aging, health and health-seeking, illness, treatment, and prevention (Jett, 2003; Spector, 2017).

Cultural perspectives are always part of health care, experienced any time the "seeker" and "giver" meet. The giver observes and analyzes cues, prioritizes hypotheses, proposes solutions, and evaluates the outcomes of nursing actions. Givers also hypothesize the way they expect seekers to respond. Many of the oldest adults in the United States today grew up during a period when paternalism was the primary principle from which health care was delivered. That is, the patient assumed that the physician would make the best decision for them, one that "he" would make for his own child. Persons in many cultures across the globe and subcultures within the United States continue to view the health care encounter from this perspective to a great extent. However, the seekers or a culturally designated authority will usually decide whether they agree with the problems identified, whether they will accept the "prescription/action," and whether it will be acted upon.

DIVERSITY

Extending the idea of culture is that of *cultural diversity* or simply the existence of more than one group with differing values and perspectives. Demographers describe the diversity of a country in several different ways; commonly used are country of origin, race, languages spoken, and religion. Regardless of the methods used, North Korea is usually described as least diverse, and those most diverse include the countries of sub-Saharan Africa. For example, there are about 40 different ethnic groups in Togo who speak at least 39 different languages and share little in common other than geography. Canada is the only "western" country in the top 20 in terms of diversity (World Population Review, 2020).

Diversity in the United Stated usually refers to the seven major ethno-racial groups: Black/African American, Asian American, Native Hawaiian/Pacific Islander, American Indian/Alaskan Native, White (of European descent)/Caucasian, multiracial, and the ethnic group who self-identify as Hispanic/Latino, regardless of race (Fig. 3.1). The category of Middle Eastern/North African has been discussed and may appear in a future US census. Of note: The most accurate use of the term African American is technically limited to the descendants of the more than 4 million people who were transported to the United States against their will between 1619 and 1860 (Spector, 2017). It does not accurately apply to individuals who have more recently migrated from the African continent.

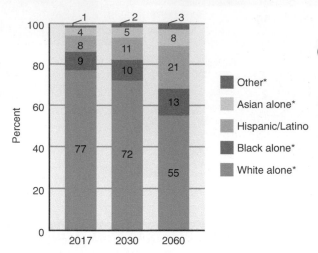

FIG. 3.1 Anticipated percentage of growth by race and ethnic group in the United States. (From https://www.prb.org/eight-demographic-trends-transforming-americas-older-population.)

It is important to recognize that within any one group, culturally similar or disparate, there is diversity of other kinds, most notably that of gender, gender identity, sexual orientation, education, power, and status. Most health care providers overlook the possibility that the 88-year-old patient may have a same-sexed next of kin. These factors greatly influence the delivery and receipt of health care in many, if not all, places in the world.

HEALTH DISPARITIES AND INEQUITIES

The terms *health inequities* and *health disparities* are often used interchangeably. Although they are somewhat different, both have implications for health outcomes. The term *health disparity* refers to differences in health outcomes between groups. It is usually discussed in terms of the excess burden of illness in one group compared with another. Most often the latter holds the majority of the power and influence, including control of the resources, such as health care. *Health inequities* refer to the excess burden of illness or the difference between an expected incidence and prevalence and that which occurs in excess in a comparison population group. The inequities are often the result of both historical and contemporary injustices. Those found to be especially vulnerable to health disparities and inequities are older adults ethnically or racially different from the majority population (Box 3.1). Health inequities most often relate to differences in the distribution of wealth and their effect on health outcomes.

One of the most dramatic examples is the 34-year discrepancy in life expectancy. A child born in the

BOX 3.1 Examples of Health Disparities Relevant to Older Adults[a]

- In 2013, Black Americans were twice as likely as non-Hispanic whites to die from diabetes.
- As reported in 2019, Black American adults were 60% more likely than non-Hispanic white adults to be diagnosed with diabetes.
- Although Black Americans are 40% more likely to have high blood pressure, they are less likely than non-Hispanic whites to have it under control.
- Between 2012 and 2016 American Indian/Alaskan Native men were twice as likely to have liver cancer and 40% more likely to have stomach cancer and twice as likely to die than non-Hispanic whites.
- In 2018 the age-adjusted percentage of American Indians/Alaska Native adults at least 18 years of age was 27.2% more likely to have hypertension than their non-Hispanic white counterparts.

[a]Most recent figure available from US Department of Health and Human Services, Office of Minority Affairs. (2019–2020). *Population profiles.* https://minorityhealth.hhs.gov/.

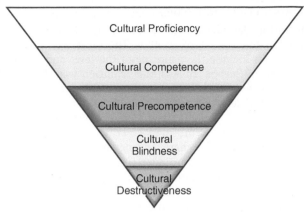

FIG. 3.2 A model for cross-cultural caring. (Adapted from Cross, T., Bazron, B., Dennis, K., et al. (1989). *Toward a culturally competent system of care,* Vol 1, Washington, DC: CASSP Technical Assistance Center, Center for Child Health and Mental Health Policy, Georgetown University Child Development Center; Goode, T. D. (2004). *Cultural competence continuum,* Washington, DC: National Center for Cultural Competence, Georgetown University Center for Child and Human Development, University Center for Excellence in Developmental Disabilities; Lindsey, R., Robins, K., & Terrell, R. (2003). *Cultural proficiency: A manual for school leaders.* Thousand Oaks, CA: Corwin Press.)

impoverished nation of Sierra Leone can only expect to live 50 years while in the high-income country of Japan the life expectancy at birth is 84 years. Yet health inequities are not limited to those between countries. In Glasgow, life expectancy ranges from 66.2 years of age in the neighborhoods of Ruchill and Possilpark to 81.7 years of age in the more affluent neighborhoods of Cathcart and Simshill. In London, there is a loss of one year of life expectancy for each train stop traveling east from Westminster in London (World Health Organization [WHO], 2017).

In any country where older adults are marginalized simply because of their age, they are especially vulnerable to health disparities. If the person has other characteristics (e.g., skin color, religion, or sexual orientation) that cause further differentiation between the person and those with power and status, the disparities are amplified. Cognitive impairment or sensory or physical disability increases the person's risk even further (Adelson, 2005; Kirmayer & Brass, 2016). While the death rate for Black Americans decreased 25% between 1999 and 2015, persons from minority groups still experience a disproportionate burden of disease (Centers for Disease Control and Prevention [CDC], 2018).

MOVING TOWARD CULTURAL PROFICIENCY TO IMPROVE HEALTH OUTCOMES

Gerontological nurses can learn to provide care more expertly as they move along a continuum from cultural destructiveness to cultural proficiency (Fig. 3.2).

This requires a willingness to become more self-aware, to observe carefully for the cues of others (i.e., "where they are coming from"), and finally to apply new skills to more effectively support rather than hinder their personal and cultural strengths in achieving healthy outcomes. (See Box 3.2 for key points in the development of cultural proficiency.)

BOX 3.2 Moving Toward Cultural Proficiency and Healthy Aging

- Become familiar with your own cultural perspectives, including beliefs about disease etiology, priorities, treatments, and factors leading to outcomes.
- Examine your personal and professional behavior for signs of bias and the use of negative stereotypes.
- Remain open to viewpoints and behaviors that are different from your expectations.
- Appreciate the inherent worth of all persons from all groups.
- Develop the skill of attending to both nonverbal and verbal communication and cues.
- Develop sensitivity to the clues given by others, indicating the paradigm from which they face health, illness, and aging.
- Learn to negotiate, rather than impose, strategies to promote healthy aging consistent with the beliefs of the persons to whom we provide care.

Cultural Destructiveness

Cultural destructiveness is the systematic elimination of the culture of another. The most well-known examples include the genocide of the Jews and others in Eastern Europe. In Australia, children were forcibly removed from their homes between 1910 and the 1970s to "assimilate" them with white Australians (Mogrady, 2019). In the United States, cultural destructiveness occurred with the removal of American Indian children to boarding schools where the language, dress, and food of their origins were forbidden (Little, 2018). American Indian healing ceremonies, performed by tribal elders, were forbidden. Practices referred to as "traditional" or "folk" healing were and continue to be discounted. Suspiciousness of Western medicine is still present among many Blacks and American Indians, especially those in their 80s and 90s today who may have first- or secondhand knowledge of the cultural destruction to which they and others were subjected (Grandbois et al., 2012) (Box 3.3).

BOX 3.3   Racism in the Boston Naming Test[a]

During a study to evaluate the cultural applicability of several standard psychological tools sometimes administered by nurses, an 82-year-old Black woman reluctantly agreed to take what is called the Boston Naming Test. This is a measure of verbal fluency used in the diagnosis of dementia and comprises a packet of pictures. The patient is asked to name the pictures. After doing so the volunteer shared, "Did you know that one of the pictures is a hangman's noose? Do you have any idea what that means to a Black person to look at that picture!" Indeed, none of the White researchers had noticed this.

[a]Personal experience of Kathleen Jett.

Cultural Blindness

It is hoped by this point the reader has begun to understand that there are multiple cultures coexisting in countries and continents and that such things as age and other factors affect the health care experience. Yet some people, including health care providers (e.g., nurses), say that they observe outward differences such as skin color and age but believe that "everyone is the same." In addition, they see no harm in applying negative stereotypes such as "all old people have a little dementia" and are blind to the fact that life experiences, such as being subjected to such stereotyping, prejudice, and historical trauma, can affect an individual's beliefs and behavior. All these experiences and the failure to recognize them frequently lead to poor health outcomes by influencing both the pursuit and the receipt of health care by older adults. It is not possible to provide cross-cultural care or to reduce health disparities in the context of cultural destructiveness or cultural blindness unless individual and community health belief paradigms consider factors such as ageism, poverty and racism (Feagin & Bennefield, 2014). Cultural blindness prevents a nurse from recognizing cues accurately and therefore from providing sensitive and, more importantly, effective care.

Cultural Pre-competence

The development of pre-competence begins with self-awareness of one's personal biases, prejudices, attitudes, and behaviors toward persons different from oneself, be it age or many other factors. It is becoming aware of one's own ageist attitudes as well as ageism found in the person's world (Box 3.4).

For persons whose culture or status places them in a position of power, cultural awareness is realizing that this alone often means special privilege and freedoms (McIntosh, 1988) (Box 3.5). Achieving cultural pre-competence requires a willingness to learn how health is viewed by others. It means playing an active role to combat ageism in society and thereby contributing to the reduction of health disparities.

Cultural Competence

A nurse who moves beyond pre-competence can step outside of biases and accept that others bring a different set of values, choices, and priorities to the health care setting. A nurse who can provide competent cross-cultural care to older adults accepts that all persons are unique

---

BOX 3.4   Unintentional Agism in Language and Its Effects

- Use of general labeling terms: sweet old lady, little old lady, geezer.
- Use of terms applied in the health care setting: fossil, bed blocker (debilitated person in the hospital awaiting a bed in a nursing home), GOMER (get out of my emergency room).
- When speaking: exaggerated pitch, demeaning emotional tone, lower quality of speech, "baby talk."
- Consequences of ageism in language: reduced sense of self, lowered self-esteem, lowered sense of self-competence, decreased memory performance.

Adapted from International Longevity Center. (2006). *Ageism in America.* http://www.graypanthersmetrodetroit.org/Ageism_In_America_-_ILC_Book_2006.pdf.

BOX 3.5   Unrecognized Privilege and Ethnocentrism

A gerontological nurse responded to a call from an older patient's room. While she was with him, he repeatedly, and without comment, dropped his watch on the floor. She calmly picked it up, handed it back to him, and continued talking. One time an aide walked in the room when the patient dropped the watch. The aide picked it up and handed it back to him just as the nurse had done. The patient immediately started yelling and cursing at the aide for attempting to steal his watch. When telling this story, the nurse thought the whole situation odd, but not too remarkable.

The patient and nurse were White, and the aide was Black. The nurse did not realize that the behavior of the patient was both ethnocentric and culturally destructive until the nurse learned these concepts while taking a formal class on cross-cultural health care.

---

and deserving of respect. It means understanding that the older the person, the more likely he or she has experience in dealing with health problems of all kinds. The nurse needs some knowledge of other cultures, particularly those she or he is most likely to encounter in the health care setting. This is especially important when the nurse and patient are of different ages or have different values, backgrounds, and cultures from each other. The acquisition of cross-cultural knowledge takes place in the classroom, at the bedside, and in the community. Cultural knowledge is both what the nurse brings to the caring situation and what the nurse learns from others (Fung, 2013).

Cultural Proficiency

It is now expected that a nurse not only demonstrates competence but also strives for cultural proficiency, which is respectful, compassionate, and relevant (see Fig. 3.2). Cultural proficiency includes applying cultural knowledge when making clinical judgments. The culturally proficient nurse moves smoothly between two worlds for the promotion of healthy aging. The nurse enters an unknown conceptual world in which time, space, religion, tradition, and wellness are expressed through a unique language that conveys the perceived nature of the health, illness, and humanity.

Culturally proficient care includes the recognition that there may be factors beyond culture to consider, such as the effects of past and current trauma, social status, and poverty, which can exacerbate health disparities and inequities. The nurse providing proficient cross-cultural care works, and builds relationships, with members from a variety of age and cultural groups

as a natural part of daily practice. The relationship building results in the ability to communicate effectively; sensitively and effectively recognize cues and generate hypotheses relative to the individual's health status; formulate and communicate mutually acceptable goals, consequences, and risks; and support and evaluate actions that are culturally acceptable, empowering, and possible within the limitations of available resources.

CULTURAL KNOWLEDGE

Cultural knowledge grows as the nurse learns about aging, older adults, their families, their communities, their beliefs, and their expectations of the health care experience. Essential knowledge includes the older person's way of life (ways of thinking, believing, and acting). This knowledge is obtained formally and informally through the individual's professional experience of nursing. It is expected that knowledge will allow the nurse to improve health outcomes more appropriately and effectively (Campinha-Bacote, 2011).

Although cultural knowledge is essential, caution must be used regarding the potential for stereotyping or the application of limited knowledge about one person with specific characteristics to other persons with some of the same characteristics. The nurse will hear that "old people just become more like children." This type of stereotyping limits the recognition of the heterogeneity of the group. At the same time, relying on knowledge of basic cultural patterns and positive stereotypes can be useful as a *starting* point, but it too can be used to limit understanding of the uniqueness of the individual and impose unrealistic expectations. For example, a common stereotype of the Black culture is that the church is a source of support. The nurse's assumption can easily have a negative outcome when working with older adults, such as fewer referrals for formal services support (e.g., home-delivered meals). This stereotype can also only be used to start conversations about discharge planning. The non-Black nurse may say to an older Black client, "I have understood that the church sometime serves as a source of support for members of the community. Is this one of the resources available to you when you return home?" If so, it is necessary to elaborate, "What kinds of help will you be able to receive and for how long?" For example, the nurse may discuss services such as parish nurses or agencies that provide meals. It is important that the nurse uses such an opening to this conversation because the person may not mention a lack of such resources to avoid embarrassment.

Orientation to Family and Self

An important concept in cross-cultural health care is orientation to self and family. Many North Americans, especially those of northern European descent, place great value on independence, that is, personal autonomy and individuality (Fung, 2013). In a classic study, Rathbone-McCune (1982) found that a large group of older American adults living in a segregated ("White") senior apartment building went to great lengths and lived with significant discomforts rather than ask for help. To seek or receive help was considered a sign of weakness and dependence, something to be avoided at all costs, including death.

In the United States, the cultural expression of autonomy was institutionalized in the passing of the Patient Self-Determination Act of 1990 wherein individuals were recognized as the sole decision-makers regarding their health. Health care providers are now legally bound to restrict access to health care information to the patient without explicit permission to do otherwise.

This orientation is in sharp contrast to that of a collectivist or interdependent culture, a norm in many parts of the world. In the Latino culture this is referred to as "familism" (Mendez-Luck et al., 2016). Self-identity is drawn from family ties (broadly defined) rather than the individual. The "family" (e.g., extended, tribe, or clan) is of primary importance; decisions are made by the group or designee based on the needs and beliefs of the group rather than those of the individual. Within families, the exchange of help and resources is both expected and commonplace. For example, older adults may care for their grandchildren or great-grandchildren in exchange for housing and assistance with their own needs, including health-related decision-making. When a nurse from a culture in which independent decision-making is expected cares for an older adult whose dominant value is interdependence, or vice versa, the potential for cultural conflict and poor outcomes is great.

Orientation to Time

Orientation to time is often overlooked as a culturally constructed factor influencing the use of health care and preventive practices. Time orientations are culturally described as future, past, or present. Conflicts between the future-oriented Westernized medical care and those with past or present orientations are many. For example, older adults who are oriented to the past may delay or omit seeking help until they have been able to correct conflicts with long-deceased parents—conflicts that are believed to be the underlying causes of the current health problems. Older adults who are present-oriented may have great difficulty with being given "the next available appointment," which could be days or months ahead. It may be very difficult to participate in preventive measures, such as a "turning schedule" for a bed-bound patient to prevent pressure injuries or immunizations to prevent future infections.

For older adults who are ill or frail and dependent on others to accompany them to appointments or provide transportation, a life-long present orientation is particularly challenging when it clashes with the capabilities of family and friends and the health care system. Members of present-oriented cultures may be those persons accused of overusing hospital emergency departments in the United States, when in fact it may be considered the only reasonable option available for today's treatment of today's problems with the help of the resources available today.

Health Beliefs

The increasing diversity of the global community increases the potential for clashes between health beliefs. Aging itself further increases diversity because of long-held beliefs about normal changes with aging, potentially extensive experience related to illness and treatment, of self, family, and others. In most cultures, older adults are likely to treat themselves and others for familiar or chronic conditions in ways they have found successful in the past, practices that are referred to as *domestic medicine,* folk medicine, or folk healing. Folk medicine is, and always has been, based on beliefs regarding the appropriate treatment for the symptoms and presumed diagnoses. Only when self-treatment fails will a person consult with others known to be knowledgeable or experienced with the problem, such as an older family member, neighbor, community, or indigenous healer. If this fails, people may (or may not) seek help within a formal system of health care.

The culture of nursing and health care in the United States advocates the *Western or biomedical model.* The health care providers within this model usually consider it to be superior to all other models, a highly ethnocentric viewpoint. However, many people have different beliefs, such as those based on *personalistic* (magicoreligious) or *naturalistic* (holistic) models (Table 3.1). Each model includes beliefs and attitudes about disease prevention, disease causation, acceptable treatment, and definitions of health. It is not uncommon for an older adult from any ethnic group to adhere to beliefs other than those used in the biomedical approach, used by most nurses in "Westernized" nations. Nonetheless, nurses who are familiar with the range of health beliefs and realize their importance will be able to provide more sensitive and appropriate care. In the absence of understanding, the potential for conflict is great.

TABLE 3.1	**Comparison of Health Belief Models**				
Model	**Illness Causation**	**Assessment and Diagnosis**	**Treatment**	**Prevention**	**Health**
Western (biomedical)	Invasion of germs or genetic mutation identified as a disease	Objective identification of pathogen or process; May include consultation with a health practitioner identified as a specialist in the subcategory of disease (e.g., oncologist)	Removing or destroying invading organism, repairing, modifying, or removing affected body part	Avoidance of pathogens, chemicals, activities, and dietary agents known to cause abnormalities	Absence of disease
Personalistic (magicoreligious)	The actions of the supernatural, such as gods, deities, or nonhuman beings (e.g., ghosts or spirits); A punishment for a breach of rules, breaking a taboo, or displeasing or failing to please the source of power	Consultation with a health practitioner associate specializing in the subcategory of practice (e.g., minister, curandero)	Religious practices, such as praying, meditating, fasting, wearing amulets, burning candles, and "laying of the hands"	Making sure that social networks with their fellow humans are in good working order; Avoid angering family, friends, neighbors, ancestors, and gods	A blessing or reward of God
Naturalistic (holistic)	Physical, psychological, or spiritual imbalance resulting in disharmony	Consultation with a health practitioner specializing in the specific subcategory of practice (e.g., Chinese physician, herbalist)	Dependent on the submodel (e.g., hot/cold practices of treating a hot illness with a cold treatment)	Life practices that maintain balance	Balance (e.g., the right amount of exercise, food, sleep)

❖ USING CLINICAL JUDGMENT TO PROMOTE HEALTHY AGING: CROSS-CULTURAL NURSING

Perhaps in cross-cultural gerontological nursing more than any other fields, skill is based on mutual respect between the nurse and the older adult: it is working "with" the person rather than "on" the person.

Contact between older patients and gerontological nurses often begins with both observing cues of the other. Several tools have been developed to accomplish this (e.g., Leininger's Sunrise Model) (Kleinman et al., 1978; Leininger, 2002; Schim et al., 2007; Shen, 2004). However, like the comprehensive instruments described in Chapter 8, a comprehensive cultural assessment takes time, often more time than is possible in today's health care setting, and somewhat objectifies the person.

An alternative is that of the LEARN Model, a negotiated plan of care that includes identification of the availability of culturally appropriate and sensitive community resources (Berlin & Fowkes, 1983) (Box 3.6). When using the LEARN Model in goal setting and care plan development with older adults, it is necessary to pay close attention to any sensory limitations that might interfere with communication; for example, hearing aids need to be both functional and used so that beneficial conversations can ensue. When others are directly involved in a person's day-to-day life, they should be present (see Chapter 27). The LEARN Model is easy to use and incorporates the collection of the most useful information needed to construct a focused, action-oriented care plan. Because it requires an interactive process, it has the highest potential for success (i.e., improved outcomes).

BOX 3.6   The LEARN Model

L Listen carefully to what the person is saying and observe cues to meaning. Attend to not just the words but to the nonverbal communication and the meaning behind the stories. Listen to the person's perception of the situation, potentially acceptable strategies, and the desired outcomes.

E Explain your hypotheses and priorities.

A Acknowledge and discuss both the similarities and the differences between your hypotheses, priorities, and desirable outcomes and those of the person.

R Recommend a plan of action that takes both perspectives into account.

N Negotiate strategies and an action plan that is mutually acceptable.

Adapted from Berlin, E. A., Fowkes, W. C. (1983). A teaching framework for cross-cultural health care: Application in family practice, *West J Med* *139*(6):934–938.

◆ L—Listen

Listening for cues includes paying attention to more than just verbal expressions. It includes physical contact, eye contact, the spoken word, and the nonverbal communication behind the words. The nurse listens carefully to the person for his or her perception about the problem at hand, the situational and cultural context, desired outcomes, and beliefs about treatment.

◆ Physical Contact

In caring for others, especially those in distress, it may seem natural for many nurses to feel that they should touch their patient in some way (such as a hug, a pat on the shoulder, or a touch of the hand) to show that they are listening. However, in the Muslim culture, cross-gender physical contact of any kind may be considered highly inappropriate or even forbidden, and care arrangements may need to be modified. Before the nurse makes physical contact with an older adult of any culture, he or she should ask the person's permission or follow the person's cue, such as an outstretched hand.

◆ Eye Contact

Eye contact is another highly culturally constructed behavior. In some cultures, direct eye contact is believed to be a sign of honesty and trustworthiness. Nursing students in the United States have been taught to establish and maintain eye contact when interacting with patients, but this behavior may be misinterpreted by persons from other cultures.

A more traditional older American Indian may not allow the nurse to make eye contact, moving his or her eyes slowly from the floor to the ceiling and around the room. During a health care encounter in most Asian cultures, direct eye contact is considered disrespectful. To impose eye contact with an elder may be particularly rude. The gerontological nurse can again follow the lead of the person by being open to eye contact but neither forcing it nor assigning it any inherent value.

◆ Verbal Communication

Respectful communication is always vital; it is essential, however, with older adults from cultures in which there are specific age-related norms. For example, in some Asian and Middle Eastern cultures children are expected to speak only when invited to do so by an elder. Respectful communication includes addressing the person in the appropriate manner (using the surname unless otherwise instructed or invited) and using acceptable body language.

In many cross-cultural health care encounters, the providers and the patients do not speak the same oral language or may not communicate with the fluency needed for the situation; some cultural traditions prevent older adults from speaking directly to the nurse (e.g., cross-gender care). To optimize the opportunity to promote healthy aging, an interpreter may be needed. *The more complex the clinical judgment needed, the more important the skills of the interpreter are, such as when determining the person's wishes regarding life-prolonging measures or the family's plan for caregiving* (Box 3.7).

BOX 3.7   When a Professional Interpreter Is Needed

An interpreter is needed whenever the nurse and the older adult speak different languages, when the person has limited proficiency in the language used in the health care setting, or when cultural tradition prevents the older adult from speaking directly to the nurse. The more complex the decision-making needed, the more important are the interpreter and their skills. These circumstances are many, such as when discussions are needed about the treatment plan for a new condition, the options for treatment, advanced care planning, or even preparation for care after discharge from a health care institution. The use of a specially trained interpreter is even more important if the person has limited health literacy.

◆ Working With Interpreters

It is ideal to engage persons who are trained medical interpreters and who are of the same age, sex, and social status as the person in need of linguistic assistance. Unfortunately, it is too often necessary to call upon strangers, such as housekeepers or younger relatives, to act as interpreters. When children and grandchildren are asked to act as interpreters, the nurse must realize that the child or the older adult may be "editing" comments because of intergenerational boundaries or cultural restrictions about the sharing of certain information (e.g., some information may not be considered appropriate to share between older and younger persons). It is increasingly common to use telephonic interpretation. The gerontological nurse recognizes that clarity of speech when listening over a phone may be very difficult with even the simplest age-related auditory losses. "Face-to-face" communication with an interpreter while using telemedicine technology will enable the older adult to hear and see the speaker to optimize communication. In the cross-cultural setting this also allows inclusion of other subtleties, such as body language discussed earlier.

E: Explain

Once the nurse has listened and observed carefully, identifying the relevant and important information, he or she must analyze this carefully and begin to generate and prioritize a hypothesis (see Box 3.8 for helpful lines

---

BOX 3.8   The Explanatory Model for Culturally Sensitive Assessment

1. How would you describe the problem that has brought you here?
   (What do you call your problem; does it have a name?)
   a. Who is involved in your decision-making about health concerns?
2. How long have you had this problem?
   a. When do you think it started?
   b. What do you think started it?
   c. Do you know anyone else with it?
   d. Tell me what happened to that person when dealing with this problem.
3. What do you think is wrong with you?
   a. How severe is it?
   b. How long do you think it will last?
4. Why do you think this happened to you?
   a. Why has it happened to the involved part?
   b. What do you fear most about your sickness?
5. What are the chief problems your sickness has caused you?
6. What do you think will help clear up this problem? (What treatment should you receive; what are the most important results you hope to receive?)
   a. If specific tests and/or medications are listed, ask what they are and do.
7. Apart from me, who else do you think can make you feel better?
   a. Are there therapies that make you feel better that I do not know? *(Maybe in another discipline?)*

Adapted from Kleinman, A., Eisenberg, L., & Good, B. (1978). Culture, illness, and care: Clinical lessons from anthropologic and cross-cultural research, *Ann Intern Med 88*(2):251–258.

---

of inquiry) from the context in which the care is being delivered. This portion of the conversation requires utmost tact and gentleness so that the nurse does not appear judgmental or exhibit any disrespect for the person's views and beliefs. Kleinman's suggestions can be used for both listening and explaining. The nurse explains to the person his or her views about the nature of the illness. The nurse must not prematurely develop action strategies or even finalize the prioritization of the hypotheses.

◆ A: Acknowledge

Achieving desired outcomes will stop at this point unless the nurses acknowledges the similarities and differences between the nurse's hypotheses and priorities and those of the older adult (and significant other if appropriate). This may be especially difficult for those on either side of the conversation who hold a preconceived cultural belief in the authority of the health care provider. When an informal interpreter is used, there is the added risk that he or she edits the conversation in a way that makes a "meeting of the minds" impossible. This mutual acknowledgment forms the basis for the next step of negotiating solutions and actions.

◆ R: Recommend

With careful and thorough consideration, the nurse can now assimilate the aforementioned cues, discussion of hypotheses, and knowledge of the person's beliefs and personal experiences with health care and develop unique, *potential* strategies. This is presented to the older adult and/or to the person(s) he or she has designated to be involved in receiving the information.

◆ N: Negotiate

Finally, cross-cultural skills include the ability to negotiate and implement an action plan that takes both perspectives into account and is mutually acceptable (Berlin & Fowkes, 1983). In many cases the nurse cannot change the person's belief system. It is difficult, if not impossible, and usually counterproductive. This is particularly true when working with older adults who carry a lifetime of beliefs about prior illness experiences and treatments. The nurse attempts to preserve helpful beliefs and practices, to accommodate beliefs that are neither helpful nor harmful, and to help persons modify beliefs or actions that are known to be harmful. A sense of caring is conveyed by giving support to the person's traditional beliefs and practices. At the same time, respectfully explaining concern about potentially harmful actions with the offer of possible alternative strategies will demonstrate that the nurse is considering the person's preferences and uniqueness.

INTEGRATING CONCEPTS

The migration of some older adults born outside the United States or other adopted countries was uneventful. They moved easily with their parents or made conscious decisions to join their child in a new country. Many others suffered horrifically in their home country before the move or during their immigration process, and for many, safety and security were never certain. Several years ago, the staff of a nursing home for Jewish residents complained that it was particularly difficult getting some of the residents with dementia to shower. Some were Holocaust survivors. It was some time before the staff realized that as the residents' dementia progressed, they were no longer able to distinguish the difference between a shower for hygiene and the fear of "going to the showers" (i.e., to the gas chamber) in the concentration camps of their youth (Weissman, 2004).

Changes are threatening the historical role of aging in families across the globe. Different degrees of assimilation between generations create a communication gap between the young and older immigrants as they join their families in new countries where the language and customs may be unknown to them. This may cause isolation and estrangement between the oldest and youngest generations (see Chapter 26).

Economic independence and mobility of the younger members of the family are chipping away at the insulation afforded by the community (Jett, 2006). Members of ethnic and sexual minorities are especially vulnerable in old age (Box 3.9). Nurses can take an active role in facilitating self-actualization by enabling expression of the uniqueness of the individual, by attending to the older adult's spiritual and cultural needs, and by taking the lead in optimizing the health and abilities of those who seek our care.

The study of aging is one of the most complex and intriguing opportunities of our day. Realistically, it will be almost impossible to become familiar with the whole range of clinically relevant cultural differences of older adults that may be encountered. Attempting to provide care holistically and sensitively is a challenge leading to personal growth for both the nurse and the person receiving care.

Skillful clinical decision-making and judgments require nurses to develop cultural proficiency through awareness of their own ethnocentricities. They must be acutely sensitive to the cues suggested (e.g., eye contact) to know how best to respond. Promoting healthy aging in cross-cultural settings includes the ability to develop actions that consider the environmental and personal factors of both the older adult/family and the nurse/health care system to negotiate an outcome that is mutually acceptable. Skillful cross-cultural communication means developing a sense of mutual respect between the nurse and the older adult. A sense of caring is conveyed in gestures of personal recognition. It is working "with" the person rather than "on" the person, and in doing so, health disparities and inequities, if they exist, can begin to be reduced and movement toward healthy aging can be facilitated.

▌KEY CONCEPTS

- Population diversity will continue to increase rapidly for many years. This suggests that nurses will be caring for a greater number of persons from a broad range of older adults than in the past.
- Nurses can contribute to the reduction of health disparities and inequities by moving toward cultural proficiency in day-to-day practice.
- Attention to cultural cues, cultural awareness, knowledge, and skills are necessary to move toward cultural proficiency.
- Nurses caring for diverse older adults must let go of their own ethnocentrism before they can give effective care.
- Many older adults hold health beliefs that are different from those of the biomedical or Western medicine used by most health care professionals in the United States and other Western countries.
- Lack of knowledge of the person's health belief model and time orientation has the potential to produce conflict regardless of the setting in which it takes place.
- The more complex the communication or decision-making needs, the greater the need for skilled interpreter services for persons with limited English proficiency.
- Programs staffed by persons who reflect the ethnic background of the participants and speak their language may be preferred by the participants.
- The LEARN Model provides a useful framework for working with persons of any ethnicity or background to develop achievable and acceptable outcomes.

BOX 3.9   Where Did the Community Go?

A middle-aged Black woman talked about her community and care of persons with dementia. She said that when she grew up, "it was expected that the neighbor would watch out for you. Like if someone saw you out and about and knew you would get lost, they would just take you home again... That just doesn't seem to be happening anymore... we don't even know each other!"

From Jett, K. F. (2006). Mind-loss in the African American community: Dementia as a normal part of aging, *J Aging Stud 20*(1):1–10.

ACTIVITIES AND DISCUSSION QUESTIONS

1. Discuss your personal beliefs regarding health and illness and explain how they fit into the three major classifications of health models. How can this affect the provision of culturally proficient care to those who hold different beliefs?
2. Explain the types of questions that would be helpful in assessing a person's health problem(s) in a way that is respectful of the person and his or her cultural background and ethnic identity.
3. Propose strategies that would be helpful in developing health promoting strategies for older adults from different ethnic and cultural backgrounds.
4. Discuss your familial and culturally determined views of aging after speaking to older family members.

NEXT-GENERATION NCLEX® EXAMINATION-STYLE QUESTIONS

Ms. Yazzie is a 78-year-old long-term care resident. She worked most of her life as a bartender. Her mother belonged to the Mescalero Apache Tribe in New Mexico. Her father was White. Her mother gave her up at birth, hoping she would be adopted, but she spent her childhood in foster care. As a young adult, Ms. Yazzie was raped and severely beaten, resulting in PTSD. She is aggressive with personal care and does not allow men to touch her; only female nurses, assistive personnel, and staff work with her. She has a history of hypothyroidism, hypertension, multi-infarct dementia, and osteoarthritis with chronic pain. She has a 66-pack-year history of smoking and typically drank liquor each night while bartending. She is 5′ 5″ tall and weighs 110 pounds (BMI 18.30 kg/m²). She is no longer ambulatory. However, she wheels herself around the facility and can often be heard crying and repeatedly asking, "Do you love me?" She engages in conversation and stops crying and talks about her childhood when asked. Ms. Yazzie never married and has no children.

Highlight the statements above that culturally proficient nurses recognize as exacerbating health disparities and inequities in this client.

REFERENCES

Adelson, N. (2005). The embodiment of inequality: Health disparities in Aboriginal Canada. *Can J Public Health, 96*, S45–S61.

Berlin, E. A., & Fowkes, W. C. (1983). A teaching framework for cross-cultural health care: Application in family practice. *West Journal Medicine, 139*(6), 934–938.

Campinha-Bacote, J. (2011). Delivering patient-centered care in the midst of a cultural conflict: The role of cultural competence. *Online Journal Nurse Issues, 16*(2), 5.

Centers for Disease Control and Prevention (CDC): *Health equity,* 2018. http://www.cdc.gov/minorityhealth/.

Feagin, J., & Bennefield, Z. (2014). Systematic racism in U.S. healthcare. *Soc Sci Med, 103*, 7–14.

Fung, H. H. (2013). Aging in culture. *Gerontologist, 53*(3), 369–377.

Grandbois, D. M., Warne, D., & Eschiti, V. (2012). The impact of history and culture on nursing care of Native American elders. *J Gerontol Nurs, 38*(10), 3–5.

Jett, K. F. (2003). The meaning of aging and the celebration of years among rural African American women. *Geriatr Nurs, 24*, 290–293.

Jett, K. (2006). Mind-loss in the African American community: A normal part of aging. *J Aging Stud, 20*(1), 1–10.

Kirmayer, L. J., & Brass, G. (2016). Addressing global health disparities among Indigenous peoples. *The Lancet, 388*(10040), 105–106.

Kleinman, A., Eisenberg, L., & Good, B. (1978). Culture, illness, and care: Clinical lessons from anthropologic and cross-cultural research. *Ann Intern Med, 88*(2), 251–258.

Leininger, M. (2002). Culture care theory: A major contribution to advance transcultural nursing knowledge and practices. *J Transcult Nurs, 13*(2), 189–192.

Little, B. (2018). Government boarding schools once separated Native American children from families. *History.* https://www.history.com/news/government-boarding-schools-separated-native-american-children-families.

McIntosh, P. (1988). *White privilege: unpacking the invisible knapsack.* https://www.racialequitytools.org/resourcefiles/mcintosh.pdf.

Mendez-Luck, C. A., Applewhite, S. R., Lara, V. E., & Toyokawa, N. (2016). The concept of familism in the lived experience of Mexican-origin caregivers. *J Marriage Fam, 78*(3), 813–829.

Mogrady, B. (2019). Historical separations still affect Indigenous children. *Nature, 570*, 423–424.

Rathbone-McCune, E. (1982). *Isolated elders: Health and social intervention.* Rockville, MD: Aspen.

Schim, S. N., Doorenbos, A., Benkert, R., et al. (2007). Culturally congruent care: Putting the pieces together. *J Transcult Nurs, 18*(2), 57–62.

Shen, Z. (2004). Cultural competence models in nursing: A selected annotated bibliography. *J Transcult Nurs, 15*(4), 317–322.

Spector, R. E. (2017). *Cultural diversity in health and illness* (9th ed). New York: Pearson.

Weissman G: Personal communication, April 10, 2004.

World Health Organization (WHO):*10 facts on health inequities and their causes,* 2017. http://www.who.int/features/factfiles/health_inequities/en.

World Population Review: *Most diverse countries 2020,* 2020. https://worldpopulationreview.com/countries/most-diverse-countries/.

4

Biological Theories and Age-Related Cues

Kathleen Jett

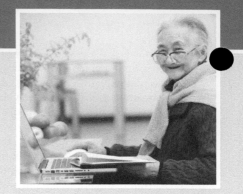

http://evolve.elsevier.com/Touhy/gerontological/

LEARNING OBJECTIVES

Upon completion of this chapter, the reader will be able to:

- Suggest ways in which normal age-related changes are supported or refuted by the major theories of aging.
- Identify the physical changes that are associated with normal aging.
- Begin to differentiate the cues suggesting normal age-related changes from those that are potentially pathological.
- Describe at least one age-related change for each body system that has the most potential to impair function.
- Utilize knowledge of the current theories of aging and age-related changes with aging to develop hypotheses based on informed cues.

THE LIVED EXPERIENCE

Until I started learning about the science of the aging process I had no idea how complicated it could be. We seem to have learned so much but still have so much more to learn.

Helena, age 20

When I was a young girl Einstein was proposing the molecular theory of matter and we had never heard of DNA or RNA. We only knew of genes in the most rudimentary theoretical sense. Now I hear that scientists believe there is a gene that is controlling my life span. I really hope they find it before I die.

Beatrice, age 72

Theories are attempts to explain phenomena, to give a sense of order, and to provide a framework from which one can interpret and simplify the world (Einstein, 1920). Although some theories of biological aging were developed in the early 1950s, more recently the focus has been on attempts to understand the cellular changes within organisms as they age. In some cases, the associations between biological processes and an organism's aging have become clearer. Physiological inflammation appears to have one of the most significant effects on aging or triggering aging, but what triggers these processes remains largely theoretical—at least for now.

Many apparent age-related changes do not happen to everyone. Others are universal but do not occur at the same chronological age (e.g., menopause). In this chapter several of the current prominent biological theories of aging and the major physical changes associated with normal aging are discussed. With this knowledge the nurse can begin to differentiate the cues related to normal aging from those associated with preventable or treatable health problems and thereby promote healthy aging.

BIOLOGICAL AGING

Biological aging, referred to as senescence, is an exceedingly complex interactive process of change, resulting in decreased physiological reserves, increased rate of cellular deterioration, and increased vulnerability to disease (Ventura et al., 2017). Aging changes are made visible in what is referred to as the "aging phenotype" that is, the physical changes that occur as we accumulate years of life. Some changes are potentially harmful (e.g., slowed reaction time) and others are harmless (e.g., graying of hair).

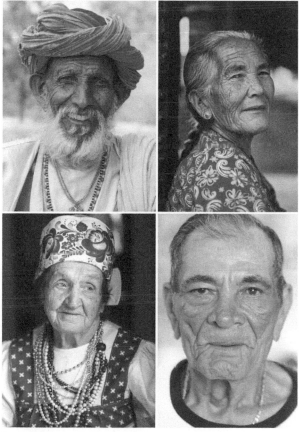

The aging phenotype. (@ iStock.com/kailash soni; Bartosz Hadyniak; De Visu; ProArtWork.)

Cellular Functioning and Aging

Survival of an organism depends on successful cellular reproduction. The genetic components of each cell (DNA and RNA) serve as templates for ensuring that, theoretically, reproduction results in new cells that are the same as the old cells in form and function. If reproduction were always perfect, the organism would never age. Instead, the ability of some cells to reproduce

decreases, errors occur in the process, and ultimately the ability to reproduce ceases altogether.

Although there is a growing body of knowledge about the genomics of aging, complex questions remain. What triggers the changes at the cellular or organ level? What are the roles of cellular mutation and epigenetics, that is, the effect of the environment on the RNA? What are the effects of lifestyle choices and how do they influence the aging phenotype?

Evolution and Aging

Evolution Theories are recognized as important tools in the understanding of the genetic influence on cellular aging and longevity. These theories draw heavily on conversations about the concept of "natural selection," that is, those who live long enough to reproduce are thought to be the fittest of a population. Since we become less fit as we age, we now must address the questions of why some persons live a very long time. What are the genetic and cellular factors influencing who survives and who does not?

The most developed of these theories is that of the "Disposable Soma [cell]." According to this theory, growth is viewed in terms of the utilization of metabolic resources. These are either spent in the preparation for and the production of offspring or in "keeping…going from one day to the next" (Kirkland, 2017, p. 23). Theoretically, those whose metabolic resources are spent almost entirely on procreation die earlier than those with fewer offspring. During procreation, fewer metabolic resources are available to repair naturally occurring cellular damage or completely meet several metabolic needs (Box 4.1). If any of these needs are completely unmet, the organism will die. Studies have shown that longevity is proportionate to an organism's ability to balance its somatic systems and metabolic needs (Kirkland, 2017).

BOX 4.1   Examples of Essential Metabolic Needs

Ability to repair damaged DNA
Ability to remove antioxidants
Ability to control stress proteins
Ability to accurately replicate DNA and proteins
Ability to suppress tumor growth
Ability to maintain a healthy immune system

Modified from Kirkwood, T. B. (2017). Theory and the mechanisms of aging. In H. M. Fillit, K. Rockwood, J. Young, (Eds.) *Brocklehurst's textbook of geriatric medicine and gerontology,* (8th ed., pp. 22–26). Philadelphia: Elsevier.

Free Radicals

Free radicals are naturally occurring molecules within the cell that are missing an electron and therefore physiologically unstable. Reactive oxygen species (ROS) are

> **BOX 4.2   Examples of Diseases Found to Be Associated With an Accumulation of Aging Cells in the Body**
>
> Diabetes
> Hypertension
> Sarcopenia
> Parkinson's disease
> Chronic skin ulcers
>
> Modified from Kirkwood, T. B. (2017). Cellular mechanisms of aging. In H. M. Fillit, K. Rockwood, J. Young (Eds.), *Brocklehurst's textbook of geriatric medicine and gerontology* (8th ed., pp. 47–52). Philadelphia: Elsevier.

also found in the cell, some of which are already free radicals or cause their formation. Both are formed spontaneously during cell metabolism. Although both free radicals and ROS are necessary for some cellular activities, they are capable of damaging lipids, proteins, and other macromolecules (Speakman & Selman, 2007). They have been found to cause mutations in mitochondrial DNA (mtDNA) (Lai et al., 2017).

The number of ROS is increased by several external factors, such as pollution and cigarette smoke, smog and ozone, pesticides, and radiation, and by internal factors, such as inflammation from many sources including emotional stress (Dato et al., 2013). A dramatic rise in the level of ROS, referred to as oxidative stress, has been well documented to lead to cell damage and an accumulation of "aging" cells. These older cells have been found to be associated with several diseases (Kirkland, 2017; Lobo et al., 2010; Speakman & Selman, 2011) (Box 4.2). This damage appears to be random and unpredictable, varying from one cell to another, from one person to another (Speakman & Selman, 2011).

For many years it was thought that the consumption of supplemental antioxidants, such as vitamins C and E, could delay or minimize the effects of aging by counteracting the damage caused by free radicals (Box 4.3). However, it is now known that the intake of supplemental antioxidants is deleterious to one's health (National Center for Complementary and Integrative Medicine [NCCAM], 2013). At the same time, diets inclusive of natural antioxidants, such as those high in fruits and vegetables or a Mediterranean diet rich with red wine and olive oil, have been found to be clearly healthful (Dato et al., 2013).

"Inflamm-aging"

The human immune system is a complex network of cells, tissues, and organs that function separately. The body maintains homeostasis through the actions of this protective, self-regulatory system. It protects the body from the invasion of exogenous substances, such as exposure to bacteria, and endogenous conditions, such as emotional stress. The function of the immune system decreases with age leading to increased risk of infection, cancers, autoimmune disorders, and associated mortality (Kirkland, 2017).

Acute inflammation is the immune system's response to a sudden insult such as trauma. When inflammation is present, several cellular mediators such as macrophages are activated. In turn, these cells release molecular mediators, which are responsible for the inflammatory cascade designed to destroy pathogens, begin tissue repair, and promote physiological homeostasis. The nurse recognizes an inflammation response in the cues suggestive of erythema, edema, pain, or emotional distress.

It has been well documented that aging is accompanied by chronic, low-level, subclinical inflammation. This has been referred to as "inflamm-aging," and there is a theory that it accelerates biological aging and increases the risk of a number of age-related diseases and cellular senescence (Chung et al., 2019; Ventura et al., 2017) (Box 4.4).

> **BOX 4.4   Aging and Inflammation: Diseases Associated with Excessive Inflammation**
>
> Dementia
> Parkinson's disease
> Atherosclerosis
> Diabetes type 2
> Sarcopenia
> Rheumatoid arthritis
> Osteoporosis
> Osteoarthritis
> Frailty syndrome
> High risk of morbidity and mortality
>
> Adapted from Ventura, M. T., Casciaro, M., Gagemi, S., et al. (2017). Immunosenescence in aging: Between immune cells depletion and cytokines up-regulation, *Clin Mol Allergy 15*(21), 1–8.

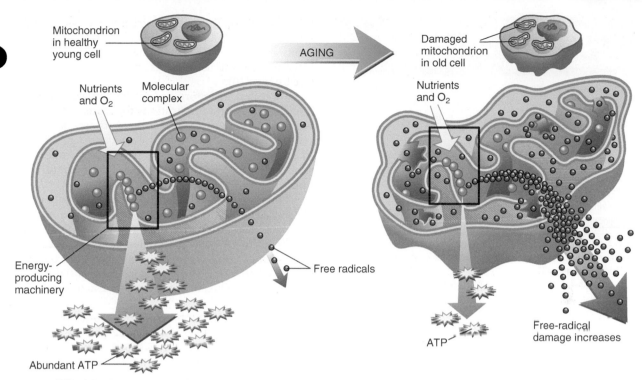

Mitochondrion in healthy young cell

AGING

Damaged mitochondrion in old cell

Nutrients and O_2

Molecular complex

Nutrients and O_2

Energy-producing machinery

Free radicals

Abundant ATP

ATP

Free-radical damage increases

FIG. 4.1 Mitochondria in young and old cells. *ATP,* Adenosine triphosphate. (From McCance, K. L., Huether, S. E. (2010). *Pathophysiology: The biologic basis for disease in adults and children* (6th ed.). St Louis: Mosby.)

Mitochondrial Dysfunction

DNA found within the cell's mitochondria (mtDNA) is key to the production of adenosine triphosphate (ATP), the precursor to the energy needed for physiological processes throughout the body (Fig. 4.1). Free radical and ROS damage to cell is in the form of mutation of the mitochondria. This leads to errors in reproduction (Kirkland, 2017; Lagouge & Larsson, 2013). mtDNA mutations have been found in both normal aging cells and those associated with neurodegenerative disorders such as Alzheimer's disease (Ventura et al., 2017).

Telomeres

Telomeres are portions of DNA found in cells at the end of each chromosome (Fig. 4.2). With each reproduction of the cell the telomeres shorten. When the telomere is short enough, the cell ages and ultimately dies (apoptosis). Length has been proposed as a potentially reliable measure of physiological age. Initial telomere length has been found to be determined by genetic factors; however, the rate of shortening is influenced by other factors, including psychosocial, environmental, and behavioral (Starkweather et al., 2014)

(Box 4.5). Shortened telomeres have been associated with decreased longevity and several chronic diseases including cardiovascular disease, hypertension, diabetes, dementia, and bipolar disorder (Lai et al., 2017;

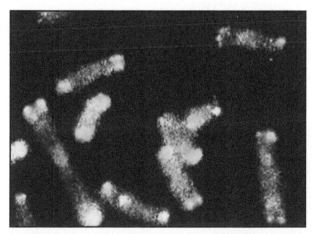

FIG. 4.2 Chromosomes with telomere caps. (Modified from Jerry Shay and the University of Texas Southwestern Medical Center at Dallas, Office of News and Publications, 5323 Harry Hines Blvd, Dallas, TX 75235.)

BOX 4.5 Examples of Factors That Have Been Suggested to Accelerate Telomere Shortening

Chronic stress (perceived)
Pessimism
Interpartner violence
Long-term caregiving (e.g., in Alzheimer's disease)
≤6 hours of sleep a night
Self-reported poor quality of sleep
Higher body mass index and lack of exercise
History of childhood neglect or adverse events
Smoking
Major depressive disorder

From Astuti, Y., Wardhana, A., Watkins, J., et al. (2017). Cigarette smoking and telomere length: A systematic review of 84 studies and meta-analysis, *Environ Re 158*, 480–489.

Starkweather, A. R., Alhaeeri, A. A., Montpetit, A. (2014). An integrative review of factors associated with telomere length and implications for biobehavioral research, *Nur Re 63*(1), 36–50.

Okazaki et al., 2020; Ventura et al., 2017) (Box 4.6). There is evidence associating this shortening with oxidative stress and inflammation. The enzyme telomerase prevents telomere shortening but is only present in human stem cells, reproductive cells, and cancer cells (Kirkland, 2017; Lai et al., 2017).

❖ RECOGNIZING AND ANALYZING CUES TO PROMOTE HEALTHY AGING: NORMAL CHANGES WITH AGING

In the application of our growing knowledge of biological aging, it appears reasonable to expect that slowing or reducing cellular damage may have the potential to promote healthy aging. Although it is not certain that this will lead to increased longevity, it may be a way ultimately to delay those diseases commonly acquired by many as they age. Helping persons reduce external factors (e.g., pollutants in the environment such as secondhand smoke) that are known to increase the development of ROS is one important approach. Levels of naturally occurring antioxidants can be increased through diet. Several studies have found either deleterious or no effects from high-dose supplemental antioxidants such as vitamin E, C, beta-carotene, etc. However, the Age-Related Eye Disease Study (ARDS) found a beneficial effect from a combination of select antioxidant supplements on reducing the risk of the development of macular degeneration for some study participants

(NCCIH, 2013). The gerontological nurse can use this knowledge to encourage persons to abandon long-held habits and beliefs and replace these with the healthiest diets and judicious use of herbs and dietary supplements (see Chapter 10).

Of significant importance in the clinical setting is inflamm-aging and implications for increased susceptibility to infections, autoimmune disorders, and cancers with aging. Observing for early cues suggestive of infections in older adults is a particularly important contribution nurses can make to facilitate a return to wellness.

With an understanding of the changes in immunity, the conscientious nurse can take an active role in promoting specific preventive strategies such as the use of immunizations, especially shingles, influenza, pneumococcus, and COVID-19, and the avoidance of exposure to others with infections. It is a nurse's responsibility not only to promote healthy lifestyles but also to serve as a role model.

Although the current biological theories provide a growing understanding of the aging process, there is still not a definitive answer to what triggers the process. However, there has been considerable progress in illuminating the association between what appears to be cellular aging and age-related diseases. Perhaps what will become more important than understanding the triggers of aging will be understanding the triggers of disease, and thereby the ability to improve health while aging.

It is important for a nurse to understand that the exact cause of aging is unknown and that there is considerable variation in the aging process from person to person and between the systems of any one person. Aging is an entirely unique and individual experience, but at the same time there are also common changes in each physical system of the body at some point and are discussed in the next section.

PHYSICAL CHANGES THAT ACCOMPANY AGING

Skin

As the largest, most visible organ of the body, the various layers of the skin mold and model the individual to give much of his or her personal and sexual identity. The skin and hair provide clues to heredity, race, and physical and emotional health.

Many age-related changes in the skin are functionally inconsequential, but others have more far-reaching implications for organs throughout the body (Table 4.1). Skin changes occur as a result of both internal factors (such

TABLE 4.1 Key Aspects of Normal Age-Related Changes With Aging: Skin and Nails

Changes	Effects
Epidermis	
Reduced number of melanocytes	Increased risk of solar damage such as skin cancers
Thinning	Bruises more easily and blood vessels more fragile
	Tears more easily
Increase time for cell renewal	Increased healing time
Dermis	
Reduced thickness	Pallor, less ability to withstand cooler temperatures
Reduced elastin	Sagging
	Increased risk of injury
Hypodermis	
Thinning	Reduced ability to modulate environmental temperatures
Reduced sebum production	Reduced ability to produce vitamin D when skin is exposed to sunlight
Nails	
Thickening of nails	Increased risk of fungal infections

as genetics) and external factors (such as wind, sun, and exposure to pollutants) to which skin is especially sensitive. Cigarette smoking causes coarse wrinkles, and the photodamage of the sun is evidenced by rough, leathery texture, itching, and mottled pigmentation. Sun damage increases the risk of skin cancer, common among older adults. Skin changes from aging include dryness, thinning, decreased elasticity, and the development of prominent small blood vessels. Skin tears, purpura (large purple spots), and xerosis (excessive dryness) are common but not normal aspects of physical aging (see Chapter 14). Visible changes of the skin—quality of color, firmness, elasticity, and texture—affirm that one is aging.

Epidermis

The epidermis is the outer layer of skin and is composed primarily of tough keratinocytes and squamous cells. Melanocytes produce melanin, which gives the skin color. With age, the production of melanin lessens, the epidermis thins, and blood vessels and bruises are much more visible. Cell renewal time increases with age and significantly more days may be necessary for skin

to repair itself after an injury when compared with a younger adult (Fendrik et al., 2019).

If the skin is injured (e.g., a cut or scrape) in a younger adult, the surrounding tissue becomes red (erythematous) almost immediately. This inflammatory response is the first step in the natural healing process. In an older adult, this inflammation may not begin for 48 to 72 hours. A laceration that becomes pink several days after the event may be misinterpreted as having become infected, when it is actually a sign of the beginning of the healing process. Evidence of a true skin infection in older adults is no different than that in younger adults, namely, odor, increasing redness, and purulent drainage.

Skin tone lightens with the aging as the number of melanocytes in the epidermis decreases, increasing the risk for skin cancer (Chapter 14). With a decrease in the amount of protection from ultraviolet rays, the importance of sunscreen and regular skin check-ups for early signs of cancer increases. However, in some body areas, melanin synthesis increases. Pigmented spots (freckles or nevi) enlarge and can become more numerous in areas exposed to ultraviolet light, such as the backs of the hands and the wrists and on the faces of those with lighter skin. Lentigines, also called age spots or liver spots, appear and are completely benign. Thick, uniformly brown, raised lesion with a "stuck on" appearance is usually seborrheic keratosis; this condition is more common in men and is of no clinical significance but may be cosmetically disturbing to the person.

All skin cancers (melanoma, squamous cell, and basal cell) are increasingly common in older adults after a lifetime of sun exposure, especially for those with very light skin or who have spent a good deal of their earlier years outdoors (e.g., in an occupation such as farming or in a sport such as tennis) (Skin Cancer Foundation, 2019). Actinic keratosis is a precancerous growth on the skin that can be easily confused with the benign seborrheic keratosis. However, on close examination, a very small red or pink ring can be seen surrounding it. This requires a visit to a dermatology office where it will probably be removed. Skin cancer is never a normal change with aging (see Chapter 14).

Dermis

The dermis, lying beneath the epidermis, is a supportive layer of connective tissue composed of a combination of yellow elastic fibers that provide stretch and recoil and white fibrous collagen fibers that provide strength. It also supports hair follicles, sweat glands, sebaceous glands, nerve fibers, muscle cells, and blood vessels, which provide nourishment to the epidermis.

Many of the visible signs of aging skin are reflections of changes in the dermis. The aging dermis loses its thickness. This thinness causes older skin to look more transparent and fragile. Dermal blood vessels are reduced, which contributes to skin pallor and cooler skin temperature. Collagen synthesis decreases, causing the skin to "give" less under stress and tear more easily. Elastin fibers thicken and fragment, leading to loss of stretch and resilience and a sagging appearance. Loss of elasticity accentuates jowls and elongated ears and contributes to the formation of a double chin. Breasts begin to sag. As will be discussed, the impact of the change in elastin also has implications for several other systems.

Hypodermis: Subcutaneous Layer

The hypodermis is the innermost layer of the skin also containing glands, connective tissues, blood vessels, and nerves, but the major component is subcutaneous fat (adipose tissue). The primary purposes of the adipose tissue are to store calories and to provide temperature regulation. It also provides shape and form to the body and acts as a shock absorber against trauma. With age, some areas of the hypodermis thin, others thicken.

Aging changes in the hypodermis increase the chance for the person to become more sensitive both to cold, because the natural insulation of fat is diminished, and to heat (overheated or hyperthermia), as a result of the reduced efficiency of the eccrine (sweat) glands. Sweat glands are located all over the body and respond to thermostimulation and neurostimulation in response to both internal (e.g., fever, menopausal hot flashes) and external causes (e.g., environmental temperatures). A younger body's response to heat is to produce moisture or sweat from these glands and thus cool the skin by evaporation. With aging, the glands become fibrotic and surrounding connective tissue becomes avascular. This leads to decreased cooling efficiency. It is not uncommon for persons to complain of being either too hot or too cold in environments that are comfortable to others.

Glands found in the hypodermis often atrophy in later life. Sebum, produced by the sebaceous (oil) gland, protects the skin by preventing the evaporation of water from the epidermis; it possesses bactericidal properties and contains a precursor of vitamin D. When the skin is exposed to sunlight, vitamin D is produced. Continuing to produce vitamin D is especially important because of the high incidence of osteoporosis (see Chapter 21). All people need limited exposure to natural ultraviolet (UV) light (with protection); therefore, vitamin D supplementation (800 international units) is recommended, especially for those who are frail or residents of care facilities and have few opportunities to be exposed to the sun. When caring for frail older adults, gerontological nurses can promote healthy aging by helping their patients avoid extremes of temperature, prevent dryness, and prevent exposure to toxic products (see Chapter 16).

Hair and Nails

Hair is part of the integument with biological, psychological, and cosmetic value. It is composed of tightly fused horny cells that arise from the dermal layer of the skin and are colored by melanocytes. Genetics, race, sex, and testosterone and estrogen hormones influence hair texture, color, distribution, and loss in both men and women.

In some persons, their genetic backgrounds related to race produce distinctive hair characteristics, which should be kept in mind when caring for the person. For example, persons of Asian descent often have sparse facial and body hair and scalp hair is dark, silky, and often straight. Persons of African descent often have slightly more head and body hair than Asians; however, the hair texture varies widely. It is always fragile and ranges from straight to spiraled and from thin to thick. Persons of European descent have the most head and body hair, with texture and form ranging from straight to curly, fine to coarse, thick to thin, and of any color.

Men and women in all racial groups have lighter, thinner, and less hair as they grow older. Scalp hair loss is prominent in men, beginning as early as the twenties. The hair in the ears, the nose, and the eyebrows of older men increases and stiffens. Women may have less pronounced scalp hair loss until after menopause. The accustomed hair color remains for some, but for most there is a gradual loss of pigmentation (melanin) and it becomes dryer and coarser. Older women develop chin and facial hair attributable to a decreased estrogen-to-testosterone level ratio. Leg, axillary, and pubic hair lessens and, in some instances, eventually disappears altogether. The absence of lower extremity hair can be misinterpreted as a sign of peripheral vascular disease in the older adult, whereas it is a normal age-related change.

Fingernails and toenails become harder and thicker, and more brittle, dull, and opaque. They change in shape, becoming at times flat or concave instead of convex. Decreasing amounts of water, calcium, and lipid in the body result in vertical ridges. Reduced blood supply slows nail growth rate. The half-moon (lunula) at the base of the fingernails may entirely disappear; the color of the nails may vary from yellow to gray. The long-term effect of the widespread use of nail acrylic and lacquer is not yet known.

The development of fungal infections of the nails (onychomycosis) is quite common but not the result of aging. Fungus invades the space between the layers of the nail, leaving a thick and unsightly appearance. The

TABLE 4.2 Key Aspects of Normal Age-Related Changes With Aging: Musculoskeletal

Changes	Effects
Dryer ligaments, tendons, and joints	Reduced flexibility
Reduced muscle mass	Reduced strength
Reduced bone mineral density	Increased risk of fractures, spontaneous and traumatic
Reduced body water	Increased risk of dehydration

slowness of growth and the reduced circulation in older nails make treatment very difficult.

Musculoskeletal

A functioning musculoskeletal system is necessary for the body's movement in space, gross responses to environmental forces, and the maintenance of posture. This complex system comprises bones, joints, tendons, ligaments, and muscles.

Although none of the age-related changes to the musculoskeletal system are life-threatening, any of them could affect one's ability to function and therefore one's quality of life (Table 4.2). Some of the changes are visible to others and have the potential to affect a person's self-esteem. As seen with the skin, changes in the musculoskeletal system are influenced by many factors, such as age, sex, race, and environment; signs of musculoskeletal changes may become obvious in a person's forties.

The musculoskeletal changes that have the most effect on function are related to the ligaments, tendons, and joints; over time these structures become dry, hardened, and less flexible. In joints that had been subjected to trauma earlier in life (injuries or repetitive movement), the changes can be seen earlier and may be more severe. If joint space is reduced, arthritis is diagnosed.

Muscle mass can continue to build until the person is in his or her fifties. However, between 40% and 50% of the skeletal muscle mass of a 30-year-old person may be lost by the time the person is in his or her eighties (Brown & McCarthy, 2015). Lack of use of skeletal muscle leading to weakening (sarcopenia) accelerates the loss of strength. The amount of muscle tissue mass decreases (atrophies) whereas levels of adipose tissue increase. The replacement of lean muscle by adipose tissue is most noticeable in men in the area of the waist and in women between the umbilicus and the symphysis pubis.

Stature, Posture, and Body Composition

Changes in stature and posture are two of the more obvious signs of aging and are associated with multiple factors involving skeletal, muscular, subcutaneous, and adipose tissue. Vertebral disks become thin as a result of both gravity and dehydration, causing a shortening of the trunk. These changes may begin to be seen as early as the fifties (Reeves et al., 2019). The person may have a stooped appearance from kyphosis, a curvature of the cervical vertebrae arising from reduced bone mineral density (BMD). Some loss of BMD in women is associated with the normal age-related lowered postmenopausal estrogen levels. With the shortened appearance, the bones of the arms and the legs may appear disproportionate in size. If a person's bone mineral density is very low, it is diagnosed as osteoporosis and a loss of 2 to 3 inches in height is not uncommon (see Chapter 21).

From 25 to 75 years of age, the fat content of the body increases slowly, altering body shape and weight as the amount of lean body mass declines. Age-related loss of body water is significant in both men and women. This water loss results in a dramatically increased risk of dehydration (Fig. 4.3).

Cardiovascular

The cardiovascular system is responsible for the transport of oxygenated and nutrient-rich blood to the organs and the transport of metabolic waste products to the kidneys and bowels. The most relevant age-related changes in this system are myocardial (heart tissue) and blood vessel stiffening and decreased responsiveness to sudden changes in cardiovascular demand (Table 4.3). Changes in the cardiovascular (CV) system are progressive and cumulative.

Cardiac

Age-related changes in the heart (presbycardia) are structural, electrical, and functional. Although the overall size of the heart remains relatively unchanged in healthy aging, the wall thickens and the shape changes somewhat. Maximum coronary artery blood flow, stroke volume, and cardiac output are decreased, putting the person at much greater risk of heart failure (Howlett, 2017). In healthy aging, the changes have little or no effect on the heart's ability to function in day-to-day life. The changes only become significant when there are environmental, physical, or psychological stresses. With sudden demands for more oxygen, the heart may not be able to respond adequately. It takes longer for the heart to both accelerate and return to a resting state.

For a gerontological nurse, this means that the increased heart rate one might expect to see when the person is in pain, anxious, febrile, or hemorrhaging may not be present or will be delayed. Similarly, an older heart may not be able to respond to other circumstances

Proportion of Body Weight Represented by Water

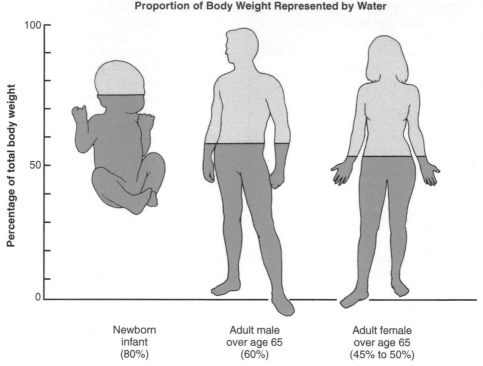

FIG. 4.3 Changes in body water distribution. (From Thibodeau, G. A., Patton, K. T. (2008). *Structure and function of the body* (13th ed.). St Louis: Mosby.)

TABLE 4.3	**Key Aspects of Normal Age-Related Changes With Aging: Cardiovascular**
Changes	**Effects**
Stiffening and thickening of the heart tissue	Decreased ability to respond to the need for increased circulation/oxygen
	Longer time for the heart to return to a resting state after stress
Decreased elasticity of the arterial walls	Increased risk for hypertension
	Reduced blood flow to some organs (e.g., kidney)

requiring increased cardiac demand, such as infection, anemia, pneumonia, cardiac dysrhythmias, surgery, diarrhea, hypoglycemia, malnutrition, drug-induced illnesses, and noncardiac illnesses such as renal disease and prostatic obstruction. Instead, the nurse must depend on other signs of distress in older patients and be diligently alert to signs of rapid decompensation both in those previously well and those who are already medically fragile, such as nursing home residents.

Heart disease is the number one cause of nonaccidental death in the world (WHO, 2020). Often the changes

associated with disease are thought to be normal, but they are not. A nurse promotes healthy aging by providing recommendations for heart-healthy life choices and urging the person to seek and receive excellent health care (see Chapter 22).

Blood Vessels

Several of the same age-related changes seen in the skin (especially loss of elastin) and muscles affect the lining (intima) of the blood vessels, especially the arteries (Howlett, 2017). As in the skin, the most significant change is decreased elasticity limiting the consistent forward movement of blood to the organs. In health, change in blood flow to the coronary arteries and the brain is minimal, but decreased blood flow to other organs, especially the liver and kidneys, has potentially significant implications for medication use (see Chapter 9). When a person already has or develops arteriosclerosis or hypertension, the age-related changes can have serious consequences (see Chapter 22).

Less dramatic changes are found in the veins, although they do stretch, but the valves, which keep the blood from flowing backward, become less efficient. This means that lower extremity edema develops more quickly and that the older adult is more at risk of deep vein thrombosis (blood clots/DVTs) because of the increased sluggishness of the venous circulation. The normal changes, when combined with long-standing but unknown weakness of the vessels, may become visible in varicose veins and explain the increased rate of stroke and aneurysms in older adults.

Respiratory

The respiratory system is the vehicle for ventilation and gas exchange, particularly the transfer of oxygen into and the release of carbon dioxide from the blood. The respiratory structures depend on the musculoskeletal and nervous systems to function fully. The respiratory system matures by the age of 20 years and then begins to decline, even in healthy individuals. Although subtle changes occur in the lungs, the thoracic cage, the respiratory muscles, and the respiratory centers in the central nervous system, the changes are small in healthy aging and, for the most part, insignificant. The specific changes include loss of elasticity resulting in stiffening of the chest wall, less efficient gas exchange, and increased resistance to air flow (Davies & Bolton, 2017) (Fig. 4.4).

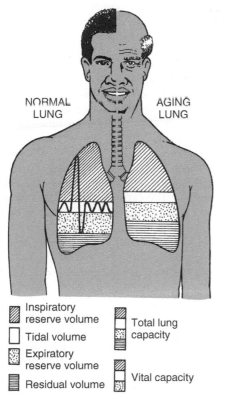

NORMAL LUNG

AGING LUNG

- ▨ Inspiratory reserve volume
- ☐ Tidal volume
- ▦ Expiratory reserve volume
- ▤ Residual volume
- ☐ Total lung capacity
- ▨ Vital capacity

FIG. 4.4 Changes in lung volumes with aging. (From McCance, K. L., Huether, S. E. (2010). *Pathophysiology: The biologic basis for disease in adults and children* (8th ed.). St Louis: Elsevier.)

Respiratory problems are common but almost always the result of past or present exposure to environmental toxins, especially cigarette smoke, rather than a consequence of the aging process (see Chapter 22).

Like the cardiovascular system, the biggest change is in the efficiency, in this case of gas exchange. Under usual conditions, this has little or no effect on the performance of customary life activities. However, a respiratory deficit may become evident when an individual is confronted with a sudden demand for increased oxygen. The body is not as sensitive to low oxygen levels or elevated carbon dioxide levels, each indicating the need to increase the rate of breathing. The changes that occur in the anatomical structures of the chest and altered muscle strength can significantly affect one's ability to cough forcefully enough to expel materials quickly that accumulate in or obstruct airways. In addition, the respiratory cilia (small fibers in the respiratory system) are less effective. Together these place the person at high risk of potentially life-threatening infections and aspiration. In the presence of impairment, such as difficulty swallowing or decreased movement of the esophagus, the risk is even more increased; this is often the case after a person has had a stroke or during end-stage dementia. All these potential complications make the promotion of health through the prevention of respiratory illnesses in older adults of the highest importance.

Renal

The renal system is responsible for regulating concentrations of water and salts in the body and maintaining the acid/base balance in the blood. Blood is filtered in the nephrons in the kidneys with each beat of the heart. The glomerulus is the key structure that controls the rate of filtering (glomerular filtration rate [GFR]). Among the many changes to the kidneys are those of blood flow, GFR, and the ability to regulate body fluids. As a result of vascular and fixed anatomical and structural changes, blood flow through the kidneys decreases by about 10% per decade, from about 1200 mL/min in young adults to about 600 mL/min by 80 years of age, (Smith & Kuchel, 2017). Yet the kidneys lose as many as 50% of the nephrons with little change in the body's ability to regulate body fluids and maintain adequate day-to-day fluid homeostasis.

Although age-related changes in the renal system are not universal, they are especially significant because of resultant heightened susceptibility to fluid and electrolyte imbalance and because of structural damage caused by medications and contrast media used in diagnostic tests. Even healthy aging kidneys have a reduced capacity to respond (renal reserve) to either salt or water overload or deficit or even a fever, and therefore older adults are at greater risk than healthy younger adult for renal insufficiency and failure.

Whereas plasma creatinine level is constant throughout life, urine creatinine level should decline even in normal aging because of the reduced lean muscle mass. The urine creatinine clearance rate, as a reflection of the ability to handle medications passing through and metabolized by the kidneys, is often calculated to determine appropriate drug therapy (Chapter 9). However, it is not always a true representation of kidney function (Smith & Kunkle, 2017).

> ⚡ **SAFETY ALERT**
>
> Persons with a reduced GFR and creatinine clearance rate usually need a reduction in the dosages of some medications to prevent potential toxicity. This is especially true for antibiotics. Caution must be used in the administration of intravenous fluids.

Endocrine

The endocrine system, working in tandem with the neurological system, provides regulation and control of the integration of body activities through the secretion of hormones from glands that can be found throughout the body. As the body ages, most glands shrink and the rate of secretion decreases. However, other than the decrease in estrogen level, leading to menopause, the impact of the changes is not clear.

Pancreas

The endocrine pancreas secretes insulin, glucagon, somatostatin, and pancreatic polypeptides. The secretion of these substances does not appear to decrease to any level of clinical significance. However, there is increased insulin resistance and accelerated aging for those with chronic inflammation and obesity, leading to diabetes mellitus type 2 (Akintola & van Heemst, 2015). Older adults have the highest rate of type 2 diabetes of any age group, with significant variation by ethnicity and region (see Chapter 20). When the pancreas is stressed with sudden concentrations of glucose, blood levels are higher for longer. These temporary levels of increased blood glucose make the diagnosis of diabetes or glucose intolerance difficult.

Thyroid

Slight changes occur in the structure and function of the thyroid gland, which may explain the increased incidence of hypothyroidism in older adults (Morley & McKee, 2017). Some atrophy, fibrosis, and inflammation occur. Diminished secretion of thyroid-stimulating hormone (TSH) and thyroxine (T4) appear to be age-related. Serum T3 levels decrease with age, perhaps as a result of decreased secretion of TSH by the pituitary gland. When thyroid replacement is needed, lower doses are usually effective and higher doses contraindicated. In addition, the therapeutic dose of thyroxine may change over time, and monitoring is required (see Chapter 20).

Collective signs, such as a slowed basal metabolic rate, thinning of hair, and dry skin, are characteristic of hypothyroidism in young people but are normal manifestations in older adults with no history of a thyroid deficiency, making the recognition of thyroid disturbances difficult (see Chapter 20). The number of persons affected by thyroid disturbances is so low that they cannot be considered normal changes with aging.

Reproductive

The reproductive systems in men and women serve the same physiological purpose—human procreation. Although both aging men and women undergo age-related changes, the changes affect women significantly more than men. Women lose the ability to procreate after the cessation of ovulation (menopause), whereas men remain fertile their entire lives. Regardless of the physical changes, the need for sexual expression remains (see Chapter 26).

Female Reproductive System

As menopause signals the end of the reproductive phase in a woman's life, several other age-related changes occur, particularly in breast tissue and urogenital structures. The testosterone-to-estrogen ratio changes, with sometimes a significant drop in a woman's relative estrogen level. Older breasts are smaller, pendulous, and less firm. Outwardly, the labia majora and minora become less prominent and pubic hair thins and may disappear altogether. The cervix, uterus, and ovaries slowly atrophy, the latter to the point where they may not be palpable on examination. The vagina shortens, narrows, and loses some of its elasticity, typical of aging muscle and skin. Vaginal walls also lose their ability to lubricate quickly, especially if the woman is not sexually active. More stimulation is needed to achieve orgasm. The vaginal epithelium changes considerably with an increase in pH and increased risk of vaginitis (Cooper & Smith, 2017). The vaginal changes result in the potential for dyspareunia (painful intercourse), trauma during intercourse, increased susceptibility to infection, and urinary incontinence.

Male Reproductive System

Although men can produce sperm throughout their lives, they also experience changes in the functioning of the reproductive and the urogenital organs in late life. The changes are usually more subtle and noticed only as they accumulate, beginning when men are in their fifties. The testes atrophy and soften. Although sperm count does not decrease, fertility may be reduced because a higher number of sperm lack motility or because of structural abnormalities such as sclerosis or fibrosis of the seminiferous tubules. More stimulation is needed to achieve a full erection, ejaculation is slower and less forceful, and refractory periods (time between erections) are longer (Rodaway & Huether, 2019). As with women, alterations in hormone balances may play a part in the age-related changes in men. Testosterone level is reduced in all men but only rarely to the level at which it would be considered a true deficiency.

By 80 years of age, more than 80% of men in the United States are likely to have some degree of prostatic enlargement (Cross & Prescott, 2017). The only time it is considered a problem is when the enlargement compresses the urethra and interferes with bladder emptying. As a result, the man may experience urinary retention leading to repeated urinary tract infections and overflow incontinence. Intervention is pursued only when the symptoms of benign prostatic hyperplasia (BPH) interfere with the man's quality of life (Cross & Prescott, 2017). In addition to aging, obesity, high glucose levels, and insulin resistance have been found to increase the risk of developing BPH (Chen et al., 2015).

Gastrointestinal

The digestive system includes the gastrointestinal (GI) tract and the accessory organs that aid in digestion. Additionally, several common health problems can have a great effect on the digestive system (Table 4.4).

Mouth

Age-related changes affect both the teeth and mouth. With the wear and tear of years of use, teeth eventually lose enamel and dentin and then become more vulnerable to decay (caries). The roots become more brittle and break more easily. The gums recede and are more susceptible to infection and chronic inflammation and may influence cardiac health (National Institute of Dental and Craniofacial Research [NIDCR], 2018). Without care, teeth may be lost. The nurse ensures the fit and cleanliness of any whole or partial dentures worn. Taste buds decline in number and salivary secretion lessens. A very dry mouth (xerostomia) is common. The sense of smell decreases and may be completely absent by 90 years of age (Feldstein et al., 2017).

Even in health, these changes combine to create the potential for decreased pleasure and comfort in eating,

TABLE 4.4 Key Aspects of Normal Age-Related Changes With Aging: Gastrointestinal

Changes	Effects
Mouth: wear and tear of teeth	Increased risk of decay
Gums recede	Increased risk of oral and cardiac disease
Esophagus: sluggish and erratic movement of muscles	Increased stress to lower end leading to discomfort and increased risk of GERD (gastroesophageal reflux disease)
Stomach: decreased motility, reduced bicarbonate and gastric mucus	Early sensation of fullness, increased risk for pernicious anemia and peptic ulcer disease
Intestines: reduced function of intestinal villi	Reduced ability to adequately absorb nutrients
Liver: reduced blood flow	Increased half-life of fat soluble medications

which in turn can lead to anorexia and weight loss. A number of medications taken for common health problems can quickly exacerbate potential problems, especially xerostomia. When a gerontological nurse administers medications to older adults or conducts medication education, he or she should warn them about this potential and how to minimize its effects (see Chapter 9).

Esophagus

In youth, food passes quickly through the esophagus to the stomach because of the strong and coordinated contractions of associated muscles and peristalsis. In aging, the contractions increase in frequency but are more disordered, and therefore propulsion is less effective. This is referred to as presbyesophagus. The sluggish emptying of the esophagus may cause the lower end of the esophagus to dilate, creating greater stress in this area and possibly causing digestive discomfort. Pathological processes that are increasingly seen as adults become older include gastroesophageal reflux disease (GERD) and hiatal hernias.

Stomach

Age-related changes in the stomach include decreased gastric motility and volume and reductions in the secretion of bicarbonate and gastric mucus. Loss of smooth muscle increases emptying time, which may lead to anorexia or weight loss as a result of distention, meal-induced fullness, and the feeling of early satiety (Feldstein et al., 2017). It will prolong the amount of time medications stay in the stomach, affecting drug metabolism (see Chapter 9). There may be a decline in hydrochloric acid and other digestive substances, leading to a decrease in the ability to produce intrinsic factor, the key component needed for the utilization of ingested vitamin B12. Without vitamin B12, pernicious anemia develops. The lessening or loss of protective gastric mucus makes the stomach more susceptible to peptic ulcer disease and atrophic gastritis, particularly when nonsteroidal anti-inflammatory medications such as aspirin and ibuprofen are used.

Intestines

The age-related changes of the small intestine include those noted earlier that involve smooth muscles as well as those related to the gastric villi, the anatomical structures in the intestinal walls where nutrients are absorbed. The villi become broader and shorter and less functional. Nutrient absorption is affected; proteins, fats, minerals (including calcium), vitamins (especially B12), and carbohydrates (especially lactose) are absorbed more slowly and in lesser amounts (Huether, 2019). Changes in motility, epithelial membranes, vascular perfusion, and gastrointestinal membrane transport may affect absorption of lipids, amino acids, glucose, calcium, and iron.

Peristalsis is slowed with aging and there is a blunted response to rectal filling; the extent of the change should not be such as to cause problems with defecation. In other words, constipation is not a normal part of aging. Instead, constipation is more often a side effect of medications, life habits, immobility, inadequate fluid intake, and lack of attention to the gastrocolic reflex (the urge to defecate after eating). The role of the gerontological nurse in addressing elimination needs is presented in Chapter 12 with suggestions on promoting healthy digestion.

Accessory Organs

The accessory organs of the digestive system are the liver and the gallbladder. The liver continues to function throughout life despite a decrease in weight (mass) and blood flow. The decreases are associated with an increased half-life of fat-soluble medications (see Chapter 9). Although slow, liver regeneration is not greatly impaired and liver function tests remain unaltered.

There does not seem to be a specific change in the gallbladder; however, the incidence of gallstones increases to about 50% (Feldstein et al., 2017). This is possibly caused by the increased lipogenic composition of bile from biliary cholesterol. Decreased bile salt synthesis increases the incidence of cholelithiasis

and cholecystitis, but these are not normal age-related illnesses.

Neurological

Contrary to popular belief, the older nervous system, including the brain, is remarkably resilient, and most changes in cognitive functioning are not a normal part of aging. Although many neurophysiological changes can occur with aging, they do not occur in all older persons and do not affect everyone the same way and therefore cannot be attributed to normal aging. For example, the presence of neurofibrillary tangles is a classic sign of dementia and is found in the brains of all persons with Alzheimer's disease, but they are also found in the brains of persons without dementia. Although it is very difficult to show a true cause and effect of age-related changes in the nervous system, several changes appear to be more common (Table 4.5).

Central Nervous System

The major changes in the aging nervous system are found in the central nervous system (CNS). With aging, the dendrites appear to be "wearing out," and the number of neurons found in several areas of the brain decreases. The older brain is smaller and weighs less than a younger brain. This change in size is seen primarily in the frontal lobe and diagnosed as normal age-related atrophy on computed tomography (CT) scans or magnetic resonance imaging (MRI). Decreased adherence of the dura mater to the skull, increased fibrosis, thickening of the meninges, narrowing of the gyri, widening of the sulcus, and an increase in the subarachnoid space also occur (Butterfield, 2019). These changes are important because

TABLE 4.5 Key Aspects of Normal Age-Related Changes With Aging: Neurological

Changes	Effects
Central nervous system: reduced number of dendrites, atrophy of brain	Decrease in brain weight and size, increased risk for trauma
Slight changes in physiology and chemistry of brain	Mild memory impairments Increased risk of slight balance difficulties
Peripheral nervous system: Significantly reduced vibratory sense in lower extremities Decreased sensory functions at the periphery Decreased proprioception	Greatly increased risk of injury (e.g., from fire or falling)

of the increased potential damage that can occur following a traumatic brain injury (see Chapter 16).

Subtle changes in cognitive and motor functioning occur in the very old. Mild memory impairments and difficulties with balance may be normal age-related changes in neurodegeneration and neurochemistry (see Chapter 23). The intellectual performance of older adults without brain dysfunction remains constant; however, the performance of tasks may take longer, which is an indication that central processing is slowed. There are also decreasing levels of the neurotransmitters choline acetylase, serotonin, and catecholamines. Reduced levels of circulating serotonin probably increase the person's risk of endogenous depression. Other enzymes such as monoamine oxidase (MAO) have increased levels. Redundancy of brain cells may forestall the effects of these changes, but the exact number of cells required for certain functions is unknown.

Peripheral Nervous System

The most important effect of the normal changes in the aging peripheral nervous system is the increased risk of injury. Vibratory sense in the lower extremities may be nonexistent. Tactile sensitivity decreases in connection with the loss of nerve endings in the skin. This is most notable in the fingertips, the palms of the hands, and the lower extremities. This decreased sensitivity is translated into delayed reactions to things such as hot surfaces, significantly increasing the risk for burns and the extent of burns should they occur. The presence of a functioning smoke detector is particularly important for safe aging.

Kinesthetic sense, or proprioception (awareness of one's position in space), is altered because of changes in both the peripheral and the central nervous systems. If one is less aware of body position and has less tactile awareness, the risk of falling is dramatically increased (see Chapter 14). For example, a person may be walking on a flat surface that suddenly becomes uneven. With reduced proprioception, it takes a little longer to realize the surface is uneven and a little longer still to realize that one has tripped (changed position in space). Whereas a younger person would be able to restore his or her body position immediately and prevent a fall, this slight delay may result in a fall in an older adult (Chapter 15). Conditions such as arthritis, stroke, some cardiac disorders, or damage to the structures of the inner ear may also affect peripheral and central mechanisms of mobility and exacerbate these changes in proprioception.

Sensory Changes

As we age, we cannot totally escape some loss of smell, sight, sound, and touch. A creative gerontological nurse

TABLE 4.6 Key Aspects of Normal Age-Related Changes With Aging: Sensory

Changes	Effects
Eyes	
Decrease in near vision (presbyopia)	Necessity of wearing reading glasses or using a magnifying glass for close work
Changes to eyelids: sagging, entropion, and ectropion	Reduced vision, excessive tearing, and scratching of cornea
Reduced efficiency of goblet cells	Uncomfortable, drying of eye
Cornea: flatter, thicker, less flexible	Increased far-sightedness
Lens and intraocular: potential thickening and yellowing, reduced flexibility	Need for increased levels of light, decreased depth and color perception
Ears	
Atrophy of cerumen glands	Thicker, dryer cerumen and increased risk of impactions that temporarily reduce hearing
Stiffening of joints within the ear (presbycusis)	Sensorineural hearing loss, permanent

can make a big difference in the quality of life for the person with sensory changes (see Chapter 19) (Table 4.6).

Eyes and Vision

Changes in vision and eyes begin very early and are both functional and structural. All the changes affect visual acuity and accommodation, that is, the ability to adjust to changes in environmental light.

Presbyopia is an age-related decrease in near vision that begins to become noticeable in midlife. Most adults older than 65 years of age wear glasses for close vision (Galvin, 2017), and may need a magnifying glass for reading and close work. Although presbyopia is first seen between 45 and 55 years of age, 80% of those older than 65 years of age have fair to adequate far vision past 90 years of age.

Extraocular. Like the skin, age-related changes affect both form and function of the extraocular structures. The eyelids lose elasticity and drooping (ptosis) results. This is either congenital or age-related. In most cases, this only affects appearance. In extreme cases the lids sag far enough to block vision and must be surgically repaired. Spasms of the orbicular muscle may cause the lower lid to turn inward. If it stays this way, it is called entropion. The lower lashes that curl inward irritate and scratch the cornea. Surgery may be needed to prevent permanent injury. Decreases in the orbicular muscle strength may result in ectropion or an out-turning of the lower lid. Without the integrity of the trough of the lower lid, tears run down the cheek instead of bathing the cornea. This and reduced ability to close the lid completely leads to dry eyes and the need for artificial tears/moisturizers. The person may need to tape the eyes shut during sleep. Exacerbating this problem, the number of goblet cells that provide mucin (essential for eye lubrication and movement) decreases. A severe deficiency of lubrication is known as dry eye syndrome.

Ocular. The cornea is the avascular transparent outer surface of the eye globe that refracts (bends) light rays entering the eye through the pupil. With aging, the cornea becomes flatter, less smooth, thicker, and duller in appearance. The result is increased far-sightedness (hyperopia). For the person who was myopic (near-sighted) earlier in life, this change may improve vision. Arcus senilis, a gray-white to silver ring or partial ring, may be observed 1 to 2 mm inside the limbus at the juncture of the iris and cornea (Fig. 4.5); it is composed of deposits of calcium and cholesterol salts. It does not appear to have any clinical significance.

The anterior chamber is the space between the cornea and the lens. The edges of the chamber include canals that control the volume and movement of aqueous fluid within the space. With aging, the chamber decreases slightly in size and capacity because of thickening of the lens. Resorption of the intraocular fluid becomes less efficient with age. If the decrease is significant, it can lead to increased intraocular pressure and glaucoma (see Chapter 19) (Huether & Rodway, 2019). Any acute

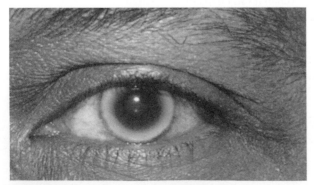

FIG. 4.5 Arcus senilis. (From Swartz, M. H. (2021). *Textbook of physical diagnosis: History and examination* (8th ed.). St Louis: Elsevier.)

changes in vision or eye pain should be considered medical emergencies and responded to accordingly.

Reduced accommodation and the need for greater levels of lighting are the result of reduced responsiveness of the pupils and changes in the lens. The lens, a small, flexible, biconvex, crystal-like structure just behind the iris, is most responsible for visual acuity; it adjusts the light entering the pupil and focuses it on the back of the retina. Age-related changes in the lens are probably universal and begin in the forties. The origins of these changes are not fully understood, although exposure to ultraviolet rays of the sun contributes to the problem, with cross-linkage of collagen creating a more rigid and thickened lens structure.

Light scattering increases and color perception decreases. As a result, glare is a problem created not only by sunlight outdoors but also by the reflection of light on any shiny object, such as a hospital floor. Eventually, people require three times as much light to see things as they did when they were in their twenties. It is more effective to place high-intensity light on the object or surface to be observed rather than increasing the intensity of the light in the entire room. For example, it would be more effective to focus a light directly on the newspaper a person was reading than turning on an overhead light.

> ## ⚡ SAFETY ALERT
>
> As a result of age-related changes in vision there is an increased sensitivity to glare. The floor in the care facility may be very clean, but if it is also shiny, it could increase an older adult's risk of falling.

Intraocular. The retina, which lines the inside of the eye globe, has less distinct margins and is duller in appearance than in younger adults. Color clarity diminishes by 25% in the sixth decade and by 59% in the eighth decade, especially that of the blues, the violets, and the greens of the spectrum; light colors such as reds, oranges, and yellows are seen more easily. Some of this difficulty is linked to the yellowing of the lens and impaired transmission of light to the retina. Finally, the number of rods and associated nerves at the periphery of the retina is reduced, resulting in peripheral vision that is not as clear or is absent (Galvin, 2017). Arteries in the back surface of the retina may show atherosclerosis and slight narrowing. Veins may show indentations (nicking) as they pass over the arteries if the person has a long history of hypertension, but this is not an age-related change in eye structure. As long as these changes are not accompanied by distortion of objects or a significant decrease in vision, they are not clinically significant.

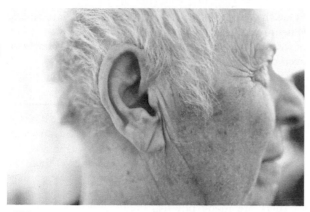

FIG. 4.6 Ear of a senior adult man. (© iStock.com/themacx.)

Ears and Hearing

Like the eye, age-related changes affect both the structure and the function of the ear. The appearance of the ear changes, especially in men (Fig. 4.6). The auricle loses flexibility and becomes longer and wider as a result of diminished elasticity. The lobe sags, elongates, and wrinkles. Together, these changes make the ear appear larger. In men, coarse, wiry, stiff hairs grow at the periphery of the auricle and the tragus enlarges. On otoscopic examination the tympanic membrane appears dull and gray.

The auditory canal narrows through inward collapse. Stiffer and coarser hairs line the canal. Cerumen glands atrophy, causing thicker and dryer wax, which is more difficult to remove. This is a substantial cause of temporary, reversible obstructive hearing loss. The gerontological nurse should be sensitive to this possibility and be skilled at safe cerumen removal. Once the cerumen is removed, the associated obstructive hearing loss is resolved (see Chapter 19).

Aging can change structures within the ear; for example, the joint between the malleus and the stapes can become calcified, causing reduced vibration of these bones and a mechanical reduction in the amount of sound transmitted to the auditory nerve, in turn impairing transmission of sound waves to the brain. This age-related hearing loss is known as presbycusis and sensorineural (SNL) in origin. The loss develops slowly and, in contrast to obstructive loss, is irreversible.

Presbycusis is primarily the loss of the ability to hear high-frequency sounds such as consonants, the chirping of birds, the rustling of leaves, and whispering. Although the person may be able eventually to decipher what is said if it is within context, this processing takes longer than usual, or language may be processed incorrectly. It is important to note that with normal age-related hearing loss the person can still hear but may not be able to make sense of the partially heard words, especially in places where there is a great deal of environmental noise, such as restaurants. Inaccurate responses too often lead to the incorrect suspicion of dementia or confusion when in fact it is a hearing loss. Hearing loss of some kind affects more than 80% of those older than 85 years of age; the major type is SNL (Wallings & Dickson, 2012).

Immune

The human immune system is a complex network of cells, tissues, and organs that function separately. The body maintains homeostasis through the actions of this protective, self-regulatory system, controlled by B lymphocytes (humoral immunity) and T lymphocytes (a type of white blood cell). Together they protect the body from the invasion of exogenous substances, such as bacteria, and endogenous conditions, such as emotional stress. The function of the immune system decreases with age leading to increased risk for infection, cancers, autoimmune disorders, and associated mortality (Kirkland, 2017).

Several age-related changes have been implicated in the increased risk for infection in the older adult (Table 4.7). For example, the skin is thinner and therefore less resistant to bacterial invasion. The reduced number of cilia in the lungs leads to the increased risk for pneumonia. The friability of the urethra increases the risk of urinary tract infections, especially in women.

In later life there is a reduction in T-cell function that results in a decrease in both innate immunity and adaptive immunity. Being alert for signs and symptoms of autoimmune changes is especially important to gerontological nursing, as part of the responsibility to promote disease prevention and protect older adults from infection. Early studies by Stengel (1983) found oral temperature norms in older adults significantly lower than those in younger adults. Older men consistently had an even lower temperature than women of comparable age. This means that a febrile response suggestive of infection is no longer restricted to a temperature greater than 98.6°F or 99°F. Instead, an older adult may have a core temperature elevation at much lower numbers. The very old

TABLE 4.7 **Key Aspects of Normal Age-Related Changes With Aging: Immune System**	
Changes	**Effects**
Reduced immunity	Increased risk of infections
Delayed immune response	Decrease in those signs of illness seen in younger adults (e.g., fever)

may have an average normal temperature of 96°F, with a range of 95°F to 97°F. These findings emphasize the need to evaluate carefully the basal temperature of older adults and recognize that even low-grade fevers (99°F) may signify serious illness. When this is combined with the age-related delay in the increases in the white blood cell count compared with younger adults, early detection of serious illness is often difficult. A lack of fever (temperature greater than 98.6°F) or initially a normal white blood count cannot be used to rule out an infection. Instead, the nurse must consider the person as a whole—mood, level of consciousness, or other cues such as a recent fall or change in level of cognitive abilities.

Based on the current biological theories of aging, with support of clinical evidence, it can be concluded that complex functions of the body decline before simple body processes; that coordinated activity, which relies on interacting systems such as nerves, muscles, and glands, has a greater detrimental loss than single-system activity; and that a loss of cell function occurs in all vital organs. Yet many older adults function effectively within the limitations of their body and continue to live to a healthy old age, capable of wisdom, judgment, and satisfaction.

The physical changes that accompany aging affect every body system and the theories of why they occur are many. Although there are numerous ways nurses can promote healthy aging in the presence of these changes, when nurses are able to begin to differentiate these normal changes from cues indicative of potential health problems, the positive effect of the nurse's interventions is multiplied.

Goals for healthy aging related to the reduction of hospitalizations due to potentially preventable infections are provided in the document *Healthy People 2030* (Box 4.6). A second immunization for the prevention of life-threatening pneumonia became available December 2014 (Prevnar). It is covered by Medicare with no copay,

as are the annual influenza and the original pneumonia (Pneumovax) vaccinations (see Chapter 7). At the time of writing, the vaccine for COVID-19 will be available to everyone, regardless of ability to pay.

KEY CONCEPTS

- The rapid advancement in understanding the biological basis of aging is in large part due to advances in genomic science.
- Although there continue to be a number of theories about aging, a commonality is in the recognition that over time the cell loses the ability to reproduce.
- There are many physical changes that accompany aging; however, a number of these are relatively insignificant in the absence of disease or unusual stress.
- There are enormous individual variations in the rate of aging of body systems and functional abilities.
- Many of the normal changes with aging may be misinterpreted as being pathological and some pathological conditions may be mistaken for normal changes of aging.
- The nurse cannot rely on the "typical" signs of infection in the older adult but must use a more holistic approach.
- Attention to the cues of any one older adult includes aging changes, lifestyle, and desires is fundamental to caring and maximizing health outcomes for persons in later life.

ACTIVITIES AND DISCUSSION QUESTIONS

1. Identify at least two normal changes that accompany aging for each body system.
2. Discuss the changes of aging you expect will be the most difficult to accept.

REFERENCES

Akintola, A. A., & van Heemst, D. (2015). Insulin, aging, and the brain: Mechanisms and implications. *Front Endocrinol (Lausanne), 6*:13. http://www.ncbi.nlm.nih.gov/pmc/articles/PMC4319489.

Brown, W. J., & McCarthy, M. S. (2015). Sarcopenia: What every NP should know. *J Nurs Practitioners, 11*(8), 753–759.

Butterfield, R. J. (2019). Structure and function of the neurologic system. In K. L. McCance, & S. E. Huether (Eds.), *Pathophysiology: The biologic basis for disease in adults and children* (ed. 8, pp. 434–467). St Louis: Elsevier.

Chen, Z., Miao, L., Gao, X., et al. (2015). Effect of obesity and hyperglycemia on benign prostatic hyperplasia in elderly patients with newly diagnosed type 2 diabetes. *Int J Clin Exp Med, 8*(7), 11289–11294.

Chung, H. Y., et al. (2019). Redefining chronic inflammation in aging and age-related diseases: Proposal of the senoinflammation concept. *Aging Dis, 10*(2), 367–382.

❤ BOX 4.6   Healthy People 2020

Goals to Reduce Potentially Preventable Infections

Objective OA-06: Reduce the rate of hospital admission for pneumonia among older adults

Baseline (2016): 713.9 hospital admissions for pneumonia per 100,000 adults aged 65 and over

Target: 642.5 admissions

Data from ODPHP (2020): *Healthy People 2030*. https://health.gov /healthypeople/objectives-and-data/browse-objectives/respiratory-disease /reduce-rate-hospital-admissions-pneumonia-among-older-adults-oa-06.

Cooper, T. K., & Smith, O. M. (2017). Gynecological disorders in older women. In H. M. Fillit, K. Rockwood, & J. Young (Eds.), *Brocklehurst's Textbook of Geriatric Medicine and Gerontology* (ed. 8, pp. 708–723). Philadelphia: Elsevier.

Cross, W., & Prescott, S. (2017). The prostate. In H. M. Fillit, K. Rockwood, & J. Young (Eds.), *Brocklehurst's Textbook of Geriatric Medicine and Gerontology* (ed. 8, pp. 689–701). Philadelphia: Elsevier.

Davies, G. A., & Bolton, C. E. (2017). Age-related changes in the respiratory system. In H. M. Fillit, K. Rockwood, & J. Young (Eds.), *Brocklehurst's Textbook of Geriatric Medicine and Gerontology* (ed. 8, pp. 101–104). Philadelphia: Elsevier.

Dato, S., Crocco, P., D'Aquila, P., et al. (2013). Exploring the role of genetic variability and lifestyle in oxidative stress response for healthy aging and longevity. *Int J Mol Sci, 14*, 16443–16472.

Einstein, A. (1920). *Relativity: The special and the general theory.* New York: Henry Holt.

Feldstein, R., Beyda, D. J., & Katz, S. (2017). Aging and the gastrointestinal tract. In H. M. Fillit, K. Rockwood, & J. Young (Eds.), *Brocklehurst's Textbook of Geriatric Medicine and Gerontology* (ed. 8, pp. 127–132). Philadelphia: Elsevier.

Fendrik, A. J., Romanelli, L., & Rotondo, E. (2019). Stochastic cell renewal process and lengthening of cell cycle. *Physical Biology, 17*(1):016004. https://iopscience.iop.org/article/10.1088/1478-3975/ab576c.

Galvin, J. E. (2017). Neurological signs in older adults. In H. M. Fillit, K. Rockwood, & J. Young (Eds.), *Brocklehurst's Textbook of Geriatric Medicine and Gerontology* (ed. 8, pp. 105–109). Philadelphia: Elsevier.

Howlett, S. E. (2017). Effects of aging on the cardiovascular system. In H. M. Fillit, K. Rockwood, & J. Young (Eds.), *Brocklehurst's Textbook of Geriatric Medicine and Gerontology* (ed. 8, pp. 96–100). Philadelphia: Elsevier.

Huether, S. E., & Rodway, G. W. (2019). Pain, temperature regulation, sleep, and sensory function. In K. L. McCance, & S. E. Huether (Eds.), *Pathophysiology: The biological basis for disease in adults and children* (pp. 468–503). St Louis: Elsevier.

Huether, S. E. (2019). Structure and function of the digestive system. In K. L. McCance, S. E. Huether, et al. (Eds.), *Pathophysiology: The biologic basis for disease in adults and children* (ed. 8, pp. 1395–1422). St Louis: Elsevier.

Kirkland, J. L. (2017). Cellular Mechanisms of aging? Mechanisms of aging. In H. M. Fillit, K. Rockwood, & J. Young (Eds.), *Brocklehurst's Textbook of Geriatric Medicine and Gerontology* (ed. 8, pp. 22–26). Philadelphia: Elsevier.

Lagouge, M., & Larsson, N.-G. (2013). The role of mitochondrial DNA mutations and free radicals in disease and aging. *J Intern Med, 273*, 529–543.

Lai, C.-Q., Parnell, L. D., & Ordovás, J. M. (2017). Genetic mechanisms of aging. In H. M. Fillit, K. Rockwood, & J. Young (Eds.), *Brocklehurst's Textbook of Geriatric Medicine and Gerontology* (ed. 8, pp. 43–46). Philadelphia: Elsevier 2017.

Lobo, V., Patil, A., Phatak, A., & Chandra, N. (2010). Free radicals, antioxidants and functional foods: Impact on human health. *Pharmacognosy Reviews, 4*(8), 118–126.

Morley, J. E., & McKee, A. (2017). Endocrinology of aging. In H. M. Fillit, K. Rockwood, & J. Young (Eds.), *Brocklehurst's Textbook of Geriatric Medicine and Gerontology* (ed. 8, pp. 138–140). Philadelphia: Elsevier.

National Center for Complementary and Integrative Health (NCCIH): *Antioxidants: in depth*, updated 2013. https://www.nccih.nih.gov/health/antioxidants-in-depth.

National Institute of Dental and Craniofacial Research (NIDCR): *Periodontal (gum) disease: Causes, symptoms, and treatments*, 2018. http://www.nidcr.nih.gov/oralhealth/Topics/GumDiseases/PeriodontalGumDisease.htm#canPeriodontal.

Okazaki, S., Numata, S., Otsuka, I., et al. (2020). Decelerated epigenetic aging associated with mood stabilizers in the blood of patients with bipolar disorder. *Transl Psychiatry, 10*(1), 129. https://www.ncbi.nlm.nih.gov/pmc/articles/PMC7198548/.

Reeves, G. C., Hopkins, L. W., & Smallheer, B. A. (2019). Structure and function of the musculoskeletal system. In K. L. McCance, & S. E. Huether (Eds.), *Pathophysiology: The biologic basis for disease in adults and children* (pp. 1395–1422). St Louis: Elsevier.

Rodway, G., & Huether, S. E. (2019). Structure and function of the reproductive systems. In K. L. McCance, & S. E. Huether (Eds.), *Pathophysiology: The biologic basis for disease in adults and children* (ed. 8, pp. 726–754), St Louis: Elsevier.

Skin Cancer Foundation. *Skin cancer facts and statistics.* http://www.skincancer.org/skin-cancer-information/skin-cancer-facts.

Smith, P. P., & Kuchel, G. A. (2017). Aging of the urinary tract. In H. M. Fillit, K. Rockwood, & J. Young (Eds.), *Brocklehurst's Textbook of Geriatric Medicine and Gerontology* (ed. 8, pp. 133–137). Philadelphia: Elsevier.

Speakman, J. R., & Selman, C. (2011). The free-radical damage theory: Accumulating evidence against a simple link of oxidative stress to ageing and lifespan. *Bioessays, 33*(4), 255–259.

Starkweather, A. R., Alhaeeri, A. A., Montpetit, A., Brumelle, J., Filler, K., Montpetit, M., et al. (2014). An integrative review of factors associated with telomere length and implications for biobehavioral research. *Nursing Research, 63*(1), 36–50.

Stengel, G. B. (1983). Oral temperature in the elderly. *Gerontologist, 23*(special issue), 306.

Ventura, M. T., Casciaro, M., Gagemi, S., & Buquicchio, R. (2017). Immunosenescence in aging: Between immune cells depletion and cytokines up-regulation. *Clinical and Molecular Allergy, 15*(21), 1–8. https://www.ncbi.nlm.nih.gov/pmc/articles/PMC5731094/pdf/12948_2017_Article_77.pdf.

Wallings, A. D., & Dickson, G. M. (2012). Hearing loss in older adults. *Am Fam Physician, 85*(12), 1150–1156.

World Health Organization (WHO) (2020). WHO reveals leading causes of death and disability worldwide: 2000-2019. https://www.who.int/news/item/09-12-2020-who-reveals-leading-causes-of-death-and-disability-worldwide-2000-2019.

5

Clinical Judgment to Promote Psychosocial, Spiritual, and Cognitive Health

Theris A. Touhy

http://evolve.elsevier.com/Touhy/gerontological/

LEARNING OBJECTIVES

Upon completion of this chapter, the reader will be able to:
- Explain the major psychosocial theories of aging.
- Discuss the importance of spirituality to healthy aging.
- Explain cognitive changes with age and strategies to enhance cognitive health.
- Discuss factors influencing learning in later life and appropriate teaching and learning strategies.
- Utilize clinical judgment to identify nursing actions to enhance cognitive health, learning, and promote spiritual well-being.

THE LIVED EXPERIENCE

If I Had My Life to Live Over

I'd dare to make more mistakes next time, I'd relax, I would limber up. I would be sillier than I've been this trip. I would take fewer things seriously. I would take more chances. I would climb more mountains and swim more rivers. I would eat more ice cream and less beans. I would perhaps have more actual troubles, but I'd have fewer imaginary ones.

You see, I'm one of those people who live sensibly and sanely hour after hour, day after day. Oh, I've had my moments, and if I had to do it over again, I'd have more of them. In fact, I'd try to have nothing else. Just moments, one after another, instead of living so many years ahead of each day. I've been one of those persons who never goes anywhere without a thermostat, a hot water bottle, a raincoat, and a parachute. If I had it to do again, I would travel lighter than I have.

If I had my life to live over, I would start barefoot earlier in the spring and stay that way later in the fall. I would go to more dances. I would ride more merry-go-rounds. I would pick more daisies.

Nadine Stair (1992)

Each individual has unique life experiences and because of this must be seen holistically, through the lens of his or her time, place, culture, gender, and personal history. The close relationship among biological, social, and psychological development that exists through childhood and adolescence varies more in adulthood because of the greater variations in life experiences and demands as one matures. This chapter provides the reader with information on the psychosocial, spiritual, and cognitive aspects of aging. The importance of the life story, reminiscence, and life review in coming to know older adults is included. Factors influencing learning in later life and appropriate teaching and learning strategies are also discussed.

PSYCHOSOCIAL THEORIES OF AGING

A person is not just a biological being but a multidimensional whole. Only when life is considered in its totality can we begin to truly understand aging. Here we discuss the psychosocial theories of aging and acknowledge that most are more accurately conceptual models or approaches to understanding. Because they are most often referred to as theories in the gerontological literature, we will do so here for ease of discussion. They can be classified as first-, second-, and third-generation theories (Hooyman & Kiyak, 2011).

First Generation

Early psychosocial theories of aging were an attempt to explain and predict the changes in middle and late life with an emphasis on adjustment. Adjustment was seen as an indication of success, at least by the academic theoreticians who developed them. The majority of these theories began appearing in the gerontological literature in the 1940s and 1950s. They were not based on extensive research; instead, they primarily developed as a consequence of "face validity," that is, emerging from the personal and professional experience of both scientists and clinicians and appearing to be reasonable explanations of aging. This set of theories has varied very little since they were first proposed. The major theories in the first generation were those of *role* and *activity*.

Role Theory

Role theory was one of the earliest explanations of how people adjust to aging (Cottrell, 1942). Self-identity is believed to be defined by a person's role in society (e.g., nurse, teacher, banker). As individuals evolve through the various stages in life, so do their roles. Successful aging means that as one role is completed, it is replaced by another one of comparative value to the individual and society. For example, the wage-earning work role is replaced by that of a volunteer, or a parent becomes a grandparent. The ability of an individual to adapt to changing roles is a predictor of adjustment to aging.

Role theory is operationalized in the phenomenon of *age norms*. They are culturally constructed expectations of what is deemed acceptable behavior in society and are internalized by the individual. Age norms are based on the assumption that chronological age and gender,

in and of themselves, imply roles; for example, one may hear, "If only they would act their age," or "You are too old to do/say/behave like that," or "That is unbecoming to a woman of your age." In each of these examples, the behavior challenged long-established age norms for White middle-aged and older individuals. With the aging of the "baby boomers," popular culture is challenging age norms; for example, from advertisements for genital lubricants featuring actors with graying hair to news of the availability of medications to treat erectile dysfunction, "older adults" are now depicted as still sexually active. These images replace the historical view that persons become asexual as they age (or so their grandchildren hope!) (Chapter 26). Both men and women are assuming roles and engaging in behaviors today that were unimaginable when role theory was first proposed.

Activity Theory

In 1953, Havighurst and Albrecht proposed that successful aging was based on the individual's ability to maintain an *active lifestyle*. It is expected that the productivity and activities of middle life are replaced with equally engaging pursuits in later life (Maddox, 1963). The theory was based on the assumption that it is better to be active (and young) than inactive (Havighurst, 1972). *Activity theory* is consistent with Western society's emphasis on work, wealth, and productivity and therefore continues to influence the perception of unsuccessful aging (Wadensten, 2006).

The first-generation theories of aging have been criticized because of their limited applicability. Problems of intersubjectivity of meaning, testability, and empirical adequacy have persisted. Consistent with the historical period of their development, they failed to consider social class, education, health, and economic and cultural diversity as influencing factors (Hooyman & Kiyak, 2011).

Second Generation

Second-generation theories expanded or questioned those of the first generation. These include the disengagement, continuity, age-stratification, social exchange, modernization, developmental, and gerotranscendence theories.

Disengagement Theory

Disengagement theory is in contrast to both role and activity theories. In 1961, Cumming and Henry proposed that in the natural course of aging the individual does, and should, slowly withdraw from society to allow the transfer of power to the younger generations. The transfer is viewed as necessary for the maintenance of social equilibrium (Wadensten, 2006). A belief in the appropriateness of disengagement provided the basis of age discrimination for many years when an older employee was replaced by a younger one. Although this practice was overtly accepted in the past, it is still present more covertly but is now being challenged socially and legally. An older adult's withdrawal is no longer an indicator of successful aging, is not *necessarily* a good thing for society, and does not take into account the needs of the individual or culture in which one lives.

Continuity Theory

Also in contrast with role theory but similar to activity theory is *continuity theory*. Havighurst and colleagues 1968) proposed that individuals develop and maintain a consistent pattern of behavior over a lifetime. Aging, as an extension of earlier life, reflects a *continuation of the patterns* of roles, responsibilities, and activities. Personality influences the roles and activities chosen and the level of satisfaction drawn from these. Successful aging is associated with a person's ability to maintain and continue previous behaviors and roles or to find suitable replacements (Wadensten, 2006).

Age-Stratification Theory

Age-stratification theory is based on the belief that aging can be best understood by considering the experiences of individuals as members of cohorts with similarities to others in the same group (Riley, 1971). The importance of the similarities exceeds that of the differences. An example of age stratification is the traditional conceptualization of "young-old," "middle-old," and "old-old" (Neugarten, 1968). The cohort of baby boomers is presenting a significant challenge to this theory in the developed world. The range of experiences and the variability in age when some of these experiences occurred to individuals within this cohort have resulted in substratifications within baby boomers themselves. The wide range of socioeconomic and educational levels furthers this diversity (Chapter 3).

Social Exchange Theory

Social exchange theory is conceptualized from an economic perspective. The presumption is that as people age, they have fewer and fewer economic resources to contribute to society. This paucity results in loss of social status, self-esteem, and political power (Hooyman & Kiyak, 2011). Only those who are able to maintain control of their financial resources have the potential to remain fully participating members of society and anticipate successful aging. Although this may have some applicability in the communities in the world that have been able to develop a stable economy for its citizens, this theory marginalizes those in communities and underdeveloped countries who struggle for the barest necessities now and into the foreseeable future.

Modernization Theory

Although not usually associated with social exchange theory, *modernization theory* can be used to consider nonmaterial aspects of exchange. This theory is an attempt to explain the social changes that have resulted in devaluing the contributions of older adults. In the United States before about 1900, material and political resources were controlled by the older members of a society (Achenbaum, 1978). The resources included their knowledge, skills, experience, and wisdom. In agricultural cultures and communities, the oldest members held power through property ownership and the right to make decisions related to food distribution. Older men and women often held valuable religious and cultural roles of instructing youth and controlling ceremonies.

According to modernization theory, the status and value of older adults are lost when their labors are no longer considered useful, their kinship networks are dispersed, their knowledge is no longer pertinent to the society in which they live, and they are no longer revered simply because of their age (Hendricks & Hendricks, 1986). Modernization has had a notable effect on cultures such as those in China and Japan where filial duty predominated as an underlying construct of eldercare. As more and more adult children enter the marketplace or emigrate for social or economic reasons, conflicts between traditional values mount (see *The Bonesetter's Daughter* by Amy Tan, 2001). It is proposed that these changes are the result of advancing technology, urbanization, and mass education (Cowgill, 1974). In some cultures or family structures and in underdeveloped areas of the world, "modernization" as described may not yet be applicable.

Developmental Theories

Psychologist Erik Erikson's theory of psychosocial development is one of the best-known theories of personality in psychology. He theorized a predetermined order of developmental and specific tasks that were associated with specific periods in the course of a person's life. The task of the last stage of life is ego integrity versus self-despair. Erikson saw the last stage of life as a vantage point from which one could look back with ego integrity or despair on one's life. Successfully completing this phase means looking back with few regrets and a general feeling of satisfaction. In later years, Erikson modified the "either-or" stance of each of the tasks. Thus ego integrity is tinged with some regrets, wisdom is balanced with frivolity, and letting go is balanced with hanging on (Erikson et al., 1986).

Another well-known theory is Maslow's Hierarchy of Needs (1954), which addresses the biopsychosocial needs of the individual. As far back as Hippocrates and Galen, the basic needs of all living people were recognized as the need for air, fluids, nutrition, hygiene, elimination, activity, and skin integrity. Along with these is the basic need for comfort or relief from suffering. The hierarchy ranks them from the most basic, related to the maintenance of biological integrity, to the most complex, associated with self-actualization. Maslow proposed that the higher-level needs cannot be met without first meeting the lower-level needs. In other words, moving toward healthy aging is an evolving and developing process. As basic-level needs are met, the satisfaction of higher-level needs is possible, with ever-deepening richness to life, regardless of age.

Gerotranscendence Theory

This theory is similar to that of disengagement, yet the reason for the withdrawal is not for societal needs but to give the person time for self-reflection, exploration of the inner self, contemplation of the meaning of life, and movement away from the material world (Tornstam, 1989, 2000, 2005). Aging is viewed as movement from birth to death and maturation toward wisdom, an ever-evolving process that alters a person's view of reality, sense of spirituality, and meaning beyond the self. Inasmuch, gerotranscendence implies achieving wisdom through personal transformation. With aging, time becomes less important, as do superficial relationships.

Transcendence is viewed as a universal goal, the highest goal any person can achieve and a marker of successful aging. This theory is based on a highly egocentric approach to aging. It is less likely to be applicable in cultures based on the quality of interpersonal relationships (Chapter 3). It also does not account for differences in economic resources, which may or may not provide the individual the "luxury" of time for introspection.

Third Generation

The third generation of theoretical development related to aging is also referred to as the "second transformation" occurring since the 1980s. The goal is "understanding the human meanings of social life in the context of everyday life rather than the explanation of facts" (Hooyman & Kiyak, 2011, p. 326). This may or may not rise to the level of a theory.

A phenomenological approach is used to achieve a qualitative understanding of the individual as an aging person. Examples include the life story, life review, and reminiscence. Aging is personally interpreted rather than socially or culturally constructed. In other words, to understand how an individual views aging, one has to come to know the individual by listening to his/her unique story rather than relying on stereotypical views of aging. This level is particularly useful in the application of nursing care and the incorporation of recognition of the aging person as unique and valuable in any circumstance and within the context of any culture. It can be used to promote healthy aging as the person is supported on the wellness continuum.

The Life Story

The life story as constructed through reminiscing, journaling, life review, or guided autobiography has held great fascination for gerontologists in the last 30 years. The universal appeal of the life story as a vehicle of culture, a demonstration of caring and generational continuity, and an easily stimulated activity has held allure for many professionals. "One of the few universals is that humans in all known cultures use language to tell stories" (Ramírez-Esparza & Pennebaker, 2006, p. 216).

The most exciting aspect of working with older adults is being a part of the emergence of the life story: the shifting and blending patterns. When we are young, it is important for our emotional health and growth to look forward and plan for the future. As one ages, it becomes more important to look back, talk about experiences, review and make sense of it all, and end with a feeling of satisfaction with the life lived.

Storytelling is a complementary and alternative therapy nurses can use with older adults to enhance communication (Moss, 2014). A nurse can learn much about an older adult's history, communication style, relationships, coping mechanisms, strengths, fears, affect, and adaptive capacity by listening thoughtfully as the life story is constructed.

Reminiscing

Reminiscing is an umbrella term that can include any recall of the past. Reminiscing occurs from childhood onward, particularly at life's junctures and transitions. Reminiscing cultivates a sense of security through recounting of comforting memories, belonging through sharing, and promotion of self-esteem through confirmation of uniqueness. Robert Butler (2003) emphasized that in the past, reminiscing was thought to be a sign of senility or what we now call Alzheimer's disease. Older adults who talked about the past and told the same stories again and again were said to be boring and living in the past. From Butler's landmark research (1963), we now know that reminiscence is the most important psychological task of older adults.

For nurses, reminiscing is a therapeutic intervention important in assessment and understanding. The work of several gerontological nursing leaders, including Irene Burnside, Priscilla Ebersole, and Barbara Haight, has contributed to the body of knowledge about reminiscence and its importance in nursing. The International Institute for Reminiscence and Life Review (University of Wisconsin, Superior, WI), an interdisciplinary organization uniting participants to study reminiscence and life review, is another valuable resource for nurses and members of other disciplines involved in research or practice. This group publishes an online journal and offers a certificate in reminiscence and life story work.

Reminiscence can have many goals. It not only provides a pleasurable experience that improves quality of life but also increases socialization and connectedness with others, provides cognitive stimulation, improves communication, facilitates personal growth, and can decrease depression scores (Chapter 24). The process of reminiscence can occur in individual conversations with older adults, can be structured as in a nursing history, or can occur in a group where each person shares his or her memories and listens to others sharing their memories. Digital storytelling is another medium that can be used with older adults to record their stories and memories across a variety of platforms including tablets and smartphones in a format that can be shared with others. Using virtual reality (VR) is also being used to stimulate reminiscence and provide pleasurable experiences such as revisiting childhood neighborhoods, travel, nature, and other experiences that trigger positive memories. The technology is also being used to allow health care staff to experience dementia, hearing loss, and other conditions American Association of Retired Persons (AARP), 2020.

Intergenerational reminiscence activities could have benefits for both older and younger individuals. In several studies, benefits include increased engagement, enthusiasm, appreciation, respect, and empathy for the older adult (Yamashita et al., 2017). Nurses in long-term care facilities who engaged in reminiscence activities reported knowing older adults better, thereby enhancing their personhood. Reminiscence can also be used by family caregivers to enhance communication and strengthen relationships with family members experiencing cognitive impairment (Karlsson et al., 2017; Latha et al., 2014). Box 5.1 provides some suggestions for encouraging reminiscence.

Reminiscing and Storytelling With Individuals Experiencing Cognitive Impairment

Cognitive impairment does not necessarily preclude older adults from participating in reminiscence or

---

BOX 5.1   Suggestions for Encouraging Reminiscence

- Listen without correction or criticism. Older adults are presenting their version of their reality; our version belongs to another generation.
- Encourage older adults to discuss various ages and stages of their lives. Use questions such as, "What was it like growing up on that farm?", "What did teenagers do for fun when you were young?", or "What was WWII like for you?"
- Be patient with repetition. Sometimes people need to tell the same story often to come to terms with the experience, especially if it was meaningful to them. If they have a memory loss, it may be the only story they can remember and it is important for them to be able to share it with others.
- Be attuned to signs of depression in conversation (dwelling on sad topics) or changes in physical status or behavior, and provide appropriate assessment and intervention.
- If a topic arises that the person does not want to discuss, change to another topic.

- If individuals are reluctant to share because they do not feel their life was interesting, reassure them that everyone's life is valuable and interesting and tell them how important their memories are to you and others.
- Keep in mind that reminiscing is not an orderly process. One memory triggers another in a way that may not seem related; it is not important to keep things in order or verify accuracy.
- Listen actively, maintain eye contact, and do not interrupt.
- Respond positively and give feedback by making caring, appropriate comments that encourage the person to continue.
- Use props and triggers such as photographs, memorabilia (e.g., a childhood toy or antique, short stories or poems about the past, favorite foods, YouTube videos, old songs).
- Use open-ended questions to encourage reminiscing. If working with a group, you can prepare questions ahead of time or you can ask the group members to pick a topic that interests them. One question or topic may be enough for an entire group session.

storytelling groups. Opportunities for telling the life story and enjoying memories should not be denied to individuals on the basis of their cognitive status. Modifications must be made according to the cognitive abilities of the person but individuals with mild to moderate memory impairment can enjoy and benefit from group work focused on reminiscence and storytelling.

Emerging evidence suggests that reminiscence is an important nonpharmacological intervention for individuals with dementia. Reminiscence and storytelling provide a structure and mechanism for communication and engaging in interaction and can enhance quality of life and improve mood (Cooney et al., 2014; O'Shea et al., 2014; Testad et al., 2014). For family caregivers, communication skills training that involves reminiscence and life review activities between the caregiver and family member with dementia can increase the quantity and quality of communication between care recipients and caregivers; lower caregiver stress and burden; and reduce behavioral problems.

When the nurse is working with a group of individuals who are experiencing cognitive impairment, the emphasis in reminiscence groups is on sharing memories; however, they may be expressed, rather than specific recall of events. There should be no pressure to answer questions such as "Where were you born?" or "What was your first job?" Rather, discussions may center on jobs people had and places they have lived. Displaying additional props, such as music, pictures, familiar objects (e.g., an American flag, an old coffee grinder) and doing familiar activities that trigger past memories (e.g., having a tea party, folding linens) can prompt many recollections and sharing. The leader of a group with participants who have memory problems must assume a more active approach.

The TimeSlips program (Basting, 2003, 2006, 2013) is an evidence-based innovation, cited by the Agency for Healthcare Research and Quality (AHRQ, 2014), that uses storytelling to enhance the lives of people with cognitive impairment. Positive outcomes associated with the program include enhanced verbal skills and provider reports of positive behavioral changes, increased communication, increased sociability, and less confusion. TimeSlips is a beneficial and cost-effective therapeutic intervention that can be used in many settings. See http://www.timeslips.org/ for more information and examples and online training and certification.

Using the TimeSlips format, group members looking at a picture are encouraged to create a story about the picture. The pictures can be fantastical and funny, such as from greeting cards, or more nostalgic, such as Norman Rockwell paintings. All contributions are encouraged and welcomed, there are no right or wrong answers, and everything that the individuals say is included in the story and written down by the scribe. Stories are read back to the participants during the session, using their names to identify their contributions. At the beginning of each session, the story from the last session is read to the participants. Care is taken to compliment each member for his or her contribution to the wonderful story. The stories that emerge are full of humor and creativity and often include discussions of memories and reminiscing.

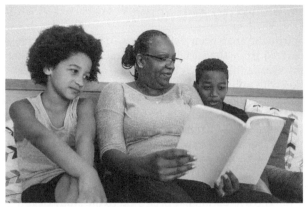

Grandmother reading a book to her grandchildren at home. (© iStock.com/IS_ImageSource.)

Life Review

Robert Butler (1963) first noted and brought to public attention the review process that normally occurs in the older adult as the realization of his or her approaching death creates a resurgence of unresolved conflicts. Butler called this process life review. *Life review* occurs quite naturally for many persons during periods of crisis and transition. However, Butler (2003) noted that in old age, the process of putting one's life in order increases in intensity and emphasis. Life review occurs most frequently as an internal review of memories, an intensely private, soul-searching activity.

Life review is a more formal therapy technique than reminiscence and takes a person through his or her life in a structured and chronological order. Life review therapy (Butler and Lewis, 1983), guided autobiography (Birren and Deutchman, 1991), and structured life review (Haight and Webster, 2002) are psychotherapeutic techniques based on the concept of life review. Gerontological nurses participate with older adults in both reminiscence and life review, and it is important to acquire the skills to be effective in achieving the purposes of both of these techniques. Life review may be especially important for older adults experiencing depressive symptoms and those facing death.

Life review should occur not only when we are old or facing death but also frequently throughout our lives. This process can assist us to examine where we are in life and change our course or set new goals. Butler (2003) commented that ongoing life review by an individual may help avoid the overwhelming feelings of despair that may surface for some individuals at the end of life when there may not be time to make changes.

SPIRITUALITY AND AGING

Spirituality has been defined as a "quality of a person derived from the social and cultural environment that involves faith, a search for meaning, a sense of connection with others, and a transcendence of self, resulting in a sense of inner peace and well-being" (Delgado, 2007, p. 230). The spiritual aspect of people's lives transcends the physical and psychosocial to reach the deepest individual capacity for love, hope, and meaning. "Spiritual health is an integral component of human well-being" (Vaineta, 2016, p. 11).

Aging as a biological process has been studied extensively. Less attention has been paid to the study of aging as a spiritual process. As people age and move closer to death, spirituality may become more important. Declining physical health, loss of loved ones, and a realization that life's end may be near often challenge older people to reflect on the meaning of their lives. Spiritual belief and practices often play a central role in helping older adults cope with life challenges and are a source of strength in the lives of older adults. Spirituality may be particularly important to healthy aging in "historically disadvantaged populations who display remarkable strength despite adversities in their lives" (Hooyman & Kiyak, 2005, p. 213).

Distinguishing between religion and spirituality is a concern for many health professionals. Religious beliefs and participation in religious obligations and rites are often the avenues of spiritual expression, but they are not necessarily interchangeable. "Religion can be described as a social institution that unites people in a faith in God, a higher power, and in common rituals and worshipful acts. A god, divinity, and/or soul is always included in the concept" (Strang & Strang, 2002, p. 858). Each religion involves a particular set of beliefs. Spirituality is a broader concept than religion and encompasses a person's values, beliefs, or search for meaning as well as their relationships with a higher power, with nature, and with other people. The concept of spirituality is found in all cultures

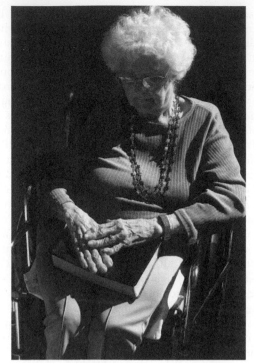

Prayer. (© iStock.com/Lisa Thornberg.)

and societies. For some people, particularly older adults, formalized religion helps them feel fulfilled.

A nursing evidence-based guideline for promoting spirituality in the older adult (Gaskamp et al., 2006) provides a framework for spiritual assessment and interventions. The guideline identifies older adults who may be at risk of spiritual distress and who might be most likely to benefit from use of the guideline (Box 5.2).

BOX 5.2   Identifying Older Adults at Risk of Spiritual Distress

- Individuals experiencing events or conditions that affect the ability to participate in spiritual rituals
- Diagnosis and treatment of a life-threatening, chronic, or terminal illness
- Expressions of interpersonal or emotional suffering, loss of hope, lack of meaning, need to find meaning in suffering
- Evidence of depression
- Cognitive impairment
- Verbalized questioning or loss of faith
- Loss of interpersonal support

Data from Gaskamp, C., Sutter, R., Meraviglia, M., et al. (2006). Evidence-based guideline: Promoting spirituality in the older adult, *J Gerontol Nurs* *32*, 8–13.

Spiritual distress or spiritual pain is "an individual's perception of hurt or suffering associated with that part of his or her person that seeks to transcend the realm of the material. Spiritual distress is manifested by a deep sense of hurt stemming from feelings of loss or separation from one's God or deity, a sense of personal inadequacy or sinfulness before God and man, or a pervasive condition of loneliness" (Gaskamp et al., 2006, p. 9).

❖ USING CLINICAL JUDGMENT TO PROMOTE HEALTHY AGING: SPIRITUAL HEALTH

◆ Recognizing and Analyzing Cues: Spiritual Health

Assessment of spirituality is as important as assessment of physical, emotional, and social dimensions. A spiritual history opens the door to a conversation about the role of spirituality and religion in a person's life (Wittenberg et al, 2017). People often need permission to talk about these issues. Without a signal from the nurse, patients may feel that such topics are not welcome. Patients welcome a discussion of spiritual matters and want health professionals to consider their spiritual needs.

Nurses may neglect to explore this issue with older adults because religion and spirituality may not seem the high priority and care focuses primarily on physical aspects (Clayton et al, 2017). The individual should be assured that religious longings and rituals are important and that opportunities will be made available as desired. Nurses need to be knowledgeable and respectful about the rites and rituals of varying religions, cultural beliefs, and values (Chapter 3). Religious and spiritual resources, such as pastoral visits, should be available in all settings where older adults reside. It is important to avoid imposing one's own beliefs and to respect the person's privacy on matters of spirituality and religion.

There are formal instruments to obtain information about spirituality, but open-ended questions can also be used to begin dialogue about spiritual concerns. Instruments are designed to elicit information about the individual's core spiritual needs and about ways the nurse and other members of the health care team can respond to them. These include the Faith or Beliefs, Importance and Influence, Community, and Address (FICA) Spiritual History (Puchalski & Romer, 2000) and the Brief Assessment of Spiritual Resources and Concerns (Koenig & Brooks, 2002; Meyer, 2003) (Box 5.3). Evaluation of spirituality is required by The Joint Commission in hospitals, nursing homes, home

---

BOX 5.3   Brief Assessment of Spiritual Resources and Concerns

Instructions: Use the following questions as an interview guide with the older adult (or caregiver if the older adult is unable to communicate).

- Does your religion/spirituality provide comfort or serve as a cause of stress? (Ask how spirituality is a comfort or stressor.)
- Do you have any religious or spiritual beliefs that might conflict with health care or affect health care decisions? (Ask the person to identify any conflicts.)
- Do you belong to a supportive church, congregation, or faith community? (Ask how the faith community is supportive.)
- Do you have any practices or rituals that help you express your spiritual or religious beliefs? (Ask the person to identify or describe practices.)
- Do you have any spiritual needs you would like someone to address? (Ask what those needs are and if referral to a spiritual professional is desired.)
- How can we (health care providers) help you with your spiritual needs or concerns?

From Gaskamp, C., Cutler, R., Meraviglia, M., et al. (2006). Evidence-based guideline: Promoting spirituality in the older adult, *J Gerontol Nurs 32*(11),10. Adapted from Meyer, C. L. (2003). How effectively are nurse educators preparing students to provide spiritual care? *Nurse Educ 28*(4), 185–190.; Koenig, H. G., Brooks, R. G. (2002). Religion, health and aging: Implications for practice and public policy, *Public Policy Aging Rep 12*, 13–19.

---

care organizations, and many other health care settings providing services to older adults. The process of understanding an individual's spirituality is more complex than completing a standardized form and must be done within the context of the nurse–patient relationship. Simply listening to patients as they express their fears, hopes, and beliefs is important.

For older adults with cognitive impairment, information about the importance of spirituality and religious beliefs can be obtained from family members. Nurses often see cognitive impairments as obstacles or excuses to providing spiritual care to individuals with dementia. Nurturing mind, body, and spirit is part of holistic nursing, and nurses must provide opportunities to all older adults, no matter how impaired, to live life with meaning, purpose, and hope.

◆ Nursing Actions: Spiritual Health

The caring relationship between nurses and persons nursed is the heart of nursing that touches and supports the spirit. Knowing persons in their complexity, responding to that which matters most to them, identifying and nurturing connections, listening with one's being, using presence and silence, and fostering connections to that

---

BOX 5.4   Spiritual Nursing Interventions

- Relief of physical discomfort, which permits focus on the spiritual
- Creating a peaceful environment
- Comforting touch, which fosters nurse-patient connection
- Authentic presence
- Attentive listening
- Knowing the patient as a person
- Listening to life stories
- Sharing fears and listening to self-doubts or guilt
- Fostering forgiveness and reconciliation
- Validating the person's life and ensuring persons they will be remembered
- Sharing caring words and love
- Encouraging family support and presence
- Fostering connections to that which is held sacred by the person
- Praying with and for the patient
- Respecting religious traditions and providing for access to religious objects and rituals
- Referring the person to a spiritual counselor

Data from Gaskamp, C., Sutter, R., Meraviglia, M., et al. (2006). Evidence-based guideline: Promoting spirituality in the older adult, *J Gerontol Nurs 32*,8.; Touhy, T., Brown, C., Smith, C. (2005). Spiritual caring: End of life in a nursing home, *J Gerontol Nurs 31*, 27–35.

---

which is held sacred by the person are spiritual nursing responses that arise from within the caring, connected relationship (Touhy et al., 2005). Suggestions for nursing actions to promote spiritual health in older adults, derived from research, are presented in Box 5.4.

Nurturing the Spirit of the Nurse

"Because spiritual care occurs over time and within the context of relationship, probably the most effective tool at the nurse's disposal is the use of self" (Soeken & Carson, 1987, p. 607). Nurses ease with their own spirituality is vital to providing spiritual care (Wittenberg et al., 2017). Thinking about what gives your own life meaning and value helps in developing your spiritual self and assists you in being able to offer spiritual support to patients. Examples of activities include finding quiet time for meditation and reflection; keeping your own faith traditions; being with nature; appreciating the arts; spending time with those you love; and journaling (Touhy & Zerwekh, 2006). Find ways to nourish your own spirit. Nurses often do not take the time to do so and become dispirited. This is especially true for nurses who work with dying patients and experience grief and loss repeatedly. Having someone to talk to about feelings is important. Practicing compassion for oneself is essential to authentic practice of compassion for others.

❖ USING CLINICAL JUDGMENT TO PROMOTE HEALTHY AGING: COGNITIVE HEALTH

◆ Adult Cognition

Cognition is the process of acquiring, storing, sharing, and using information. Components of cognitive function include language, thought, memory, executive function (planning, organizing, remembering, paying attention, solving problems), judgment, attention, and perception. The determination of intellectual capacity and performance has been the focus of a major portion of gerontological research. Emerging research suggests that cognitive function and intellectual capacity is a complex interplay of age-related changes in the brain and nervous system and many other factors such as education, environment, nutrition, life experiences, physical function, emotions, biomedical and physiological factors, and genetics (Agency for Healthcare Research and Quality, 2017).

Before the development of sophisticated neuroimaging techniques, conclusions about brain function as we age were based on autopsy results (often on diseased brains) or results of cross-sectional studies conducted with older adults who were institutionalized or had coexisting illnesses. Changes seen were considered unavoidable and the result of the biological aging process rather than disease. As a result, the bulk of research has focused on the inevitable cognitive declines rather than on cognitive capacities. There are many old myths about aging and the brain that may be believed by both health professionals and older adults. It is important to understand cognition and memory in late life and dispel the myths that can have a negative effect on wellness and may, in fact, contribute to unnecessary cognitive decline (Box 5.5).

Changes in the aging nervous system (Chapter 4) cause a general slowing of many neural processes, but they are not consistent with deteriorating mental function, nor do they interfere with daily routines. Age-related changes in brain structure, function, and cognition are also not uniform across the whole brain or across individuals. Recent research suggests that the reason older brains respond more slowly is because they take longer to process constantly increasing amounts of information (Ramscar et al., 2014).

Cognitive functions may remain stable or decline with increasing age. The cognitive functions that remain stable include attention span, language skills, communication skills, comprehension and discourse, and visual perception. The cognitive skills that decline are verbal fluency, logical analysis, selective attention, object naming, and complex visuospatial skills. Overall cognitive abilities remain intact, and it is important to remember that if brain function becomes impaired in old age, it is the result of disease, not aging (Crowley, 1996).

BOX 5.5 Myths About Aging and the Brain

MYTH: People lose brain cells every day and eventually just run out.

FACT: Most areas of the brain do not lose brain cells. Although you may lose some nerve connections, it can be part of the reshaping of the brain that comes with experience.

MYTH: You cannot change your brain.

FACT: The brain is constantly changing in response to experiences and learning and it retains this "plasticity" well into aging. Changing our way of thinking causes corresponding changes in the brain systems involved; that is, your brain believes what you tell it.

MYTH: The brain does not make new brain cells.

FACT: Certain areas of the brain, including the hippocampus (where new memories are created) and the olfactory bulb (scent-processing center), regularly generate new brain cells.

MYTH: Memory decline is inevitable as we age.

FACT: Many people reach old age and have no memory problems. Participation in physical exercise, stimulating mental activity, socialization, healthy diet, and stress management helps maintain brain health. The incidence of dementia does increase with age, but when there are changes in memory, older adults need to be evaluated for possible causes and receive treatment.

MYTH: There is no point in trying to teach older adults anything because "you can't teach an old dog new tricks."

FACT: Basic intelligence remains unchanged with age and older adults should be provided with opportunities for continued learning. Minimizing barriers to learning such as hearing and vision loss and applying principles of geragogy enhance learning ability.

Modified from American Association of Retired Persons (April 10, 2006). *Myths about aging and the brain.* https://www.aarp.org/health/brain-health/info-2017/common-myths-aging-brains-fd html.

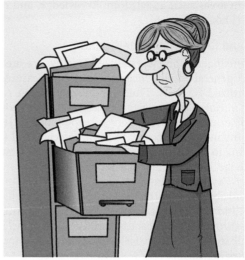

Alex Comfort, an early gerontologist, described the slower response time of an older adult: "By the time you are 80, you have a lot of files in the file cabinet. Your secretary is 80, so it also takes her a lot longer to locate the files, go through them, find the one you want, and bring it to you."

◆ Neuroplasticity

It is very important to know that the aging brain maintains resiliency or the ability to compensate for age-related changes. Developing knowledge refutes the myth that the adult brain is less plastic than the child's brain and less able to strengthen and increase neuronal connections. We now know that the brain has the capacity for neuronal replacement (Fick, 2016). The old adage "use it or lose it" applies to cognitive and physical health. Stimulating the brain increases brain tissue formation, enhances synaptic regulation of messages, and improves the development of cognitive reserve (CR).

CR is based on the concept of neuroplasticity and refers to the strength and complexity of neuronal/dendrite connections from which information is transmitted and cognition/mentation emerges. The greater the strength and complexity of these connections, the more the brain can absorb damage before cognitive functioning is compromised. Individuals vary in the amount of CR they have and this variability may be because of differences in genetics, overall health, education, occupation, lifestyle, leisure activities, or other life experiences. To maximize brain plasticity and CR, it is important to engage in challenging cognitive, sensory, and motor activities, as well as meaningful social interactions, on a regular basis throughout life.

Changes in the brain with aging, once seen only as compensation for declining skills, are now thought to indicate the development of new capacities. These changes include using both hemispheres more equally than younger adults, greater density of synapses, and more use of the frontal lobes, which are thought to be important in abstract reasoning, problem solving, and concept formation (Davis et al., 2017). Later adulthood is no longer seen as a period when growth has ceased and cognitive development halted; rather, it is seen as a life stage programmed for plasticity and the development of unique capacities. The renewed emphasis on the development of cognitive capabilities that can develop with age provides a view of aging that reflects the history of many cultures and provides a much more hopeful view of both aging and human development. While "some areas experience decline (e.g. memory and processing speed), improvements are noted in areas such as wisdom, knowledge, and resilience" (Fick, 2016, p. 6).

◆ Fluid and Crystallized Intelligence

Fluid intelligence and crystallized intelligence are factors of general intelligence and can be measured in standardized IQ tests. Fluid intelligence (often called *native intelligence*) consists of skills that are biologically determined, independent of experience or learning. It involves the capacity to think logically and solve problems in novel situations, independent of acquired knowledge. Fluid intelligence has been likened to "street smarts." Crystallized intelligence is composed of knowledge and abilities that the person acquires through education and life ("book smarts") and is demonstrated largely through one's vocabulary and general knowledge. Crystallized intelligence is long-lasting and improves with experience.

Older adults perform more poorly on performance scales (fluid intelligence), but scores on verbal scales (crystallized intelligence) remain stable. This is known as the classic aging pattern. The tendency to do poorly on performance tasks may be related to age-related changes in sensory and perceptual abilities, as well as psychomotor skills. Older adults need more time to process the knowledge they have gained from experiences. "In other words, you get slower when you're older because you're smarter" (Hill, 2017). Testing methods also affect performance.

◆ Memory

Memory is defined as the ability to retain or store information and retrieve it when needed. Memory is a complex set of processes and storage systems. Three components characterize memory: immediate recall; short-term memory (which may range from minutes to days); and remote or long-term memory. Biological, functional, environmental, and psychosocial influences affect memory development throughout adulthood. Recall of newly encountered information seems to decrease with age and memory declines are noted in connection with complex tasks and strategies. Even though some older adults show decrements in the ability to process information, reaction time, perception, and capacity for attentional tasks, the majority of functioning remains intact and sufficient. Familiarity, previous learning, and life experience compensate for the minor loss of efficiency in the basic neurological processes.

In unfamiliar, stressful, or demanding situations (e.g., hospitalization), however, these changes may be more marked. Healthy older adults may complain of memory problems, but their symptoms do not meet the criteria for

---

BOX 5.6   Memory and Thinking: What's Normal and What's Not?

Normal Aging/ARCD
Making a bad decision once in a while
Missing a monthly payment
Forgetting which day it is and remembering it later
Sometimes forgetting names or what word to use
Losing things from time to time

Dementia
Making poor judgments and decisions a lot of the time
Problems taking care of monthly bills/managing finances
Losing track of the date, year, or time of year
Trouble having a conversation
Misplacing things often and being unable to find them

ARCD, Age-related cognitive decline.
From National Institute on Aging: *Memory and thinking: what's normal and what's not?* https://www.nia.nih.gov/health/memory-and-thinking-whats-normal-and-whats-not.

---

mild or major neurocognitive impairment (Chapter 23). The term *age-related cognitive decline (ARCD)* has been used to describe memory loss that is considered normal in light of a person's age and educational level. This may include a general slowness in processing, storing, and recalling new information, as well as difficulty remembering names and words. However, these concerns can cause great anxiety in older adults who may fear dementia (Box 5.6). Many medical or psychiatric difficulties (delirium, depression) also influence memory abilities and it is important for older adults with memory complaints to have a comprehensive cognitive evaluation (Chapters 8 and 23).

Healthy cognitive aging (healthy brain aging) is comprehensive and proactive; it implies that cognitive health is much more than simply a lack of decline with aging. A healthy brain is "one that can perform all mental processes that are collectively known as cognition, including the ability to learn new things, intuition, judgment, language, and remembering" (Centers for Disease Control and Prevention [CDC], 2017). Attention to cognitive health, beginning at conception and continuing throughout life, is just as important as attention to physical and emotional health. Many of the behaviors influencing physical and emotional health also promote cognitive health.

◆ Nursing Actions: Cognitive Health

Nurses need to educate people of all ages about effective strategies to enhance cognitive health and vitality and to promote cognitive reserve and brain plasticity (Box 5.7). Blood pressure management, particularly in

---

BOX 5.7 Tips for Best Practice

Cognitive Health

- Dispel myths about brain aging and teach about cognition and aging.
- Educate people of all ages about factors that influence cognitive health.
- Be aware of cultural differences in perceptions of cognitive health and adapt education accordingly.
- Advise older adults to have comprehensive assessment if they are experiencing cognitive decline.
- Encourage socialization and participation in intellectually stimulating activities, exercise, healthy diets (e.g., Mediterranean diet, DASH diet).
- Teach chronic illness prevention strategies and ensure good management of chronic illnesses.
- Share resources for cognitive training (memory enhancing techniques, puzzles, card games).

---

midlife, physical activity (Chapter 13), adherence to a Mediterranean diet (MetDiet) and a combined MetDiet and Dietary Approaches to Stop Hypertension (DASH) diet plan (Chapter 10), social engagement, and cognitive stimulation may reduce the risk of ARCD. The CDC and the National Institute on Aging have large-scale programs focused on healthy brain aging and provide resources nurses can use in health-promotion education.

Learning in Later Life

Basic intelligence remains unchanged with increasing years and older adults should be provided with opportunities for continued learning. Adapting communication and teaching to enhance understanding requires knowledge of learning in late life and effective teaching learning strategies with older adults. *Geragogy* is the application of the principles of adult learning theory to teaching interventions for older adults. The older adult demands that teaching situations be relevant; new learning must relate to what the person already knows and should emphasize concrete and practical information. Aging may present barriers to learning, such as hearing and vision losses and cognitive impairment. Pain and discomfort can also interfere with learning. Moreover, the process of aging may accentuate other challenges that had already been factors in a person's life, such as cultural and cohort variations (Chapter 3) and education. Some older adults may have special learning needs based on educational deprivation in their early years and consequent anxiety about formalized learning.

Health literacy is defined as the degree to which individuals have the capacity to obtain, process, and understand basic health information and services needed to make appropriate health decisions (Center for Disease Control, 2017). Health literacy is not about reading skills or having a college degree. It means the individual knows how to ask a health care provider the right questions, read a food label, understand what they are signing on a consent form, and has the numeric ability to analyze relative risks when making treatment decisions. Limited health literacy has been linked to increased health disparities, poor health outcomes, inadequate preventive care, increased use of health care services, higher health care costs, higher risk of mortality for older adults, and several health care safety issues, including medical and medication errors (Cutilli et al., 2018).

Some older adults may be disproportionally affected by inadequate health literacy. Older adults have lower health literacy scores than all other age groups and more than half of individuals over 65 years of age are at the below-basic level (MacLeod et al, 2017). Older adults are a heterogeneous group in their characteristics and literacy skills, therefore strategies to enhance understanding of health information need to be individualized. However, as the major consumers of health care in this country, many are at risk of poor outcomes related to understanding health care information and navigating the health care system. Box 5.8 presents Tips for Best Practice in guiding older learners, and Box 5.9 presents additional resources for cognitive health and health literacy.

Learning Opportunities

Opportunities for older adults to learn are available in many formal and informal modes: self-teaching, college attendance, participation in seminars and conferences, public television programs, CDs, Internet courses, and countless others. In most colleges and universities, older adults are taking classes of all types. Fees are usually lower for individuals older than 60 years of age and older adults may choose to work toward a degree or audit classes for enrichment and enjoyment. Senior centers and local school districts often provide a wide array of adult education courses. The Road Scholar (formerly Elderhostel) program is an example of a program designed for older adults that combines continued learning with travel. The program offers trips to all 50 states and 150 countries. Road Scholar offers intergenerational programs for grandparents and grandchildren aged 4 years and older (https://www.roadscholar.org/). "Skip gen" travel (travel with grandchildren alone) is experienced by a third of grandparents (Ianzito, 2019).

BOX 5.8 Tips for Best Practice

Strategies to Improve Health Literacy in Older Adult Learners

Manage the Teaching Environment
- Schedule appointment when individual is rested
- Ensure comfort (appropriate seating, room temperature, pain medication if needed)
- Limit session to 10 to 15 minutes
- Observe for signs of fatigue, discomfort during session

Improve Oral Communication
- Pay attention to vision and hearing deficits (face individual, speak slowly, keep pitch of voice low, eliminate background noise)
- Adapt materials for culture, language, health literacy
- Limit content to three to five points and repeat key points frequently
- Be specific and concrete; use plain language
- Connect new learning to past experiences
- Conclude with brief summary of essential points

Modify Written Communication
- Use 16–18 point Arial font for written material with both upper-case and lowercase letters
- Use high contrast on printed materials (dark colors for text and lighter for background, black print on white)
- Use gestures, demonstrations, and pictures in addition to printed material
- Bold key points
- Avoid charts with rows and columns
- Use lots of white space

Evaluate Comprehension
- Use "teach-back" methods to ensure understanding, e.g., "Can you show me how to use your inhaler?"
- Have individual paraphrase instructions
- Have individual demonstrate and provide feedback
- Encourage individual to teach family/caregivers in your presence

BOX 5.9 Resources for Best Practice

- **Centers for Disease Control and Prevention:** The Healthy Brain Initiative: A National Public Health Road Map to Maintaining Cognitive Health: https://www.cdc.gov/aging/pdf/thehealthybrain initiative.pdf.
- **Agency for Healthcare Research and Quality (AHRQ):** Health literacy universal precaution toolkit. https://www.ahrq.gov/sites /default/files/publications/files/healthlittoolkit2_3.pdf.

◆ Information Technology and Older Adults

Older adults comprise the fastest growing population using computers and the Internet. More than half of Internet users age 65 and older use Facebook (Pew Research Center, 2018). More than any other age group, older adults perceive the Internet as a valuable resource to help them more easily obtain information and connect to loved ones. This could range from using a cell phone to set medication reminders to using Skype and FaceTime to interact with long-distance grandchildren. Many individuals are also using email to communicate with their health care providers. Organizations such as Cyber-Seniors and AARP provide basic computer and Internet training for older adults.

With the aging of the baby boomers and the young tech-savvy adults, the future of technology in care and services for older adults can only be imagined. Technology has the potential to improve the quality of life for older adults across settings by enhancing access to health information and resources, making communication with family and friends easier, providing cognitive stimulation and enjoyable activities, and alleviating isolation among community-dwelling older adults and those in nursing homes (Chapter 16).

◆ Nursing Actions: Learning in Later Life

Traditional ways of providing health information and services are changing and both public and private institutions are increasingly using the Internet and other technologies. This presents challenges for individuals with limited experience using computers and for those with limited literacy. Nurses can share resources available for older adults who want to learn computer skills and adaptations that can be made to make computers as user-friendly as possible (e.g., touch screens, voice systems) for those who may have limitations.

Nurses and other health professionals need to develop skills in the understanding and use of consumer health information and teach clients how to evaluate the reliability and validity of health information on the Internet. Using social media as a platform for health promotion and health education presents exciting possibilities. Continued attention to access to technology, especially among disadvantaged groups, and also efforts to enhance culturally and language-appropriate materials are important. *Healthy People 2020* (USDHHS, 2012) has set goals for information technology that include improving health literacy and access to the Internet, increasing the proportion of reliable health-related websites, and encouraging use of the Internet to organize health data and communicate with health care providers. The increase in use of telehealth technology and coverage of cost by Medicare and other insurers that began with the COVID pandemic will significantly change traditional care practices (Chapter 16).

KEY CONCEPTS

- The impact of gender, culture, and cohort must always be considered when discussing the validity of psychosocial theories of aging.
- Spirituality must be considered a significant factor in understanding healthy aging. Using clinical judgment to implement and evaluate nursing actions to promote spiritual health is an important nursing role.
- Late adulthood is no longer seen as a period when growth ceases and cognitive development halts; rather, it is seen as a life stage programmed for plasticity and the development of unique capacities.
- Cognitive stimulation and attention to brain health is just as important as attention to physical health.
- Learning in late life can be enhanced by utilizing principles of geragogy and adapting teaching strategies to minimize barriers such as hearing and vision impairment and health literacy challenges.

ACTIVITIES AND DISCUSSION QUESTIONS

1. How well do the psychological and sociological theories of aging "fit" within your own cultural perspective?
2. Review the myths about aging and the brain (Box 5.5). Were any of the facts surprising to you?
3. Discuss some ways that nurses can respond to the spiritual needs and concerns of older adults.
4. What types of health teaching would you provide to a young adult to enhance brain health in aging? How would the teaching differ for an older adult with ARCD?
5. How would you respond to the following myth of aging: "You can't teach an old dog new tricks"?

NEXT-GENERATION NCLEX® EXAMINATION-STYLE QUESTIONS

Mr. Stanton, an 88-year-old widower, is preparing for discharge following hospitalization for community acquired pneumonia. He has a history of hypertension and osteoarthritis but is otherwise healthy. He lives by himself in a split-level home, in an established neighborhood. He has two grown children who live in neighboring cities. He worked most of his life as a laborer, having dropped out of school in the eighth grade to help provide for his family. Mr. Stanton states he never did well in school and was happy to leave the classroom to work in the fields to help his parents put food on the table. He wears bifocal glasses and a hearing aid on the right ear. He admits to not wearing the hearing aid all the time as his arthritis makes it difficult to adjust. His blood pressure is 138/86 mmHg, respirations are 18 breaths per minutes, heart rate is 92 beats per minute, and temperature is 98.4°F. His oxygen saturation is 94% on room air. He becomes short of breath and begins to cough, bringing up thick sputum, with exertion. The nurse comes to Mr. Stanton's room to go over his discharge instructions, prepares his room to facilitate teaching and reviews the teaching materials with him. His discharge medications include:

Levofloxacin 750 mg daily
Prednisone Taper:
  Day 1: 10 mg PO before breakfast, 5 mg after lunch and after dinner, and 10 mg at bedtime
  Day 2: 5 mg PO before breakfast, after lunch, and after dinner and 10 mg at bedtime
  Day 3: 5 mg PO before breakfast, after lunch, after dinner, and at bedtime
  Day 4: 5 mg PO before breakfast, after lunch, and at bedtime
  Day 5: 5 mg PO before breakfast and at bedtime
  Day 6: 5 mg PO before breakfast
Lisinopril/hydrochlorothiazide 20 mg/25 mg daily
Acetaminophen 500 mg every 4 hours as needed for pain
Multivitamin daily

Which strategies should the nurse take to improve health literacy for the client? (Select all that apply)

1. Schedule discharge teaching for a time when the client is rested and ready to learn.
2. Ensure the client is wearing glasses and hearing aids.
3. Use proper medical terminology
4. Limit the teaching session to 15 minutes.
5. Use bright colored paper for handouts to gain the client's attention
6. Use charts to organize content on printed materials
7. Use 12-point Times New Roman font
8. Ensure the teaching environment is free from background noise

REFERENCES

Achenbaum, W. A. (1978). *Old age in a new land*. Baltimore: Johns Hopkins University Press.

Agency for Healthcare Research and Quality (AHRQ): Weekly group storytelling enhances verbal skills, encourages positive behavior change, and reduces confusion in patients with Alzheimer's and related dementias, 2014, AHRQ Innovations Exchange. https://innovations.ahrq.gov/profiles/weekly-group-storytelling-enhances-verbal-skills-encourages-positive-behavior-change-and/.

American Association of Retired Persons (AARP). (Jan 7 2020). "Virtual travel" with real friends is combating isolation. https://www.aarp.org/home-family/personal-technology/info-2020/vr-social-connections/#:~:text=Senior%20living%20communities%20and%20experts,of%20their%20homes%20but%20also.

Basting, A. (2003). Reading the story behind the story: Context and content in stories by people with dementia. *Generations, 27*, 25–29.

Basting, A. (2006). Arts in dementia care: "This is not the end… it's the end of this chapter". *Generations, 30*, 16–20.

Basting, A. D. (2013). Time Slips: creativity for people with dementia. *Age Action, 28*(4), 1–5.

Birren, J. E., & Deutchman, D. E. (1991). *Guiding autobiography groups for older adults: Exploring the fabric of life.* Baltimore: Johns Hopkins University Press.

Butler, R. (1963). The life review: An interpretation of reminiscence in the aged. *Psychiatry, 26*, 65–76.

Butler, R. (2003). Age, death and life review. In K. Doka (Ed.), *Living with grief: Loss in later life.* Washington, DC: Hospice Foundation.

Butler, R., & Lewis, M. (1983). *Aging and mental health: Positive psychosocial approach* (ed. 3). St Louis, MO: Mosby.

Centers for Disease Control and Prevention (CDC): *Healthy brain initiative*, 2017a. https://www.cdc.gov/aging/healthybrain/index.htm.

Centers for Disease Control and Prevention (CDC): *Health literacy*, 2017b. https://www.cdc.gov/healthliteracy/index.html.

Clayton, M., Hulett, J., Kapur, K., Reblin, M., Wilson, A., & Ellington, L. (2017). Nursing support of home hospice caregivers on the day of patient death. *Oncol Nurs Forum, 44*, 457–464.

Cottrell, L. (1942). The adjustment of the individual to his age and sex roles. *Am Sociol Rev, 7*, 617–620.

Cooney, A., Hunter, A., Murphy, K., et al. (2014). 'Seeing me through my memories': a grounded theory study on using reminiscence with people with dementia living in long-term care. *J Clin Nurs, 23*, 3564–3574.

Cowgill, D. (1974). Aging and modernization: A revision of the theory. In J. Gubrium (Ed.), *Late life communities and environmental policy.* Springfield, IL: Charles C Thomas.

Crowley, S. L. (1996). Aging brain's staying power. *AARP Bulletin, 37*(1).

Cumming, E., & Henry, W. (1961). *Growing old.* New York: Basic Books.

Cutilli, C. C., Simko, L. C., Colbert, A. M., & Bennett, I. M. (2018). Health literacy, health disparities, and sources of health information in U.S. older adults. *Orthop Nurs, 37*(1), 54–65.

Davis, S. W., Luber, B., Murphy, D. L. K., Lisanby, S. H., & Cabeza, R. (2017). Frequency-specific neuromodulation of local and distant connectivity in aging and episodic memory function. *Hum Brain Mapp, 38*(12), 5987–6004.

Delgado, C. (2007). Sense of coherence, spirituality, stress and quality of life in chronic illness. *J Nurs Scholarsh, 39*(3), 229–234.

Erikson, E. H., Erikson, J. M., & Kivnick, H. Q. (1986). *Vital involvement in old age: The experience of old age in our time.* New York: WW Norton.

Fick, D. M. (2016). Promoting cognitive health. *J Gerontol Nurs, 42*(7), 4–6.

Gaskamp, C., Sutter, R., Meraviglia, M., et al. (2006). Evidence-based guideline: Promoting spirituality in the older adult. *J Gerontol Nurs, 32*(11), 8–11.

Haight, B., & Webster, J. (2002). *Critical advances in reminiscence work: From theory to application.* New York: Springer.

Havighurst, R. J. (1972). *Developmental tasks and education* (ed. 3). New York: Longman.

Havighurst, R. J., & Albrecht, R. (1953). *Older people.* New York: Longmans, Green.

Havighurst, R. J., Neugarten, B. L., & Tobin, S. S. (1968). Disengagement and patterns of aging. In B. L. Neugarten (Ed.), *Middle age and aging.* Chicago: University of Chicago Press.

Hendricks, J., & Hendricks, C. D. (1986). *Aging in mass society: Myths and realities.* Boston: Little, Brown.

Hill, N. L. (2017). Person-centered technology for older adults. *J Gerontol Nurs, 43*(4), 3–4.

Hooyman, N., & Kiyak, H. (2005). *Social gerontology* (ed. 7). Boston: Pearson.

Hooyman, N., & Kiyak, H. (2011). *Social gerontology* (ed. 9). Boston: Pearson.

Ianzito C: New trend: grandparents vacationing with grandchildren. April 10, 2019. https://www.aarp.org/travel/vacation-ideas/family/info-2019/skip-generation-travel.html.

Karlsson, E., Zingmark, K., Axelsson, K., & Savenstedt, S. (2017). Aspects of self and identity in narrations about recent events: communication with individuals with Alzheimer's disease enabled by a digital photograph diary. *J Gerontol Nurs, 43*(6), 25–31.

Koenig, H. G., & Brooks, R. G. (2002). Religion, health and aging: Implications for practice and public policy. *Public Policy Aging Rep, 12*, 13–19.

Latha, K., Bhandary, P., Tejaswini, S., et al. (2014). Reminiscence therapy: An overview. *Middle East J Age Ageing, 11*(1), 18–22.

Maddox, G. (1963). Activity and morale: A longitudinal study of selected elderly subjects. *Soc Forces, 42*, 195–204.

Meyer, C. L. (2003). How effectively are nurse educators preparing students to provide spiritual care? *Nurse Educ, 28*(4), 185–190.

MacLeod, S., Musich, S., Gulyas, S., et al. (2017). The impact of inadequate health literacy on patient satisfaction, healthcare utilization, and expenditures among older adults. *Geriatr Nurs, 38*(4), 334–341.

Maslow, A. H. (1954). Motivation and personality. New York: Harper and Row.

Moss, M. (2014). Storytelling. In R. Lindquist, M. Snyder, & M. Tracy (Eds.), *Complementary and alternative therapies in nursing* (ed. 7, pp. 215–228). New York: Springer.

Neugarten, B. L. (1968). *Middle age and aging.* Chicago: University of Chicago Press.

O'Shea, E., Devane, D., Cooney, A., et al. (2014). The impact of reminiscence on the quality of life of residents with dementia in long-stay care. *Int J Geriatr Psychiatry, 29*, 1062–1070.

Pew Research Center: *Social media fact sheet*, 2018. http://www.pewinternet.org/fact-sheet/social-media/.

Puchalski, C., & Romer, A. (2000). Taking a spiritual history allows clinicians to understand patients more fully. *J Palliat Med, 3*, 129–137.

Ramírez-Esparza, N., & Pennebaker, J. (2006). Do good stories produce good health? Exploring words, language and culture. *Narrat Inq, 16*(11), 211–219.

Ramscar, M., Hendrix, P., Shaoul, C., et al. (2014). The myth of cognitive decline: Non-linear dynamics of lifelong learning. *Top Cogn Sci, 6*(1), 5–42.

Riley, M. W. (1971). Social gerontology and the age of stratification of society. *Gerontologist, 11*, 79–87.

Soeken, K., & Carson, V. (1987). Responding to the spiritual needs of the chronically ill. *Nurs Clin North Am, 22*, 603–611.

Stair, N. (1992). If I had my life to live over. In S. Martz (Ed.), *If I had my life to live over I would pick more daisies.* Watsonville, CA: Papier Mache Press.

Strang, S., & Strang, P. (2002). Questions posed to hospital chaplains by palliative care patients. *J Palliat Med, 5*, 887.

Tan, A. (2001). *The bonesetter's daughter* (1). New York: Putnam Adult.

Testad, I., Corbett, A., Aarsland, D., et al. (2014). The value of personalized psychosocial interventions to address behavioral and psychological symptoms in people with dementia living in care home settings: a systematic review. *Int Psychogeriatr, 26*, 1083–1098.

Tornstam, L. (1989). Gerotranscendence: A meta-theoretical reformulation of the disengagement theory. *Aging Clin Exper Res, 1*, 55–64.

Tornstam, L. (2000). Transcendence in later life. *Generations, 23*, 1014.

Tornstam, L. (2005). *Gerotranscendence: A developmental theory of positive aging.* New York: Springer.

Touhy, T., Brown., C., & Smith., C. (2005). Spiritual caring: End of life in a nursing home. *J Gerontol Nurs, 31*, 27–35.

Touhy, T., & Zerwekh, J. (2006). Spiritual caring. editor. In J. Zerwekh (Ed.), *Nursing care at the end of life: Palliative care for patients and families.* Philadelphia: FA Davis.

U.S. Department of Health and Human Services (USDHHS). *Office of Disease Prevention and Health Promotion: Healthy People 2020*, 2012. http://www.healthypeople.gov/2020.

Wadensten, B. (2006). An analysis of the psychosocial theories of ageing and their relevance to practical gerontological nursing in Sweden. *Scand J Caring Sci, 20*, 347–354.

Vaineta, J. (2016). Spiritual health as an integral component of human well-being. *Appl Res Health Soc Sciences: Interface and integration, 13*(1), 3–13.

Wittenberg, E., Ragan, S. L., & Ferrell, B. (2017). Exploring nurse communication about spirituality. *Am J Hosp Palliat Med, 34*(6), 566–571.

Yamashita, T., Hahn, S., Kinney, J., Yamashita, T., Hahn, S., Kinney, J., & Poon, L. (2018). Impact of life stories on college students' positive and negative attitudes toward older adults. *Gerontol Geriatr Educ, 39*(3), 326–340.

6

Gerontological Nursing Across the Continuum of Care

Theris A. Touhy

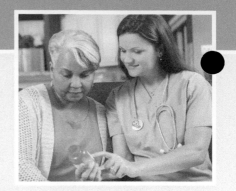

LEARNING OBJECTIVES

Upon completion of this chapter, the reader will be able to:

- Compare the major features, advantages, and disadvantages of several residential options available to the older adult.
- Discuss long-term care as a component of health care systems.
- Understand the role of nursing in quality improvement and culture change in LTC.
- Utilize clinical judgment skills to identify and evaluate nursing actions to improve outcomes for older adults in LTC and during transitions between health care settings.

THE LIVED EXPERIENCE

We are dealing with some really tough decisions for my parents. They insist on staying in their own home but I don't think it's safe anymore. They need quite a bit of help and I cannot do it all. We talked about assisted living and nursing home but they don't want that and would have to use all of their savings to pay for care. Coming to my home is not an option with three active teenagers and only three small bedrooms. I worry constantly about what to do.

Marianne, age 50

This chapter discusses residential and long-term care options across the continuum and transitions between health care settings with related implications for nursing practice. Long-term care (LTC) as a component of the health care system and the role of skilled nursing facilities (SNFs) in the provision of post–acute care are also discussed.

Most people would prefer to stay in their own home (age in place), but there are many factors that can affect decision-making about where to live as one ages (Chapter 16). Some older adults, by choice or by need, move from one type of residence to another. A number of options exist, especially for those with the financial resources that allow them to have a choice. Residential options range along a continuum from remaining in one's private house or apartment to senior retirement communities; to shared housing with family members,

friends, or others; to residential care communities such as assisted living settings; to nursing facilities for those with the most needs. It is important for nurses in all practice settings to be knowledgeable about the range of options so that they can assist older adults and their families who may need to make decisions about relocation.

COMMUNITY CARE

Program for All-Inclusive Care for the Elderly (PACE)

This program is a Medicaid and Medicare program that provides community services to individuals who would otherwise need a nursing home level of care. Participants must meet the criteria for nursing home admission, prefer to remain in the community, and be eligible for

Medicare/Medicaid. It is a full service model that covers the cost of primary care, hospitalization, emergency department visits, approved specialty services, rehabilitation, home care, medication and treatment, and social and recreational services in a community center environment. The PACE program has been the only Medicare program that has required and paid for interdisciplinary team care using a capitated payment. Nursing has been central to the PACE care model since its inception. Outcomes of PACE include increased use of ambulatory services, lower rates of nursing home use and in-patient hospitalization, lower rates of functional decline, and better reported health status than among a comparison population (Cortes & Sullivan-Marx, 2016).

PACE is recognized as a permanent provider under Medicare and a state option under Medicaid. Currently, there are 123 PACE programs operating 250 PACE centers in 31 states serving over 45,000 participants. PACE has been approved by the US Department of Health and Human Services (USDHHS) Substance Abuse and Mental Health Services Administration (SAMHSA) as an evidence-based model of care. Models such as PACE are innovative care delivery models, and continued development of such models is important as the population ages (National PACE Association, 2019).

Adult Day Services

Adult day services (ADSs) are community-based group programs designed to provide social and some health services to adults who need supervised care in a safe setting during the day. They also offer caregivers respite from the responsibilities of caregiving and most provide educational programs, support groups, and individual counseling for caregivers. Adult day centers are serving populations with higher levels of physical disability and chronic disease.

Increasingly, ADSs are being utilized to provide community-based care for conditions such as Alzheimer's disease and for transitional care and short-term rehabilitation following hospitalization. Nearly half of all ADS participants have some level of dementia. Staff ratios in ADS are one direct care worker to six clients. Almost 80% of centers have professional nursing staff, 50% have a social worker, and 60% offer case management services. Most also offer transportation services.

Some ADSs are private pay and others are funded through Medicaid home and community-based waiver programs, state and local funding, and the Veterans Administration (Table 6.1). ADSs hold the potential to meet the need for cost-efficient and high-quality LTC services and continued expansion and funding are expected. ADSs are an important part of the long-term post–acute care (LTPAC) continuum and a cost-effective

TABLE 6.1 Costs of US Long-Term Care Services and Support Programs

Service	Cost
Homemaker services	National median hourly rate: $22.50
Home health aide	National median hourly rate: $23.00
Adult day health	National median daily rate: $75
Assisted living facility	National median monthly rate: $4051; Annually $48,612
Skilled nursing facility	National median daily rate: $247 (semi-private room); $280 (private) Annually semi-private: $90,155; Private: $102,200

From Genworth (2019) Genworth launches cost of care survey. https://www.multivu.com/players/English/8625551-8625551-genworth-cost-of-care-survey-2019/.

alternative or supplement to home care or institutional care. Although further research is needed on patient and caregiver outcomes of ADS, findings suggest that they improve health-related quality of life for participants and improve caregiver well-being. Local area agencies on aging are good sources of information about ADSs and other community-based options.

Continuing Care Retirement Communities (CCRCs)

Life care communities, also known as CCRCs, provide the full range of residential options, from single-family homes to skilled nursing facilities all in one location. Most of these communities provide access to these levels of care for a community member's entire remaining lifetime and for the right price, the range of services may be guaranteed. Having all levels of care in one location allows community members to make the transition between levels without life-disrupting moves. For married couples in which one spouse needs more care than the other, life care communities allow them to live nearby in a different part of the same community. Most CCRCs are managed by not-for-profit organizations. Entrance fees can range from as low as $20,000 for a non-purchase (rental) agreement to buy-in fees among the most expensive CCRCs of up to $500,000 or more depending on the size and location of the unit and the community. Monthly costs can be as low as $500 at some communities and as high as $3000 or more depending on type of contract and service plan. Costs of CCRCs are paid out-of-pocket and not covered by Medicare or Medicaid.

Residential Care/Assisted Living

Residential care/assisted living (RC/AL) facilities are non-medical facilities that provide room, meals, housekeeping, supervision and distribution of medication, and personal care assistance with basic activities such as hygiene, dressing, eating, bathing, and transferring. This level of care is for individuals who are unable to live by themselves but who do not need 24-hour nursing care. RC/AL are known by more than 30 different names across the country, including adult congregate facilities, foster care homes, personal care homes, domiciliary care homes, board and care homes, rest homes, family care homes, retirement homes, and assisted living facilities (ALFs).

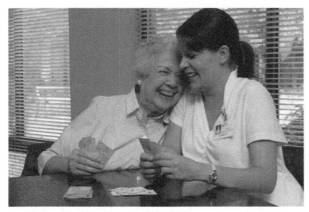

Providing nursing services in assisted living facilities promotes physical and psychosocial health. (From Potter, P. A. (2010). *Basic nursing: Essentials for practice* (7th ed.). St Louis: Mosby.)

RC/AL facilities are viewed as more cost-effective than nursing homes while providing more privacy and a homelike environment. Medicare does not cover the cost of care in these types of facilities. The majority of individuals in RC/AL pay for their care from their personal resources and 47% of facilities accept Medicaid. Private and LTC insurance may also cover some costs. The rates charged and the services those rates include vary considerably, as do regulations and licensing. States are responsible for regulating RC/AL, and there are no federal quality standards or mandatory reporting on quality similar to requirements for skilled nursing facilities.

Assisted Living

A popular type of RC/AL is the assisted living facility (ALF), also called *board and care homes* or *adult congregate living facilities*. Box 6.1 presents information about the typical ALF resident. ALF settings may be a shared room or a single-occupancy unit with a private bath, kitchenette, and communal meals. They all provide some support services, but if care needs increase, there is usually a charge for services.

Assisted living is more expensive than independent living and less costly than skilled nursing home care, but it is not inexpensive (Table 6.1). Costs vary by

> **BOX 6.1   Profile of a Resident in an Assisted Living Facility**
>
> - 32% 75 years to 84 years; 51% over 85 years
> - Female (72%)
> - 38% need help with 3–5 activities of daily living; 61% need help with bathing; 45% need help dressing; 37% need help with toileting; 18% need help with eating; 25% need help with bed transfer
> - About 52% are cognitively impaired
> - The median length of stay is about 22 months
> - 59% move to a nursing facility
> - 33% die while a resident of an assisted living facility
>
> From National Center for Assisted Living: https://www.ahcancal.org/ncal/Pages/index.aspx.

geographical region, size of the unit, and relative luxury. Forty-two percent of ALFs are small with 4 to 10 beds, and 33% have between 26 and 100 beds. Most ALFs offer two or three meals per day, light weekly housekeeping and laundry services, and optional social activities. Each added service increases the cost of the setting but also allows individuals with resources to remain in the setting longer as functional abilities decline. Consumers are advised to inquire as to exactly what services will be provided and by whom if a resident of an ALF becomes frailer and needs more intensive care.

Many older adults and their families prefer ALFs to nursing homes because they cost less, are more homelike, and offer more opportunities for control, independence, and privacy. However, many residents of ALFs have chronic care needs and over time may require more care than the facility is able to provide. Services (e.g., home health, hospice, homemakers) can be brought into the facility, but some question whether this adequately substitutes for 24-hour supervision by registered nurses (RNs). Only 17% of residential care facilities (RCFs) reported having registered, licensed practical, or vocational nurses on staff. RCFs are not required to provide licensed nursing on a 24-hour basis, even though there is evidence that many residents in some facilities are frail, with many chronic illnesses, impaired self-care needs and cognition, and unmet care needs (Harrington et al., 2017). In the ALF there is no organized team of providers such as that found in skilled care facilities (i.e., nurses, social worker, therapists, pharmacists, dieticians).

With the growing numbers of older adults with dementia residing in ALFs, many are establishing dementia-specific units. It is important to investigate services available and staff training, when making decisions about the most appropriate placement for older adults with dementia. Continued research is needed on best-care practices and outcomes of care for people with dementia in both ALFs and nursing homes. The Alzheimer's Association has issued a set of dementia care practices for ALFs and nursing homes (Alzheimer's Association, 2009).

The nonmedical nature of ALFs is a primary factor in keeping costs more reasonable than those in nursing facilities, but costs are still high for those without adequate funds. Appropriate standards of care must be developed and care outcomes monitored to ensure that residents are receiving quality care in this setting, which is almost devoid of professional nursing. Available data about facility to resident ratios raise questions about care quality (Harrington et al., 2017). "The absence of oversight and regulations requires families to do extra due diligence before choosing a facility" (Gleckman, 2018). Further research is needed on care outcomes of residents in ALFs and the role of unlicensed assistive personnel and RNs in these facilities.

Advanced practice gerontological nurses are well suited to the role of primary care provider in ALFs and many have assumed this role. The American Assisted Living Nurses Association has established a certification mechanism for nurses working in these facilities and has also developed a *Scope and Standards of Assisted Living Nursing Practice for Registered Nurses.* The Assisted Living Federation of America and the National Center for Assisted Living provide a consumer guide for choosing an AL residence (Box 6.2).

NURSING FACILITIES (NURSING HOMES)

Nursing homes are the settings for the delivery of around-the-clock care for those needing specialized care that cannot be provided elsewhere. Nursing homes are a complex health care setting that is a mix of hospital, rehabilitation facility, hospice, and dementia-specific units, and they are a final home for many older adults. When used appropriately, nursing homes fill an important need for families and older adults. The settings called *nursing homes* or *nursing facilities* most often include up to two levels of care: *skilled nursing care* (also called *subacute care*) and chronic care (also called long-term or custodial).

Skilled nursing care facilities are required to have licensed professionals with a focus on the management of complex medical needs, and a *chronic care* facility is required to have 24-hour personal assistance that is supervised and augmented by professional and licensed nurses. Often, both kinds of services are provided in one facility. There are significant differences in focus of care, staffing, level of reimbursement, and regulatory guidelines between these two kinds of services.

BOX 6.2   Resources for Best Practice

Alzheimer's Association: Dementia Care Practice Recommendations for assisted living facilities (ALFs) and Nursing Homes

American Assisted Living Nurses Association: Certification, Scope and Standards of Practice

American Healthcare Association/National Center for Assisted Living: Information, educational resources, guide to choosing an assisted living facility and skilled nursing facility

Argentum (formerly the Assisted Living Federation of America): Information, educational resources, guide to choosing an ALF

Centers for Medicare and Medicaid Services: Guide to choosing a nursing home; Nursing Home Compare; Nursing Home Quality Care Collaborative (NHQCC) Learning; Partnership to Improve Dementia Care in Nursing Homes; Quality Assurance and Performance Improvement (QAPI)

Eden Alternative

National Adult Day Services Association

National Programs of All-Inclusive Care for the Elderly (PACE) Association

The Green House Project

The National Nursing Home Quality Improvement Campaign: Evidence-based and model-practice resources to support quality improvement

National Consumer Voice for Long-Term Care: National voice representing consumers in issues related to long-term care; information and resources to help insure quality care; Guide to Choosing a Nursing Home

Pioneer Network: Culture change information and toolkit

There are approximately 15,655 certified nursing homes in the United States with 1.7 million beds. Of the 3.9 million individuals needing care, 22% have stays of less than 100 days and 78% have stays of 100 days or more (CDC, 2020). The majority of nursing homes (70%) are for-profit organizations (American Healthcare Association/National Center Assisted Living [HCA/NCAL], 2020). The number of nursing home beds is decreasing in the United States as a result of the increased use of RCFs and more reimbursement by Medicaid programs for community-based care alternatives. However, in most areas of the country, the supply and use of nursing homes is still greater than those of other LTC service options.

Subacute Care (Short Term)

The old concept of nursing homes has dramatically changed with the increase in the number of patients with complex medical needs being cared for in this setting. Skilled nursing facilities are the most frequent site of post–acute care in the United States. Subacute care is more intensive than traditional nursing home care and several times more costly, but far less costly than care in a hospital. The expectation is that the patient will be discharged home or to a less intensive setting. Length of stay is usually less than 1 month and is largely reimbursed by Medicare. In addition to skilled nursing care, rehabilitation services are an essential component of subacute units. Patients in subacute units are usually younger and less likely to be cognitively impaired than those in traditional nursing home care. Generally, higher levels of professional staffing are found in the subacute setting because of the acuity of the patient's condition. Roles for professional nursing in this setting are increasing. Nurses with expert skills in rehabilitation nursing and acute and long-term care will be needed (Chapter 1).

Skilled nursing facilities (both post–acute and long-term chronic) utilize interprofessional teams, working with the individual and family to assess, plan, and implement care. Rehabilitation and restorative care is increasingly important in light of shortened hospital stays that may occur before conditions are stabilized and the individual is able to function independently. The opportunity to work with an interprofessional team is one of the most exciting aspects of nursing practice in long-term care facilities (Box 6.3).

The setting provides opportunities for learning and practice in areas that are core to 21st-century nursing: managing chronic illness and palliative care in ways that are patient-centered and evidence-based, working with interdisciplinary teams, supervising unlicensed caregivers, and developing systems for quality improvement. LTC should be marketed as a bright future career for young nurses that requires excellent technical and critical thinking skills and is more autonomous than other areas of nursing (Sherman & Touhy, 2017). Nursing education programs and facility orientation and training programs must prepare nurses to practice competently in this important and growing care setting.

Chronic Care (Long Term)

Nursing homes also care for patients who may not need the intense care provided in subacute units but still need ongoing 24-hour care. This may include individuals with severe strokes, dementia, or Parkinson disease, and those receiving hospice care. Residents of long-term chronic care facilities are predominantly women, 80 years or older, widowed, and dependent in activities of daily living (ADLs) and instrumental activities of daily living (IADLs). About 50% of these residents are cognitively impaired and these types of facilities are increasingly caring for people at the end of life. Twenty-three percent of Americans die in nursing homes and this figure is expected to increase to 40% by 2040 (Stanford School of Medicine, 2019). While the percentage of older adults living in nursing homes at any given time is low (4% to 5%), those who live to 85 years of age will have a one in two chance of spending some time in a nursing home. This could be for subacute care, ongoing LTC, or end-of-life care. Individuals needing long-term chronic care in nursing homes represent the frailest of all older adults. Their needs for 24-hour care could not be met in the home or RC setting or may have exceeded what the family was able to provide.

Many people still believe that Medicare and Social Security protect them from the costs of long-term care, until "they discover otherwise when their first family member needs long-term care. Then they realize that Medicaid is their safety net, but Medicaid requires both severe poverty and substantial illness and disability, and often provides less appealing nursing homes" (Lynn, 2019). Medicare only pays for long-term care if there is a skilled need. The cost of long-term chronic nursing home care is largely paid by Medicaid (57%), Medicare (14%), and 29% by private insurance plans, other payers, and the individuals and families themselves (Chapter 7).

LONG-TERM CARE AND THE US HEALTH CARE SYSTEM

The term long-term care (LTC) is often only associated with nursing homes and with care of older adults. However, LTC describes a variety of services, including medical and nonmedical care, provided on an ongoing basis to people of all ages who have a chronic illness or physical, cognitive, or developmental disabilities. LTC can be provided informally or formally in a range of environments, from an individual's home to the home of a friend or relative, an adult day health center, independent and assisted living facilities, continuing care retirement communities, skilled nursing facilities, and hospice.

BOX 6.3   Interprofessional Teams in Nursing Homes

Patient
Family/significant others
Nurse
Primary care provider: physician, nurse practitioner
Physical, occupational, speech therapists
Social worker
Dietitian
Discharge planner/case manager
Psychologist
Prosthetist and orthotist
Audiologist

Long-term services and supports (LTSS) consist predominantly of assistance or supervision with ADLs, such as bathing, dressing, toileting, or eating, or with IADLs, such as shopping or cleaning. Older adults receive the majority of LTSS (80%) on a yearly basis, but children and younger adults also receive this type of care. Children younger than age 18 are a small percentage of the total population requiring LTSS but can have substantial needs that will last a lifetime. Most people with LTSS needs live in their own home with family, friends, and volunteers (as well as hired personnel) providing most of the care.

However, the bulk of LTC throughout the developed world is informal unpaid care provided by friends and relatives. The nature of family caregiving is changing as more individuals are discharged early from acute settings with increasingly complex medical care needs to be met in the home. Without family caregivers, the present level of LTC could not be sustained (Chapters 26 and 27). In the coming years, most families will have a member with a need for LTC services and supports. However, with shrinking family sizes, there will be fewer potential caregivers and reliance on formal care services can be expected to expand. Estimates are that spending on LTC will increase fivefold by 2045 in the United States.

The US health care system has been focused on delivering acute care and addressing time-limited and specific illnesses and injuries as they occur in episodes. Such a system does not address the increasingly complex and long-term needs of people with chronic conditions. There has been little recognition of LTC as an integral part of the continuum of care. Today, the spectrum of care has been expanded to include LTPAC, which includes nursing facilities, assisted living facilities, home care, and hospice (Fig. 6.1).

The LTC system is complex and fragmented, isolated from other service providers, and poorly funded; it is confusing for the individual and the caregiver to access and negotiate. There is no comprehensive approach to care coordination, which results in unmet needs, risk of injuries, and adverse outcomes. There is also a critical shortage of well-prepared health care professionals and direct care staff to provide LTC, putting the individual who needs this care at further risk of poor outcomes (Chapter 1).

Health care professionals who have not had experience in the long-term care system are often unaware of the many differences between acute and long-term care. Unless they have experienced the problems in their own families, they may be unaware of the challenges associated with obtaining quality care for individuals with long-term needs. It is important for health care professionals, especially nurses, to understand the total spectrum of care and the differences between acute and long-term care (Boxes 6.4 and 6.5).

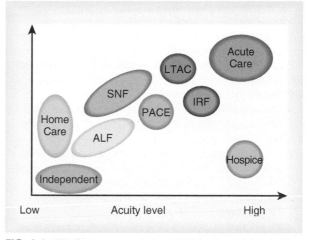

FIG. 6.1 LTPAC spectrum of care. *ALF,* Assisted living facility; *IRF,* inpatient rehabilitation facility; *LTAC,* long-term acute care; *PACE,* Program of All-Inclusive Care for the Elderly; *SNF,* skilled nursing facility. (From John F. Derr, RPh; JD and Associates Enterprises, Inc., https://www.jd-associatesenterprises.com/ltpac-health-it-collaborative.html.)

Costs of LTC

LTC is expensive and becoming more expensive; costs have outpaced inflation since 2003. The number of older adults needing long-term care services and support is dramatically increasing year after year. Worldwide, the number of individuals older than age 80, those most

---

BOX 6.4   Focus of Acute and Long-Term Care

Acute Care Orientation
- Illness
- High technology
- Short term
- Episodic
- One-dimensional
- Professional
- Medical model
- Cure

Long-Term Care Orientation
- Function
- High touch
- Extended
- Interdisciplinary model
- Ongoing
- Multidimensional
- Paraprofessional and family
- Care

BOX 6.5   Goals of Long-Term Care

1. Provide a safe and supportive environment for chronically ill and functionally dependent individuals.
2. Restore and maintain highest practicable level of functional independence.
3. Preserve individual autonomy.
4. Maximize quality of life, well-being, and satisfaction with care.
5. Provide comfort and dignity at the end of life for individuals and their families.
6. Provide coordinated interdisciplinary care to subacutely ill individuals who plan to return home or to a less restrictive level of care.
7. Stabilize and delay progression, when possible, of chronic medical conditions.
8. Prevent acute medical and iatrogenic illnesses, and identify and treat them rapidly when they do occur.
9. Create a homelike environment that respects the dignity of each individual.

likely to need long-term care services, will increase by 233% between 2008 and 2040 (Applebaum et al., 2013). A fivefold increase in spending on LTC is projected by 2045 in the United States (Frank, 2012). Long-term care coverage in the United States is overly reliant on institutional care (the most expensive) and primarily financed by Medicaid and individuals themselves. The United States and the United Kingdom (excluding Scotland) are the only two countries in the developed world that do not have some system for universal long-term care.

LTC is the largest expenditure for older adults in the United States. Finding a way to pay for LTC is a growing concern for people of all ages (Chapter 7). Most people have not planned for their LTC needs and are not knowledgeable about resources. Health care reform measures will continue to address rising health care costs across the continuum and develop programs to decrease costs while enhancing quality. Medical (health) homes and accountable care organizations (ACOs) are examples of these types of programs.

QUALITY OF CARE IN SKILLED NURSING FACILITIES

Nursing homes are one of the most highly regulated industries in the United States. The Omnibus Budget Reconciliation Act (OBRA) of 1987 and the frequent revisions and updates are designed to improve the quality of resident care and have had a positive impact. Some of the requirements of OBRA and subsequent

legislation include the following: comprehensive resident assessments (Minimum Data Set [MDS]) (Chapter 8), increased training requirements for nursing assistants, elimination of the use of medications and restraints for the purpose of discipline or convenience, higher staffing requirements for nursing and social work staff, standards for nursing home administrators, and quality assurance activities. The Quality Assurance Performance Improvement (QAPI) requires all nursing homes participating in Medicare or Medicaid programs to implement a QAPI program to assess quality of care provided to residents and to improve outcomes. Box 6.6 presents quality measures.

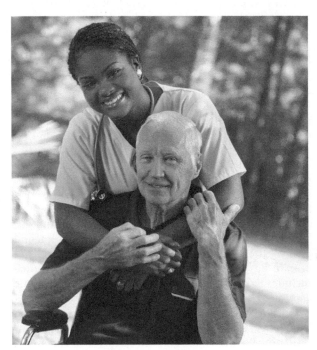

Caring relationships between staff and residents in long-term care enhance quality of care. (© iStock.com/Pamela Moore.)

The National Nursing Home Quality Improvement Campaign provides free, easy access to evidence-based and model-practice resources to support continuous quality improvement (Box 6.2). The Skilled Nursing Facility Value-Based Purchasing Program (SNF VBF), beginning in 2019, rewards skilled nursing facilities with incentive payments for the quality of care they give to individuals with Medicare (CMS, 2018).

Nursing homes undergo regular unannounced surveys every 9 to 15 months and surveys are also conducted in response to complaints. Detailed inspection data and penalties for violations for individual nursing homes are reported on CMS's Nursing Home Compare

---

BOX 6.6   Quality Measures for LTC Facilities

Short Stay Quality Measures

- Percentage of short-stay residents who were re-hospitalized after a nursing home admission.
- Percentage of short-stay residents who have had an outpatient emergency department visit.
- Percentage of short-stay residents who got antipsychotic medication for the first time.
- Percentage of SNF residents with pressure injuries that are new or worsened (SNF QRP).
- Rate of successful return to home and community from a SNF (SNF QRP).
- Percentage of short-stay residents who improved in their ability to move around on their own.
- Percentage of short-stay residents who needed and got a flu shot for the current flu season.
- Percentage of short-stay residents who needed and got a vaccine to prevent pneumonia.
- Percentage of SNF residents who experience one or more falls with major injury during their SNF stay (SNF QRP).
- Percentage of SNF residents whose functional abilities were assessed and functional goals were included in their treatment plan (SNF QRP).
- Rate of potentially preventable hospital readmissions 30 days after discharge from a SNF (SNF QRP).
- Medicare Spending Per Beneficiary (MSPB) for residents in SNFs (SNF QRP).

Long Stay Quality Measures

- Number of hospitalizations per 1000 long-stay resident days.
- Outpatient emergency department visits per 1,000 long-stay resident days.
- Percentage of long-stay residents who got an antipsychotic medication.
- Percentage of long-stay residents experiencing one or more falls with major injury.
- Percentage of long-stay high-risk residents with pressure injuries.
- Percentage of long-stay residents with a urinary tract infection.
- Percentage of long-stay residents who have or had a catheter inserted and left in their bladder.
- Percentage of long-stay residents whose ability to move independently worsened.
- Percentage of long-stay residents whose need for help with daily activities has increased.
- Percentage of long-stay residents who needed and got a flu shot for the current flu season.
- Percentage of long-stay residents who needed and got a vaccine to prevent pneumonia.
- Percentage of long-stay residents who were physically restrained.
- Percentage of long-stay low-risk residents who lose control of their bowels or bladder.
- Percentage of long-stay residents who lose too much weight.
- Percentage of long-stay residents who have symptoms of depression.
- Percentage of long-stay residents who got an antianxiety or hypnotic medication.

From Centers for Medicare and Medicaid Services (2020). https://www.cms.gov/Medicare/Quality-Initiatives-Patient-Assessment-Instruments/NursingHomeQualityInits/NHQIQualityMeasures. Accessed January 2021.

---

website (www.medicare.gov/NHCompare). Nursing homes were the first to publish online quality information, which is now available for hospitals and other health care organizations. Nursing homes also receive an overall quality rating using CMS's Five-Star Rating System based on annual inspection and complaint investigation data provided by state agencies; facility-reported nurse staffing hours/resident day; and quality measures based on MDS resident data.

Most nursing home quality measures have improved over time. Between 2011 and 2016, the use of physical restraints and antipsychotic medications, pressure injuries among high-risk residents, the percentage of residents experiencing pain and urinary tract infections, and the proportion of residents with ADL impairments who got worse declined. In 2014, 23.9% of long-stay nursing home residents were receiving an antipsychotic medication; since then there has been a decrease of 35.4% to a national prevalence of 15.4%

(CMS, 2019). The prevalence rate of antipsychotic use declined in nursing homes as a result of several proactive measures but rates of antipsychotic use among individuals with dementia living in the community are rising (Chapter 25). Recommendations are to expand the efforts to curb the use of these drugs beyond nursing homes (Carter, 2018).

Disparities in care quality are associated with resident race/ethnicity; for profit/nonprofit status (higher quality is associated with the nonprofit status); and staffing levels. In spite of the benefits of using report cards, a recent study found that most hospital patients do not receive data about nursing home quality and receive only lists of nursing homes. Nurses involved in discharge planning are encouraged to use the CMS report cards so that a patient's choices are based on quality data. Additionally, patient and family education should include information on the role of skilled nursing facilities in rehabilitation, roles of members of the interprofessional team; interpretation of five-star ratings; and other information on how to choose a facility. CMS provides a nursing home checklist on its website and the National Consumer Voice for Quality Long-Term Care also provides resources for choosing a nursing home and understanding quality measures (Box 6.2).

Resident Bill of Rights

Quality is also promoted through regulations to protect the rights of the residents of nursing homes. Residents in long-term care facilities have rights under both federal and state laws. The staff of the facility must inform residents of these rights and protect and promote their rights. The rights to which the residents are entitled should be conspicuously posted in the facility (Box 6.7). Also, the Long-Term Care Ombudsman Program is a nationwide effort to support the rights of both the residents and the facilities. In most states, the program provides trained volunteers to investigate residents' rights and to examine quality complaints or conflicts. All reporting is anonymous. Each facility is required to post the name and contact information of the ombudsman assigned to the facility.

BOX 6.7 Bill of Rights for Long-Term Care Residents

- The right to voice grievances and have them remedied
- The right to information about health conditions and treatments and to participate in one's own care to the greatest extent possible
- The right to choose one's own health care providers and to speak privately with one's health care providers
- The right to consent to or refuse all aspects of care and treatments
- The right to manage one's own finances, if capable, or to choose one's own financial advisor
- The right to be transferred or discharged only for appropriate reasons
- The right to be free from all forms of abuse
- The right to be free from all forms of restraint to the extent compatible with safety
- The right to privacy and confidentiality concerning one's person, personal information, and medical information
- The right to be treated with dignity, consideration, and respect in keeping with one's individuality
- The right to immediate visitation and access at any time for family, health care providers, and legal advisors; the right to reasonable visitation and access for others

Note: This list of rights is a sampling of federal and several states' lists of rights of residents or participants in long-term care. Nurses should check the rules of their own state for specific legal rights.

The Culture Change Movement

Across the United States and internationally, the movement to transform nursing homes from the typical medical model into "homes" that nurture quality of life for older adults and support and empower front-line caregivers is changing the face of LTC. Begun by the Pioneer Network, a national not-for-profit organization that serves the culture change movement, many facilities are changing from a rigid institutional approach to one that is person centered. CMS has endorsed culture change in the federal nursing home regulations and has also released a self-study tool for nursing homes to assess their own progress toward culture change.

Culture change is the "process of moving from a traditional nursing home model—characterized as a system unintentionally designed to foster dependence by keeping residents, as one observer put it, 'well cared for, safe, and powerless'—to a regenerative model that increases residents' autonomy and sense of control" (Brawley, 2007, p. 9). The ultimate vision of culture change is to improve the lives of residents and staff by centering facility's philosophies, organizational structures, environmental designs, and care around practices that support residents' needs and preferences.

Older adults in need of LTC want to live in a homelike setting that does not look and function like a hospital. They want a setting that allows them to make decisions they are used to making for themselves, such as when to get up, take a bath, eat, or go to bed. They want caregivers who know them and understand and respect their individuality and their preferences. Box 6.8 presents some of the differences between an institution-centered culture and a person-centered culture.

Although further research is needed, some results suggest that the culture change movement has a positive effect on resident satisfaction and autonomy (Duan et al., 2020). Examples of philosophies and programs of culture change are the Eden Alternative (companion animals, indoor plants, frequent visits by children, involvement with the community), the Green House Project (small homes designed for 10 to 12 residents), and the Wellspring Model. The Eden Alternative is best known for the addition of animals, plants, and visits from children to nursing homes. However, cats and dogs are not the heart of culture change. Truly transforming a nursing home starts at the top requires involvement of all levels of staff and changes in values, attitudes, structures, and management practices. The principles central to culture change are presented in Box 6.9. Strategic and cost-efficient methods of assisting nursing homes to implement culture change are needed and will require strong nursing leadership.

BOX 6.8   Institution-Centered Versus Person-Centered Culture

Institution-Centered Culture

- Schedules and routines are designed by the institution and staff and residents must comply.
- Focus is on tasks that need to be accomplished.
- Rotation of staff among units occurs.
- Decision-making is centralized with little involvement of staff or residents and families.
- There is a hospital environment.
- Structured activities are provided to all residents.
- There is little opportunity for socialization.
- Organization exists for employees rather than residents.
- There is little respect for privacy or individual routines.

Person-Centered Culture

- Emphasis is on relationships between staff and residents.
- Individualized plans of care are based on residents' needs, usual patterns, and desires.
- Staff members have consistent assignments and know the residents' preferences and uniqueness.
- Decision-making is as close to that of the resident as possible.
- Staff members are involved in decisions and plans of care.
- Environment is homelike.
- Meaningful activities and opportunities for socialization are available around the clock.
- There is a sense of community and belonging—"like family."
- There is involvement of the community—children, pets, plants, outings.

Adapted from the Pioneer Network. http://www.pioneernetwork.net.

BOX 6.9   Principles of Culture Change

- Care and activities are directed by the residents.
- The environment and care practices support a homelike atmosphere.
- Relationships among staff and residents are supported and fostered.
- Increased attention to respect of staff and the value of caring are promoted.
- Staff is empowered to respond to the residents' needs and desires.
- The organizational hierarchy is flattened to support collaborative decision-making for staff.
- Comprehensive and continuous quality improvement underscores all activities and decisions to sustain a person-directed organizational culture.

Adapted from Mueller, C., Burger, S., Rader, J., et al. (2013). Nurse competencies for person-directed care in nursing homes, *Geriatr Nurs 34*, 101–104.

TRANSITIONS ACROSS THE CONTINUUM

Care transition refers to the movement of patients from one health care practitioner or setting to another as their condition and care needs change. Older adults may have complex health care needs and often require care in multiple settings across the health-wellness continuum. This makes them and their families and/or caregivers vulnerable to poor outcomes during transitions (Naylor, 2012). An older adult may be treated by a family practitioner or internist in the community and by a hospitalist and specialists in the hospital; discharged to a post–acute care setting and followed by another practitioner; and then discharged home or to a less care-intensive setting (e.g., assisted living facilities/residential care settings) where their original providers may or may not resume care.

The lack of coordinated care often contributes to serious consequences and frequent readmissions. Approximately one in four patients experiences an adverse event from medical mismanagement within

3 weeks of discharge from the hospital; 66% of those events are drug-related (Jusela et al., 2017). Most health care providers practice in only one setting and are not familiar with the specific requirements of other settings. Each setting is seen as a distinct provider of services and little collaboration exists (Jones et al., 2017). The purpose of health care reform initiatives (ACOs, medical homes, bundled care) is to improve coordination and communication among providers so that a person receives the most appropriate care in the most appropriate setting.

Readmissions: The Revolving Door

Avoidable readmissions are one of the leading problems facing the US health care system. Hospital readmission is a critical event for both the patients and the health care system with extraordinary associated costs. One in four Medicare patients is readmitted to the hospital within 30 days of discharge. Readmissions have been a critical quality indicator for more than two decades because they cost the health care system money and because they indicate incomplete discharge planning (Carnahan et al., 2016; Horney et al., 2017; Jones et al., 2017).

To address the concern of hospital readmission, the Hospital Readmission Reduction Program (HRRP) was established in 2013 as a permanent component of Medicare's inpatient hospital payment system. The HRRP requires Medicare to reduce payments to hospitals with relatively high readmission rates for selected conditions for patients in traditional Medicare (Box 6.10). Under the HRRP, hospitals with readmission rates that exceed the national average are penalized by a reduction in payments from the CMS across all of their Medicare admissions, not just those that resulted in readmissions.

Since the HRRP, readmission rates for the selected conditions have dropped nationwide but about 82%

BOX 6.10 **Conditions Included in the Hospital Readmission Reduction Program**

- Acute myocardial infarction
- Heart failure
- Pneumonia
- Total hip and knee replacement
- Chronic obstructive pulmonary disease
- Coronary artery bypass surgery

of hospitals still incurred a penalty in 2019, a minor increase from 2018 (Advisory Board, 2018). The HRRP has been the impetus for many hospitals to institute system-wide interventions to prevent readmissions that have also contributed to the decline in readmission rates. Readmission concerns have encouraged the development of closer alliances (e.g., accountable care organizations) and communication between hospitals and posthospital care providers, including SNFs, home health, and primary care. Hospital readmission rates are posted on the CMS Hospital Compare website (Boccuti & Casillas, 2017; Zuckerman et al., 2016).

Additionally, 30-day readmissions for patients at skilled nursing facilities are common and preventable. Medicare patients discharged to an SNF have a 25% likelihood of readmission within 30 days with a quarter readmitted to the hospital in the first week (Mendu et al., 2018). Individuals with dementia are an especially high-risk group for readmissions. Challenges unique to this population include the need for dementia care expertise among the team, the reliance on the caregiver as an essential member of the team, the need for caregiver education and preparation, and the challenges of behavioral symptom management (Hirschman & Hodgson, 2018).

Interventions to Reduce Acute Care Transfers (INTERACT) is an exemplary program for reducing the frequency of transfers to the acute hospital from SNFs. INTERACT is a quality improvement program with communication tools, care paths or clinical tools, and advance care planning tools to assist nursing homes in identifying and managing acute changes in condition without hospital transfer when safe and feasible (https://pathway-interact.com/). Other successful interventions include the use of nurse practitioners working in collaborative teams with physicians, standardized admission assessments, palliative care consultations for residents with recurrent hospitalizations, and interprofessional case conferences.

Multiple factors contribute to poor outcomes during transitions: patient, provider, and system (Boxes 6.11

BOX 6.11 **Story of Mr. Jordan**

Mr. Jordan is a 68-year-old retired farm laborer who was readmitted for heart failure 10 days after hospital discharge. He lives alone in a rural community and has no friends or family to assist in his care and was not given a referral for home health care follow-up. His medical records document teaching about medication usage and his ability to repeat back the instructions correctly. On his first post-discharge medical visit, he brought all of his pill bottles in a bag; all of the bottles were full, not one was opened. When questioned why he had not taken his medication, he looked away and began to cry, explaining he had never learned to read and could not read the instructions on the bottles.

Suggested Interventions: Adequate discharge planning is essential upon hospital discharge. Risk factors for this readmission include low literacy, living alone, complex chronic illness. Suggested interventions are assessment of literacy and adaptations of health teaching, collaboration with pharmacist to develop a person-centered plan of care for medication administration; medication reconciliation; determination of most appropriate setting for post-hospital care; inform patient about symptoms that should be reported after discharge; social work collaboration for identifying community resources and other forms of assistance and support (e.g., Meals on Wheels, transportation).

Adapted from Center for Patient Safety (2020). Hot Topics in Healthcare: Transitions of Care: The need for a more effective approach to continuing patient care. https://www.centerforpatientsafety.org/resource/hot-topics-in-healthcare-transitions-of-care-the-need-for-a-more-effective-approach-to-continuing-patient-care/.

and 6.12). Coordination and communication between settings contribute to poor outcomes during transitions (especially between acute care and SNFs) as does medication management (Ouslander et al., 2016). Contributing factors related to medication management include complex medication regimes; a lack of recognition by health professionals of the medication activities performed by families; haphazard and disorganized medication plans of care; inappropriate medications; and a lack of shared decision-making (Manias et al., 2019; see also Chapter 9).

⚡ SAFETY ALERT

Medication discrepancies are the most prevalent adverse events following hospital discharge and the most challenging component of a successful hospital-to-home transition (Hain et al., 2012; Tong et al., 2017). Nurses' attention to an accurate prehospital medication list, medication reconciliation during hospitalization, at discharge and after discharge, and patient and family education about medications are required to enhance safety.

BOX 6.12 Story of Mr. Jones

Mr. Jones is an 87-year-old ambulatory male who presents to the emergency department (ED) with altered mental status and unwitnessed fall in the skilled nursing facility (SNF) where he was admitted after being discharged one week ago from an acute care facility. While in the hospital, his food and fluid intake was deficient and remained poor during the SNF stay. After undergoing an extensive evaluation, it was determined that Mr. Jones had acute kidney injury (AKI) related to dehydration.

Suggested Interventions: This visit to the ED could, potentially, have been prevented. The first step in prevention is performing a comprehensive history and physical upon admission to the SNF to discover possible risk factors: (1) identification of risk factors such as decreased food and fluid intake, polypharmacy (he was prescribed 10 medications including a diuretic), decreased mobility (he was unable to obtain fluids without assistance), preexisting chronic disease (he has diabetes mellitus and chronic kidney disease stage 3b); (2) develop person-centered, evidence-based nursing interventions; (3) provide more intensive monitoring of high risk patients upon admission to SNF (more frequent vital signs including weight in patients with congestive heart failure (CHF), pulse oximetry in patents at risk for hypoxia, specific monitoring for high-risk conditions in this patient population including volume depletion, bleeding, hypo or hyperglycemia in diabetics); (4) facilitate effective communication at the time of discharge between health care facilities and/or other health care professionals involved in Mr. Jones' care.

BOX 6.13 Factors Associated With Readmission Risk

- The presence of complex comorbidities
- Sensory impairment
- Functional decline
- Cognitive dysfunction
- Poor communication between disciplines and across sites of care
- Inadequate discharge planning and involvement of caregivers
- Shorter hospital stays
- Increasing acuity of patients in skilled nursing facilities (SNFs)
- Scarcity of geriatric trained health care professionals
- Inadequate knowledge and use of evidence-based protocols for geriatric care
- Certain disease states such as cancer and respiratory diseases
- Social concerns (isolation, living situation, lack of caregiver support)
- Language and literacy
- Culture
- Socioeconomic factors
- Place of residence and the health care available
- Inadequate funding for post–acute care (PAC) and staff shortages.
- Patients who are clinically unstable at time of transfer
- Patients hospitalized in the last 30 days or within the last year
- Inadequate end-of-life planning/advance directives

Other factors contributing to poor outcomes identified in the literature are presented in Box 6.13.

Improving Transitional Care

Transitional care "refers to a broad range of time-limited services to ensure health care continuity, avoid preventable poor outcomes among at-risk populations, and promote the safe and timely transfer of these patient groups from one level of care (e.g., acute to subacute) or setting (e.g., hospital to home) to another" (Naylor, 2012, p. 116). National attention to improving patient safety during transfers and preventing avoidable readmissions is increasing, and a growing body of evidence-based research provides data for design of care to improve transition outcomes. Working with the patient and the caregiver to provide education to enhance self-care abilities and to facilitate linkages to resources is important to promote safe discharges and transitions to home and other care settings.

Nurse researchers Dorothy Brooten and Mary Naylor, along with their colleagues, have significantly contributed to knowledge in the area of transitional care and the critical role of nurses in transitional care improvement. The Transitional Care Model (TCM) is a rigorously tested comprehensive advanced practice model of care that starts in the hospital and continues through skilled nursing facilities and back to the community. The TCM focuses on person-centered care; education and promotion of self-managed care; continuity, collaboration, and care coordination with all members of the interprofessional team (Hirschman and Hodgson, 2018). TCM has been one of the most rigorously studied transitional care approaches and has demonstrated reductions in preventable hospital readmissions, improvements in health outcomes, improved care transitions for individuals with dementia and their caregivers, enhancement in patient satisfaction, and reductions in total health care costs (Garcia, 2017; Hirschman & Hodgson, 2018).

Nurses in acute and long-term care are uniquely positioned to play a lead role in transitional care to improve outcomes and form a "bridge across settings" (Jones et al., 2017, p. 18). This will require closer collaboration and knowledge of the settings and valuing the different nursing practice roles. In addition to roles as care managers and transition coaches, nurses play a key role in many of the elements of successful transitional care models, such as medication management, patient and family caregiver education, comprehensive discharge planning, and adequate and timely communication between providers and sites of service.

The nursing role in discharge planning and patient and family education is critical. Engaging patients and families in learning about care required after discharge contributes to improved outcomes. Teaching must be based on a complete assessment of the unique needs of the individual and adapted to ensure understanding (Chapter 5). Patients who lack the knowledge, skills, and confidence to manage their own care after discharge have nearly twice the rate of readmissions as patients with the highest level of engagement (Kangovi et al., 2014; Schneidermann & Critchfield, 2012–2013). Box 6.14 presents Resources for Best Practice and Box 6.15 gives Tips for Best Practice for Nursing Roles in Preventing Readmissions.

❖ USING CLINICAL JUDGMENT TO PROMOTE HEALTHY AGING: TRANSITIONAL CARE

Nurses in all practice settings play a key role in improving care for older adults across the continuum. New roles for nurses are emerging in the era of health care reform and heightened attention to improved patient outcomes. Nursing education must prepare graduates to develop the clinical judgment skills to practice effectively in roles across the continuum and work collaboratively to improve care outcomes, particularly during

---

BOX 6.14 Resources for Best Practice: Transitional Care

Transitional Care Model: http://evidencebasedprograms.org/1366-2/transitional-care-model-top-tier; https://www.nursing.upenn.edu/ncth/transitional-care-model/

Agency for Healthcare Research and Quality: Taking Care of Myself: A Guide for When I Leave the Hospital. https://www.ahrq.gov/patients-consumers/diagnosis-treatment/hospitals-clinics/goinghome/index.html

Interventions to Reduce Acute Care Transfers (INTERACT): Program to reduce frequency of transfers to the acute care hospital from skilled nursing facilities when feasible. Nursing home capabilities list, stop and watch early warning tool. https://pathway-interact.com/

Go to the Hospital or Stay Here: A Decision Guide for Residents, Families, Friends, and Caregivers. http://decisionguide.org/

BOX 6.15 Tips for Best Practice
Nursing Roles in Preventing Readmissions

- Identify patients at high risk of poor outcomes (e.g., low literacy, living alone, frequent or recent hospitalizations, complex chronic illness, cognitive impairment, socioeconomic deprivation)
- Adapt patient teaching for health literacy, language, culture, cognitive function, and sensory deficits
- Determine most appropriate setting for post-hospital care and educate discharge planners and family about capacity of skilled nursing facility (SNF) to care for high-risk patients
- Timely transfer of accurate information between hospital and SNF including direct communication of time-sensitive information critical to care of high-risk patients (phone, secure text, or other form of protected health information technology
- More intensive monitoring of high risk patients upon admission to SNF (more frequent vital signs including weight in patients with heart failure, pulse oximetry in patents at risk for hypoxia, specific monitoring for high-risk conditions in this patient population including volume depletion, bleeding, hypo or hyperglycemia in adults with diabetes
- Obtain complete history that includes more than this episode of illness and other risk factors
- Discussion of goals of care and advance directive status; palliative/hospice care consultations as appropriate
- Provide a complete and updated medication record; explain purpose of all medications, side effects, correct dosing, and how to obtain more medication. Evaluate barriers to successful medication management (delirium, financial, transportation)
- Perform a medication reconciliation
- Assist in establishing regimen for proper administration of medication (consider patient's usual routine when developing a plan of care)
- Discuss symptoms that should be reported after discharge and how to contact provider; provide follow-up plan for how outstanding diagnostic tests and follow-up appointments will be completed
- Coach patient/family in self-care skills and encourage active involvement in care
- Be aware of community resources in your area to assist with needs following discharge and how to link patient to resources

---

times of transition. We can no longer work in our individual "silos" and not be concerned with what happens after the patient is out of our particular unit or institution. Nurses are well positioned "to create services and environments that embrace values that are at the core of this profession—patient/caregiver centered care, communication and collaboration, and continuity" (Naylor, 2012, p. 140).

KEY CONCEPTS

- Nurses need to develop the clinical judgment skills to identify and evaluate nursing actions to improve outcomes for older adults in LTC and during transitions between health care settings.
- Nurses must be knowledgeable about the range of residential options for older adults so that they can assist the individual and the family to make appropriate decisions.
- The old concept of nursing home has dramatically changed with the increase in the number of patients with complex medical needs being cared for in this setting. Skilled nursing facilities are the most frequent site of post–acute care in the United States.
- Quality of care in skilled nursing facilities is improving. Nationwide, the average performance has improved in 12 of the 15 reported clinical outcome quality measures over the past 5 years.
- Culture change in nursing homes is a growing movement to develop models of person-centered care and improve care outcomes and quality of life.
- LTC can be provided informally or formally in a range of environments, from an individual's home to the home of a friend or relative, an adult day health center, independent and assisted living facilities, continuing care retirement communities, skilled nursing facilities, and hospices.
- LTC coverage in the United States is expensive and fragmented, overly reliant on institutional care, and primarily financed by individuals or their families or by Medicaid.
- Professional nursing involvement is an essential component in models to improve transitions across the continuum.

ACTIVITIES AND DISCUSSION QUESTIONS

1. Identify three objects in your living space that are important to you and explain why these are significant. Would you take these with you whenever you relocate?
2. Ask an older relative about the items or conditions in his or her home that make him or her feel secure and comfortable.
3. Discuss with the older adult from Question 2 the various moves he or she has made and how he or she felt about them.
4. How might the care needs of an older adult in assisted living, sub–acute care, and a nursing home differ? What is the role of the professional nurse in each of these settings?
5. Select three websites of assisted living facilities in your area and make inquiries regarding possible placement of an older adult parent. What questions did you ask? Suggestions include: What is the cost? What are the provisions for health care? What types of activities and assistance are available? After your review, which would you select for your grandmother and why?
6. In your experience in the acute care setting, what improvements would you suggest to improve transitions to other care settings? Discuss any experience you or your friends or family may have had with transitions after hospital discharge.
7. If you were the director of nursing, what would your nursing home be like (design, staffing, quality of care, training)?

NEXT-GENERATION NCLEX® EXAMINATION-STYLE QUESTIONS

Mrs. Adams is an 87 year old widowed female. She is being admitted to a rural long-term care (LTC) facility following hospitalization for uncontrolled hypertension. Prior to hospitalization, she had been living alone and it was determined she had not been taking her medications for hypertension, osteoporosis, depression, and coronary artery disease. The nurse completing her admission interview concludes by asking Mrs. Adams what time she usually eats, stating the facility serves food cafeteria style between 0600 and 0800 hours for breakfast, 1100 and 1300 for lunch, and 1700 and 1900 hours for dinner. Residents are assisted to bed by 2200 hours. Her bath days would be Tuesday, Thursday, and Saturday mornings. The nurse gives Mrs. Adams an activity schedule with the daily offerings and states that if she did not like any of them, they would try to find something else she enjoyed.

Highlight the statements above that correspond to a patient-centered culture.

REFERENCES

Advisory Board. (2018). Map: See the 2,599 hospitals that will face readmissions penalties this year. https://www.advisory.com/daily-briefing/2018/09/27/readmissions.

American Health Care Association, National Center for Assisted Living (2020). *Assisted Living*. https://www.ahcancal.org/Assisted-Living/Pages/default.aspx. Accessed January 2020.

Applebaum, R., Bardo, A., & Robbins, E. (2013). International approaches to long-term services and supports. *Generations, 37*(1), 59–65.

Boccuti, C., & Casillas, G. (2017). Aiming for fewer hospital U-turns: The Medicare hospital readmission reduction program. *Issue*

Brief. https://www.kff.org/medicare/issue-brief/aiming-for-fewer-hospital-u-turns-the-medicare-hospital-readmission-reduction-program/.

Brawley, E. (2007). What culture change is and why an aging nation cares. *Aging Today, 28*, 9–10.

Carnahan, J., Unroe, K., & Torke, A. (2016). Hospital readmission penalties: Coming soon to a nursing home near you!. *JAGS, 64*(3), 614–618.

Carter, S. E. (2018). *Off-label antipsychotic use in older adults with dementia: not just a nursing home problem.* https://www.healio.com/psychiatry/alzheimers-disease-dementia/news/online/%7Bfd3bb4c1-2b69-472c-895f-d7a303636f3f%7D/off-label-antipsychotic-use-rising-among-community-dwelling-dementia-patients.

Centers for Disease Control and Prevention (CDC) (2020). *Fast Facts: nursing home care.* https://www.forbes.com/sites/howardgleckman/2018/02/05/what-we-dont-know-but-should-about-assisted-living-facilities/?sh=15b5ecf7e043. Accessed January 2020.

Centers for Medicare and Medicaid Services (CMS). (2018). *The skilled nursing facility value-based purchasing program (SNF VBP).* https://www.cms.gov/Medicare/Quality-Initiatives-Patient-Assessment-Instruments/Value-Based-Programs/SNF-VBP/SNF-VBP-Page.

Cortes, T., & Sullivan-Marx, E. (2016). A case exemplar for national policy leadership. *J Gerontol Nurs, 2*(3), 9–14.

Duan, Y., Mueller, C. A., & Yu, F. (2020). The effects of nursing home culture change on resident quality of life in U.S. nursing homes: an integrative review. *Res Gerontol Nurs*, (22), 1–15.

Frank, R. (2012). Long-term care financing in the United States: sources and institutions. *Appl Econ Perspect Poligy, 34*(2), 333–345.

Garcia, C. (2017). A literature review of heart failure: Transitional care interventions. *Am J Accountable Care.* http://www.ajmc.com/journals/ajac/2017/2017-vol5-n3/a-literature-review-of-heart-failure-transitional-care-interventions.

Gleckman, H. (2018). What we don't know—but should—about assisted living facilities. *Forbes.* https://www.forbes.com/sites/howardgleckman/2018/02/05/what-we-dont-know-but-should-about-assisted-living-facilities/?sh=15b5ecf7e043. Accessed January 2020.

Hain, D., Tappen, R., Diaz, S., & Ouslander, J. G. (2012). Characteristics of older adults rehospitalized within 7 and 30 days of discharge: Implications for nursing practice. *J Gerontol Nurs, 38*(8), 32–44.

Harrington, C., Wiener, J. M., Ross, L., & Musumeci, M. (2017). Key issues in long-term services and supports quality. *The Henry J Kaiser Family Foundation Issue Brief.* https://www.kff.org/report-section/key-issues-in-long-term-services-and-supports-quality-appendix/. Accessed January 2020.

Hirschman, K., & Hodgson, N. (2018). Evidence-based interventions for transitions in care for individuals living with dementia. *Gerontologist, 58*(Issue suppl_1), S129–S140.

Horney, C., Capp, R., Boxer, R., & Burke, R. E. (2017). Factors associated with early readmission among patients discharged to post-acute care facilities. *J Am Geriatr Soc, 65*(6), 1199–1205.

Jones, J., Lawrence, E., Ladebue, A., Leonard, C., Ayele, R., & Burke, R. E. (2017). Nurses' role in managing "the fit" of older adults in skilled nursing facilities. *J Gerontol Nurs, 43*(12), 11–19.

Jusela, C., Struble, L., Gallagher, N., et al. (2017). Communication between acute care hospitals and skilled nursing facilities during care transitions: a retrospective chart review. *Jour Gerontol Nurs, 43*(3), 19028.

Kangovi, S., Barg, F. K., Carter, T., et al. (2014). Challenges faced by patients with low socioeconomic status during post-hospital transition. *J Gen Intern Med, 29*(2), 283–289.

Lynn, J. (2019). The 'fierce urgency of now': geriatrics professionals speaking up for older adult care in the United States. *JAGS, 67*(10), 2001–2003.

Manias, E., Bucknall, T., Hughes, C., et al. (2019). Family involvement in managing medications of older patients across transitions of care. *BMC Geriatrics, 19*(95).

Mendu, M., Michaelidis, C., Chu, M., Sahota, J., et al. (2018). Implementation of a skilled nursing facility readmission review process. *BMJ Open Quality, 7*(3), Article e000245.

National PACE Association. (2019). What is PACE?. http://www.npaonline.org/website/article.asp?id=12&title=Who,_What_and_Where_Is_PACE.

Naylor, M. (2012). Advancing high value transitional care: The central role of nursing and its leadership. *Nurs Admin Q, 36*(2), 115–126.

Omnibus Reconciliation Act (OBRA) (1987). https://www.gapna.org/omnibus-budget-reconciliation-act-obra.

Ouslander, J., Naharci, I., Engstrom, G., et al. (2016). Hospital transfer of skilled nursing facility (SNF) patients within 48 hours and 30 days after SNF admission. *JAMDA, 17*:839–845.

Schneidermann, M., Critchfiel, J. (2012–2013). Customizing the "teachable moment": ways to address hospital transitions in a culturally conscious manner, *Generations, 36*(4), 94–97.

Sherman, R., & Touhy, T. (2017). An exploratory descriptive study to evaluate Florida nurse leader challenges and opportunities in nursing home settings. *SAGE Open Nurs, 3*, 1–7.

Stanford School of Medicine (2019). *Palliative care.* https://palliative.stanford.edu/home-hospice-home-care-of-the-dying-patient/where-do-americans-die/. Accessed January 2020.

Tong, M., Thomas, J., Patel, S., Hardesty, J. L., & Brandt, N. J. (2017). Nursing home medication reconciliation: A quality improvement initiative. *J Gerontol Nurs, 43*(4), 9–14.

Zuckerman, R., Sheingold, S., Orav, J., Ruhter, J., & Epstein, A. M. (2016). Readmissions, observation, and the hospital readmissions reduction program. *N Engl J Med, 374*, 1543–1551.

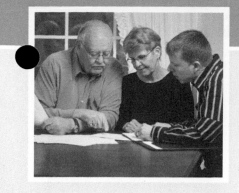

7

Economic and Legal Issues Affecting Clinical Judgment

Kathleen Jett

http://evolve.elsevier.com/Touhy/gerontological/

LEARNING OBJECTIVES

Upon completion of this chapter, the reader will be able to:

- Describe the major sources of late-life income for older adults living in the United States.
- Describe the major methods of financing health care for older adults in the United States.
- Explain the fundamentals of Medicare, Medicaid, and TRICARE sufficiently to assist older adults in accessing the services needed.
- Discuss the potential impact of health care financing in long-term and home health care.
- Compare the major forms of legal protection for persons with limited capacity such as dementia.

THE LIVED EXPERIENCE

When I was growing up life was hard. We were so poor we couldn't do much but to hold on tight. When I was lucky I could get work plowing a field and make $1.00 an acre. You work hard, and you make do. When I turned 65 I got a little check from the government and a red, white, and blue insurance [Medicare] card. The check isn't much, only about $564 a month, but you know I just consider myself blessed. And now I don't worry about my health, I will be taken care of.

Aida, age 74

People living in the United States represent all levels of income and experience with the health care system. Obtaining health care in the face of skyrocketing costs, especially during the COVID pandemic, has become increasingly difficult. An exceptional number of older adults needing care has taxed all of the current systems.

This chapter reviews the major mechanisms by which eligible adults 65 years and older in the United States receive both a basic income and health insurance at the time of this writing.

The chapter concludes with a discussion of common key legal issues related to a person's capacity to make informed health care decisions.

LATE-LIFE INCOME

Until the early 1900s, most families lived in agricultural areas. People usually worked in some way until death. If care was needed, an extended network of family, friends, and community members provided whatever support was necessary (Achenbaum, 1978).

The social and financial basis of the family changed when people moved from rural areas to cities, seeking work in factories. Whole families worked to survive, including very young children. The work was onerous and fraught with demands that became increasingly difficult to meet as one aged. The family was no longer available to provide care or support for older and disabled family members.

In 1935, the Social Security Act was passed and has been considered by many to be one of the most successful federal programs. Its primary function was to provide monetary benefits to eligible older adults in an attempt to lighten the burden on families.

Social Security

Social Security was designed as a pay-as-you-go system. Although individually deposited, the revenues are not reserved for any one individual; that is, no one has an account reserved in their name. Payroll taxes collected from employees and employers are immediately distributed to beneficiaries (retirees, the disabled, eligible spouses, or dependent children). All funds that are not immediately paid to beneficiaries are "borrowed" by the federal government for regular operating expenses.

At the time of its inception, the system was constructed to transfer funds from those believed to be relatively prosperous (workers) to those believed to be relatively poor (older adults). Social Security and a number of services that followed were established as "age-entitlement" programs. This meant that they are available to eligible persons at a certain age regardless of other sources of personal income or assets. They were and are, however, limited to US citizens and legal residents or a dependent of someone who is eligible. Beneficiaries must have earned a maximum of 40 "work credits" during their work years. In 2020 one credit was equivalent to $1410 in earnings during one calendar year which was subject to Social Security taxes. A maximum of four credits can be earned in a year. Special rules apply for earnings of less than $400. Eligibility further takes into account a number of factors, including date of birth, disability, spousal income, and dependent parents Social Security Administration (SSA, 2020a).

The amount of Social Security received is calculated in part on the person's average salary during their working years. If one did not earn the requisite credits, the "nonworking years" count as zero in the calculation. This formula has been most beneficial to older White men, who are more likely to have worked the most consistently at higher salaries than any other group. It has been most disadvantageous for persons of color, those paid in cash, and for those who took time off for child or parent care. The Social Security monthly stipend is further dependent on age at the time of retirement.

Except under special circumstances, 62 years is the earliest age when one may begin receiving Social Security. However, the amount received is only 75% than it would be at "full retirement age" of 65 years of age for those

TABLE 7.1   Full Retirement Age

Year of Birth[a]	Full (Normal) Retirement Age
1937 or earlier	65
1938	65 and 2 months
1939	65 and 4 months
1940	65 and 6 months
1941	65 and 8 months
1942	65 and 10 months
1943–1954	66
1955	66 and 2 months
1956	66 and 4 months
1957	66 and 6 months
1958	66 and 8 months
1959	66 and 10 months
1960 and later	67

[a]Persons whose birthday is January 1 should refer to the previous year.
Data from Social Security Administration. (n.d.). *Full Retirement age.* https://www.ssa.gov/planners/retire/retirechart.html.

born in 1937 or earlier, with age of eligibility for full benefits slowly increasing (Table 7.1). For those who want or need to work beyond the age of full retirement, the benefit increases 8% every year one delays receiving Social Security until the age of 70. The benefit also has the potential to increase each year on January 1 in the form of a cost-of-living adjustment (COLA) based on the consumer price index (CPI) for the previous year (SSA, 2020b.).

A person's highest median income usually occurs between ages 45 and 55 years, after which it declines each decade to age 65 years. However, there is great variation by gender, race, and ethnic group, with those of Asian descent having the highest median income and Blacks the lowest. Compared with wages paid to White male employees for a specific occupation, older White female workers earn 49–81 cents for every dollar. There is more of a disparity among women of color. Although there is less of a gap among young men and women, the disparity among older women translates into lower Social Security upon retirement (PayScale, 2020).

Supplemental Security Income (SSI)

Not all older persons living in the United States have Social Security benefits adequate enough to provide even the most basic necessities of life. This has been especially true for many of today's oldest adults, particularly if they spent their lives employed in the agricultural industry, as domestic workers, in the service industry and were paid very low wages, if Social Security taxes were not withheld by their employers, or if they were paid on a cash basis. SSI was established in 1965 to provide a minimum level of economic support to older adults and select others.

Among the eligibility requirements are a very low income and few resources (variable amounts and exclusions) excluding one's home and prepaid burial expenses. The maximum SSI benefit to persons at least 65 years of age was $783 per month for an individual and $1175 for an eligible couple in 2020. Unlike Social Security, the amount is reduced by any countable income such as cash or in-kind contributions, including housing or food provided by others (SSA, 2020c).

In the first quarter of 2020, the median income of working women between 55 and 64 years of age was $922 a week and $1082 for men with considerable variation by race/ethnicity (US Bureau of Labor Statistics, 2020). This lowered income has significant implications for a person's future calculation of Social Security benefits. In 2020, 45% of unmarried persons (primarily) older women depended on Social Security for 90% of their income (SSA, 2020d).

Other Late-Life Income

Finally, late-life income may come from private retirement investments or employer pensions. Monies are held for the beneficiary until such a time when he or she must begin to "withdraw" all or a portion of it at the age determined by the fund. Usually the beneficiary may elect to take their pension in one lump sum or in a monthly amount based on their own anticipated life expectancy or based on the life expectancy of a spouse or partner. In other words, a person may establish a plan so that he or she receives all or most of the benefit during their expected lifetime rather than providing for any survivor benefit. Notification of the potential survivor of such a choice is now required but was not always so in the past. This may still affect some older survivors (Box 7.1).

BOX 7.1   A Surprising Change of Income

Mrs. Jones lived in a small rural community. Her husband had worked for the same company from the time he was 18 until he died. His pension and Social Security benefits were small because of a lifetime of low wages. When Mr. Jones died suddenly, Mrs. Jones was informed that she would no longer receive support from his pension. When he enrolled, he had opted for the "no survivor benefit," meaning that all benefits would cease upon his death.[a] Because she had never worked outside of the home, Mrs. Jones was dependent solely on her husband's Social Security as his widow. She was in danger of losing her home because she could not afford her taxes.

[a]Note: For new retirees, this is no longer legal without express permission of spouse.

HEALTH CARE INSURANCE PLANS IN LATER LIFE

Until 1965, there were only a few successful insurance plans for wealthier working people in the United States. In most cases health care was on a fee-for-service basis. This meant that each health care service could only be obtained if bartered or purchased for cash (or "out-of-pocket"). Health care in the United States has never been a "right." In 1934, President Franklin D. Roosevelt tried to create a plan to provide universal health insurance for US citizens. This was met with unbeatable opposition from groups such as the American Medical Association and, by poll, the majority of the American public (Cantril, 1951). When costs were reasonable, many could continue to pay for their care. However, as people began to live longer with more chronic health problems, advances in technology escalated, costs for health care increased, and paying out-of-pocket became harder and even impossible for many older adults who were entirely dependent on limited incomes. In 1965, through the efforts of President Lyndon B. Johnson, legislation (the Social Security Act) was passed creating an insurance plan for all persons eligible for Social Security, SSI, or railroad retirement benefits. The US Department of Health and Human Services created the Centers for Medicare and Medicaid Services (CMS) to administer these benefits. In 2019, 52.9 million people over 65 years of age were enrolled in Medicare (CMS, 2020).

The federal government is the major insurer of health care. In the United States through its insurance plans (Medicare, Railroad Medicare, Medicaid, and TRICARE) or through direct care provided by Veterans and Indian Health Services. The major plan available to and used by eligible older adults (≥65 years of age) living in the United States is Medicare. Those with very low incomes may also be eligible for Medicaid, an insurance plan that is jointly funded by state and federal resources (referred to as "joint eligibility").

Medicare

Medicare covers select medically necessary services. This means that the prescribed treatments and services are needed for the prevention, diagnosis, or treatment of a medical condition; meet the standards of good medical practice; and are not performed for the convenience of the health care provider. The costs are paid by the beneficiary in the form of premiums, deductibles, and co-pays and subsidized by the federal government.

Medicare is an insurance plan consisting of four parts. Part A, covering some of the costs associated with a hospitalization, is free to all eligible beneficiaries at the age of 65. Medicare Part B is a plan to cover the costs of seeing health care providers and several other services. Due to

TABLE 7.2   **Major Components of the Affordable Care Act That Affect Older Adults**

Component	Description
Primary care	Incentives to providers based on quality and not just quantity of care ("evaluation of quality-based indicators")
Bundled payments	Payment to hospital for entire "bundle of care," which will include both the hospital stay and the medical needs for a period of time after discharge
Demonstration projects	Welcoming of creative proposals to improve quality and control cost
Five-star programs	Yearly evaluation and ranking of Medicare Parts C and D plans, nursing homes and acute care hospitals, home health agencies, and a growing number of other sources for health care
No co-pays for many preventive services[a]	Increased access to preventive services

[a]See http://www.medicare.gov/coverage/preventive-visit-and-yearly-wellness-exams.html for "Is my test, item, or service covered?"

BOX 7.2   **The "Welcome to Medicare" Examination**

Must be obtained within 12 months of enrolling in Medicare Part B and includes:
- Review of medical record
- Review of social history related to your health
- Education and counseling about preventive services
- Health screenings, immunizations, or referrals for other care as needed
- Height, weight, and blood pressure measurements
- Calculation of body mass index
- Simple vision test
- Review of risk for depression and level of safety
- An offer to discuss advance directives
- Written preventive health plan

Data from https://www.medicare.gov/coverage/welcome-to-medicare-preventive-visit.

the COVID pandemic, visits to providers may be in person or via telehealth. Medicare Part C (Advantage Plans) was created as an alternative to Medicare Part B. The costs of outpatient medications were not covered by Medicare until 2006, when an elective drug plan (Medicare Part D) was created under President G. W. Bush's administration. Elective supplementary plans (Medigap) cover some of the costs not covered by Medicare A and B. Medicare D is offered by private insurers in cooperation with CMS.

Further services, several of which are relevant to older adults, have been added (Table 7.2). The "Welcome to Medicare Visit" was established under President G. W. Bush (Box 7.2). A subsequent "Annual Wellness Visit" (Box 7.3) was added through the Affordable Care Act under the Obama administration.

Between October 15 and December 7 (open enrollment) of each year, persons with Medicare may make changes to any of the component Parts B, C, or D. Medicare Part A does not change. If new coverage is chosen, it will begin on January 1 of the next year (e.g., a change made by December 6, 2020 becomes effective January 1, 2021).

Medicare Part A

Medicare Part A is a plan covering some of the costs associated with an acute hospital stay, short-term acute rehabilitative care, and costs associated with hospice and home health care under certain circumstances. It is free to those who are 65 years of age and eligible for Social Security. As an "age entitlement" program, it provides insurance to eligible beneficiaries regardless of their personal financial status. Unless already a Medicare recipient for some other reason (e.g., end-stage renal disease), a person must enroll in Medicare Part A and it becomes effective on the first day of the month of their 65th birthday. The deductible and copayments vary by setting and community and can be quite high (Box 7.4).

For any Part A coverage in skilled *nursing homes* or acute rehabilitation hospitals, the transfer must be directly from an acute care facility after at least a 72-hour *admission* (day of discharge not included), enter a SNF within 30 days of discharge, and require skilled nursing or therapy at least 5 days a week. Extended hours spent in an emergency department or even on a hospital unit for the purpose of *observation* do not apply (Medicare Interactive, 2020). As a result of the significant financial

BOX 7.3   **Annual "Wellness" Visit[a]**

MUST be at least 12 months from "Welcome to Medicare" examination or last wellness examination.
- A review of medical and family history
- Developing or updating a list of current providers and prescriptions
- Height, weight, blood pressure, and other routine measurements
- Detection of any cognitive impairment and depression
- A list of person-specific health advice risk factors and treatment options
- A screening schedule for appropriate preventive services

[a]This is a component of the Affordable Care Act and therefore subject to change. Data from https://www.medicare.gov/coverage/yearly-wellness-visits.

BOX 7.4 Health Services Provided Through Medicare Part A (Original Medicare)

1. Acute care
   a. Coverage of varying amounts 1–150 days.
   b. Deductibles and copays increase every year.
   c. The deductibles and copays are either paid out-of-pocket or reimbursed by Medicaid or Medigap policies.
2. Skilled rehabilitative nursing care in a health care facility (only when care by a registered nurse or physical or occupational therapist is needed):
   a. Only after a minimum 72-hour acute care hospital admission
   b. The first 20 days are covered at 100%.
   c. Days 21 to 100 daily copay
   d. No coverage after 100 days
   e. Coverage ceases the day skilled care is no longer needed.
3. Home health services requiring skilled care (only when care by a registered nurse or physical or occupational therapist is needed):
   a. Intermittent skilled care for the purpose of rehabilitation provided in the home
   b. The person must be ill enough to be considered homebound.
   c. Medicare pays 80% of allowable costs.
4. Hospice care (provided for terminally ill persons expected to live less than 6 months who elect to forgo traditional medical treatment for the terminal illness):
   a. Replaces Medicare Parts A and B for all costs associated with the terminal condition
5. Inpatient psychiatric care:
   a. Deductible for each stay
   b. Day 1–60: no copay
   c. Day 61–90: daily copay
   d. After day 90 start using lifetime reserves of 60 days with copay

BOX 7.5 Health Services Provided Through Medicare Part B (Original Medicare)

Designed to cover some of the costs associated with outpatient or ambulatory services. Deductibles and copays are required in most cases.

1. Physician, nurse practitioner, or physician assistant medically necessary services
2. Limited prescribed supplies
3. Medically necessary diagnostic tests
4. Physical, occupational, and speech therapy for the purpose of rehabilitation
5. Limited durable medical equipment if prescribed by a physician and documented medical necessity
6. Outpatient hospital treatment, bloodwork, and ambulatory surgical services
7. Some preventive services (many with no copay or deductible)
8. Diabetic supplies (excluding insulin and other medications) (see Chapter 20)
9. Ambulance (medically necessary)
10. Mental health services

From Medicare. (n.d.). *What Part B covers?* https://www.medicare.gov/what-medicare-covers/what-part-b-covers.

ramifications of observation stays, this important distinction should be made very clear so that the individual and/or caregivers can plan accordingly. When the assistance needed is limited to personal care or medication supervision, it is not covered by Medicare at all.

There are no prehospitalization requirements for the receipt of skilled *home* health care. To be considered a covered service, however, nursing care or physical, occupational, or speech therapy must be required on an intermittent basis with the goal of restoring the person to a prior level of functioning and preventing the necessity of 24-hour care. The care must be provided by a Medicare-certified agency at the written direction of a physician or nurse practitioner.

Medicare Part B

A person who is eligible for Part A must apply for Part B through the local Social Security Administration office

in the 6 months surrounding their 65th birthday (from 3 months before to 3 months after the birth month) or at the time when the person is no longer covered by an employer's comparable plan. At the time of enrollment, the person will be asked to choose either the *"Original"* Medicare Part B plan (Box 7.5) or one of the alternative plans available in the person's geographical area. If beneficiaries do not apply during their initial eligibility period, they must wait for the next "open enrollment period" and significant penalties may be levied.

The *Original Medicare Part B plan* is based on a traditional fee-for-service arrangement. The patient buys the insurance policy and receives services from a provider, a bill for the costs of care is sent to Medicare, and the patient is billed for the associated copays and deductible. Medicare reimburses physicians at a rate of 80% of what it considers an "allowable charge" for medically necessary services. The patient is responsible for the remaining 20%. A provider who "accepts assignment" cannot charge a patient any more than the 20% of the "allowable charge." The number of physicians and nurse practitioners who accept assignment is decreasing rapidly. Providers who do not accept assignment may charge the patient up to 15% more than the allowable charge ("excess charge") and are not required to bill Medicare directly. As the "allowable" for mental health services is very low, those who accept assignment are rare.

With the Original Medicare Part B plan, the patient is responsible for a monthly premium (usually deducted directly from the monthly Social Security check), an annual deductible, and copays. The premium is now based on income and marital status and was $144.60–$491.60 a month in 2020 (Medicare, 2020).

The advantages of the Original Medicare plan include choice and access. The person can seek the services of any provider of choice and without a referral from their primary care provider. Some providers are members of Accountable Care Organizations (ACOs). The only difference when a person uses an ACO in conjunction with the Original Medicare Part B plan is that a group of providers have elected to work together and are able to share information about the patient to help provide the most coordinated care possible while maintaining patient choice. There is no penalty for seeking care outside of the ACO (Medicare, n.d.).

Medicare Part C

Medicare Part C (also referred to as *Medicare Advantage Plans* or *MAP*) replaces both Medicare Part A and Medicare Part B, and in some cased Part D, the prescription drug plan. Part C plans are privately managed health maintenance organizations (HMOs), preferred provider organizations (PPOs), private fee-for-service plans and special need plans. The type and availability of such plans depend on location. All Part C plans are required to provide at least all those benefits provided by Part A and the original Medicare Part B and may include extra benefits as well. Copays and deductibles, if any, vary considerably, and extra premiums may be required for added services. All Medicare Part C plans have special rules that must be followed or services are only covered partially (PPOs) if at all (HMOs).

The PPO plans work like the Original Medicare except that only specific providers can be used (those in the network) and the allowable charges are preset. Any additional services and fees or copays vary by plan. If a patient chooses to be seen by a provider outside the network, the services received may not be covered by the plan.

In HMOs, the consumer "enrolls" to receive services at specific locations and from assigned primary health care providers. There are fewer out-of-pocket costs, but care received from providers outside of the network is not covered. Specialists cannot be seen without a referral from one's primary care provider. Medicare contracts with the private HMO to provide comprehensive services, financed by Medicare premiums paid directly to the company. The best of these are complete health care systems with highly trained physicians, nurse practitioners, and other health care professionals working out of single or regional completely equipped medical centers. Medical services are expected to emphasize preventive medicine, comprehensive care, periodic physical examinations, and immunizations.

Capitation is imposed on HMOs by Medicare; this means that the plan is paid a fixed amount each day for each enrollee regardless of the amount of care needed and provided. Although the intention of this design was to increase preventive care, in some cases it created abuse and there were horror stories in which older adults were denied necessary treatments, presumably motivated by the plan's desire to lower its costs. Patient protection laws now allow consumers to lodge complaints and initiate legal action against an HMO as appropriate. The Center for Patient Advocacy supported a much needed bill that became law in October 1999 allowing appeals when a managed care plan (MCP) denies care, guarantees access to specialists, ensures that health-related decisions are made by health care providers rather than administrators, and holds MCPs legally accountable for medical decisions that cause harm.

The supplemental services offered may save the participant a considerable amount in the costs of medications, assistive devices, and professional consultation charges. Some HMOs provide extensive health education services, support groups, and telephone support and other services to homebound persons. The potential negative aspects of HMOs and PPOs include limited choice of, and access to, providers.

Alternatives to Medicare Part C. Health care finance is changing in the United States and several new programs have emerged. One of these is the Medicare Medical Savings Account. The federal government makes monthly payments directly into the person's bank account, and when health services are obtained, the individual pays for them directly. The fees charged by the providers are predetermined on a contractual basis between the provider and Medicare. Although no contracted provider can deny services at the agreed rate, noncontracted providers are under no obligation to accept the rate. For information about the range of existing and pending plans, see http://www.medicare.gov.

Medicare Part D

Medicare Part D was created as part of the Medicare Modernization Act of 2003 and is an optional prescription coverage plan. Those interested in purchasing this plan must enroll within the same 6 months of Medicare B eligibility to prevent paying possible late enrollment penalties and waiting until the next open enrollment period. Medicare Part D is not one plan but is a designation for dozens of private plans that have met certain criteria and are

BOX 7.6 **Medicare Prescription Drug Plans (PDPs)**

Most PDPs are organized in a similar way with deductibles and co-pays; however, to be a provider in Medicare Part D, the insurance plan must meet the following specific guidelines:
1. Premiums based on the plan
2. Annual deductible as low
3. Co-pay of medications dependent on plan and how much has been spent that year

From *Medicare: Medicare and You 2021* CMS Product No. 10050.

approved by the CMS (Box 7.6). The premiums vary by company and reflect the range of medications covered and the person's income. A Part D income-related monthly adjustment amount (IRMAA) is added to the premium. There were four different periods potentially affecting drug cost each year: (1) payment of out-of-pocket until the annual deductible is paid; (2) some insurance coverage along with a copay up to $4020 out of pocket and insurance premiums (2020 figures); (3) a period of a much larger copay (the donut hole); and (4) finally "catastrophic" coverage with very small copays beginning when $5100 out of pocket has been spent. Which medications are covered, the premiums, amount of the deductible, and copays are determined solely by the insurance company.

As with Medicare Parts B and C plans, there is an open enrollment period every year. Recipients should be encouraged to examine their current plan annually to ensure they are enrolled in the plan that provides the best coverage for their medications. Most plans change to some extent every year. There is a calculator comparing the medications needed, the plans available, and the associated costs at http://www.medicare.gov/part-d.

Medicare Supplement Insurance/Medigap Policies

Those who enrolled in the *Original* Medicare B plan will have copayments and deductibles like any other insurance plan. With aging, medical expenses often rise as more and more chronic diseases are accumulated. People who have the financial resources to do so often purchase commercial supplemental insurance plans, referred to as Medigap (A-N). A monthly premium is paid and in exchange all or part of the co-pays and deductibles not covered by the "primary insurance" (e.g., *Original* Medicare) are paid. The gerontological nurse can refer persons searching for an appropriate plan to a SHINE (Serving Health Insurance Needs of Elders) volunteer in their state. Volunteers are specially trained and can assist with Medicare questions.

Medicaid

Another amendment to the Social Security Act of 1965 created a second form of insurance for those 65 years of age and older, the disabled, and children with very low incomes, known as *Medicaid*. Medicaid was designed to help states defray expenses of the very poor; this included those who did not qualify for or could not afford to purchase Medicare Parts B/C and Medicare Part D or to pay the required deductibles or copayments. Medicaid is used by only a relatively small number of older adults, and nearly all of these people are "dually eligible" or qualify for both Medicare and Medicaid.

Many who need long-term nursing home care qualify for special Long-Term Care Medicaid at some point in their stay when their personal resources are exhausted. In 1988, Congress enacted provisions to protect a spouse who can remain in the community "spousal impoverishment." Depending on the spouse's income, burial funds and only a certain amount of the joint assets are counted as belonging to the patient, are used to determine eligibility, and are expected to be used to pay for care. On the death of community-living spouses, it is expected that the amount that Medicaid has spent on the care (and only up to that point) be reimbursed with any remaining funds in the couple's estate (Medicaid, n.d.).

Within the broad guidelines established by the federal government, each state establishes its own eligibility criteria, determines the types and extent of services to be covered, sets the payment rates to providers, and administers its own programs. States pay about 40% of the costs with the federal government paying the remainder. This means that the Medicaid services available to the poorest older adults are dependent on the affluence and the policy of a given state. Alabama, with one of the highest percentages of poor residents, also has one of the lowest state incomes and therefore one of the lowest levels of Medicaid services. In most cases, Medicaid covers more services than Medicare, including custodial care in nursing homes.

In some states there are "Medically Needy" programs, with month-to-month Medicaid coverage provided only during the months the older adults' medical expenses exceed a preset threshold. With the financial crisis that states have been experiencing, many of these programs have been abandoned and services under Medicaid have been reduced.

More states are turning to Medicaid MCPs and HMOs and requiring persons who are dually eligible to enroll in these plans in an attempt to control costs. Waiver programs (that is, alternative and sometime innovative models) are used in some states to control costs further by providing extra support to help keep Medicaid-eligible beneficiaries in their own homes and out of nursing homes. Medicaid does not help the near-poor: those who cannot qualify for aid but cannot afford basic or long-term health care.

The premise of Medicaid MCPs is that better outcomes will result from systems of care that integrate professionals in responsive teams, maximize the use of sub–acute care, and provide incentives to reduce the reliance on institutional acute care. Managed care systems are most effective for individuals enrolled over a long period who use ongoing primary care and preventive strategies to maintain health and avoid high-cost emergency services and intensive treatment.

Other Means to Finance Health Care

In some parts of the country (and for some persons), alternative plans have been developed to finance and provide health care.

Indian Health Services

The Indian Health Service (IHS) is a federal health program for and with American Indians and Alaskan Natives (http://www.ihs.gov). Services are provided both at the Tribal level and through Urban Indian Health Programs. Traditional IHS is available to documented members of one of the Indian Nations who have no other source of care (e.g., Medicare, Medicaid, TRICARE). The very high rate of COVID infections in many tribal groups have taxed the IHS more than ever seemed possible (see http://www.ihs.gov/ElderCare).

Care for Veterans

The Veterans Health Administration (VA) system has long held a leadership role in gerontological research, medical care, and extended care. Veteran's services have been models for continuity of care. Since their inception, these included VA-run nursing homes, home care and community-based primary care programs, respite care, blindness rehabilitation, mental health, and numerous other services in addition to acute medical-surgical hospitals. As a result of a combination of budget cuts and an increasing number of veterans in need of care, services have become more restricted, but the needs of veterans, especially those who served in a war zone, have remained a priority.

At one time, veterans' hospitals and services were available on an as-needed basis for anyone who had served at any time. It was not necessary for individuals to use their Medicare benefits. However, this system has undergone significant change. One of the first changes was the placement of restrictions on the use of veterans' hospitals and services. Instead of coverage for any health problem, priorities were set for those problems that were in some way deemed "service-connected"; in other words, the problem had to be linked to the time the person was on active duty. In addition, those receiving Medicare benefits are expected to apply for and use that payment mechanism first before the VA will cover medical expenses. American Indians and Alaska Natives who are also veterans can receive care from INS and the cost of the care is paid for by the Veterans Association.

TRICARE for life. TRICARE for Life (TFL) is a no-premium Medigap insurance program provided by the Department of Defense. This plan requires that the person enroll in both Medicare Part A and Medicare Part B and pay the premiums for Part B. Dependent parents or parents-in-law may be eligible for pharmacy benefits if they turned 65 years of age on or after April 1, 2001, and are already enrolled in Medicare Part B. For more information, see http://www.tricare.mil.

Veteran aid and dependence. For those veterans who served at least 90 consecutive days and at least 1 full day in a war zone and receive a military pension (i.e., have retired), additional monetary support is available if they need assistance with daily personal needs or are homebound. The application process to the program, which is called "Aid and Attendance Pension," is quite cumbersome but may be especially helpful for those who need custodial care at home or in a long-term care facility. The veteran may qualify for monetary help for their own care or for care of a spouse, depending on circumstances. Other benefits change over time, such as the recent availability of funds to reimburse a veteran for travel to and from a physician's office. For those living in rural areas or dependent on companion transport services, this can be quite helpful. The nurse is encouraged to learn more about these services to promote care for military-retired veterans (VeteranAid, 2019).

Long-Term Care Insurance

Some persons are electing to purchase additional insurance (long-term care insurance [LTCI]) for their potential long-term care needs. Ideally these policies cover the expenses related to copays both for nursing home and home care and for what is called custodial care, which is help with activities of daily living (ADLs). Traditionally these policies were limited to care in long-term care facilities and provided a flat-rate reimbursement to residents to help cover their costs. However, these policies have become more comprehensive and innovative and may cover home care costs instead or both LTC costs and home care costs under some circumstances. Because they do not receive any governmental subsidies, the premiums can be prohibitive.

Although many do not reach the ideal benefits, many plans are being marketed at present. The purchaser must be cautioned to read the policy carefully and understand all the details, limitations, and exclusions. There are particular concerns related to Alzheimer's disease because many policies exclude these individuals from home benefits and include very limited institutional benefits. The best LTCI packages have been negotiated by a large employer or state organization or association. A useful resource for persons considering the purchase of long-term care insurance can be found at http://longtermcare.gov/costs-how-to-pay/what-is-long-term-care-insurance/.

❖ USING CLINICAL JUDGMENT TO PROMOTE HEALTHY AGING

Gerontological nurses have long been helping their older patients deal with financial issues, such as the following: Are adequate funds available for needed food and medication or for the copayments for needed health care? Does the Medicare plan in which they are currently enrolled (Part B, C, or D) best meet their needs, or can the nurse refer them to a community organization to help them find a plan that will be more appropriate for their needs (Box 7.7)? These questions may be part of the comprehensive assessment as described in Chapter 8 or be a specific issue under special circumstances. Nurses are able to use their well-known expert advocacy and negotiation skills in these situations to help older persons reach the highest level of wellness possible.

BOX 7.7 Tips for Best Practice
Helping Your Patients Enroll in Medicare Plans That Best Suit Their Needs

When it is time for the person to enroll in Medicare, he or she can be referred to the Medicare website (http://www.madicare.gov). At this website, the person will find not only information about plans available in their area but also information about the procedures for changing from one plan to another according to personal choice or change in needs. If the person needs additional help, he or she should be referred to the nearest Area Agency on Aging for guidance (for locations, see http://www.n4a.org).

LEGAL ISSUES IN GERONTOLOGICAL NURSING

In the day-to-day practice of caring for older adults, gerontological nurses face questions and situations that have legal components. Although nurses (unless they are also attorneys) cannot provide any legal advice, it is imperative that they are aware of several key legal issues frequently encountered in their work. Legal concerns are most often related to an individual's capacity

to make health care decisions and consent to treatment or research. Although this section is not intended to provide legal advice or to encourage nurses to do so, it is intended to provide background regarding common protective issues the gerontological nurse will be exposed to in caring for older persons, especially those who are vulnerable.

Decision-Making
In the Western model of health care, decisions are expected to be based on the ethical concepts of autonomy (self-determination) and informed consent. The provider has a responsibility to inform the individual of the decision needed and the individual has the right and responsibility to make his or her own decisions. In many cultures, decision-making responsibilities, including decisions related to health care, are shared or delegated (see Chapter 3).

Regardless of the culture or circumstances, the responsibility to obtain informed consent often falls on the nurse. In most circumstances consent is implied, such as when the person accepts a medication that is offered or cooperates with a dressing change. Obtaining consent can also be difficult and complex because of a multitude of factors but can be made easier through advance planning if this is acceptable in the person's culture (Box 7.8).

BOX 7.8 Factors Affecting the Responsibility of Nurses in Obtaining Informed Consent

1. Impaired sensory functioning
2. Low educational level
3. Low or limited health literacy
4. Low literacy of any kind
5. Questionable cognitive status
6. Complexity of procedure (e.g., surgery of any kind)
7. Participation in research

Capacity
Informed consent in health care is only possible with the assumption that adults have decision-making capacity. Decisional capacity means that a person is able to understand a problem, the risks and benefits of a decision, the alternative options, and the consequences of the decision. Most courts require information to be provided in such a way that an average person would understand it before a decision is made. *Capacity is presumed when the legal age of "adult" is reached, unless the person has been adjudicated (decided by a court) to lack such capacity.* However, even in the absence of such adjudication, it

is sometimes necessary to make professional judgments that influence accepting consent from a person, especially those with limited cognitive capacity or advanced frailty for any other reason.

Capacity is multifaceted. It ranges from the ability to accomplish IADLs (instrumental activities of daily living, e.g., handle finances and daily business), to the capacity to complete ADLs (one's most basic personal needs), to the capacity to make medical and specific health-related decisions. Capacity includes the ability to accept or decline health care treatments and procedures (e.g., consent to a surgical procedure). Giving consent to participate in research is more complex because it may or may not directly benefit the individual.

When the capacity of an individual to make informed decisions is believed to be impaired, only the courts can declare the person "incapacitated" (formerly referred to as "incompetent"). They may be determined to have no or limited capacity in one area of their life but to have ability in others. For example, a person may be unable to take care of day-to-day personal business, such as bill paying, adequately but may still be able to make personal health care decisions. For those who are unable to speak for themselves or are unable (for any reason) to understand the consequences of their decisions, legal protection may be needed. Guiding principles are that protection is provided to those with questionable capacity in a manner that ensures that the person's needs are met, personal rights are protected to the extent possible, and the least restrictive type of protection necessary is used.

These types of protection include power of attorney, appointment of a health care proxy, conservatorship, and guardianship. It is important that nurses understand the meaning of each and the differences between them.

Advance Care Planning

Gerontological nurses have the responsibility to encourage their patients, neighbors, and family members to discuss their wishes regarding potential incapacity, otherwise referred to as advance care planning. It is always advisable to appoint a legal surrogate or proxy (see following sections) and formally document one's wishes. The use of living wills is addressed in Chapter 28.

Power of Attorney

A *power of attorney* (POA) is a legal document in which one person designates another person (e.g., family member, friend) to act on their behalf. The two types are a general POA and a durable POA. The person named in a general POA usually has rights to make financial decisions in defined circumstances, but not necessarily to make decisions related to health care. The person appointed in a durable POA usually has additional rights and responsibilities to make health-related decisions for persons when they are unable to do so themselves. This person is known as the *health care surrogate* or *proxy*.

POAs are in effect only at the specific request of the person or, in the case of the durable POA, if the person is unable to act on their own behalf. As soon as the person regains capacity, the POA is no longer in force unless the individual requests it to continue. The individual retains all the rights and responsibilities afforded by usual law. This is the least restrictive form of protection and assistance, providing decision-making for persons with impaired capacity. An important aspect of the POA is that persons who are given decision-making rights are those who have been chosen by the individual rather than by a court. Because gerontological nurses work with people who are making decisions about the selection of a surrogate, they can encourage persons to consider carefully someone who is willing to uphold their wishes and holds similar values.

Health Care Proxy

Most state statutes and cultures provide a "hierarchy" of those who have the authority to act on a person's behalf when capacity has been either temporarily or permanently lost and preferences have not been documented or expressed in advance. For example, in the state of Florida, this is written into Statute 765.401, and all health care facilities have the legal responsibility to follow this "order of decision-maker" (Box 7.9). The decision-making responsibilities proceed down the list until a willing proxy is found.

Both surrogates and proxies are expected to use "substituted judgment": that is, decisions are made on the basis of what they believe the person would decide if able to do so and not the surrogate's choice in a similar situation (Zorowitz, 2014). The gerontological nurse can support the surrogate in following the person's wishes (Box 7.10).

BOX 7.9 Hierarchy of Appointments of Health Care Proxy by Florida State Statute, From First to Last

Guardian
Spouse
Majority of adult children
Parents
Majority of adult siblings reasonably available for consultation
Adult relative who has exhibited special care and has regular contact
Close friend
Licensed clinical social worker appointed by a bioethics committee

BOX 7.10   "I Know That Is What She Would Want But That Is Not What I Want"

Mr. and Mrs. Jones had been married for 60 years. She had developed Alzheimer's disease a number of years earlier and reached a point where she did not always know what to do with food in her mouth. She no longer recognized her husband and did not respond in any verbal way. In almost daily distress, her husband intermittently pleaded that a "feeding tube" be placed into her so that she could "eat." However, Mrs. Jones had made it very clear to her husband and to all who knew her that she "never wanted artificial nutrition" or to do anything to stop a natural death when she worsened. When Mr. Jones asked for a feeding tube, the only thing we could say was that we were very sorry, but her wishes had been made very clearly and that is what we were bound to follow. He agreed that those indeed were her wishes and started to cry.

Guardians and Conservators

Guardians and conservators are individuals, agencies, or corporations that have been appointed by the court to have care, custody, control of a disabled person (ward) and manage their personal or financial affairs (or both), and assure that all needs are met, when the person has been found (adjudicated) to lack capacity.

Whereas a *conservator* is appointed specifically to control the finances of the ward, the person appointed to be responsible for the ward is usually called the *guardian,* although these terms are sometimes used interchangeably. The conservator or guardian continues in that role until the court rescinds the order. The appointment is made at a court hearing in which a person demonstrates the incapacity of the older adult (who may not be present) and he or she is declared *incapacitated* (formerly called *incompetent*). How this is handled differs by state. In many states the ward is unable to petition the courts to have their rights restored.

In some states, limits are set according to the degree of protection needed. Total dependency means the person cannot meet basic needs for survival and is unable to manage the environment in any self-sustaining way. Some dependency means the person may be able to manage certain challenges of life; health or judgment may interfere with management of other needs. In the latter situation, a limited guardian may be appointed to protect the person in very specific ways.

There are considerable pros and cons in the use of conservatorships and guardianships, especially risk of exploitation. The use of these mechanisms of care is the most restrictive, and in most cases the person loses all rights to self-determination; therefore, appointment of conservators and guardians should only be considered

in cases of severe impairment, such as advanced dementia. Nurses working with older adults and their families can encourage the use of advance planning to find alternatives that are less restrictive, noting that the definitions and rules vary among states.

❖ RECOGNIZING AND ANALYZING CUES: RELATED TO CAPACITY

Nursing has long recognized the need for gerontological specialization, and lawyers have done so as well. The National Academy of Elder Law Attorneys and the National Elder Law Foundation (NELF) are two of the few specialty organizations that certify lawyers who have demonstrated knowledge pertinent to the legal needs of older adults (http://www.naela.org).

Nurses and nurses' aides may be the first persons to notice the subtle cues suggesting a potential change in capacity, indicating the need for an evaluation for reversible causes and then consideration of the extent of impairment. These concerns are first discussed with the individual; only when this is not possible are those legally designated as decision-makers involved. It is vital for the nurse to work within the applicable statutes of their state, province, or country. Nurses who are consulted by older adults or their families about legal issues should not attempt to provide legal advice, but instead refer them to a NELF-certified attorney.

KEY CONCEPTS

- Health care and its systems are undergoing profound changes, including an increase in the number of managed care organizations and changes in the roles of health care providers. All of these changes affect the care of the older adult.
- A combination of Social Security and Supplementary Security Income payments provides eligible persons with a regular income after the age of 65 years, or earlier if the person is disabled. The total amount varies greatly and is dependent on qualified income earned during the working years.
- There may be substantial out-of-pocket costs associated with the receipt of health care today.
- In order for Medicare to pay for the expenses related to long-term care or home health care, strict criteria of medical necessity must be met.
- The nurse can encourage and to some extent guide the person toward advance care planning.
- In the Western culture of health care, informed consent is based on the ethical principle of autonomy, which requires the capacity to understand a situation,

the choices that are available, and the consequences of a decision.

- In the health care setting, an individual may be legally competent but have diminished or varying levels of capacity to make health-related decisions.
- Varying levels of protection are available to protect persons with diminished capacity to ensure their previously expressed wishes are followed.
- The nurse has a responsibility to ensure the safety and security of those persons to whom care is provided. This responsibility does not change with a change in the person's legal status or capacity.
- The nurse has the responsibility to observe for sometimes subtle cues that a person's capacity should be questioned.

ACTIVITIES AND DISCUSSION QUESTIONS

1. Describe the role of the nurse advocate in relation to health and consumer protection.
2. Explain the fundamentals of Medicare and Medicaid sufficiently to assist older adults in obtaining more specific information.
3. Interview an older resident in a rehabilitation center or a participant in an adult day health or senior center and ask about their experience in the setting and across settings.
4. Identify a person at least 70 years of age who has Medicare. Ask the person how Medicare does or does not meet their needs. Write a brief summary and present it to the class.

NEXT-GENERATION NCLEX® EXAMINATION-STYLE QUESTIONS

Mr. Carter, 65 years old, comes to the senior health center for his "Welcome to Medicare" preventive visit. He tells the nurse he is generally healthy and only takes a multivitamin and valsartan/hydrochlorothiazide 160 mg/12.5 mg daily. He is a widower and has only recently entered the dating scene again. He quit smoking 15 years ago and has a 60-pack/year history. Mr. Carter is 6'1" and weighs 195 pounds (BMI 25.72). He states he has three brothers and a sister who are all in good health. His father died from a heart attack at age 70 years; his mother is still alive and lives next door to him so that he can keep an eye on her because she has mild cognitive impairment. His vital signs include a blood pressure of 132/84 mmHg, pulse of 86 beats per minute, respiratory rate of 14 breaths per minute, and a temperature of 97.4°F. His oxygen saturation is 98% on room air. After completing Mr. Carter's history, the nurse explains that advance directives describe "how you want medical decisions to be made when you are too ill to speak for yourself." Mr. Carter states that he does not have any of these documents completed. On discharge from the office, he is provided a written health plan that includes paperwork for his advance directives; the nurse tells him that in addition to completing the paperwork, he should discuss his wishes and preferences with his relatives. He also has appointments for vision and hearing screening and an ultrasound for abdominal aortic aneurism screening.

Which statements indicate the client understood teaching about advance directives? (Select all that apply).

1. "My mother has the right to make decisions for me."
2. "I can name my sister in the general power of attorney and she becomes my health care proxy."
3. "If I name one of my brothers in the durable power of attorney, he can make health care decisions for me."
4. "The person named in my durable power of attorney can only act as my proxy if I am unable to act."
5. "My brother, named in the durable power of attorney, can substitute his judgment and change my living will."
6. "If I don't create a durable power of attorney, my brothers and sisters would consult with the health care provider and make decisions on my behalf."
7. "I should tell all of my family my wishes, so that they can use substituted judgment if asked to act on my behalf."
8. "The person named in my general power of attorney can ask the health care provider to change my living will."

REFERENCES

Achenbaum, W. A. *Old age in a new land,* Baltimore (1978), Johns Hopkins University Press.

Cantril, H. *Public-opinion 1935-1946.* Princeton, New Jersey (1951), Princeton University Press.

CMS: *CMS fast facts* (2020). https://www.cms.gov/Research-Statistics-Data-and-Systems/Statistics-Trends-and-Reports/CMS-Fast-Facts.

Medicaid.gov. (n.d.). *Spousal impoverishment.* https://www.medicaid.gov/medicaid/eligibility/spousal-impoverishment/index.html.

Medicare. *Accountable care organizations,* n.d. https://www.medicare.gov/manage-your-health/coordinating-your-care/accountable-care-organizations.

Medicare. *Medicare costs at a glance* (2020). https://www.medicare.gov/your-medicare-costs/medicare-costs-at-a-glance.

Medicare Interactive: *SNF basics.* https://www.medicareinteractive.org/get-answers/medicare-covered-services/skilled-nursing-facility-snf-services/snf-basics.

PayScale: *The state of the gender pay gap 2020* (2020). https://www
.payscale.com/data/gender-pay-gap.

Social Security Administration (SSA). *How you earn credits* (2020a).
https://www.ssa.gov/pubs/EN-05-10072.pdf.

Social Security Administration (SSA). *Cost-of-living adjustment
(COLA) information for 2020* (2020b). https://www.ssa.gov
/news/cola/.

Social Security Administration (SSA). *Supplemental security income
(SSI)* (2020c). https://www.ssa.gov/oact/cola/SSI.html.

Social Security Administration (SSA): *Fact sheet* (2020d). https://
www.ssa.gov/news/press/factsheets/basicfact-alt.pdf.

US Bureau of Labor Statistics: *Economic New Release* (2020). https://
www.bls.gov/news.release/wkyeng.t03.htm.

VeteranAid. *Find senior care options for veterans* (2019). http://www
.veteranaid.org.

Zorowitz, R. A., et al. (2014). Ethics. In R. J. Ham, D. Sloane, &
G. A. Warshaw et al. (Eds.), *Primary care geriatrics: A case-based
approach* (ed. 6, pp. 77–91). Philadelphia: Elsevier.

8

Recognizing and Analyzing Cues in Gerontological Nursing

Kathleen Jett

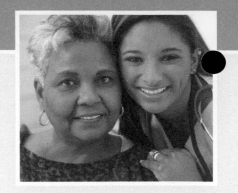

LEARNING OBJECTIVES

Upon completion of this chapter, the reader will be able to:
- Identify key differences in recognizing and analyzing cues and prioritizing hypotheses when working with older and younger adults.
- Describe the range of tools that may be used in gerontological nursing which assist in achieving the highest level of clinical judgment.
- Discuss the advantages and disadvantages of the use of standardized instruments in gerontological nursing.
- Discuss the impact of common normal changes with aging on each aspect of clinical judgment.
- Identify ways in which errors in documentation and communication are especially dangerous when caring for older adults.
- Compare the major documentation methods used in acute, long-term, and home care.
- Describe the methods that can be used in the recognition and analysis of cues leading to the expert clinical judgments.

THE LIVED EXPERIENCE

I was so happy to be able to make a big difference in Mrs. Jones' life. She was 97 and had grown slowly confused over the years. She was also profoundly hard of hearing. She spent the majority of time calling for "Mary," her deceased sister. We really could not communicate effectively with her; we could only show her we cared and keep her safe. Eventually she became acutely ill and a decision had to be made about CPR (cardiopulmonary resuscitation). When we tried to find out what her wishes were, we could not immediately find any record of them, and she had no living relatives or friends, just an attorney. I searched and searched and finally found documentation of her wishes. We were able to provide her the comfort she wanted because of a nurse's careful documentation years before.

Kathleen, GNP, at age 45

Gerontological nurses make skilled and detailed clinical judgments relating to and with persons who entrust themselves to their care. Although many of the techniques used with younger and older adults are the same, the overall process of working with the latter is strikingly different primarily because of the medical, psychological, and social complexity of late life. Older adults vary greatly in their health and function, from active and independent to medically fragile and dependent.

Generating solutions and taking action to promote healthy aging requires special abilities: to listen patiently, to allow for pauses, to optimize communication, to recognize and analyze cues from all sources and to understand that not all positive findings will require nursing actions. The nurse must be able to recognize cues indicating normal changes of aging (see Chapter 4) and those associated with atypical presentation of illness to appropriately develop hypotheses and generate solutions where needed and possible. The search for cues must be paced to the stamina of both the person and the nurse. If an older adult is physically frail or cognitively impaired, is unable to speak, or does not speak the same language as the nurse, this becomes particularly difficult and the quality of the ultimate clinical judgment is even more important.

The quality and efficiency of a nurse's clinical judgments when working with complex older adults are reflections of experience. Novice nurses should expect improvement in their ability over time. However, an experienced nurse is not always available. By following some basic guidelines and learning how to use the wide range of instruments and resources now available, a more consistent level of the highest quality of clinical judgment is possible.

Ultimately all actions are evaluated and documented. Nursing documentation is an age-old practice of making a permanent record of the conditions of our patients, our actions, and the patients' responses to our actions or those of others. Probably all of today's nurses know the mantra, "If you didn't document it—you didn't do it!" Further, if you did not document both your hypotheses and actions then you cannot determine their outcomes, appropriateness and efficacy.

In this chapter, the basic concepts of recognizing and analyzing cues involved in making clinical judgments as they apply to working with older persons are reviewed. The chapter further provides the reader with basic information about documentation in specific care settings. The instruments included are those most nurses may encounter at some time in their day-to-day practice. Those used in specialty situations can be found elsewhere in the text.

❖ USING CLINICAL JUDGMENT TO PROMOTE HEALTHY AGING: CLINICAL CUES

Clinical judgment begins with the recognition and analysis of clinical cues through the observation of physical data and the integration of spiritual and psychosocial factors within the context of an individual's cultural orientation. When working with older adults, these cues also include functional and cognitive status, caregiver stress or burden, patterns of health and health care utilization, advance care planning, and the presence or absence of any of the *geriatric syndromes* (Box 8.1). Areas or problems frequently not addressed by the care provider or mentioned by the older adult that should be addressed are sexual function, depression, alcoholism, hearing loss, oral health, and environmental safety. Although not usually conducted by a nurse, a driving assessment may

---

BOX 8.1 Geriatric Syndromes[a] and Relevant Chapter

Falls and gait abnormalities, Chapter 15
Frailty, Chapter 17
Delirium, Chapter 25
Urinary incontinence, Chapter 12
Sleep disorders, Chapter 13
Pressure injuries, Chapter 14

[a]Note that there is considerable discussion about the exact "conditions" that are considered "geriatric syndrome." There is agreement that a syndrome is something that does not neatly fit into another disease category. From Brown-O'Hara, T. (2013). Geriatric syndromes and their implications for nursing. *Nursing 43*(1), 1–3.

---

be recommended any time there is a question of ability. Questions regarding genetic background in this age group, especially for those in the younger range, have most relevance as they relate to Alzheimer's disease, stroke, diabetes, and several types of cancer.

The recognition of cues begins with establishing rapport. It is never appropriate to address the patient by their first name unless invited to do so. The assumption of familiarity of any kind including the use of the first name in addressing an older adult can easily be perceived as condescending, especially when the nurse is younger than the patient or of a different racial/ethnic background (Box 8.2) (see Chapter 3).

There are three initial approaches used in recognizing the cues needed to develop working hypotheses: self-report, report-by-proxy, and direct observation. In the self-report format, either questions are asked directly or the person is expected to respond to written

---

BOX 8.2 Key Points to Consider in Observing Cultural Rules and Etiquette

- Be aware of potentially traumatic past experiences in the health care setting.
- Ask whether there are persons (e.g., males in the family) who need to be present or involved in some way with the examination.
- Respect the communication style used, especially in the health care setting.
- Do not intrude into personal space without permission.
- Be aware of general health orientation related to time (past, present, future).
- Inquire as to appropriate wording in reference to the person; presume using last name unless otherwise welcomed.
- Inquiry as to acceptable level of touch and gender of provider.

questions about his or her health status. Older adults may overestimate their own abilities and under-report symptoms, often because of the erroneous belief that these are normal parts of aging. When information is obtained indirectly (report-by-proxy), the nurse asks another person to report his or her observations. This approach is used extensively with persons who are cognitively impaired; abilities and health are often underestimated. In the observational approach, the nurse collects and records both objective and subjective cues in the determination of performance-based function (e.g., the distance the person can walk) and physical and psychological health.

THE HEALTH HISTORY

Recognition of cues found in the health history is often the beginning of the process leading to clinical judgment. It begins with a review of what the *person* reports as problems, known as the "chief complaints." These are considered subjective data that are documented in the patient's own words. In older populations, the "complaint" is often very vague because the interaction of the numbers of chronic diseases, medications used, and other factors which obscure what may be a simple or multifactorial problem. For example, it is not unusual for the older adult to say, "I just don't feel well."

The health history is best collected either verbally in a face-to-face interview or using the interview to review a written history completed by the patient or by the patient's trusted proxy beforehand. A written format should never be used if the person has limited vision, questionable reading level, limited health fluency, or if it is written in a language or at a level in which the patient does not have reading fluency. Although it takes more time for persons to complete written formats, they are more advantageous for nurses because they may afford the nurse time to review the information that is most important and then concentrate on specific information when meeting the patient. Whether collecting the history verbally or reviewing a previously written document, the nurse uses techniques that optimize communication. If the older adult has limited language proficiency, a trained medical interpreter is needed and about twice the typical time may be needed. If the person has limited health fluency, special attention will need to be paid to wording of questions and answers to the patient's questions. In either case it is especially important to avoid generating solutions until hypotheses have been tested as thoroughly as possible. If the person is cognitively impaired, additional information obtained from a proxy, such as an aide, who knows the person well should be included (Box 8.3).

> **BOX 8.3   Speaking to the Wrong Person**
>
> Madame DuBois came to the clinic for a checkup related to her diabetes and hypertension, both of which were out of control. She spoke no English. At the first visit the nurse spent a long time explaining the plan of care through an interpreter, making the interaction especially time-consuming for the patient, the nurse, and the person accompanying Mme DuBois. Few questions were asked. A different person accompanied Mme DuBois at her next visit and asked the same questions that had been addressed in the first visit. The nurse then discovered that the woman at the second visit was actually the person who helped Mme DuBois. The person at the first visit was a neighbor who happened to have time to accompany Mme DuBois and held the cultural belief that it was not polite to question the nurse.

Any health history form or interview includes a list of allergies, a patient profile, a medical history, a review of systems (Box 8.4), a medication history (see Chapter 9), and a nutritional history (see Chapter 10) as well as any other factors that influence the person's health-related quality of life. In gerontological nursing, prioritization of cue-seeking is paramount. The nurse should be aware that with an older adult the traditional review of systems may be quite lengthy because of the number of years the person has had the opportunity to be affected by illness or disease. It may be easier and more appropriate to begin with reviewing the symptoms the person is currently having and then guide the review accordingly. In the oldest older adults, family history in and of itself becomes less important as they outlive siblings and live longer than any other relatives or parents.

Social history increases in importance when compared with younger adults. This includes current living arrangements, economic resources to meet current health-related or food expenses, level of family and friend support, and community resources available if needed. Tools to measure social networks have been in development for many years. However, the many nuances and configurations of social support networks make standardized measurements difficult.

Finally, to meet the needs of our increasingly diverse aging population, the use of the LEARN Model, modified specifically for clinical judgment in gerontological nursing, is highly recommended to complement the health history (see Chapter 3) The responses will better enable the nurse to understand the person's perception of the problem and to plan culturally and individually appropriate and effective solutions.

BOX 8.4   Tips for Best Practice

Areas of Emphasis When Conducting a Review of Systems With an Older Adult

Constitutional
- Change in the level of energy

Senses
- Changes in vision or hearing acuity and situations in which changes occur or others make comments related to these changes
- Increase in dental caries, changes in taste, presence of bleeding gums, level of current dental care
- Changes in smell

Respiratory
- Shortness of breath and, if present, circumstances in which this occurs
- Frequency of respiratory problems
- Need to sleep in chair or with head elevated on pillows

Cardiac
- Chest, shoulder, or jaw pain and circumstances in which pain occurs
- If already taking antianginal medication such as nitroglycerin, how often is it needed
- Sense of heart palpitations
- If using anticoagulants, any evidence of bruising or bleeding

Vascular
- Cramping of extremities, decreased sensation (see also Neurological), edema (including time of day and amount)
- Change of color to the skin, especially increased pigmentation of the lower extremities, cyanosis, or any other change in color

Urinary
- Changes in urine stream and length of time condition has been present; difficulty starting stream

- Incontinence and, if present, under what circumstances and to what degree; personal strategies used to address this (e.g., pads)

Sexual
- Desire and ability to continue physical sexual activity
- Ability to express other forms of intimacy
- Changes with aging that may affect sexual functioning (e.g., vaginal dryness, erectile dysfunction)

Musculoskeletal
- Pain in joints, back, or muscles
- Changes in gait and sense of safety in ambulation
- If stiffness is present, when it is the worst and when it is relieved by activity
- If mobility is limited, effect on day-to-day life

Neurological
- Changes in sensation, especially in extremities
- Changes in memory other than very minimal
- Ability to continue usual cognitive activities
- Changes in sense of balance or episodes of dizziness
- History of falls, trips, slips

Gastrointestinal
- Incontinence, constipation, bloating, anorexia
- Changes in appetite
- Loss of smell or taste

Integument
- Dryness, frequency of injury, and speed of healing
- Itching, history of skin cancer, sun exposure

❖ RECOGNIZING AND ANALYZING CUES: PHYSICAL HEALTH

Nurses learn to conduct a complete "head-to-toe" examination when collecting physical cues. Although this is usually done with younger persons, it is rarely possible when working with an older adult, especially one who is medically complex or fragile. To do so would be excessively time-consuming and burdensome to all involved. Instead the focus is first directed to that which is most likely associated with the presenting problem or major diagnoses. The gerontological nurse must be able to prioritize quickly which information is the most necessary to generate hypotheses (based on the chief complaint) and proceed to what would be "nice to know."

If the chief complaint is not known, such as in persons with moderate to advanced dementia, in persons who are unable to express themselves (such as those with expressive aphasia), or in the presence of any other type of language barrier, a more detailed search for cues is always necessary. When the focus is on health promotion and disease prevention, the emphasis is on the major preventable health problems, especially obesity, cardiovascular disease, and other illnesses associated with smoking as appropriate.

The recognition and analysis of physical cues begins the moment the nurse sees the person, noting such things as skin color and texture and presence or absence of lesions. If the person "looks ill," this should be documented with a detailed explanation of this observation. Is the person able to ambulate alone or does he or she hold on to the walls along the way to the examination room, dining room, or bathroom? Are assistive devices used? Is the person able to follow directions when the nurse uses a normal voice volume or is an elevated voice needed? If unable to follow directions at all or only with difficulty, it will be necessary to determine whether this is related to sensory losses or cognitive impairments.

While considering the expected findings related to normal age changes discussed in Chapter 4, the manual techniques used in the physical examination are applicable to any age group and the reader is referred to any number of excellent textbooks solely dedicated to this. However, extra time is usually needed for dressing and undressing older patients and some positions (e.g., lying flat for an abdominal examination) may not be possible. Several modifications may be necessary because of common changes seen in later life (Table 8.1).

TABLE 8.1 **Considerations of Common Changes in Late Life During the Search for Physical Cues in Older Adults**	
Height and weight	Monitor for changes in weight. *Weight gain:* Especially important if the person has any heart disease; be alert for early signs of heart failure. *Weight loss:* Be alert for indications of malnutrition from dental problems, depression, cancer, or advancing dementia. Check for mouth lesions from ill-fitting dentures.
Temperature	Even a low-grade fever could be an indication of a serious illness. Temperatures as low as 100°F may indicate pending sepsis.
Blood pressure	Positional blood pressure readings should be obtained because of the high occurrence of orthostatic hypotension. Both arms should be checked (at heart level) and the arm with the highest measurement should be recorded. Isolated systolic hypertension is common.
Skin	Check for indications of solar damage, especially among persons who worked outdoors or lived in sunny climates. Because of thinning of skin, "tenting" cannot be used as a true measure of hydration status.
Ears	Cerumen impactions are common. These must be removed before hearing can be adequately assessed or tympanic membrane visualized. Common site for skin cancers.
Hearing	High-frequency hearing loss (presbycusis) is common. The person often complains that he or she can hear but not understand because some, but not all, sounds are lost. The person with severe but unrecognized hearing loss may be incorrectly thought to have dementia. Ensure nurse's lips can be seen when speaking if possible.
Eyes	Lids sag. Reduced pupillary responsiveness (miosis) occurs (normal if equal bilaterally). Gray ring around the iris (arcus senilis) may develop. Artificial lens are common due to cataract surgery.
Vision	Person exhibits increased glare sensitivity, decreased contrast sensitivity, and need for more light to see and read. Ensure that waiting rooms, hallways, and examination rooms are adequately lit. Decreased color discrimination may affect ability to self-administer medications safely.
Mouth	Excessive dryness is common and exacerbated by many medications. Cannot use mouth moisture to estimate hydration status. Periodontal disease is common. Decreased sense of taste occurs. Tooth surface may be abraded.
Neck	Because of loss of subcutaneous fat it may appear that carotid arteries are enlarged when they are not.
Chest	Any kyphosis will alter the location of the lobes, making careful assessment more important. Risk of aspiration pneumonia is increased, increasing the importance of the lateral examination and the need for measurement of oxygen saturation. Evidence of pneumonia may not be evident if the person is dehydrated. Third heart sound indicative of pathology.
Heart	Listen carefully for third and fourth heart sounds. Faint fourth heart sounds may be heard. Determine whether this was present in the past or is new. Up to 50% of persons have a heart murmur.
Extremities	Dorsalis pedis and posterior tibial pulses are very difficult or impossible to palpate. Slight dependent edema is common. Must look for other indications of vascular integrity. Check temperature.
Abdomen	Because of deposition of fat in the abdomen, auscultation of bowel sounds may be difficult.
Musculoskeletal	Osteoarthritis is very common and pain is often undertreated. Ask about pain and function in joints. Conduct very gentle passive range of motion if active range of motion not possible. Do not push past comfort level. Observe for gait disorders. Observe the person get in and out of chair in order to assess independent function and fall risk.
Neurological	Although there is a gradual decrease in muscle strength, it should still remain equal bilaterally. Greatly diminished or absent ankle jerk (Achilles) tendon reflex is common and normal. Decreased or absent vibratory sense of the lower extremities is common, making testing unnecessary.
Genitourinary: male	Men have pendulous scrotum with less rugae. Have thin and graying pubic hair.
Genitourinary: female	Women have nonpalpable ovaries; short, dryer vagina; decreased size of labia and clitoris; sparse pubic hair. **Note:** Use utmost care with internal examination to avoid trauma to the friable tissues.

Most often the physical cues are only one piece of the information needed to take action to promote healthy aging. Because of the complexity of life and health in later life, this elevates the responsibility of the nurse. The nurse working in the geriatric setting must have a considerable repertoire of skills and be able to draw upon these as the circumstance arises; in some cases under a great deal of time pressure. In most circumstances the quality of care older adults receive is dependent on the quality of the hypotheses generated.

Comprehensive Information Gathering: Frail and Medically Complex Older Adults

The mnemonic FANCAPES stands for Fluids, Aeration, Nutrition, Communication, Activity, Pain, Elimination, and Socialization. The guide was developed by Barbara Bent (2005) in her work as a geriatric resource nurse at Missouri Hospital in Asheville, North Carolina, with broad applicability in any setting. It is a model for a comprehensive, yet prioritized, recognition of physical cues and especially useful when working with those who are frail or hospitalized. It emphasizes the determination of very basic needs and the individual's functional ability to meet these needs independently. It can be used in all settings, may be used in part or whole depending on the need, and is easily adaptable to functional pattern grouping if nursing diagnoses are used.

F—Fluids

What is the current state of hydration (see Chapter 11)? Does the person have the functional capacity to consume adequate fluids to maintain optimal health? This includes the abilities to sense thirst, mechanically obtain the needed fluids, swallow them, and excrete them. Medications are reviewed to identify those with the potential to affect intake or affected by intake. This is especially important when working with older adults who are taking psychotropic medications, not able to independently access fluids because of functional limitations, or for anyone with a reduced sense of thirst, a common change with aging (see Chapter 4).

A—Aeration

Because of the close relationship between pulmonary function (aeration) and cardiovascular function, cues are analyzed simultaneously. Is the person's oxygen exchange adequate for full respiratory functioning (see Chapter 22)? Measurement of the oxygen saturation rate is a part of this examination and easily done in any setting with a small, inexpensive fingertip device, familiar to most nurses. Persons with any amount of peripheral cyanosis will have artificially low readings. Is

supplemental oxygen required and, if so, is the person able to obtain it and use it properly? What is the respiratory rate and depth at rest and during activity, talking, walking, exercising and while performing activities of daily living? Which sounds are auscultated, what is learned from palpation and percussion, and what do they suggest? For the older person, it is particularly important to carefully assess all lung fields including the lateral and apical.

N—Nutrition

What mechanical and psychological factors affect the person's ability to obtain and benefit from adequate nutrition (see Chapter 10)? What is the type and amount of food consumed? Does the person have the ability to bite, chew, and swallow? What is the oral health status and what is the impact of periodontal disease if present? For edentulous persons, do their dentures fit properly and are they worn? If a special diet is recommended, has it been designed so that it is consistent with the person's eating and cultural patterns? Is the person able to obtain the special foods needed? Is the person at risk of aspiration? Have preventive strategies been taught or provided, including meticulous oral hygiene?

C—Communication

Is the person able to communicate his or her needs adequately? Do the persons who provide care understand the patient's form of communication? What is the person's ability to hear in various environments? Are there any situations in which understanding of the spoken word is inadequate? If the person depends on lipreading, is his or her vision adequate? If hearing aides are needed, are they functional and used? Is the person able to clearly articulate words that are understandable to others? Does the person have either expressive or receptive aphasia (see Chapter 23) and if so, has a speech therapist been made available to the person and significant others? What is the person's reading and comprehension levels? The impoverished childhoods of some individuals and the racist educational practices for others, even in developed countries, may have resulted in very low or no literacy levels in these groups. It is best to assume that a person's literacy is no greater than at a fifth-grade level in most settings. Inadequate recognition of communication needs will lead to erroneous hypotheses and significantly reduce the quality of health outcomes.

A—Activity

The ability to continue to participate in enjoyable activities is an important part of healthy aging. However, establishing useful hypotheses related to activity level is exceedingly complex. As more baby boomers age, this complexity increases as a result of the range of abilities among those referred to as "older adults." Nursing actions may result from the analysis of the consequences of fall risk (Chapter 15) and the need for, and correct use of, assistive devices or the degree to which one can participate in aerobic exercises. Collection of information regarding activity abilities may be accomplished by the combined efforts of nurses, physical therapists, and personal trainers (see Chapters 13 and 16).

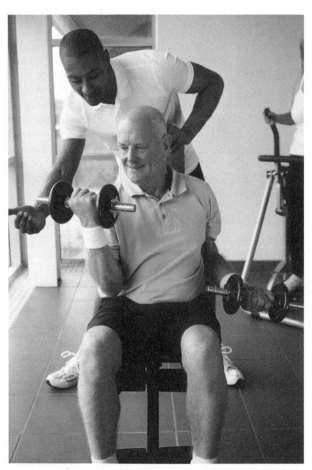

(© iStock.com/Dean Mitchell.)

P—Pain

Is the person experiencing physical, psychological, or spiritual pain? Rarely does one type of pain occur in isolation. Is the person able to communicate both the presence of pain and the relief of pain? Are there cultural barriers between the nurse and the patient that make the communication of pain difficult? Do cognitive limitations provide further barriers? How does the person

customarily attain pain relief (see Chapter 18)? As a result of the increasing amount of pain common with each decade of life (e.g., progression of arthritis or number of losses through death or change), this deserves particular attention by gerontological nurses.

E—Elimination

Although difficulties with bowel and bladder functioning are not normal parts of aging, they are more common than they are in younger adults and can be triggered by such things as immobility attributable to physical limitations (e.g., following a stroke) and medications (e.g., diuretics). Incontinence can result from cognitive changes that may cause reduction, or even absence, of the sensation indicating a need to void or defecate. Altered elimination is often among the risks and consequences of older adults living in institutional settings when they are dependent on others for assistance to maintain continence (e.g., getting to the toilet in time). Cues include: Is the person having difficulty with bladder or bowel elimination (see Chapter 12)? Is there a lack of control? Does the environment interfere with elimination and related personal hygiene (e.g., are toileting facilities adequate and accessible)? Are any assistive devices used, such as a high-rise toilet seat or bedside commode and if so, are they available and functioning? If there are problems, how are they affecting the person's social functioning and self-esteem?

S—Socialization and Social Skills

Socialization and social skills include the individual's ability to function in society, to give and receive love and friendship, and to feel self-worth. The selection of persons included in a social network is highly culturally influenced (Box 8.5). Cues to be recognized and analyzed include the individual's ability to deal with loss and to interact with other people in give-and-take situations. It is addressed in more detail in Chapters 26 and 28.

BOX 8.5 Culturally Constructed Support

Helen, Age 82

I grew up in a large extended Catholic family. As a child, all our activities and even lives, revolved around the Church and the family. Now my family members are grown and have families of their own. While we have been able to hold on to our affection, we live scattered across the country. Over the years I have also been apart from the Church. Now that I need support, I don't really have any experience reaching out for it—it was "just always there." I stay connected with my family through Facebook, but it is not the same.

❖ RECOGNIZING AND ANALYZING CUES: COGNITIVE ABILITY

With increases in age there is an increased rate of neu-rocognitive illnesses, such as Alzheimer's disease and Lewy body dementia. Cognitive ability is also easily threatened by any disturbance in physical health, such as an electrolyte disturbance. Altered or impaired men-tal status may be the first cue of anything from a heart attack to a urinary tract infection. The gerontological nurse must be aware of the high level of need to develop careful and accurate hypotheses and clinical judgments related to mental status, especially in light of changes in cognitive abilities and mood, whenever there is a change in an older adult's condition or safety. Several of the most commonly used instruments used to direct the attainment of reliable cues are described here, with more details in Chapters 24 and 25. The nurse work-ing in a geriatric setting is often expected to be profi-cient in their use. To ensure validity and reliability, the nurse must be able to administer them correctly each time they are used while minimizing distractions and interruptions.

Mini-Mental State Examination

For many years the 30-item Mini-Mental State Examination (MMSE) had been the mainstay for the gross recognition and analysis of cues to cognitive abil-ity (Folstein et al., 1975). It has not been found useful as an independent tool for the diagnosis of dementia but does indicate a need for further evaluation (Arevalo-Rodriquez et al., 2015). It is used to screen and monitor orientation, short-term memory and attention, calcula-tion ability, language, and visuospatial proficiency (abil-ity to correctly copy a figure). There are reports that this instrument has a sensitivity of 78%–84% (Norris et al., 2016). Considerable adjustment for educational level is necessary. There is now a revised 16-item instrument, the *MMSE-2,* and a slightly longer *Expanded Version.* Both are reported to be equivalent to the original instru-ment and have been translated into multiple languages. The instruments, permission for use, and instructions for use are available from a number of sources and can be found easily with an Internet search.

Montreal Cognitive Assessment

The Montreal Cognitive Assessment (MoCA) was designed as a brief screening instrument to provide cues leading to the hypothesis of mild cognitive impairment. It provides information about the same aspects of cog-nition as does the MMSE (Nasreddine, 2010). However, the MoCA has proven to be more sensitive (Ciesielska et al., 2016; Nasreddine et al., 2005) but slightly less

sensitive when used with Blacks (Sink et al., 2015). It has been found to be applicable in several countries (Memoria et al., 2013; Fujiwara et al., 2010). Because of the complexity of the tests within each category, under-standable speech, past math abilities, vision, functional hearing, and ability to use a pencil or pen are necessary. Like the MMSE it is available on the internet.

Clock Drawing Test

In use since 1992, the *Clock Drawing Test* is not appro-priate for use with those who are blind or who have limiting conditions such as tremors or who have had a stroke that has affected their dominant hand. Although reading fluency is not necessary, completion of the Clock Drawing Test requires number fluency, adequate vision and hearing, manual dexterity sufficient to hold a pencil, and experience with analog clocks (Box 8.6). This tool cannot be used as the sole measure for dementia, but it does test for constructional apraxia, an early indicator (Shulman, 2000) (Fig. 8.1). Since it was created, other tools have been developed, all with varying levels of use-fulness and sensitivity (Norris et al., 2016). However, the Clock Drawing Test is an evidence-based instrument that has been found to be useful across cultures and lan-guages and is a sensitive instrument to provide the cues needed to develop hypotheses differentiating those with and without some level of dementia (Borson et al., 1999; Tuokko et al., 1992).

BOX 8.6   Clock Drawing Test

Instructions

Provide the person with a blank piece of paper. Ask the person to:
1. Draw a circle for a clock (may be pre-drawn circle) and draw a clock in the circle.
2. Place the hands so that the clock reads a time such as 10 minutes after 11.

Scoring[a]

Draws closed circle	1 point
Places numbers in correct position	1 point
Includes all 12 correct numbers	1 point
Places hands in correct position	1 point

Interpretation

[a]There are at least 15 different methods of scoring the Clock Test. All methods consider the following:
1. Executive functioning: The symmetry of the numbers, indicating ability to plan ahead: Are all numbers included? Are any numbers repeated or missed? Are the numbers inside or outside of the circle? Do they look like numbers?
2. Abstract thinking: Are there hands on the clock? Are they in the correct place relative to the numbers?

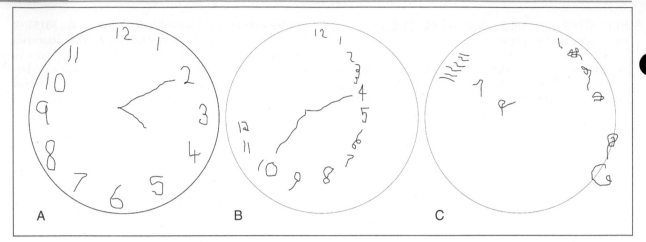

FIG. 8.1 Examples of results of a clock drawing test (of ten minutes after 4:00). (A) Unimpaired. (B and C) Impaired. (From Stern, T. A., Rosenbaum, J. F., Fava, M., et al. (2008). *Massachusetts General Hospital comprehensive clinical psychiatry*, St Louis: Mosby.)

The Mini-Cog

The Mini-Cog combines the test of short-term memory in the original MMSE with the Clock Drawing Test (Box 8.7) (see also www.mini-cog.com). In a few studies it has been found to be as accurate and reliable as the MMSE but less biased, easier to administer, and possibly more sensitive to dementia (Norris et al., 2016). It has been found to be equally reliable with English-speaking and non–English-speaking individuals (Borson et al., 2003). Although it is sensitive to cues of cognitive impairment, the analysis can only be used to develop hypotheses and indicate the need for more detailed testing leading to potential medical diagnoses (Seitz et al., 2018). It requires the same skills as the *Clock Drawing Test*.

The Global Deterioration Scale

The *Global Deterioration Scale* (Reisberg et al., 1982) is a classic measure of the levels of cognitive changes as one passes through the process of dementia (Table 8.2). It uses an ordinal scale from stage 1 (no cognitive decline, i.e., no dementia) to stage 7 (late-stage dementia, i.e., very severe cognitive decline) and provides cues to a person's ability to perform increasingly complex tasks. It is sensitive enough to show changes in outcomes (Reisberg, 2007). It has remained a useful instrument for cue recognition for many years (Sheehan, 2012). It is commonly used in the United States, Canada, and many other countries (Alzheimer Society of Canada, 2019). It is useful to both the nurse and the family in the development of appropriate strategies and actions to help the person optimize his or her health and anticipate future needs and changes.

❖ RECOGNIZING AND ANALYZING CUES: MOOD

Mood Measures

Assessment of mood is especially important because of the high rate of depression in late life; it can occur as a side effect of a medication or develop in association with several health conditions, including stroke and Parkinson's disease. Persons with untreated depression are more functionally impaired and will have prolonged hospitalizations and nursing home stays, lowered quality of life, and shortened length of life. They may appear as if they have dementia, and many persons with dementia are also depressed. The interconnection

---

BOX 8.7   The Mini-Cog

1. Tell the person that you are going to name three objects (e.g., apple, table, coin) and ask the person to repeat the objects after you and remember them (maximum of three tries).
2. Administer the Clock Drawing Test (see Box 8.6).
3. Ask the person to repeat the objects back to you.
4. Give 1 point for each recalled word, 2 points for a normal clock, and 0 points for an abnormal clock.

Score

0	Indication of dementia
1–2	No Indication of dementia if clock is normal
3–5	No indication of dementia but does not rule out some level of cognitive impairment

Adapted from Borson, S. (2003). The mini-cog as a screen for dementia: Validation in a population-based sample. *J Am Geriatr Soc 51*,1451–1454.

TABLE 8.2 **The Global Deterioration Scale**

Diagnosis	Stage	Signs and Symptoms
No dementia	Stage 1: no cognitive decline	In this stage the person functions normally, has no memory loss, and is mentally healthy. People with no dementia would be considered to be in Stage 1.
No dementia	Stage 2: very mild cognitive decline	This stage is used to describe normal forgetfulness associated with aging; for example, forgetfulness of names and where familiar objects were placed. Symptoms are not evident to loved ones or the physician.
No dementia	Stage 3: mild cognitive decline	This stage includes increased forgetfulness, slight difficulty concentrating, decreased work performance. People may get lost more often or have difficulty finding the right words. At this stage, a person's loved ones will begin to notice a cognitive decline. Average duration: 7 years before onset of dementia.
Early stage	Stage 4: moderate cognitive decline	This stage includes difficulty concentrating, decreased memory of recent events, and difficulties managing finances or traveling alone to new locations. People have trouble completing complex tasks efficiently or accurately and may be in denial about their symptoms. They may also start withdrawing from family or friends because socialization becomes difficult. At this stage a physician can detect clear cognitive problems during a patient interview and exam. Average duration: 2 years.
Midstage	Stage 5: moderately severe cognitive decline	People in this stage have major memory deficiencies and typically require some assistance to pick out the proper clothing to wear for the season and/or the activities of the day. Memory loss is more prominent and may include major relevant aspects of current life; for example, people may not remember their address or phone number and may not know the date or where they are. Average duration: 1.5 years.
Midstage	Stage 6: severe cognitive decline (middle dementia)	People in Stage 6 require assistance to carry out daily activities. They start to forget names of close family members and have little memory of recent events. Many people can remember only some details of earlier life. They may also have difficulty counting down from 10 and finishing tasks. Incontinence (loss of bladder or bowel control) is a problem in this stage. Ability to speak declines. Personality changes such as delusions (believing something to be true that is not), compulsions (repeating a simple behavior, such as cleaning), or anxiety and agitation may occur. Average duration: 2.5 years.
Late stage	Stage 7: very severe cognitive decline (late dementia)	People in this stage have little or no ability to speak or communicate. They require assistance with most activities (e.g., using the toilet, eating). They eventually lose psychomotor skills, for example, the ability to walk. Average duration: 2 to 7 years.

Original tool in Reisberg, B., Ferris, S. H., de Leon, M. J., et al. (1982). The Global Deterioration Scale for assessment of primary degenerative dementia, *Am J Psychiatry 139*,1136–1139. Revised as written per personal communication with Dr. Reisberg. Copyright © 1983 Barry Reisberg, MD. Reproduced with permission.

between depression and dementia necessitates skill and sensitivity in the nurse to ensure that elders receive the assessment and care they need (see Chapter 24).

Geriatric Depression Scale

The instrument used most commonly to recognize and analyze cues related to depression in both middle-aged and older adults is the *Geriatric Depression Scale (GDS)*, developed by Yesavage and colleagues (1982). The GDS has been extremely successful in hypothesizing the possibility of depression because it deemphasizes physical complaints, sex drive, and appetite—those things most affected by medications (Table 8.3). It has been tested extensively with translations in multiple languages (Sheehan, 2012). The instrument can be completed on an iPhone or ANDROID with an automatic calculation of the results, which can then be downloaded to a computer. It cannot be used in persons with dementia or other cognitive impairment. Dr. Yesavage may be contacted directly at Stanford University for more information and a description of the free, associated products he has available. See also http://www.stanford.edu/~yesavage/GDS.html.

TABLE 8.3   Geriatric Depression Scale (Short Form)

Are you basically satisfied with your life?	Yes	No*
Have you dropped many of your activities and interests?	Yes*	No
Do you feel that your life is empty?	Yes*	No
Do you often get bored?	Yes*	No
Are you in good spirits most of the time?	Yes	No*
Are you afraid that something bad is going to happen to you?	Yes*	No
Do you feel happy most of the time?	Yes	No*
Do you often feel helpless?	Yes*	No
Do you prefer to stay at home, rather than going out and doing new things?	Yes*	No
Do you feel you have more problems with memory than most?	Yes*	No
Do you think it is wonderful to be alive?	Yes	No*
Do you feel pretty worthless about the way you are now?	Yes*	No
Do you feel full of energy?	Yes	No*
Do you feel that your situation is hopeless?	Yes*	No
Do you think that most people are better off than you?	Yes*	No

*Each answer indicated by an asterisk counts as 1 point. Scores greater than 5 indicate need for further evaluation. Contact Dr. Yesavage directly at Stanford University in Palo Alto, CA, or see http://www.stanford.edu/~yesavage/GDS.html.

From Brink, T.L., Yesavage, J., Lum, O., et al. (1982). Screening tests for geriatric depression. *Clinical Gerontologist 1*, 37–44.

❖ RECOGNIZING AND ANALYZING CUES: FUNCTIONAL ABILITY

Recognizing and analyzing cues of functional ability is part of the clinical judgment needed when working with older adults, especially those who are vulnerable to frailty. If the person is healthy and active, a simple observation may be all that is needed, such as "Patient is active and independent; denies functional difficulties." However, if early cues suggest potential limitations, such as Parkinson's disease or for a person who recently fell, detailed information is gathered to minimize any untoward consequences.

A thorough analysis of functional ability should lead to hypotheses and potential solutions and actions including the following:

- Specific areas in which help is needed
- Changes in abilities from one period of time to another
- Specific service(s) needed
- Safety of the current living situation

Functional abilities have been divided between those associated with the ability to perform the tasks needed for self-care (i.e., needed to maintain one's health), referred to as activities of daily living (ADLs), and those tasks needed for independent living, referred to as instrumental activities of daily living (IADLs). ADLs are most often identified as eating, toileting, ambulation, bathing, dressing, and grooming. Three of these tasks (grooming, dressing, and bathing) entail higher cognitive function than the others. The IADLs such as cleaning, yard work, shopping, and money management are considered to be more complex activities necessitating higher physical and cognitive functioning than the ADLs. For persons with dementia, the progressive loss of abilities begins with IADLs and progresses to the higher-level ADLs. The nurse must keep in mind that both the willingness and the ability to perform skills are influenced by sociocultural factors unique to the person.

Numerous instruments are available that help elucidate, monitor, and predict functional ability. They are also used to evaluate outcomes. Like the health history, cues to functional ability are obtained by observation, self-report, or report-by-proxy. The analysis of the cues obtained through the use of most of the instruments results in an arbitrary score of some kind—a rating of the person's ability to do the task alone, with assistance, or not at all. When functional information is needed, the use of existing and established tools is recommended. However, most do not divide a task into its component parts, such as picking up a spoon or cup and swallowing when considering the task of eating; instead, eating is not seen as the complex task that it is. The instruments are useful in that they serve the purposes noted earlier. However, the analyses are not usually sensitive enough to show small changes in function and are more global in nature.

Activities of Daily Living

ADLs were first classified by Sidney Katz and colleagues in 1963 (Katz et al., 1963). The *Katz Index* has served as a basic framework for most of the subsequent measures (Box 8.8). On the Katz Index, the ADLs are considered

BOX 8.8   Examples of Activities of Daily Living

- Bathing
- Dressing
- Using the toilet
- Transferring oneself
- Feeding oneself
- Controlling bowel and bladder function (continence)

From Katz, S., Down, T. D., Cash, H. R., et al. (1970). Progress in the development of the index of ADL, *Gerontologist 10*(1):20–30.

only in dichotomous terms: the ability to complete the task independently (1 point) or the complete inability to do so (0 points). Over the years this instrument has been refined to afford more sensitivity to the nuances of, and changes in, functional ability (Nikula et al., 2003). Despite these limitations, the tool is useful because it creates a common language about patient function for all caregivers involved in clinical judgment, planning actions and evaluating overall outcomes. It can be found at www.consultgeri.org.

Barthel Index

The *Barthel Index* (BI) (Mahoney & Barthel, 1965) is a quick and reliable instrument used to obtain information about both mobility and the ability to perform ADLs. The cues are rated in various ways, depending on the item. The BI has been found to be sensitive enough to identify when a person first needs help and to evaluate outcomes of nursing actions, especially for those who have had a stroke (Quinn et al., 2011). It is available in multiple locations on the Internet.

Functional Independence Measure

The *Functional Independence Measure* (FIM) was designed to provide cues regarding a person's need for assistance with ADLs and for the evaluation of rehabilitation outcomes during inpatient rehabilitation and skilled nursing home stays, especially following a stroke or traumatic injury (Uniform Data Systems, 1999-2020). In some studies, the BI and FIM were found to be comparable. In other studies, the FIM was deemed preferable (Cech & Martin, 2012). The FIM is a highly sensitive instrument and includes cues related to ADLs, mobility, cognition, and social functioning. The tasks are rated using a seven-point scale that ranges from totally independent to totally dependent. The FIM is commonly used in acute rehabilitation and Veteran's Administration health care facilities in the United States and several other countries (Lundgren-Nilsson et al., 2005). For information about licensing, training, certification, and purchasing see https://www.udsmr.org/products/snf-subacute.

Instrumental Activities of Daily Living

The original tool for the assessment of IADLs was developed by Lawton and Brody (1969) (Box 8.9). Both the original tool and the subsequent variations use the self-report, report-by-proxy, and observed formats with three levels of functioning (independent, assisted, and unable to perform). The advantages and disadvantages of using these instruments are the same as those for the measures of ADLs. A copy of this instrument for individual use is available at www.consultgeri.org.

BOX 8.9 Examples of Instrumental Activities of Daily Living

- Ability to use the telephone (look up numbers, make phone calls)
- Ability to travel (alone [e.g., drive], with another, unable)
- Ability to shop for necessities (alone even if needs someone to provide transportation, cannot do without help, unable)
- Ability to prepare meals (plan and prepare full meals safely, can prepare light meals but cannot cook full meals, unable)
- Ability to do housework (heavy housework, limited to light housework, unable)
- Ability to self-administer medication (independently take medications in the right dose at the right time, able to take medications but needs reminding or someone to prepare them, unable)
- Ability to manage money (independently manage money [e.g., write checks, pay bills], needs some help, unable)

From Lawton, M. P. & Brody, E. M. (1969). Assessment of older people: Self-maintaining and instrumental activities of daily living, *Gerontologist* 9(3):179–186.

❖ RECOGNIZING AND ANALYZING COMPREHENSIVE CUES

In some cases, a comprehensive approach is used rather than a collection of separate instruments when collecting cues, analyzing them, prioritizing hypotheses, generating solutions, and taking actions to foster healthy aging. The original integrated instrument was probably the *Older American's Resources and Services* (OARS) and later refined as the *Older American's Resources and Services Multidimensional Functional Assessment Questionnaire* (OMFAQ) developed at Duke University (Duke, n.d.). It has been translated into other languages and found valid and reliable outside of the United States (Falahati, 2018). All comprehensive instruments are quite lengthy and completion often requires a collaborative and interdisciplinary approach and training. When completed, they serve as a resource for the development of care strategies and nursing actions and the evaluation of outcomes. Related instruments discussed herein are the Fulmer SPICES (Fulmer, 2007), the Minimum Data Set used in skilled nursing facilities; and OASIS, used in certified home care agencies.

The OARS Multidimensional Functional Assessment Questionnaire (OMFAQ)

When the OMFAQ is completed, the nurse will have cues related to social and economic resources, mental and physical health, and ADLs. The person's functional capacity in each area is rated on a scale of 1 (excellent functioning) to 6 (totally impaired functioning). At the conclusion, a cumulative impairment score (CIS) is calculated ranging from the most capable (6) to total disability (30). Cue analysis results in hypotheses related to (1) the ability, disability, and capacity level at which the person is able to function, and (2) the extent and intensity of utilization of resources.

The OMFAQ and training materials can be purchased for a nominal fee from the Center for the Study of Aging and Human Development at Duke University at https://sites.duke.edu/centerforaging/?s=OMFAQ&submit=.

Fulmer SPICES

The *Fulmer SPICES* is a simple comprehensive instrument focusing on geriatric syndromes (Fulmer, 2007) (see Chapter 17). It has proved reliable and valid when used with older persons either in health or illness, regardless of the setting. The acronym *SPICES* refers to the sometimes vague but nonetheless very important cues that require nursing action: Sleep disorders, Problems with eating or feeding, Incontinence, Confusion, Evidence of falls, and Skin breakdown. Nurses are encouraged to use this acronym as a reference when caring for older adults (see https://consultgeri.org/try-this/general-assessment/issue-1). It is a system that alerts the nurse to attend to cues related to the most common problems that occur in the health and well-being of older adults, particularly those who have one or more medical conditions.

Resident Assessment Instrument (RAI)/Minimum Data Set (MDS 3.0)

In 1986, what was then referred to as the Institute of Medicine, completed a study indicating that although considerable variation existed, residents in skilled nursing facilities in the United States were receiving an unacceptably low quality of care (IOM, 1986). As a result, nursing home reform was legislated as part of the Omnibus Budget Reconciliation Act (OBRA) of 1987. The creators of OBRA recognized the challenging work of caring for increasingly ill persons discharged from acute care settings to nursing homes and, along with this, the need for comprehensive assessments, complex clinical judgment, and documentation regarding the interdisciplinary care/action that was needed, planned, implemented, and evaluated.

In 1990, a Resident Assessment Instrument (RAI) was created and mandated for use in all skilled nursing facilities that receive compensation from either Medicare or Medicaid (see Chapter 7). The documents included in the RAI are many with the major portion being the MDA or Minimum Data Set. Now in its third version, the 450-item *Minimum Data Set* (MDS 3.0) is the basis for the assessment within the RAI. As the cues generated by the MDS are analyzed, specific areas of need are hypothesized that guide the development of actions and subsequent repeated evaluations of outcomes. The most recent revision has been found to be more reliable, efficient, and clinically relevant than previous versions; evidence-based tools are included whenever possible. In a significant change from MDS 2.0, care recipient interviews are included.

Quality Measures are now included to provide standardized information about outcomes. These have been updated and revised and now considered in terms of "Meaningful Measures" or those indicators with the potential for the most impact of quality of care (Box 8.10)

BOX 8.10 **Examples of Quality Measures Highly Relevant to Persons Receiving Care in Skilled Nursing Facilities**

Short-Stay Residents	Long-Term Stay Residents
Medicare spending per patient	Number of hospitalizations per 1000 resident days
Rate of successful return to home or community	Emergency room visits per 1000 resident days
Rate of potentially preventable hospital re-admission 30 days after discharge	Percentage of residents:
Percentage of residents with:	• Experienced one or more falls with a major injury
• Improved independent mobility	• High-risk residents who develop pressure-injuries
• Self-report of moderate to severe pain	• Developed a urinary tract infection
• Pressure injuries: new or worsened	• Developed bowel or bladder incontinence
• One or more falls with major injury	• Has/had catheter inserted and left in into bladder
• Assessed for/given seasonal influenza vaccination	• Are physically restrained
• Assessed for/given pneumococcal vaccine	• Have increased need for assistance with ADLs
• New antipsychotic medication	• Ability to move independently worsened
• Re-hospitalized after an admission	• Has/had excessive weight loss
• Had an emergency room visit	• Shows depressive symptoms
• Functional abilities assessed and goals part of treatment plan	• Received an antipsychotic, antianxiety or hypnotic medication
	• Needs and got flu or pneumonia vaccine

From CMS. (2020a). *Quality measures.* http://www.cms.gov/Medicare/Quality-Initiatives-Patient-Assessment-Instruments/NursingHomeQualityInits/NHQIQuality Measures.html.

(CMS, 2020a). The Quality Indicators, along with the RAI, are used in several countries outside the United States, including provinces in Canada, and have been found to provide a foundation for quality care/actions.

The RAI/MDS provides a comprehensive health, social, and functional profile of persons as they enter skilled nursing facilities and at designated times thereafter. The initial assessment serves as the framework for the initial goals and outcomes for the individual. As outcomes are evaluated, the nurse and other members of the care team can track the progress toward the solution of identified problems and make changes to the action plan as appropriate. As goals are met and resources are made available, the RAI/MDS leads to the goal of discharge to a lower level of care, such as returning home or to an assisted living facility. For a person whose condition is one of progressive decline, the RAI leads to actions focused on comfort. The RAI process is dynamic and outcome oriented. It is used to gather definitive information and promote healthy aging in a specific care setting and in a holistic manner. The RAI is coordinated by a nurse and requires his or her signature attesting to its accuracy.

Outcome and Assessment Information Set

The skilled care provided in the home, usually following a hospitalization, is based on, and documented in, the Outcome and Assessment Information Set (OASIS). The fifth revision OASIS-D became effective on January 1, 2019 (CMS, 2020b). A further revision (OASIS-E) has been delayed until the January 1st that follows a full 12 months after the end of the COVID-19 public health emergency (CMS, 2020b). The information collected is very comprehensive and focuses on the development of prioritized hypotheses, generated solutions, and specific actions designed to address the most relevant needs and prevent rehospitalization and ensure safety in the home setting (Box 8.11). The majority of the documentation takes place in the patient's home and is entered into a laptop or tablet for transmission to the agency database, and ultimately to the Centers for Medicare and Medicaid Services. Completion is required for all care that is compensated by Medicare or Medicaid and forms the basis for the level of reimbursement. As with other instruments, it is completed at the time the care is begun and at intervals thereafter. Nurses supplement the cues based on OASIS with information necessary to generate solutions within the context of existing environmental and personal factors. Clinical judgment at this level is exceedingly complex. Training is required for the accurate use of the OASIS instrument. For the latest information, see http://www.cms.gov and search OASIS.

BOX 8.11   Risk of Hospitalization From the OASIS Assessment

- ☐ 1. History of falls (two or more falls—or any fall with an injury—in the past 12 months)
- ☐ 2. Unintentional weight loss of a total of 10 pounds or more in the past 12 months
- ☐ 3. Multiple hospitalizations (two or more) in the past 6 months
- ☐ 4. Multiple emergency department visits (two or more) in the past 6 months
- ☐ 5. Decline in mental, emotional, or behavioral status in the past 3 months
- ☐ 6. Reported or observed history of difficulty complying with any medical instructions (e.g., medications, diet, exercise) in the past 3 months
- ☐ 7. Currently taking five or more medications
- ☐ 8. Currently reports exhaustion
- ☐ 9. Other risk(s) not listed in 1–8
- ☐ 10. None of the above

❖ USING CLINICAL JUDGMENT TO PROMOTE HEALTHY AGING: DOCUMENTATION

Clinical documentation chronicles, supports, and communicates the information needed to make clinical judgments. It provides the information needed for the careful development of the individualized solutions and actions and the evaluation of outcomes. Good documentation will help the nurse identify, monitor, and evaluate actions. It also provides a means of the communication needed to ensure continuity of care—from one shift to another, from one caregiver to another, and across care settings. The nurse who cares for a patient for whom the previous nurse did not document is very familiar with the potential consequences and the added risk to the patient and legal liability for the nurse. At the same time, documentation is the major means for the nurse to demonstrate the quality of care he or she provides.

Since the Patient Self-Determination Act was passed in 1991, all persons entering a health care facility or who begin to receive skilled home care are asked if they have an advance directive and, if not, are provided information about them (see Chapters 7 and 28). The nursing records supplement this documentation with more details regarding a person's wishes and include the names of people that person wants involved in their care, who he/she wants to have access to their records, and their wishes related to everything from organ donation to the use of cardiopulmonary resuscitation (CPR) to the handling of their bodies after death. Patients often discuss these issues with nurses during quiet moments. By noting these conversations in the clinical record, nurses can both officially document this important information and share it with other members of the health care team to ensure that the patient's wishes are respected.

Documentation in Acute Care and Acute Rehabilitation Care Settings

Documentation in the acute care setting has undergone a significant change in recent years with mandates for upgrading to the electronic medical record (EMR). Computers can be found at the bedside, in nurses' pockets, and in strategic locations around the unit. Nurses are given passwords that may be more important than their name tags or the bar codes on their name tags. In some settings, fingerprints are scanned for anything from access to records and supplies, to administration of treatments and medications, to identification of patients. The use of checklists, flow sheets, and standardized tools has become the norm, all documented electronically. A care map of some kind is used to predict the nursing actions within a preestablished trajectory to anticipate the day of discharge as far as possible.

Documentation in Long-Term Care Facilities

The term long-term care facility is applied to a number of settings, including family care homes, assisted living facilities (board and care homes), nursing facilities, skilled nursing facilities (SNFs), and "swing beds" in rural hospitals (beds that serve for either acute or long-term care, depending on the patient's needs) (see Chapter 6). The level of documentation required varies by setting and is prescribed by state or jurisdiction statutes and payors. In family care homes and assisted living facilities, documentation generally occurs only if a licensed nurse has been hired or is under contract with the facility. This service is usually limited to administration of medications or the delegation of this act to certified nursing assistants.

Both nursing facilities and skilled nursing facilities are making the transition to the electronic medical record but still lag behind acute care facilities. In addition to documentation of patient cues (e.g. vital signs) in these facilities, the documentation encompasses the recording of daily care/actions (such as eating status and presence or absence of bowel movements), mandated periodic re-analyses of cues, medication and treatment administration, and any unusual event or change in condition. Documentation in SNFs includes narrative progress notes, flow sheets, checklists, and the RAI as already discussed. The RAI data are transmitted to Medicare electronically and subsequently into a national database. When a resident's care is not considered "skilled" and therefore no longer covered by Medicare, narrative notes are reduced to "problem-oriented only" and are completed on an "as-needed" and weekly or monthly basis depending on the

facility and licensing body. Good documentation and analysis of such is an expectation of all care staff. Licensed nurses are ultimately responsible for the quality and accuracy of the hypotheses generated and the evaluation of outcomes. The completeness and accuracy of the documentation of the care is a means of monitoring the whole person in the promotion of healthy aging.

Documentation in Home Care

The majority of the care provided in the home is by informal caregivers such as family members and hired "private duty attendants." They will often develop documentation systems of their own to track appointments, medication administration, and health care provider instructions. If used, this system increases the continuity of care. Nurses may need to assist the family in developing and using effective systems.

The Association Between Documentation and Reimbursement

When care is paid for by Medicare, Medicaid, or another insurer (see Chapter 7) reimbursement is based on the analysis of care needs and the documentation of nursing actions and outcomes. In skilled nursing facilities this is through the analysis of the MDS and the subsequent calculation of resources needed for care when Medicare is the payor. Reimbursement is similarly calculated in skilled home care through the documentation found on the OASIS instrument.

Initial reimbursement in acute care settings (hospitals and acute rehabilitation) is preset by diagnosis codes (diagnosis-related groups [DRGs]) and analyses of cues at the time of admission and with any change in condition. Specific preventable events (hospital-acquired condition [HAC]) (Box 8.12) and readmission for the

---

BOX 8.12   Hospital-Acquired Conditions (HACs)

- Hospital acquired infections
- Pressure injury rate
- Iatrogenic pneumothorax rate
- In-hospital fall with hip fracture
- Perioperative Hemorrhage or Hematoma rate
- Postoperative acute kidney injury requiring dialysis rate
- Postoperative respiratory failure rate
- Perioperative pulmonary embolism or DVT rate
- Postoperative sepsis rate
- Postoperative wound dehiscence rate
- Unrecognized abdominopelvic accidental puncture/laceration rate.

Information from CMS (2020). *Hospital-acquired condition reduction program (HACRP).* https://www.cms.gov/Medicare/Medicare-Fee-for-Service-Payment/AcuteInpatientPPS/HAC-Reduction-Program.html.

same problem within 30 days of discharge have negative financial consequences for the facility. No payment is made for the presumed HAC when the cues were not present or not documented at the time of admission. *Documentation is necessary to determine if they were present* (CMS, 2020a).

EVALUATING OUTCOMES

Communication of both cues/information needed in day-to-day actions through documentation has become critical to ensure patients' rights, maximize outcomes, and the economic survival of providers. It is the responsibility of the nurse to make sure that communication and documentation are of the highest quality to provide seamless, error-free and appropriate care and continuity and to maximize both patient outcomes and appropriate reimbursement.

Whether the nurse is working with a standardized instrument or creating a new one, the goal of the solutions generated by gerontological nurses is to promote healthy aging. To accomplish this, it is necessary to collect the most accurate cues in the most efficient, yet caring manner possible. The use of instruments serves as a way to organize the information and makes it possible to compare outcomes from one time to another. As noted earlier, each tool has strengths and weaknesses. Multiple factors complicate the determination of healthcare needs of the older adult. These include the difficulty of differentiating the effects of aging from those originating from disease, the coexistence of multiple diseases, the under-reporting of symptoms by older adults, the atypical presentation or nonspecific presentation of illnesses, and the increase in iatrogenic illnesses.

Overdiagnosis or underdiagnosis occurs when the cues associated with normal aging are not considered; these include physical, psychosocial, and spiritual cues. Underdiagnosis is far more common in gerontological nursing. Many observed and reported cues are ascribed to normal aging rather than to the possible development of a health problem.

Working with the medically complex older adult is a challenge. Cues related to one condition can mask those of another. Yet the gerontological nurse is expected to provide assurance that the health outcomes are at the highest level of effectiveness possible. If an instrument will facilitate the achievement of this goal, it should be used. If it serves little purpose or is burdensome to either the nurse or the patient, it should be avoided or replaced. Without appropriate documentation the recognition and analysis of cues cannot fully contribute to the well-being of those who entrust themselves to our care.

KEY CONCEPTS

- Recognition and analysis of physical, cognitive, psychosocial, spiritual, and environmental cues are essential when developing the solutions and taking action in the care of older adults.
- The quality and quantity of the information gathered when using a collection instrument are affected by the manner used and whether self-report, report-by-proxy, or nurse observation is used.
- Skill in the use of an instrument is needed in order to assure accuracy in the information collected.
- Anticipate that compensation may be necessary for older adults with hearing or visual impairments when seeking cues.
- Expect findings that are different from those for a younger adult and anticipate the need to begin to differentiate normal age-related changes from potential pathological conditions.
- For those with cognitive impairments, obtaining some health-related information from a proxy may be necessary but can only be done with the permission of the legal representative.
- Excellence in documentation sets the stage for excellence in care outcomes.
- Standardized instruments for use in the observation of cues related to the health status of patients are integral to consistent and appropriate reimbursement for care provided.
- Documenting patient health status and evaluating the effectiveness of actions is a key responsibility of licensed and registered nurses.

ACTIVITIES AND DISCUSSION QUESTIONS

1. What is the importance of the determination of the ability of an older adult to perform ADLs and IADLs?
2. What makes an information collection instrument useful?
3. Discuss problems you have experienced with incomplete cues or poor documentation in a health facility.
4. Discuss the potential uses of MDS 3.0 and OASIS-D.
5. Explain why documentation is critical to insuring optimal outcomes.

NEXT-GENERATION NCLEX® EXAMINATION-STYLE QUESTIONS

The home health nurse is completing the intake assessment for Mr. Agens, an 85-year-old male. When responding to question, he replies in clear, complete sentences without dyspnea. He lives on his own in a small one story, two-bedroom home. He has been a widow for 10 years. His two adult children live in a neighboring state. They call him once a month and visit twice a year. He has a 60-pack per year history of smoking; he has been using portable oxygen for the past 10 years. He states he has shortness of breath with exertion at times. He receives Meals-on-Wheels each weekday. His neighbor's wife buys his groceries when she goes shopping once a week. He can cook simple meals without difficulty. Mr. Agens ambulates using a walker; he has used it for the past 3 years. He no longer drives. He attends the local senior center bingo night each month and attends the local church on Sundays. He wears bilateral hearing aids and has no difficulty hearing the questions he is asked. Mr. Agens also wears bifocal glasses. He states he dropped out of school in the 8th grade to go to work. His vital signs include a blood pressure of 132/82 mmHg, pulse of 80 beats per minute, respiratory rate of 14 breaths per minute, a temperature of 97.6°F, and pulse oximetry reading of 92% on O_2 at 2 L per nasal canula.

Medications

Lisinopril 25 mg/hydrochlorothiazide 25 mg daily
Sennosides 8.6 mg/docusate sodium 50 mg at bedtime
Tamsulosin 0.8 mg daily
Fluticasone furoate 100 µg/umeclidinium 62.5 µg/ vilanterol 25 µg daily

Highlight the cues that correspond to the "C" in the FANCAPES assessment mnemonic.

REFERENCES

Alzheimer Society of Canada: *Stages of Alzheimer's disease,* 2019. http://www.alzheimer.ca/en/About-dementia/Alzheimer-s -disease/Stages-of-Alzheimer-s-disease.

Arevalo-Rodriquez, I., Smailagic, N., Rogue, I., et al. (2015). Mini-Mental State Examination (MMSE) for the detection of Alzheimer's disease and other dementias in people with mild cognitive impairment (MCI). *Cochrane Syst Rev, 2015*(3), CD010783.

Bent, B. (2005). FANCAPES assessment: Increases in longevity lead to need for expertise in geriatric care. *Adv Healthcare Network Nurses, 7*(14), 10.

Borson, S., Brush, M., Gil, E., et al. (1999). The Clock Drawing Test: Utility for dementia detection in multiethnic elders. *J Gerontol A Biol Sci Med Sci, 54*(11), M534–M540.

Borson, S., Scanlan, J. M., Chen, P., et al. (2003). The Mini-Cog as a screen for dementia: Validation in a population-based sample. *J Am Geriatr Soc, 51*(10), 141–144.

Cech, D. J., & Martin, S. (2012). Evaluation of function, activity, and participation. In D. J. Cech, & S. Martin (Eds.), *Functional movement development across the lifespan* (3rd edition). St. Louis: Elsevier.

Centers for Medicare and Medicaid Services (CMS): *Quality measures,* 2020a. https://www.cms.gov/Medicare/Quality-Initiatives -Patient-Assessment-Instruments/QualityMeasures/index .html?redirect=/QUALITYMEASURES/.

Centers for Medicare and Medicaid Services (CMS): *OASIS data sets,* 2020b. https://www.cms.gov/Medicare/Quality-Initiatives -Patient-Assessment-Instruments/HomeHealthQualityInits /OASIS-Data-Sets.

Ciesielska, N., Sokołowski, R., Mazur, E., et al. (2016). Is the Montreal Cognitive Assessment (MoCA) test better suited than the Mini-Mental State Examination (MMSE) in mild cognitive impairment (MCI) detection among people aged over 60? Meta-analysis. *Psychiatria Polska, 50*(5), 1039–1052.

Duke University Center for the Study of Aging and Human Development: *Older Americans resources and services,* n.d. https://sites.duke.edu/centerforaging/?s=OMFAQ&submit=.

Falahati, A., Sabaf, R., Kamrani, A. A. A., et al. (2018). Validity and reliability of OARS Multidisciplinary Functional Assessment Questionnaire in Iranian elderly. *Iranian Rehabilitation Journal, 16*(2), 169–176.

Folstein, M. F., Folstein, S. E., & McHugh, P. R. (1975). Mini-mental state: A practical method for grading the cognitive state of patients for the clinician. *J Psychiatr Res, 12*(3), 189–198.

Fujiwara, Y., Suzuki, H., Yasunaga, M., et al. (2010). Brief screen tool for mild cognitive impairment in older Japanese: Validation of the Japanese version of the Montreal Cognitive Assessment. *Geriatrics & Gerontology International, 10*(3), 225–232.

Fulmer, T. (2007). How to try this: Fulmer SPICES. *AJN, 107*(10), 40–48.

Institute of Medicine (IOM): *Improving the quality of care in nursing homes: Consensus report,* 1986. https://www.nap.edu/catalog/646 /improving-the-quality-of-care-in-nursing-homes.

Katz, S., Ford, A. B., Moskowitz, R. N., et al. (1963). Studies of illness in the aged: The index of ADL: A standardized measure of biological and psychosocial function. *JAMA, 185*, 914–919.

Kidd, D., Stewart, G., Baldry, J., et al. (1995). The Functional Independence Measure: A comparative validity and reliability study. *Disabil Rehabil, 17*, 10.

Lawton, M. P., & Brody, E. M. (1969). Assessment of older people: Self-maintaining and instrumental activities of daily living. *Gerontologist, 9*(3), 179–186.

Lundgren-Nilsson, A., Grimby, G., Ring, H., et al. (2005). Cross-cultural validity of Functional Independence Measure items in stroke: A study using Rasch analysis. *J Rehabil Med, 37*, 23–31.

Mahoney, F. I., & Barthel, D. W. (1965). Functional evaluation: The Barthel index. *Md State Med J, 14*, 61–65.

Memória, C. M., Yassuda, M. S., & Nakano, E. Y. (2013). & Brief screen for mild cognitive impairment: Validation of the Brazilian version of the Montreal cognitive assessment. *International Journal of Geriatric Psychiatry, 28*(1), 34–40.

Nasreddine, Z.: *Montreal cognitive assessment: Administration and score instructions,* 2010. www.mocatest.org.

Nasreddine, Z. S., Phillips, N. A., Bédirian, V., Charbonneau, S., Whitehead, V, et al. (2005). Montreal Cognitive Assessment, MoCA: A brief screen tool for mild cognitive impairment. *Journal of the American Geriatrics Society, 53*(4), 695–699.

Nikula, S., Jylha, M., Bardage, C., et al. (2003). Are ADLs comparable across countries? Sociodemographic associates of harmonized IADL measures. *Aging Clin Exp Res, 15*(6), 451–459.

Norris, D. R., Clark, M. S., & Shipley, S. (2016). The mental status examination. *Am Fam Physician, 94*(8), 635–641.

Quinn, T. J., Langhorne, P., & Stott, D. J. (2011). Barthel Index for stroke trials: Development, properties and application. *Stroke, 42*, 1146–1151.

Reisberg, B. (2007). Global measures: Utility in defining and measuring treatment response in dementia. *Int Psychogeriatr, 19*, 421.

Reisberg, B., Ferris, S., de Leon, M. J., et al. (1982). The global deterioration scale for assessment of primary progressive dementia. *Am J Psychiatry, 139*(9), 1136–1139.

Seitz, D. P., Chan, C. C., Newton, H. T., Gill, S. S., Hermann, N., et al. (2018). Mini-Cog for the diagnosis of Alzheimer's disease dementia and other dementias within a primary care setting. *Cochrane Database Syst Rev, 2018*(2), CD011415.

Sheehan, B. (2012). Assessment scales in dementia. *Therapeutic advances in neurological disorders, 5*(6), 349–358.

Shulman, K. I. (2000). Clock drawing: Is it the ideal cognitive screening test? *Int J Geriatr Psychiatry, 15*, 545.

Sink, K. M., Craft, S., Smith, C., et al. (2015). Montreal cognitive assessment and modified mini mental state examination in African Americans. *Journal of Aging Research* (ID 872018): 6 pages on-line. https://www.hindawi.com/journals/jar/2015/872018/.

Tuokko, H., Hadjistavropoulos, T., Miller, J., et al. (1992). The clock test: A sensitive measure to differentiate normal elderly from those with Alzheimer disease. *J Am Geriatr Soc, 40*(6), 579–584.

Uniform Data System for Medical Rehabilitation: *SNF/Subacute*, 1999–2020. https://www.udsmr.org/products/snf-subacute.

Yesavage, J. A., Brink, T. L., Rose, T., et al. (1982). Development and validation of a geriatric depression screening scale: A preliminary report. *J Psychiatr Res, 17*(1), 37–49.

9

Clinical Judgment to Promote Safe Medication Use

Kathleen Jett

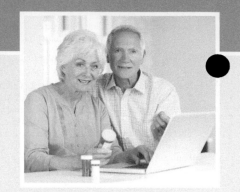

LEARNING OBJECTIVES

Upon completion of this chapter, the reader will be able to:
- Explain age-related pharmacokinetic and pharmacodynamics changes.
- Discuss potential use of chronotherapy.
- Explain the roles of older adults, their caregivers, and social network in reducing medication misuse and polypharmacy.
- List nursing actions that can reduce medication misuse by older adults and their health care providers.
- Identify the cues and hypotheses that may indicate a need for psychotropic medications.
- Identify environmental and individual factors that increase the complexity of the use of all medications management in older persons.

THE LIVED EXPERIENCE

It is so hard to keep track of my medications. I try arranging them in little cups to take with each meal, but then there are the ones that I take at odd times. Those are the easiest to forget. I think sometimes that I have taken them twice and then it feels like I must be going crazy. I really wish I didn't have to take so many pills, but I'm not sure what would happen if I stopped all of them. I don't even know why I'm taking most of them.

Geraldo, with hypertension, diabetes, and cardiac disease

In the United States, persons 65 years of age and older are prescribed more medications than any other age group. Although the exact statistics vary among studies, all findings indicate that as people age, the number of prescribed medications, dietary supplements, and herbal products taken increases. When used appropriately, the outcomes of using such products and prescription medications may include improved survival and enhanced quality of life for those with chronic conditions and disabilities. When they are used inappropriately, they threaten even the most basic level of physiological stability. However, at times, even when drugs are used appropriately, they may adversely affect health outcomes. Many factors influence how and when prescribed medicines and other bioactive products are used.

Gerontological nurses have a responsibility to help minimize the risks and maximize the safety of medication use in the persons who receive their care. They must watch for the very earliest cues that suggest either misuse or adverse events. A review of the effects of aging on drug pharmacokinetics and pharmacodynamics and the occurrence of medication-related problems in older adults is presented in this chapter. The final section addresses the use of psychotropic agents. These are frequently prescribed to those who are frail and have the potential for both great benefit and significant risk, thereby requiring special attention.

PHARMACOKINETICS

The term *pharmacokinetics* refers to the movement of a medication in the body from the point of administration to excretion. During this process they are absorbed, distributed, and metabolized. There is no conclusive evidence of an appreciable change in overall pharmacokinetics with aging; however, several normal age-related physiological changes have implications for safe drug use in later life (Fig. 9.1). These changes significantly increase the risk of adverse reactions or unpredictable effects.

This chapter is not intended to replace a pharmacology text, but to supplement it for the key associations between safe medication use and the aging process.

Absorption

For a drug to be effective it must be absorbed into the bloodstream. The amount of time between the administration of the drug and its absorption depends on several factors, including the route of introduction (i.e., intravenous, oral, parenteral, transdermal, or rectal) and the bioavailability and dose of the medication. The drug is delivered immediately to the bloodstream when administered by the intravenous route and is quickly delivered when using parenteral and transdermal routes

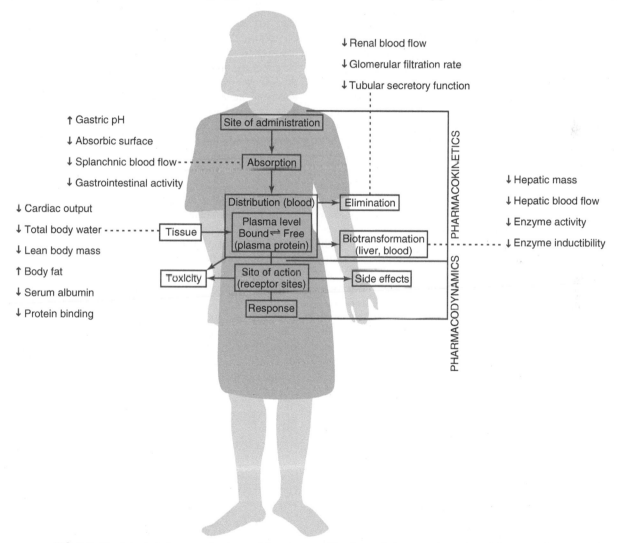

FIG. 9.1 Physiological changes of aging and the pharmacokinetics and pharmacodynamics of drug use. (Data from Kane, R. L., Ouslander, J. G., Abrass, I. B. (1984). *Essentials of clinical geriatrics.* New York: McGraw-Hill; Lamy, P. P. (1984). Hazards of drug use in the elderly: Commonsense measures to reduce them, *Postgrad Med 76*(1),50–53; Vestal, R. E., Dawson, G. W. (1985). Pharmacology and aging. In C. E. Finch, E. L. Schneider, (Eds). *Handbook of biology and aging.* New York: Van Nostrand Reinhold; Roberts, J., Tumer, N. (1988). Pharmacodynamic basis for altered drug action in the elderly, *Clin Geriatr Med 4*(1),127–149.; Montamat, S. C., Cusack, B. J., Vestal, R. E. (1989). Management of drug therapy in the elderly, *N Engl J Med 321*(5), 303–309.)

or when mucous membranes, such as the rectum and the oral mucosa, are utilized. Compared with other routes of administration, orally administered drugs are absorbed the most slowly, especially those with enteric coatings.

The increased gastric pH of the aging stomach retards the action of acid-dependent medications. Delayed emptying diminishes or negates the absorption and therefore the effectiveness of short-lived drugs; they could become inactivated before reaching the small intestine. Enteric-coated medications such as aspirin are specifically designed to bypass the stomach and be absorbed in the small intestine. If absorption of these products is delayed, gastric irritation or nausea may result. Absorption in the older body is also influenced by changes in gastrointestinal motility. If there is increased motility in the small intestine, the effect of the drug is diminished because of shortened contact time, resulting in decreased absorption and effectiveness. Conversely, slowed intestinal motility, common in aging, increases the contact time, amount absorbed, and effect.

Distribution

When a drug is absorbed it must be transported to the receptor site on a targeted organ to have the desired effect. Distribution depends on the availability of plasma protein in the form of lipoproteins, globulins, and especially albumin. As drugs are absorbed, they bind with the protein and are distributed throughout the body. Normally, a predictable percentage of the absorbed drug is inactivated as it binds to a protein. The remaining free drug is available in the blood and has a therapeutic effect when an adequate concentration is reached in the plasma. Most older adults have an insignificant reduction of serum albumin. However, the presence of albumin may become dramatically reduced in those who are frail, have an inadequate diet, or have reduced protein intake. Low serum albumin levels are found in many adults needing long-term care, have dementia, or are socially isolated. When this occurs, toxic levels of available free drug may accumulate in the blood-stream unpredictably, especially highly protein-bound medications (because protein is not available) with narrow therapeutic windows, such as levothyroxine, phenytoin (Dilantin), and warfarin (Ruscin & Linnebur, 2018).

Potential alterations of medication distribution in late life are also related to changes in body composition, particularly decreased lean body mass, increased body fat, and decreased total body water (see Fig. 9.1). Decreased body water leads to higher relative serum levels of water-soluble drugs, such as lithium, digoxin, ethanol, and aminoglycosides. With extended diarrhea, vomiting, or other conditions leading to dehydration, increased serum levels can quickly lead to toxicity.

Adipose tissue nearly doubles in older men and increases by one-half in older women. Drugs that are highly lipid-soluble are stored in the fatty tissue, extending and possibly elevating their effect. This affects drugs such as lorazepam, diazepam, chlorpromazine, phenobarbital, and haloperidol. If the medication accumulates in excess, it may result in an accidental and potentially fatal overdose (Hughes & Beizer, 2014).

Metabolism

Metabolism (biotransformation) is the process by which the body modifies the chemical structure of the drug. The compound is converted to a metabolite that is later more easily excreted. A drug will continue to exert a therapeutic effect as long as it remains either in its original state or as an "active" metabolite. Active metabolites retain the ability to have a therapeutic effect, as well as the same or a greater chance of causing adverse effects. For example, the metabolites of acetaminophen (e.g. Tylenol) can cause liver damage with higher dosages (>4 g/24 h or more than eight extra-strength products in any 24-hour period). The duration of drug action is determined by the metabolic rate and is measured in terms of half-life, or the length of time one-half of the drug remains active in the body. Because of the unpredictable nature of drug metabolism in the older body, it is probably safer to consider 3 g of acetaminophen in 24 hours (from all sources) as the maximum dosage. This is reached rapidly with the popular formulations of "extra strength" 500-mg tablets.

A number of enzymes play an active part in drug metabolism with one of these (CYP2D6) acting on one-quarter of all medications. An individual's age, weight, sex, and liver and kidney function affect the availability of enzymes and metabolism (Box 9.1).

The liver is the primary site of drug metabolism. With aging, the liver's activity, mass, volume, and blood flow are reduced and hepatic clearance may decrease by up to

BOX 9.1   Focus on Genomics

Pharmacogenomics (also called pharmacogenetics) is a field of research focused on understanding how genes affect the body's response to medications. Genes may explain why some people have side effects from some medications and others do not. They may even determine why one medication works on one person and not another. One gene, CYP2D6, has been found to act on 25% of all prescription drugs, including the painkiller codeine, which it converts into the drug's active form, morphine. The long-term goal of pharmacogenomics is to provide information ensuring that both the medication and the dosage best suit the individual.

From National Institute of General Medical Sciences. (2020). *Pharmacogenomics.* https://www.nigms.nih.gov/education/fact-sheets/Pages/pharmacogenomics.aspx.

TABLE 9.1 Drugs to Watch: Examples of Commonly Used Medications Affected by Normal Changes With Aging

Class or Category	Affected by Decreased Hepatic Metabolism	Affected by Decreased Renal Excretion
Analgesic/ anti-inflammatory	Nonsteroidal anti-inflammatories such as naproxen and ibuprofen[a] Morphine	
Antibiotics		Cipro Macrobid
Cardiovascular	Amlodipine (Norvasc) Diltiazem (Cardizem) Verapamil (Calan)	Captopril (Capoten) Digoxin (Lanoxin) Enalapril (Vasotec) Lisinopril (Zestril)
Diuretics		Furosemide (Lasix) Hydrochlorothiazide (HCTZ)
Others	Levodopa	Glyburide Ranitidine (Axid)
Psychoactive drugs	Alprazolam (Xanax) Diazepam (Valium) Trazodone	Risperidone

[a]See Box 9.14 for FDA warning related to the use of NSAIDs.

30% to 40% (Ruscin & Linnebur, 2018). These changes result in a potential decrease in the liver's ability to metabolize drugs such as benzodiazepines (e.g., the tranquilizer lorazepam [Ativan]) (Table 9.1). This reduction in liver function results in a significant increase in the half-life of these drugs. For example, the half-life of diazepam (Valium) in a younger adult is about 37 hours, but in an older adult it may extend up to 96 hours (Ruscin & Linnebur, 2018). If the dose and timing are not adjusted, drugs can accumulate and the administration of a single dose can have significantly more effects (and longer) than those found in a younger person. It is never appropriate to prescribe Valium to anyone older than 65 years (American Geriatrics Society [AGS], 2019).

Excretion

Drugs and their metabolites are excreted in sweat, saliva, and other secretions, but their primary site of excretion is through the kidneys. However, because kidney function declines significantly with aging (up to a 50% decrease by the time one is 80 years old), so does the ability to excrete or eliminate drugs in a timely manner.

The considerably decreased glomerular filtration rate (GFR) further prolongs the half-life of drugs and the amount of time required to eliminate the drug, adding to the risk of accumulation and increasing the potential for toxicity or other adverse events. Renal function can be estimated through the calculation of the serum creatinine clearance rate (CrCl). Reductions in dosages for drugs excreted by the kidneys (e.g., allopurinol, vancomycin) are needed when the CrCl is reduced. Reductions in dosages may also be necessary when the patient is very ill or dehydrated. Although there are several nomograms and algorithms available to estimate CrCl, the Cockcroft-Gault equation is thought to be the most reliable tool to use for those at the extremes of age or with active diseases (Hughes & Beizer, 2014).

Estimated creatinine clearance rate (the Cockcroft-Gault equation):

$$\frac{(140 - age) \times wt(kg)(\times 0.85 \text{ only if female})}{(serum creatinine \times 72)}$$

For automatic calculators, see http://www.nephron.com/cgi-bin/CGSI.cgi or search "CrCl calculator."

PHARMACODYNAMICS

Pharmacodynamics refers to the interaction between a drug and the body (see Fig. 9.1). The older the person becomes, the more likely there will be an altered or unreliable response of the body to the drug. Although it is not always possible to explain the change in response, several mechanisms are known. For example, the aging process causes a decreased response to beta-adrenergic receptor stimulators and blockers; decreased baroreceptor sensitivity; and increased sensitivity to a number of medications, especially anticholinergics, benzodiazepines, narcotic analgesics, warfarin, and the cardiac drugs diltiazem and verapamil (Rochon et al., 2020).

CHRONOPHARMACOLOGY

The relationship between the biological rhythms of the body and variations in pharmacokinetics and pharmacodynamics is referred to as chronopharmacology (Dallmann et al., 2014). For example, if a cortisone tablet (e.g., from a Medrol dose pack) is taken in the early morning, it may have little or no effect on the adrenocortical system. If the same dose is taken in divided amounts over the day as labeled, unwanted effects of the drug may suppress the hormonal activities stemming from the hypothalamus-pituitary-adrenal axis.

As noted earlier, absorption is influenced by the pH of gastric acid, the level of motility of the gastrointestinal tract, and the degree of blood flow. All have been shown to have biorhythmical variations. Distribution of protein-bound drugs depends on levels of albumin and glyco-proteins produced by the liver. During the day, albumin levels are high, but they are low in the early morning. Drug metabolism is also biorhythmical because of changes in the liver over the course of the day. Renal elimination depends on kidney perfusion, glomerular filtration, and urine acidity and has shown rhythmi-cal variation. The brain, the heart, and blood cells have also been found to have varied rhythmicity, resulting in a cyclical response for beta blockers, calcium channel blockers, angiotensin-converting enzyme (ACE) inhibi-tors, nitrates, and other similar drugs (Table 9.2).

TABLE 9.2 Chronopharmacology: Rhythmical Influences on Disease and Physiological Processes

Disease or Process	Rhythmical Influence
Allergic rhinitis	Symptoms worse in the morning
Arterial blood pressure	Circadian surge in the morning hours
Asthma	Greatest respiratory distress overnight (during sleeping) Symptoms peak in early morning (4–5 a.m.)
Blood plasma volume	Plasma volume falls at night; thus, hematocrit increases
Cancer	Tumor cells proliferate when normal cell miosis is low
Cardiac disease	Angina, myocardial infarction, thrombolytic stroke most often occur in the first 4 hours after waking (peak 9–10 a.m.) (Prinzmetal's angina—during sleep)
Catecholamines	Increase in early morning
Fibrinolytic activity	Increases in early morning
Gastric system	Gastric acid secretion peaks every morning (2–4 a.m.); annual pattern—incidence of gastric ulcers greater in winter
Osteoarthritis	Pain more severe in morning
Platelet activation	May result from abnormality in circadian rhythm, which affects cortisol levels, body temperature, sleep–wake cycle
Potassium excretion	Lowest in morning; highest in late afternoon
Rheumatoid arthritis	Pain more severe in late afternoon
Systemic insulin level	Highest in afternoon

As more is learned about chronotherapeutics, the potential for decreasing individual doses of medications and/or the frequency of administration is present. When we can do so we will be able to decrease the potential for adverse drug events significantly, while maximiz-ing therapeutic effects. Research has begun to produce promising results of understanding potential changes in circadian rhythm in aging (Li et al., 2018).

MEDICATION-RELATED PROBLEMS AND OLDER ADULTS

Polypharmacy

Polypharmacy has been defined as the use of approx-imately five or more medications or the use of mul-tiple medications for the same problem (Fig. 9.2). In a representative American sample of 2206 adults 62–85 years of age and living in the community, 87% used at least one prescription item and 36% used five or more and 38% also used over the counter medica-tions (Rochon et al., 2020). Kim and Parish (2017) concluded that when five or more medications were taken, for each additional medication there was a sig-nificantly increased risk for the development of frailty, disability, death, and falls. If the patient has multiple

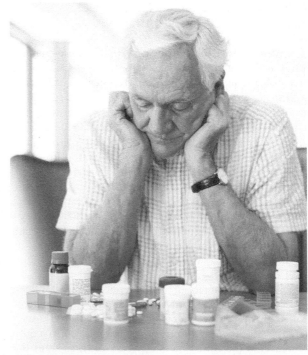

FIG. 9.2 Polypharmacy. (From © iStock.com/Squaredpixels.)

chronic conditions, simple polypharmacy may be necessary, even if the prescribing provider is following evidence-based guidelines. It may occur unintentionally, especially if an existing medication regimen is not considered when new prescriptions are given or if any number of the hundreds of over the counter (OTC) preparations, supplements, and herbs are added to those prescribed. Polypharmacy may occur "accidentally" if an existing drug regimen is not considered when new medications are prescribed.

The likelihood of polypharmacy is exacerbated by the combination of multiple health care specialists and a reluctance of prescribers to discontinue potentially unnecessary medications that have been prescribed by someone else. This can lead to the continued use of medications that may no longer be necessary (Rochon et al., 2020). When communication between patients, nurses, other health care providers, and caregivers becomes fragmented, the risk of duplicative medications, inappropriate medications, potentially unsafe dosages, and potentially preventable interactions is heightened. The two major concerns with polypharmacy are the increased risk of drug interactions and the increased risk of adverse events.

Drug Interactions

An interaction may result in altered pharmacokinetic activity, that is, alterations in the absorption, distribution, metabolism, or excretion of one or any of the medications. Absorption can be delayed by drugs exerting an anticholinergic effect, a particular danger for frail older adults. More than one drug may compete to occupy the necessary binding receptors simultaneously, preventing one of the drugs from reliably reaching the target organs and creating a varied bioavailability of one or both drugs.

The more medications a person takes, the greater the possibility that one or more of them will interact with each other, with an herbal product, with a nutritional supplement, with food, or with alcohol. When two or more medications or foods are taken together or close together, the drugs may potentiate one another; that is, one may increase the effectiveness of the other.

Medication–Herb/Supplement Interactions

As the popularity of medicinal herbs and other dietary supplements rises, so does the risk of interactions with prescribed medications. In a study of 369 persons 60–99 years of age, 10 of the 22 supplements used had potential interaction with their prescription medications (Rochon et al., 2020). Although much remains unknown, new knowledge is added almost daily to that which the gerontological nurse uses in the observation of cues and analyses. For example, many herbs and some vitamins have a direct effect on coagulability. When these are taken with warfarin (Coumadin or Jantoven), the risk of bleeding increases significantly. The interactions presented in Table 9.3 represent only a small fraction of the many real and potential problems in prescribing medications and caring for persons who take an herb or a dietary supplement in addition to prescribed medications.

Medication–Food Interactions

Many foods interact with medications, producing increased, decreased, or variable effects such as inhibiting absorption (Table 9.4). For example, the calcium in dairy products will bind to levothyroxine, ferrous sulfate, tetracycline, and ciprofloxacin, greatly decreasing their absorption; lovastatin absorption is increased by a high-fat, low-fiber meal. All of these are medications frequently prescribed to older adults. Grapefruit juice contains substances that inhibit CYP3A4-mediated metabolism in the gut and bind with the statins used for cholesterol-lowering medications, clopidogrel, and many antibiotics. When a bisphosphonate (e.g., Fosamax) is taken with food of any kind, the absorption is reduced to only a few milligrams, and therefore the drug has no effect on the target organ, the bones.

The vitamin K in leafy green vegetables antagonizes (decreases) the anticoagulant effects of warfarin and may have a significant effect on the coagulability of the blood reducing its effect of decreasing strokes. It is recommended that patients taking warfarin pay close attention to the regularity of their diet and especially green vegetables to avoid variations in their warfarin levels (Box 9.2).

Spironolactone, prescribed for end-stage heart failure, increases potassium (K^+) reabsorption. If a patient's diet is high in potassium (e.g., KCl salt substitute, molasses, oranges, bananas) or if other potassium-sparing agents (e.g., Lisinopril) are taken at the same time, K^+ levels can rise significantly and quickly reach toxic levels.

BOX 9.2 Top 10 Foods to Avoid When Taking Warfarin

Kale	Turnip greens
Spinach	Parsley
Collards	Broccoli
Swiss chard	Brussels sprouts
Mustard greens	

For expanded list and patient information, see https://www.mayoclinic.org/diseases-conditions/thrombophlebitis/expert-answers/warfarin/faq-20058443.

TABLE 9.3 Selected[a] Herb–Medication and Herb–Disease Interactions Especially Relevant in the Lives of Older Adults

Herb	Medication	Complication	Nursing Action
Garlic	Antihypertensives	Increased hypotensive effect	Advise provider approval with use
	Antivirals, such as ritonavir	Altered drug effect	Advise against use
	Antimetabolites such as cyclosporine	Risk of less effective response	Advise against use
	Insulin or oral hypoglycemic agent such as pioglitazone or tolbutamide	Serum glucose level control may improve; less antidiabetic drug needed	Monitor blood glucose levels
Ginkgo	Antidiabetic drugs: insulin, oral DMT2 drugs such as metformin	May alter blood glucose levels	Monitor blood glucose level closely
	Antidepressants, MAOIs, SSRIs	May cause abnormal response or decrease effectiveness	Advise not to take with these drugs
	Antihypertensives	May cause increased effect	Monitor blood pressure
	Antiseizure drugs	Risk for seizure if history of seizure	Advise against use
	Insulin and oral antidiabetic drugs	Blood glucose levels may be altered	Monitor blood glucose levels closely
Ginseng	MAOIs such as isocarboxazid	Headaches, tremors, mania	Advise against use
St John's Wort	Antihypertensives, cardiac drugs such as calcium channel blockers	May alter effects of drug	Advise against use unless provider monitors closely
	Immunosuppressants	May interfere with action	Advise against use
	Stimulants	May cause additive effect	Advise against use
	Digoxin	Decreases effects of the drug	Advise against use
	Alprazolam	May decrease effect of drug	Advise against use
	Tramadol and some SSRIs	May increase risk of serotonin syndrome	Advise against use
	Olanzapine	May cause serotonin syndrome	Advise against use
	Paroxetine	Sedative-hypnotic intoxication	Advise against use
	Theophylline or Albuterol	Increases metabolism; decreases drug blood level	Monitor drug effects
	Amlodipine	Lowers efficacy of calcium channel	Advise against use
	Antivirals	May alter drug effects	FDA advises avoidance of this herb for patients taking these drugs
	Warfarin	Potential for increased bleeding	Advise against use

[a]The interactions listed represent only a few of the possible herb-drug interactions.

AIDS, Acquired immunodeficiency syndrome; *DMT2,* diabetes mellitus type 2; *FDA,* US Food and Drug Administration; *HIV,* human immunodeficiency virus; *HMG-CoA,* 3-hydroxy-3-methylglutaryl coenzyme-A; *MAOIs,* monoamine oxidase inhibitors; *NSAIDs,* nonsteroidal anti-inflammatory drugs; *SSRIs,* selective serotonin reuptake inhibitors.

Data from Asher, G. N., Corbett, A. H., & Hawke, R. L. (2017). Common herbal dietary supplement-drug interactions, *Am Fam Physician,* 96(2), 101–107. Websites for NIH: Office of Dietary Supplements ods.od.nih.gov; National Center for Complementary and Integrative Health nccih.nih.gov.

TABLE 9.4 Common Drug–Food Interactions

Food	Drug	Potential Effect
Fiber	Digoxin	Absorption of drug into fiber, reducing drug action
Foods with vitamin K	Warfarin	Decreased effect of drug
Any food	Many antibiotics	Reduced absorption rate of drug
Grapefruit juice	Multiple medications	Altered metabolism and elimination can increase concentration of drug
Citrus juice	Calcium channel blockers	Gastric reflux exacerbated

BOX 9.3 Tips for Best Practice

Examples of Potential Medication–Medication Adverse Interactions

ACE inhibitors and potassium-sparing diuretics
ACE inhibitors or ARBs and Septra (Bactrim)
Macrolide antibiotics (e.g., Cipro) and either calcium channel blockers or digoxin
Warfarin and any of the antibiotics or NSAIDs

ACE, Angiotensin-converting enzyme; *ARB*, alpha-receptor blocker; *NSAIDs*, nonsteroidal anti-inflammatory drugs.
From Hines, L. E., Murphy, J. E. (2011). Potentially harmful drug-drug interactions in the elderly. A review, *Am J Geriatr Pharmacother 9*(6), 364–377.

Drug–Drug Interactions

Many medications commonly prescribed to older adults can affect the absorption of other drugs. Antacids or iron preparations affect the availability of some drugs for absorption by binding the drug with elements and forming chemical compounds.

The polypharmacy that may be a necessary part of health care in later life significantly increases both the risk and the frequency of medication–medication or medication–herb interactions (Boxes 9.3 and 9.4). These may occur at any time from preparation to excretion. This can be especially dangerous for older adults when two or more drugs with the same effect are additive; that is, together they are more potent than when taken separately. Unless attention is paid to the components of the overall drug list, the time when each drug is administered, and the other products that are taken (such as OTC medications, herbs, vitamins, and other supplements), an adverse drug event can occur.

For example, persons who cannot swallow after a stroke may receive all feedings and medications via the enteral route. Medications intended for oral administration must be converted to a soluble form for unobstructed passage through the tube and yet also remain in their original form. When several medications are crushed, mixed together, and then dissolved in water for administration, a new product is created, and medication–medication interactions may have already begun. The nurse decreases the likelihood of this happening by monitoring the medications he or she administers and encouraging persons to do the same.

BOX 9.4 Herbs to Avoid When Taking Any Anticoagulant

Echinacea	Ginseng
Garlic	Green tea
Gingko	

Adverse Drug Reactions

Polypharmacy, reduced organ function and physiological reserve (Chapter 5), and varying levels of skills of health care providers put older adults at greater risk than younger adults of adverse drug reactions (ADRs) and adverse drug events (ADEs) (Barclay et al., 2018). An ADR is an unwanted pharmacological effect such as a minor rash or nausea. When a reaction reaches the level of harm, it is referred to as an *adverse drug event* and includes adverse drug withdrawal and therapeutic failures. Many of these must be reported to the US Food and Drug Administration or other regulatory bodies.

ADRs are most common in those over 65 years of age. People in this age group are at greater risk of both ADE and ADR because of age-related changes in metabolism and decreased drug clearance. The signs and symptoms are both typical and atypical. They can sometimes be predicted from the pharmacological action of the drug (e.g., bleeding from warfarin) and can also occur when a patient is started on a drug at a dosage that is inappropriately high. ADRs can also occur when a patient takes a medication that necessitates laboratory monitoring (e.g., lithium, Coumadin) and adjustment of dosage is needed but this is not done for whatever reason. Between 2007 and 2009, nearly two-thirds of the hospitalizations among persons 65 years and older were related to accidental overdoses. Four medications made up 67% of the hospitalizations: warfarin, insulins, antiplatelet medications, and oral hypoglycemic agents (Rochon et al., 2020).

One of the most troublesome ADRs for older adults is drug-induced delirium. Polypharmacy with several psychoactive drugs exerting anticholinergic actions is perhaps the greatest precipitator of delirium. Too often it is unrecognized as an ADR and instead is viewed as a worsening of preexisting dementia or even new-onset dementia (see Chapter 25). Any time there is a change in a person's cognitive abilities or mental status, the possibility of a drug effect must be thoroughly evaluated (Box 9.5).

Another common adverse effect seen in older adults is lethargy, especially with the use of a number of the cardiovascular agents and antidepressants. Like confusion, lethargy can also be misinterpreted as a symptom

BOX 9.5 Examples of Medications That Can Easily Impair Cognitive Function in Older Adults

Analgesics	Benzodiazepines
Those with anticholinergics properties	Antiparkinsonian medications
Antihistamines	Beta blockers
	Lanoxin

of decline in cardiac, respiratory, or neurological conditions rather than as an ADR.

Although ADRs and ADEs continue to occur, there has been considerable progress in the development of strategies to reduce their likelihood, especially in the recognition of the age-related pharmacokinetic and pharmacodynamic changes in later life. We now know that an older adult should be prescribed lower dosages of several medications, especially when they are first prescribed. To minimize the likelihood of an ADR, the dose can be slowly increased until it safely reaches a therapeutic level. A common adage related to medication dosing in older adults is "Start low, go slow, but go." There has also been a recognition that the risk of ADEs is so high with some medications that the drugs are simply not recommended for use in persons as they age.

Misuse of Drugs

The more drugs taken, the more likely misuse will occur. Forms of drug misuse include overuse, underuse, erratic use, and contraindicated use. Misuse can occur for any number of reasons, from inadequate skills of the nurse or the prescriber to inadequate funds to purchase prescribed medications. It is likely if there is inadequate patient/caregiver education. Although this is often referred to as noncompliance or nonadherence, "misuse" is a term that is more descriptive of what is happening. For older adults without medication insurance coverage, such as older recent immigrants, the cost of necessary medication may be prohibitive.

Misuse by patients may be accidental, which often occurs through misunderstanding or inability to read labels or understand instructions (Box 9.6). It may be deliberate, such as in an attempt to make a prescription last longer for financial reasons or because of beliefs that the dose is either too low or too high or that the medication prescribed is the wrong/inappropriate treatment (see Chapter 2).

When a patient is labeled as noncompliant, the nurse and other health care personnel may become exasperated

and angry at the individual for his or her failure to follow the established plan of care. In an attempt to help and do what they think is best for the patient, the nurse and other care providers tend to forget or ignore that some people cannot and will not comply with a prescription or treatment plan under certain circumstances, such as when it is incompatible with the person's daily life. For example, the individual cannot follow the instruction "take medication three times per day with meals" if he or she eats only two meals each day.

Memory failures affect drug misuse in two major ways: forgetting how to take medications correctly and forgetting the correct time(s) to take medications, which is called "prospective" recall failure. The more frequently a medication must be taken, the less anyone will comply. With an increasing number of medications available in once-daily dosing rather than three or four times each day, we can expect more people to take their medications as instructed.

Problems with health literacy also limit the ability to take medications correctly. Many older adults, especially those from minority groups or new immigrants, are more likely to have low levels of literacy or no English literacy; written instructions should be at the third-grade level or below (see http://www.pfizerhealthliteracy.com). Limitations in vision will interfere with reading instructions, especially of bottle labels. The pharmacist can be asked to use large type or symbols. The tendency of nurses and physicians to give rapid-fire directions is not effective when addressing most persons, especially those with hearing impairments or with the normal age-related need for slightly slower verbalizations. In addition, the use of ambiguous terms such as "slowly increase" or "only in moderation" leads to further opportunities for misuse.

Unfortunately, it is also common for nurses to explain the treatment and give directions concerning medications when the patient is physically uncomfortable or is about to be discharged from a care facility; to explain in English even when the person has limited English proficiency; or to explain in a noisy or busy place. Background noise or an unfamiliar accent of the nurse can significantly reduce comprehension for those with normal age-related hearing loss (see Chapter 19).

BOX 9.6   A Potentially Lethal Misunderstanding

I was making a visit to Mrs. Helena to enroll her in a research study. As we were reviewing her health and current medications, she shared that she had not been feeling well and thought it was her heart, and that she had been told to "take the little white pills" until she felt better. When I looked at her pill bottle, she had already taken five or more digoxin in the space of about 2 hours. I called an ambulance.

Potentially Inappropriate Medications: The "Beers Criteria"

The appropriate use of medications in older adults means that such products are used only as needed, at the minimum dose necessary to achieve the desired effects, and in a way the risks relative to benefits have been considered within the greater context of the person's life expectancy, health, lifestyle, and values. Beers published a list of "potentially inappropriate medications (PIMs)" for the nursing home setting in 1997 (Beers, 1997). It was expanded several times to cover all care settings and most recently by the American Geriatrics Society (Box 9.7) (AGS, 2019).

The Beers Criteria list is the result of an exhaustive analysis of medications frequently prescribed to older adults. The 2019 list includes medications that (1) are potentially inappropriate for use with all older adults, (2) are potentially inappropriate for older adults with certain conditions, (3) should only be used with caution, (4) should be avoided or have their dose changed for people with impaired renal function, and (5) are on a list of drug–drug interactions documented to be especially harmful to older adults. The most common potentially inappropriate medications are the NSAIDS (Rochon et al., 2020). The American Geriatric Society has created a list of alternatives that is intended to be used along the use of the Beers List (HealthinAging, 2019).

Although the Beers Criteria have been incorporated into regulatory policy, the authors of the 2019 document emphasize the need to use it as a guide rather than absolute direction. The Beers Criteria are a part of the quality measures for the National Committee for Quality Assurance (NCQA) and the Healthcare Effectiveness Data and Information Set (HEDIS) (NCQA, 2019). When a potentially inappropriate medication is prescribed in the long-term care setting without documentation of an overwhelming benefit of its use, it can be considered a form of medication misuse by the prescribing practitioner. In a study of primary care, a prevalence was found in more than one-third of the over 5 million participants, explaining between 7.7 and 17.3% of adverse outcomes (Liew et al., 2020). The use of PIMs has been found to be associated with confusion, falls, other syndromes, and death.

At the same time, in a study of 6427 older adults seen in emergency rooms in Germany for ADR, 1253 were preventable. Although risk factors were identified (especially age 70 years and over), the use of PIMs list was found to be of limited value in increasing safety for the patient (Schmiedl et al., 2018).

PSYCHOACTIVE MEDICATIONS

Psychoactive medications are those that affect neuropsychiatric function, which in turn affects behavior and how the world is experienced. A gerontological nurse, especially one working in a long-term care setting, is likely to be responsible for older adults who are receiving psychoactive medications, especially those for the treatment of depression, anxiety, and psychosis (see Chapter 24).

Medications with psychoactive properties have a higher than usual risk of adverse events in older adults and must be prescribed and administered with an acute awareness of how age-related changes in absorption, distribution, excretion, and hepatic function affect their overall serum concentration. When the person is frail or has multiple comorbidities, the risk of accidental injuries and other adverse effects is even higher (Box 9.8). Some studies indicate that 17% of those admitted to a long-term care facility were prescribed an antipsychotic within 100 days of admission and 24% within one year (Rochon et al., 2020).

In 1987, the Health Care Financing Administration mandated that residents of long-term care settings may only be prescribed psychotropic drugs for specific diseases or symptoms and that the use be monitored,

BOX 9.8   Tips for Best Practice
Psychotropic Drugs

Mrs. Jones suffered from dementia that was progressing rapidly. She eventually had to be moved to a "Memory Unit" where she could be cared for closely. She began attempting to hit other residents for "stealing her things" and the staff when they paid attention to anyone else. When these behaviors began to be accompanied by hallucinations, she was in danger of retaliation by other residents and they were in danger of being injured. She stopped eating because she felt that she was being poisoned. Her provider determined that a prompt response was needed to assure the safety of all. While we were waiting for the urine analysis, CMP, and CBC, she was given the antipsychotic Seroquel beginning at a slightly higher starting dose than usual. She quickly "calmed down," sleeping soundly after several nights and days awake. On the second day she fell and fortunately did not have an injury. Her laboratory findings indicated slight dehydration and anemia but no infection. Her Seroquel was held for several days and restarted at the lowest dose possible. She returned to her baseline, highly argumentative but without the delusions.

reduced, or eliminated when possible. Prescribing physicians and nurse practitioners may use them only if documentation reasonably explains the rationale for the benefit with a goal of restoring function or preventing dangerous behavior (Omnibus Budget Reconciliation Act [OBRA], 1987). Since that time, the concern over the potential misuse of psychotropic medications or their effects continues to grow. For example, at one time an atypical antipsychotic such as risperidone was commonly prescribed for the patient with dementia who exhibited neuropsychiatric symptoms, especially agitation.

A patient should be prescribed a psychotropic medication only after thorough medical, psychological, and social assessments (Chapter 8). Nursing assessment before pharmacological intervention contributes knowledge and baseline information that can optimize the patient's medical and psychological improvement and perhaps minimize the duration of the need for the psychotropic. At the same time, assessments should be done quickly to enable the patient to receive the appropriate treatment as soon as possible when nonpharmacological approaches have not worked adequately (Chapter 24). The hypotheses leading to the use of a psychotropic medications will include information drawn from the medical record and medication review as well as the analyses of cues regarding health status, mental status, ability to carry out activities of daily living, and ability to participate in social activities and maintain satisfying relationships with others, as well as the potential for patient or caregiver compliance with any pharmacological or nonpharmacological recommendations.

Gerontological nurses, especially those working in a long-term care setting, are very likely to care for older adults with psychiatric and cognitive problems, especially dementia, depression, anxiety, and psychosis. The rate of depression in older persons living in the community is significant and even more so for those living in long-term care facilities (see Chapter 24). Anxiety is also common and when anxiety is treated with benzodiazepines, plasma levels are higher than seen in younger adults increasing an older person's risk of adverse effects and drug interactions. These should never be used with opioids (Rochon et al., 2020).

Finally, a small group of older adults, especially those with neurological conditions such as any one of the dementias, may develop psychosis at some time in their illnesses. Psychosis is also seen in delirium from an infection or from an ADR and in older adults with schizophrenia. Persons with psychoses are often treated with antipsychotics that require special attention and skills from the gerontological nurse in cooperation with a psychiatrist or a psychiatric nurse practitioner specializing in geriatrics (see Chapter 24).

BOX 9.9   Potential Anticholinergic Side Effects in Older Adults

Memory impairment	Nausea
Confusion	Urinary retention
Hallucinations	Impaired sweating
Dry mouth	Tachycardia
Blurred vision	Hospitalization
Constipation	Falls

Antidepressants

Antidepressants, as the name implies, are medications used to treat depression. In the past, the major drugs used were monoamine oxidase inhibitors (MAOIs) and tricyclic antidepressants (TCAs) (e.g., amitriptyline, doxepin). These drugs required high doses to be effective and had significant anticholinergic side (Box 9.9). Since the development of the selective serotonin reuptake inhibitors (SSRIs), serotonin-norepinephrine reuptake inhibitors (SNRIs), and several other medications, the MAOIs and TCAs are rarely prescribed for the treatment of depression in older adults. They may still be prescribed to those who have taken them since earlier in their lives.

The SSRIs (e.g., Zoloft, Prozac, Lexapro, Celexa) have been found to be highly effective, with minimal or manageable side effects, and are the drugs of choice for older adults. Most of these medications cause initial problems with nausea or dry mouth. Although often effective, these must be used with caution, especially with regard to serum sodium levels. The SSRIs should also be used with caution in persons with a history of falls because of the potential to produce ataxia or dizziness (AGS, 2019). One side effect of the SSRIs that does not resolve with time, if experienced, is sexual dysfunction. For older adults who are sexually active, alternatives to the SSRIs are more appropriate, such as bupropion. When sleep is a problem, the patient may be prescribed a low dose of the tetracyclic antidepressant mirtazapine (Remeron), which is often well tolerated in older adults and may also increase appetite. It can increase agitation and when stopped the nurse must observe carefully for cues related to side effects related to withdrawal. Trazodone is an antidepressant that also has sedating qualities that may be helpful. But it can cause orthostatic hypotension, has anticholinergic side effects, and interacts with several other medications. Many older adults are sensitive to these medications and may find significant relief from depression at low doses. Although it sometimes takes time to find the optimal dose, the nurse can help the person or caregiver to monitor target symptoms and advocate for continued dose adjustments or changes until relief is obtained rather than simply reducing the depression.

Antianxiety Agents

Drugs used to treat anxiety are referred to as *anxiolytics* or *antianxiety agents*. These agents include benzodiazepines, buspirone (BuSpar), and beta blockers. Antihistamines, especially diphenhydramine (Benadryl), are often self-administered (e.g., Tylenol PM) but *not recommended* because of their significant and highly dangerous anticholinergic effects. The decision to treat anxiety pharmacologically is based on the degree to which the anxiety interferes with the person's ability to function and subjective feelings of discomfort.

Older adults metabolize these drugs slowly and renal excretion is compromised. Even in health they persist in the bloodstream for long periods and can easily reach toxic levels more quickly than anticipated. Side effects include drowsiness, dizziness, ataxia, mild cognitive deficits, and memory impairment. Signs of toxicity include excessive sedation, unsteady gait, confusion, disorientation, cognitive impairment, memory impairment, agitation, and wandering. Because these symptoms resemble dementia, people can easily be misdiagnosed when they start taking benzodiazepines.

Benzodiazepines are highly addicting yet very popular with patients and nurses because of their quick sedating effects for the highly anxious or agitated person. However, because of the problems noted earlier they should be avoided except in extreme cases. If necessary, lorazepam (Ativan) appears to be the least problematic, when prescribed in very low doses and for short periods. It has the shortest half-life of the benzodiazepines and no active metabolites.

BuSpar (buspirone) is a safer alternative. Although dizziness is a side effect, it is often dose-related and resolves with time. It is not addictive and may have an additive effect to some of the SSRIs and lower doses can therefore be used. No therapeutic effect may be felt by the patient or observed by the nurse for 5 to 7 days and the drug may be mistakenly discontinued because of its apparent lack of effect. BuSpar is best used for chronic anxiety and is not indicated for acute needs.

Mood Stabilizers

Mood stabilizers are the group of agents used for the treatment of a bipolar disorder, which is uncontrollable fluctuations in mood. The most common mood stabilizers include lamotrigine (Lamictal), lithium, and valproic acid (Depakote). Along with these, the anticonvulsants carbamazepine (Tegretol) and gabapentin (Neurontin) are used as well as several of the atypical antipsychotics (e.g., Abilify, Zyprexa, and Seroquel) even when psychosis is not present. Each drug has a very individualized drug–drug interaction profile and several medications require blood level monitoring. A nurse who is caring for a patient with a bipolar disorder or for a patient who is taking a mood stabilizer should seek guidance from the person's psychiatrist regarding specific strategies to enhance the person's quality of life and information regarding the drug's need for laboratory testing and dosage monitoring. If the patient is taking lithium, this is especially important because lithium interacts with other medications and certain foods and has a narrow therapeutic window. For example, a low-salt diet will elevate the lithium level and a high-salt diet will decrease it; dehydration can occur quickly and result in life-threatening toxicity. Likewise, thiazide diuretics and nonsteroidal anti-inflammatory drugs (NSAIDs) will elevate the serum lithium level. Side effects include the following: confusion, disorientation, and memory loss; flattening of T waves on the electrocardiogram; polyuria and polydipsia; nausea, vomiting, and diarrhea; fine resting tremor; benign goiter; tardive dyskinesia; and ataxia. Lithium should only be prescribed by psychiatric nurse practitioners or psychiatrists who have special skills in caring for older adults.

Antipsychotics (Neuroleptics)

The term *psychosis* covers a range of cognitive and behavioral disorders that are based on responses of the ill person to a private reality—a reality that may be distressing and problematic for the patient and those around him or her. Characteristically, psychosis occurs in schizophrenia but can also occur in mania, depression, delirium, dementia, and paranoid states. When psychosis occurs in a person with dementia, it is often seen in a cluster of neuropsychiatric symptoms, especially agitation, physical aggression, and wandering.

Antipsychotics, formerly known as major tranquilizers are used to treat both psychosis, mood stabilization, and in situations where an older adult or those around them are at risk of injury (Pathak and Duff, 2018). They have been used "off-label" to reduce anxiety, depression, and agitation. Second-generation antipsychotics are referred to as atypical antipsychotics (e.g., risperidone [Risperdal], quetiapine [Seroquel], olanzapine [Zyprexa]). Because of their danger, especially risk of cardiovascular events, stroke, and even death, they are used as drugs of last resort and can only be prescribed following a careful assessment and search for any potential underlying cause of the problem. Inappropriate use of antipsychotic medications is a significant problem in long-term care settings. In addition to the risk of ADEs, they may mask a reversible cause for the problem, such as a thyroid disturbance, infection, dehydration, fever, electrolyte imbalance, an ADR, or a sudden change in the environment.

However, when no other approaches have been successful, they may be necessary and must be used very cautiously in true psychiatric disorders. Antipsychotics can provide a person with relief from what may be frightening and distressing symptoms. When they are used, the medications with the lowest side effects' profile, at the lowest dose possible, and for the shortest length of time should be prescribed. In most states the prescribing and use of antipsychotics in long-term care settings is carefully monitored. They can only be withdrawn slowly.

There are different classes and potencies of antipsychotics. First-generation antipsychotics (chlorpromazine [Thorazine], fluphenazine [Prolixin], thioridazine [Mellaril], and haloperidol [Haldol]) are less sedating than some of the second-generation drugs. However, they are considered inappropriate medications and are rarely used except in emergencies (AGS, 2019). Patients who take first-generation antipsychotic medications are more susceptible to developing extrapyramidal reactions, particularly neuroleptic-induced Parkinsonian symptoms and orthostatic hypotension. In older adults this means an increased risk of falls, sedation, orthostatic hypotension, medication-induced psychosis, and weight gain (Pathak & Duff, 2018). A permanent side effect for this class of antipsychotics is tardive dyskinesia (see later section).

Neuroleptic Malignant Syndrome

A rare but potentially life-threatening ADE to antipsychotics is neuroleptic malignant syndrome (NMS). The most typical physical cues are temperature greater than 100.4°F, muscle rigidity, autonomic instability (e.g., labile blood pressure, tachycardia), and altered mental status. Onset is rapid and unless treated appropriately death can occur quickly. The drug most associated with NMS is haloperidol (Haldol) but it has also developed when a person is taking chlorpromazine (Compazine) and promethazine (Phenergan) used for nausea. It occurs most often in the first 2 weeks of the start of treatment but must also be considered whenever a dose is increased. NMS may also be seen if anti-Parkinson's medications are stopped abruptly. In most instances the person is hospitalized in an intensive care unit while being treated. The immediate response is to recognize the cues that an adverse event is occurring, with the priority action being to help the person obtain emergency medical assistance, and gently begin cooling the person. Actions to reduce the risk of NMS include ensuring adequate hydration, performing activities in a cool area away from direct sunlight, and using a fan or sponge bath

if overheating should occur. An older adult, especially one who has dementia, may or may not communicate their discomfort from the heat, therefore observation of signs and symptoms may be left to the nurse or other caregiver. Any circumstance resulting in dehydration greatly increases the risk of heatstroke, with morbidity and mortality increasing with age. Diuretics, coffee, alcohol, lithium, and uncontrolled diabetes decrease vascular volume, thereby decreasing the body's ability to handle antipsychotics.

> ⚡ **SAFETY ALERT**
>
> Concurrent use of medications with anticholinergic properties or more than one antipsychotic significantly increases the risk of ADEs and ADRs.

Extrapyramidal Reactions

Although neuroleptic malignant syndrome is not commonly seen, the most significant potential side effects of antipsychotics (especially first generation) are movement disorders, also referred to as *extrapyramidal syndrome* (EPS) reactions. These include acute dystonia, akathisia, parkinsonian symptoms, and tardive dyskinesia.

Acute dystonia. An acute dystonic reaction is an abnormal involuntary movement consisting of a slow and continuous muscular contraction or spasm. Involuntary muscular contractions of the mouth, jaw, face, and neck are common. The jaw may lock (trismus), the tongue may roll back and block the throat, the neck may arch backward (opisthotonos), and the eyes may close. In an oculogyric crisis, the eyes are fixed in one position. This often creates a feeling of needing to look up constantly without the ability to make the eyes shift downward. Dystonia can be painful and frightening. An acute dystonic reaction may occur hours or days following antipsychotic medication administration or after dosage increases and may last minutes to hours. It is considered a medical emergency.

Caregivers or others unfamiliar with these EPS reactions often become alarmed. Although frightening, acute dystonia is usually not dangerous and is quickly relieved by anticholinergic medication, such as benztropine (Cogentin), trihexyphenidyl (Artane), or diphenhydramine (Benadryl), providing relief within minutes if given intravenously, within 10 to 15 minutes if given intramuscularly, and within 30 minutes if given orally. These medications should be readily available to treat an EPS reaction for all persons taking antipsychotics. Although they are not recommended for use in persons more than 65 years of age, anticholinergics and amantadine (Symmetrel), a dopamine agonist, are sometimes prescribed to prevent dystonic reactions, but because of slow onset of action, they are not used for acute treatment.

Akathisia. Akathisia refers to the compulsion to be in motion and may occur at any time during therapy. Patients describe feeling restless, being unable to be still, having an unrelenting desire to move, and feeling "like crawling out of my skin." Often this symptom is mistaken for worsening psychosis instead of the ADR that it is. Pacing, aimless walking, fidgeting, shifting weight from one leg to the other, and marked restlessness are characteristic behaviors for a person experiencing akathisia. Safety is the immediate concern.

Parkinsonian symptoms. The use of neuroleptics may cause a collection of symptoms that mimic Parkinson's disease. A bilateral tremor (as opposed to a unilateral tremor in true Parkinson's), bradykinesia, and rigidity may be seen, which may progress to the inability to move. The patient may have an inflexible facial expression and appear bored and apathetic and mistakenly be diagnosed as depressed. More common with the higher-potency antipsychotics (e.g., Haldol), Parkinsonian symptoms may occur within weeks to months of the initiation of antipsychotic therapy.

Tardive dyskinesia. When antipsychotics, especially typical antipsychotics (TAP) have been used continuously for 3 to 6 months, patients are at risk of the development of the irreversible movement disorder of tardive dyskinesia (TD). Symptoms of TD usually appear first as wormlike movements of the tongue; other facial movements include grimacing, blinking, and frowning. Slow, maintained, involuntary twisting movements of limbs, trunk, neck, face, and eyes (involuntary eye closure) have been reported. Aging and being a female are two of several risk factors (Cornett et al., 2017). There is no treatment that reverses the effect of TD, therefore it is essential that the nurse is attentive for early cues so that the health care provider can make prompt changes to the psychotropic regimen.

Response to treatment is the most important consideration when psychotropic medications are given. Subjective patient comments about feelings and symptoms and observation of both subtle and gross cues in a patient's behavior are important data for evaluating the effectiveness of a medication. Several tools are available to help the nurse monitor the patient taking antipsychotics. The Abnormal Involuntary Movement Scale (AIMS) was designed to quantify changes in movement. Other tools include the Barnes Rating Scale for Drug-Induced Akathisia (Barnes, 1989) and the Simpson-Angus Rating Scale for EPS (Simpson & Angus, 1970). All of these can be found on the Internet.

❖ USING CLINICAL JUDGMENT TO PROMOTE HEALTHY AGING: MEDICATION USE

Nurses in all inpatient and outpatient settings are responsible for ensuring safe outcomes when medications are prescribed to older adults either for routine or "as needed" (PRN) use.

◆ Recognizing and Analyzing Cues

Conducting a comprehensive drug review is the initial step in ensuring that older adults are using medications safely and effectively. Although a clinical pharmacist may collect the medication history, it is more often completed through the combined efforts of the licensed practical or registered nurse and the prescribing health care provider. This includes a careful reconciliation during transitions of care from one setting to another (Cook et al., 2019).

In the outpatient, ambulatory care setting, it is best to use a "brown bag approach" or to ask the person to bring all medications and other products he or she is currently taking to all health care encounters. As each container is removed from the bag, the person is asked how he or she actually takes the medicine rather than depending on how the prescription is written. This provides an opportunity not only to determine whether there is a misunderstanding but also to begin reconciliation between the labeling and any adjustments that may have been made by other clinicians. This is an important change in approach from what is too often used when the person is asked, "Has anything changed since you were last seen?"

An alternative strategy is based on the "review of systems" discussed in Chapter 8. To increase the quality of information received, questions will be something like, "What do you take for your heart, circulation, and breathing?" Collection of information always ends with questioning if there are any other medications/supplements taken, such as a vitamin, regular use of an antihistamine, or St. John's wort (commonly taken) (Box 9.10).

BOX 9.10   We Finally Solved the Mystery

Mr. Samuels had been taking warfarin for several years and it had stayed within normal limits (INR of 2–3) for some time. During a routine check, his INR was very low to the point of no longer therapeutic at 1.2. Although he denied any medication or herbal product changes, he admitted to being on a diet and was consuming one "Atkins" shake a day. On reading the label, we found it to have a high vitamin K content and therefore it was contraindicated for someone taking warfarin.

Without the bag of medications or a list of some kind, patients often answer some of the preceding questions with descriptions (e.g., "a little blue pill" or "a bad-tasting one"), which provides little information upon which the nurse can develop hypotheses relating to medication use.

In other settings, obtaining accurate information is considerably more difficult. A person may arrive at an emergency department with no medication information. In transitions from one care setting to another such as from a skilled nursing center to the hospital or the hospital back to home, medication "reconciliation" has been found to be highly fraught with errors in part because of the number of medications an older person is likely to be prescribed. Nonetheless the nurse is responsible for medication reconciliation comparing the previously prescribed medications with the newly prescribed ones or clarifying the new orders in the Long Term Care setting. This is often a laborious process, from records not arriving with patients to physicians and nurse practitioners being asked to "approve" orders for unfamiliar patients without having access to patients' medical records.

Similar problems occur in the transfer between long-term care settings and home when the patient may have difficulty deciphering changes to previous drug regimens and may take his or her former medications instead of the new ones or both at the same time (Box 9.11). When electronic medical records become universal, the interface between settings may become seamless and a significant number of errors are expected to decrease and the ease and accuracy of the assessment to increase.

All of these actions help the nurse improve outcomes by determining discrepancies between the prescribed dosage and the actual dosage, potential drug–drug and food–drug interactions, and potential or actual ADRs. When potentially inappropriate products are identified, the prescriber can be notified and changes made. Box 9.12 gives examples of the information that is particularly important when conducting a medication assessment with older adults.

BOX 9.11 Polypharmacy Gone Wild

Mr. Greene asked to speak with the clinic nurse about his medications. He had recently had a short stay in a skilled nursing facility. When he left, he was given the "cards" they were kept on when he was there with the left-overs for him to take. At home he resumed those he was taking at home and one from each of the cards he was given. In the end he was only supposed to be taking three different medications and instead he was taking eight, three of which were duplicates.

BOX 9.12 Tips for Best Practice
Components of a Medication Assessment With Special Emphasis for Older Adults

Ability to pay for prescription medications
Ability to obtain medications and refills
Persons involved in decision-making regarding medication use
Medications obtained from others
Recently discontinued medications or "left-over" prescriptions
Strategies used to remember when to take medications and when it has already been taken
Recent medication blood levels as appropriate
Recent measurement of liver and kidney functioning
Ability to remove packaging, manipulate medication, and store supply

---

◆ Nursing Actions

Another common strategy used by nurses to improve outcomes is health education. However, the complex needs of the older patient can make this particularly challenging. The following may be helpful when the nurse's goal is to promote healthy aging related to safe medication use:

Key persons: Find out who, if anyone, assists the person with decision-making and administration and make sure that the helper is present when any teaching is done (Box 9.13).

Environment: Minimize distraction and avoid competition with television, grandchildren, or others demanding the person's attention; make sure the person is comfortable and is not hungry, thirsty, tired, too warm or too cold, in pain, or in need of the toilet.

BOX 9.13 Knowing Who You Are Talking To

M. François came to the clinic as a new patient with uncontrolled hypertension. The nurse practitioner, through an interpreter, spent a lot of time with M. François explaining how to take his medications, the purpose of the medications, and so on. M. François and his caregiver sat quietly and appeared to understand. When M. François returned a month later his blood pressure was still out of control. There was a different person with him and the new person asked all of the questions that were addressed at the first appointment. On further inquiry it was determined that the person who accompanied M. François to his first appointment was just a neighbor helping out and not involved in his day-to-day life at all! M. François' niece, who "takes care of things," had been unavailable during the previous appointment.

Timing: Provide the teaching during the best time of the day for the person, when he or she is most engaged and energetic. Keep the education sessions short and succinct.

Communication: Communicate the information in a way that compensates for language differences and physical-sensory and cognitive changes so that the person understands to the extent possible. Use simple and direct language and avoid medical or nursing jargon (e.g., "intake" "voiding" etc.). Speak clearly, face the person at eye level and with light on the speaker's face. Make sure the person is wearing reading glasses or hearing aids if they are needed. If the person has limited health fluency, plan for extra time. If the person has limited language proficiency in the country where care is delivered, a trained medical interpreter is needed and up to twice the amount of time should be planned for the encounter.

Reinforce teaching: Although there is a wide array of teaching tools and medication reminders available on the market today, many older adults continue to use the strategies they have developed over the years to remember to take their medications. These may be as simple as a commercially available storage box or turning a bottle upside down once the medication has been taken for the day, or as intense as having a family member or friend call the person at designated times. Encourage the person to use techniques that have worked in the past or to develop new strategies to ensure correct and timely medication use when needed. All education is supported by written or graphic material in the language that the person can read (if literate) or in the language of the person who helps.

Most older adults who live in the community self-administer their own medications; others receive help from family, friends, or health care professionals. Without a dependable system it may be very difficult to take the 5–9 medications prescribed appropriately. In nursing homes and other institutional settings, the administration of medications occupies nearly all of the "medication" nurses' time. In assisted living facilities, medication administration is an optional service and available only if permitted by local laws. Regardless of the setting or the persons involved, several skills are needed for safe administration.

Because of the high rate of arthritis and other debilitating conditions, it may be difficult or impossible for the person to remove a cap or break a tablet. If no children will have access to the medications, alternative bottle caps that are easier to open can be requested. Either the person or the nurse can also ask the pharmacist to pre-break the pills or if possible, dispense a dose that does not require this. Pill cutters are commercially available but still call for fine motor dexterity to place the pill for cutting in the correct place. Only pills that are "scored" can be cut. Some persons, especially those of low fixed incomes, will attempt to break unscored pills to have them last longer, resulting in inconsistent dosing.

Most medications are taken orally but many tablets and capsules are difficult to swallow because of their size or because they stick to the tongue, especially if the mouth is dry because of anticholinergic effects or dehydration. The person can be advised to first moisten the mouth and then place the pill or capsules on their tongue and swallow a fluid or semisolid food, such as applesauce, chocolate syrup, or peanut butter—as long as the substances do not interact.

Enteric-coated, extended-release, or sustained-release products are all used to allow absorption at different places in the gastrointestinal tract. They can *never* be crushed because this will interfere with their pharmacological effects (causing either underdose or toxicity) or create problems in administration, such as injuring the mouth or gastrointestinal tract. However, since the formulation of medications is rapidly changing, the nurse or older adult is advised to contact a pharmacist or consult the package insert (found in the most recent edition of the *Physicians' Desk Reference* [PDR]) for the changing list of "do-not-crush" products. The person must be taught that any medication ending in terms such as SR, XL, or SR can never be crushed without risking an ADE.

Administration of a drug in liquid form is sometimes preferable and allows flexible dosing especially in a person with dementia. Concentrations can be varied so that quantities of solution can be prepared and taken by the teaspoon, tablespoon, or ounce, with simple and commonly used household tools. Household spoons vary greatly in actual volume and the home health nurse should ensure that an accurate measurement is used. Liquid self-administration is not an option for the person with any type of tremor.

An increasing number of medications are becoming available in a transdermal route of delivery. Transdermal patches are not recommended for persons who are noticeably underweight because absorption is unpredictable owing to the reduced body fat. They are helpful for persons who have difficulty swallowing, such as those with end-stage dementia. The patches may not be cut or altered in any way; gloves must be worn when they are being applied and the expired patch must be removed at the same time.

When medications are being administered directly into the stomach or duodenum via a feeding tube, special precautions are needed. Safe administration is a time-consuming task resulting in a high risk for medication errors. To administer enteral medications safely, a detailed knowledge of their formulation is needed along with the skills required to prepare them appropriately. The outcomes of the errors include occluded tube, reduced drug effect, drug toxicity, patient harm, or patient death. The three most common errors are incompatible route, improper preparation, and improper administration (see Safety Alert).

⚡ SAFETY ALERT

Administration of Medications Through Enteral Feeding Tubes: The Three Most Common Errors

Incompatible route: Medications must be appropriate for the oral route for immediate action. Watch for extensions such as CD, CR, ER, LA, SA, SE, TD, TR, XL, and XR as warnings for not crushable formulation of drugs (this list is not inclusive). See the "do-not-crush" lists available from the pharmacy or on-line (http://www.ismp.org/Tools/DoNotCrush.pdf).

Improper preparation: Medications administered via an enteral feeding tube must be fully dissolved in a liquid or in semiliquid form in order to pass through the tube and not clog the tube by adhering to its lining. Drug remaining on tubing means a reduced dose has been administered. This is a special concern when administering oral suspensions and tinctures.

Improper administration: Be sure to know where the distal end of the tube is resting. A drug that requires partial absorption in the stomach cannot be used if it will be administered directly into the duodenum or jejunum. Do not combine with a feeding product unless directions are to "administer with food." When more than one tablet is crushed (or more than one capsule is opened) and the contents are mixed before administration, a new "product" has been prepared and may not have the same pharmacotherapeutic effect as the two products taken separately. Find "compatibility information" from pharmacists to determine which medications may be mixed in this way.

◆ Evaluating Outcomes

A significant part of a nurse's responsibilities is to monitor and evaluate the outcomes and effectiveness of prescribed treatments and observe for cues indicative of problems (e.g., ADRs) either from a change in condition or from iatrogenic complications (i.e., problems that are the result of something the health care provider has done), especially misuse, interactions, or early and unreported adverse events (Table 9.5).

Monitoring involves making astute recognition and analyses of cues and documenting these, noting changes in physical and functional status (e.g., vital

TABLE 9.5	**Indications of Toxicity**
Medication(s)	**Signs and Symptoms**
Benzodiazepines (e.g., Ativan)	Ataxia, restlessness, confusion, depression, coma, lethargy, drowsiness
Beta blockers	Acidosis, bradycardia, coma, hyper or hypoglycemia, hyperkalemia, hypotension, respiratory depression, seizures
Furosemide (Lasix)	Electrolyte imbalance, hepatic changes, pancreatitis, leukopenia, thrombocytopenia
Levodopa (L-Dopa)	Muscle and eye twitching, disorientation, asterixis, hallucinations, dyskinetic movements, grimacing, depression, delirium, ataxia
Nonsteroidal anti-inflammatory medications (NSAIDs) such as Advil and Naprosyn	Photosensitivity, fluid retention, anemia, nephrotoxicity, visual changes, bleeding, blood pressure elevations
Sulfonylureas—first generation (e.g., Diabinese)	Coma, decreased appetite, hypoglycemia, lethargy, seizures, weakness, coma

From Frithsen, I. L., Simpson, W. M. (2010). Recognition and management of acute medication poisoning, *American Family Physician 81*(3), 316–323.

signs, performance of activities of daily living, sleeping, eating, eliminating) and mental status (e.g., attention and level of alertness, memory, orientation, behavior, mood). This is particularly important in gerontological nursing because of the medical complexity of the patient combined with age-related changes and the polypharmacy that often exists. Monitoring for iatrogenic effects means ensuring that blood levels are measured when they are needed, such as scheduled thyroid-stimulating hormone (TSH) levels for all persons taking thyroid replacement therapy, international normalized ratios (INRs) for all persons taking warfarin, and periodic hemoglobin A1c levels for all persons with diabetes. Care of a patient also means that nurses promptly communicate their findings of potential problems to the patient's primary care provider.

The gerontological nurse is a key person in ensuring that the medications are used as safely as possible, are appropriate, effective, and health outcomes are monitored. The nurse determines whether side effects are minimal and tolerable or serious. The knowledgeable nurse is alert for cues indicating potential drug interactions and ADRs. The nurse promotes the strategies

BOX 9.14 FDA Warning: NSAIDs and Stroke

In July 2015, the US Food and Drug Administration (FDA) published a new, stronger alert related to the use of over-the-counter nonsteroidal anti-inflammatory medications (NSAIDs), such as ibuprofen and naproxen sodium. In detailed studies the following information has been found:

- The risk of heart attack or stroke can occur as early as the first weeks of using an NSAID. The risk may increase with longer use of the NSAID.
- The risk appears greater at higher doses.
- NSAIDs can increase the risk of heart attack or stroke in patients with or without heart disease or risk factors for heart disease.
- Patients with heart disease or risk factors for heart disease have a greater likelihood of heart attack or stroke following NSAID use than patients without these risk factors because they have a higher risk at baseline.
- Patients treated with NSAIDs following their first heart attack were more likely to die in the first year after the heart attack compared with patients who were not treated with NSAIDs after their first heart attack.
- There is an increased risk of heart failure with NSAID use.
- Patients taking NSAIDs should seek medical attention immediately if they experience symptoms such as chest pain, shortness of breath or trouble breathing, weakness in one part or side of their body, or slurred speech.

From FDA drug safety communication (2018). *FDA strengthens warning that non-aspirin nonsteroidal anti-inflammatory drugs (NSAIDs) can cause heart attacks or strokes.* https://www.fda.gov/drugs/drug-safety-and-availability/fda-drug-safety-communication-fda-strengthens-warning-non-aspirin-nonsteroidal-anti-inflammatory.

necessary to prevent drugs from becoming toxic and treats toxicity promptly should it occur. The nurse must give prompt attention to cues indicating changes in physiological function that either are the result of the medication regimen or are affected by the regimen, such as use of nonsteroidal anti-inflammatories (Box 9.14). The nurse is often the person to initiate assessment of medication use, provide the teaching needed for safe drug use and self-administration, and evaluate outcomes.

In most settings the nurse is also in a position to influence the timing of prescribed doses; therefore, some patients might benefit by understanding some of the findings emerging from the science of chronopharmacology (Dallmann et al., 2014). In all settings, a vital nursing function is to educate patients, to ensure that they understand the purpose and the side effects of medications, and to help the person develop strategies to address questions and concerns as they arise. The development of hypotheses leading to actions by the licensed practical nurse (LPN), registered nurse (RN), or advanced practice nurse (APN) should be centered on identifying unnecessary or inappropriate medications, establishing safe usage, determining the patient's self-medication management ability, monitoring the effect of current medications and other products (e.g., herbals), and evaluating the effectiveness of any education provided. Ideally, the nurse should be aware of the resources available for teaching about medications, such as access to a clinical pharmacist. The nurse is well situated to coordinate care, identify the patient's goals, determine what the patient needs to learn in order to understand his or her medications, and arrange for follow-up care to monitor the outcome of medication teaching.

Medications occupy a central place in the lives of many older persons; cost, acceptability, interactions, unacceptable side effects, and the need to schedule medications in the context of their lives all combine to create many difficulties. Although nurses, with the exception of advanced practice nurses, do not prescribe medications, we believe that having a basic understanding of issues specific to the safe administration and consumption of medications by persons in later life will reduce the use of inappropriate medications and allow the nurse to observe more closely for cues of adverse side effects and interactions. In the roles of educator and advocate the nurse might promote safe medication use through personally and culturally appropriate guidance.

KEY CONCEPTS

- As we age, the way our body responds to medication changes.
- All medications have side effects. The therapeutic goal is to reduce the targeted symptoms without undesirable side effects.
- Drug–drug, drug–herb/supplement, and drug–food interactions are increasing problems that require the nurse to be aware of the cues as appropriate.
- Polypharmacy is one of the most serious problems for older adults today and this is usually the first area to investigate when adverse physiological or psychiatric cues are recognized.
- Drug misuse may be triggered by prescriber practices, individual self-medication, individual physiology, altered biodegradability, nutritional and fluid states, and inadequate assessment before prescribing, administering, or monitoring.
- Nurses must consider the occurrence of a possible adverse medication effect immediately if a cue indicative of change in the person's condition is observed, including mental status changes in an individual who is normally alert and aware, or increasing confusion.

Many drugs cause temporary cognitive impairment in older persons.

- The side effects of psychotropic medications vary significantly; thus, these medications must be carefully selected and prescribed for older adults. This increases the nurse's responsibility in the actions associated with administration and monitoring outcomes of these medications.
- The cues indicating that an older adult is having positive outcomes related to the use of psychotropic medications should show reduced distress, clearer thinking, and more appropriate behavior.
- It is always expected that pharmacological approaches augment rather than replace nonpharmacological approaches.
- Older adults are particularly vulnerable to developing movement disorders (extrapyramidal symptoms, Parkinsonian symptoms, akathisia, and dystonia) with the use of antipsychotics.
- The Omnibus Budget Reconciliation Act (OBRA) restricts the use of psychotropic drugs in the long-term care setting unless they are truly needed for specific disorders and to maintain or improve function. It is expected that they are discontinued as soon as possible.
- Any time a behavior change is observed in a person, reversible causes must be sought and treated before medications are used.
- Dosages of medications must be carefully titrated for the individual and the individual's responses must be accurately and consistently recorded.

ACTIVITIES AND DISCUSSION QUESTIONS

1. What are the age-related changes that occur in the pharmacokinetics of older adults?
2. What are the drug use patterns of older adults and what can be done to correct or improve them?
3. Explain the roles of older adults, care providers, and the social network in reducing medication misuse.
4. List a variety of strategies that the nurse can suggest to assist older adults with their medication use and adherence to a medication regimen.
5. Which side effects of antipsychotic medications are suggestive of poor or very poor outcomes and require immediate nursing action?
6. Mrs. J. is repeatedly asking for a nurse; other patients are complaining and you simply cannot be available to Mrs. J. soon or repeatedly. Considering the setting and the OBRA guidelines, what would you do to manage the situation?

NEXT-GENERATION NCLEX® EXAMINATION-STYLE QUESTIONS

A nurse is performing the first home visit for Mr. Ortiz, an 86-year-old male, following his discharge from the hospital after community-acquired pneumonia. Assessment findings include blood pressure of 110/60 mmHg, heart rate of 75 beats per minute, respirations 14 breaths per minute, temperature 97.3°F, and oxygen 94% on room air. His heart has regular rate and rhythm; lungs with rhonchi in the left lower lobe; abdomen with normoactive bowel sounds, soft and non-tender; no peripheral edema; skin warm and pale. He reports feeling fatigued but unable to sleep. He has pain in his back and ribs with coughing; he denies shortness of breath. Mr. Ortiz states his appetite has not yet returned, but he is trying to eat. He also states his last bowel movement was yesterday; it was soft. The hospital discharge summary notes a HbA1c of 7.2%, creatinine 1.8 mg/dL, BUN 32 mg/dL, sodium 134 mEq/L, potassium 4.2 mEq/L, glucose of 150 mg/dL, and hemoglobin/hematocrit of 10.2 mg/dL and 30%. When asked to show his medications, Mr. Ortiz brings out the following bottles:

Levofloxacin 750 mg daily
Lisinopril/hydrochlorothiazide 20/25 mg daily
High-Potency Multivitamin 400 µg daily
Calcium carbonate 500 mg daily
Vitamin D3 400 units daily
Aspirin 81 mg daily
Metformin 850 mg twice daily
Glipizide 5 mg twice a day
Gemfibrozil 600 mg daily
Glucosamine and chondroitin 2 tabs daily
Melatonin 300 µg daily
CoQ10 200 mg daily
Odorless Garlic 1000 mg daily
Probiotics 2 caps daily
Pantoprazole 20 mg daily
Paroxetine 10 mg every evening
Percogesic Extra Strength 2 tabs every 6 hours as needed
Tylenol Extra Strength 2 tabs every 8 hours as needed

Which medication should the nurse clarify with the provider? Select all that apply.

1. Levofloxacin 750 mg daily
2. Metformin 850 mg twice daily
3. Glipizide 5 mg twice a day
4. Odorless Garlic 1000 mg daily
5. Pantoprazole 20 mg daily
6. Paroxetine 10 mg every evening
7. Percogesic Extra Strength 2 tabs every 6 hours as needed
8. Tylenol Extra Strength 2 tabs every 8 hours as needed

REFERENCES

American Geriatrics Society (AGS). (2019). American Geriatrics Society 2019 updated expert panel: American Geriatrics Society 2019 updated Beers Criteria for potentially inappropriate medication use in older adults. *J Am Geriatr Soc, 67*(4), 674–694.

Barclay, K., Frassetto, A., Robb, J., & Mandell, E. (2018). Polypharmacy in the elderly: How to reduce adverse drug events. *Clinician Reviews, 28*(2), 38–44.

Barnes, T. R. (1989). A rating scale for drug-induced akathisia. *Br J Psychiatry, 154,* 672–676.

Beers, M. (1997). Explicit criteria for determining potentially inappropriate medication use by the elderly. An update. *Arch Intern Med, 157,* 1531–1536.

Cook, H., Parson, J., & Brandt, N. (2019). Identifying potential medication discrepancies during medication reconciliation in the post-acute long-term care setting. *J Geron Nurs, 45*(7), 5–10.

Cornett, E. M., Novitch, M., Kaye, A. D., Kata, V., & Kaye, A. M. (2017). Medication-induced tardive dyskinesia: a review and update. *Ochsner J, 17*(2), 162–174.

Dallmann, R., Brown, S. A., & Gachon, F. (2014). Chronopharmacology: New insights and therapeutic implications. *Annu Rev Pharmacol Toxicol, 6*(54), 1–25.

HealthinAging.org. Alternatives for medications listed in the AGS Beer Criteria® for potentially inappropriate medication use in older adults, 2019. https://www.healthinaging.org/tools-and-tips/alternatives-medications-listed-ags-beers-criteriar-potentially-inappropriate.

Hughes, G. J., Beizer, J. L., et al. (2014). Appropriate prescribing. In R. J. Ham, P. D. Sloane, & G. A. Warshaw et al. (Eds.), *Primary care geriatrics: A case-based approach* (ed. 6, pp. 67–76). Philadelphia: Elsevier.

Kim, J., & Parish, A. L. (2017). Polypharmacy and medication management in older adults. *Nurs Clin North Am, 52*(3), 457–468.

Li, J., Vitiello, M. V., Gooneratne, N. S. (2018). Sleep in normal aging. *Sleep Med Clin, 13*(1), 1–11.

Liew, T. M., Lee, C. S., Goh, S. K. L., & Chang, Z. Y. (2020). The prevalence and impact of potentially inappropriate prescribing among older persons in primary care: Multilevel meta-analysis. *Age Aging, 49*(4), 570–579.

NCQA Measuring quality. Improving health care: HEDIS and performance measurement, 2019. https://www.ncqa.org/hedis/.

Omnibus Budget Reconciliation Act (OBRA) of 1987, House of Representatives, 100th Congress, 1st Session, Report 100-391, Washington, DC, 1987, US Government Printing Office.

Ortiz-Tudela, E., Martinez-Nicolas, A., Diaz-Mardomingo, C., et al. (2014). The characterization of biological rhythms in mild cognitive impairment. *Biomed Res Int,* (Article ID 524971), 1–7.

Pathak, S., & Duff, F. (2018). Antipsychotic use in older adults: Canadian best practices. *The Nurse Practitioner, 43*(6), 50–54.

Rochon, P. A., Schmader, K. E., Givens, J. Drug prescribing for older adults, 2020. UpToDate. http://www.uptodate.com/contents/drug-prescribing-for-older-adults.

Ruscin, J. M., Linnebur, S. A. Overview of drug therapy in the elderly, 2018. http://www.merckmanuals.com/professional/geriatrics/drug-therapy-in-the-elderly/introduction-to-drug-therapy-in-the-elderly.

Schmiedl, S., Rottenkolber, M., Szymanski, J., et al. (2018). Preventable ADRs leading to hospitalization – results of a long-term prospective safety study with 6,427 ADR cases focusing on elderly patients. *Expert Opinion Drug Safety, 17*(2), 125–137.

Simpson, G. M., & Angus, J. W. S (1970). A rating scale for extrapyramidal side effects. *Acta Psychiatr Scand, 212,* 11–19.

10

Clinical Judgment to Promote Nutritional Health

Theris A. Touhy

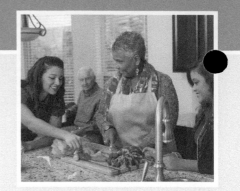

http://evolve.elsevier.com/Touhy/gerontological/

LEARNING OBJECTIVES

Upon completion of this chapter, the reader will be able to:
- Discuss nutritional requirements and factors affecting nutrition for older adults.
- Describe a nutritional screening and evaluation.
- Utilize clinical judgment to identify and evaluate nursing actions to promote adequate nutrition for older adults.
- Utilize clinical judgment to recognize and analyze cues and identify and evaluate nursing actions for older adults with dysphagia.

THE LIVED EXPERIENCE

If I do reach the point when I can no longer feed myself, I hope that the hands holding my fork belong to someone who has a feeling for who I am. I hope my helper will remember what she learns about me and that her awareness of me will grow from one encounter to another. Why should this make a difference? Yet, I am certain that my experience of needing to be fed will be altered if it occurs in the context of my being known. I will want to know about the lives of the people I rely on, especially the one who holds my fork for me. If she would talk to me, if we could laugh together, I might even forget the chagrin of my useless hands. We could have a conversation rather than a feeding.

From Lustbader (1999)

NUTRITIONAL HEALTH

Adequate and affordable food supplies and improved nutrition are concerns worldwide with some differences between developed and developing countries. Although issues vary among different areas of the globe, nutrition as a major contributor to health is a significant concern for all nations. The link between healthy eating patterns and healthy aging is well documented. The quality and quantity of diet are important factors in preventing, delaying the onset of, and managing chronic illnesses associated with aging. About half of all American adults have one or more preventable diet-related chronic diseases, including cardiovascular disease, type 2 diabetes, and overweight and obesity (US Department of Health and Human Services [USDHHS] and US Department of Agriculture [USDA], 2015–2020).

Proper nutrition means that all of the essential nutrients (i.e., carbohydrates, fat, protein, vitamins, minerals, and water) are adequately supplied and used to maintain optimal health and wellness. Although some age-related changes in the gastrointestinal (GI) system do occur (Chapter 4), these changes are rarely the primary factors in inadequate nutrition. Fulfillment of nutritional needs in older adults is more often affected by numerous other factors, including chronic disease, lifelong eating habits, ethnicity, socialization, income, transportation, housing, mood, food knowledge, functional impairments, health, and dentition.

This chapter discusses the dietary needs of older adults, the risk factors contributing to inadequate nutrition, and the effects of obesity, diseases, functional and cognitive impairments, and dysphagia on nutrition. Several conditions warrant further discussion because they are frequently encountered in older adults and are related to adequate diet and nutritional status. Dehydration and oral health are discussed in Chapter 11, and the effect of neurocognitive disorders on nutrition is discussed in Chapter 25. Readers are referred to a nutrition text for more comprehensive information on nutrition and aging and disease.

United States Dietary Guidelines

The *2010 Dietary Guidelines for Americans,* published by the federal government of the United States, are designed to promote health, reduce the risk of chronic diseases, and decrease the prevalence of overweight and obesity through improved nutrition and physical activity. The guidelines focus on balancing calories with physical activity; encouraging Americans to consume more healthy foods such as vegetables, fruits, whole grains, fat-free and low-fat dairy products, and seafood; and urging Americans to consume less sodium, saturated and trans fats, added sugars, and refined grains. In addition to the key recommendations, there are recommendations for specific population groups including older adults (USDHHS and USDA, 2015). *Healthy People 2020* also provides goals for nutrition (Box 10.1).

MyPlate for Older Adults

Choose MyPlate is a visual depiction of daily food intake. The USDA Human Nutrition Research Center on Aging

♥ BOX 10.1 *Healthy People 2020*
Nutrition and Weight Status

- Promote health and reduce chronic disease through the consumption of healthful diets and achievement and maintenance of body weight.
- Increase the proportion of primary care physicians who regularly measure the body mass index in their adult patients.
- Increase the proportion of physician office visits made by adult patients who are obese that include counseling or education related to weight reduction, nutrition, or physical activity.
- Increase the proportion of physician visits made by all child and adult patients that include counseling about nutrition or diet.
- Increase the proportion of adults who are at a healthy weight.
- Reduce household food insecurity and in so doing reduce hunger.

From US Department of Health and Human Services, Office of Disease Prevention and Health Promotion. (2012). *Healthy People 2020.* http://www.healthypeople.gov/2020.

at Tufts University provides a *MyPlate for Older Adults* emphasizing the nutritional needs of older adults in a framework based on the *2015–2020 Dietary Guidelines for Americans* (Fig. 10.1). The *MyPlate for Older Adults* depicts a colorful plate composed of approximately 50% fruits and vegetables; 25% grains, many of which are whole grains; and 25% protein-rich foods such as nuts,

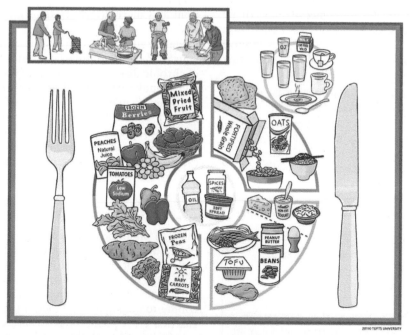

FIG. 10.1 MyPlate for Older Adults. (From the Jean Mayer USDA Human Nutrition Research Center on Aging, Tufts University. (2011). *MyPlate for older adults.* http://hnrca.tufts.edu/myplate/.)

beans, fish, lean meat, poultry, and fat-free and low-fat dairy products such as milk, cheeses, and yogurts. Images of good sources of fluids, heart-healthy fats such as vegetable oils and soft margarines; and herbs and spices to be used in place of salt to lower sodium intake are also included (Tufts University, 2016).

Generally, older adults have lower energy requirements and need fewer calories because they may not be as active and metabolic rates decline. However, they still require the same or higher levels of nutrients for optimal health outcomes. The recommendations may need modification for individuals who have illnesses. The Dietary Approaches to Stop Hypertension (DASH) eating plan is a recommended eating plan to assist with maintenance of optimal weight and management of hypertension. This plan consists of fruits, vegetables, whole grains, low-fat dairy products, poultry, fish, and restriction of salt intake.

The Mediterranean diet (MedDiet) has also been associated with a lower incidence of chronic illness, weight gain, and impaired physical function and with improved cognition. This diet is characterized by a greater intake of fruits, vegetables, legumes, whole grains, and fish; a lower intake of red and processed meats; higher amounts of monosaturated fats, mostly provided by olive oil from Mediterranean countries; and lower amounts of saturated fats. The MIND (Mediterranean-DASH diet Intervention for Neurodegeneration Delay) combines the MedDiet with the DASH diet. In a large representative sample of older adults, greater adherence to the MedDiet and the MIND diet was independently associated with better cognitive function and lower risk of cognitive impairment (McEvoy et al., 2017). When evaluating

---

BOX 10.2   Resources for Best Practice

Consultgeri.org: Assessing Nutrition in Older Adults (includes video of administration of MNA); Mealtime Difficulties, Preventing Aspiration in Older Adults with Dysphagia (includes video)

Mediterranean-DASH diet Intervention for Neurodegenerative Delay (MIND) Diet: http://www.healthline.com/nutrition/mind-diet

Mini Nutritional Assessment: https://consultgeri.org/try-this/general-assessment/issue-9.pdf

MyPlate: http://hnrca.tufts.edu/myplate/

National Council on Aging: Benefits Checkup for Seniors: https://www.benefitscheckup.org/

National Heart, Lung, and Blood Institute: Dietary Approaches to Stop Hypertension (DASH) diet

National Institute on Aging: Healthy Eating: Choosing healthy meals as you get older. Self MNA: http://www.mna-elderly.com/mna_forms.html

---

different options for healthy eating, a balanced, unprocessed diet, rich in very colorful fruits and vegetables, lean meats, fish, whole grains, nuts, seeds, olive oil, and lots of water seems to have the best evidence for a long, healthier, vibrant life. Further research and clinical trials are needed to understand the role of dietary patterns in cognitive aging and brain disease (Box 10.2).

Other Dietary Recommendations

Fats

Similar to other age groups, older adults should limit intake of saturated fat and trans fatty acids. High-fat diets cause obesity and increase the risk of heart disease and cancer. Less than 10% of calories per day should come from saturated fats.

Protein

The current protein reference nutrient intake (RNI) is 0.8 g protein/kg body weight in healthy adults of all ages. However, emerging evidence-based studies suggest that an increased protein intake may be beneficial to fulfill the needs of vulnerable older adults, particularly those with chronic disease. Additionally, more protein, calcium, and vitamin D are recommended to prevent bone loss and maintain existing bone density, thereby reducing the risk of falls and fractures (Chapter 21).

Inadequate protein intake contributes to poor nutritional status; reduced muscle mass, strength, and function; and increased mortality. Intakes above the RNI of certain nutrients, such as protein, vitamin D, antioxidants, vitamin E, and selenium, are associated with beneficial effects on physical function and prevention of chronic diseases in older age (Baugreet et al., 2017). Older adults who are ill are the most likely segment of society to experience protein deficiency. Those with limitations affecting their ability to shop, cook, and consume food are also at risk of protein deficiency and malnutrition. In a study conducted by Gropper et al. (2019), protein intake differed among ethnic/racial groups, but all groups studied were below recommendations for protein intake.

Fiber

Fiber is an important dietary component that some older adults do not consume in sufficient quantities. A daily intake of 25 g of fiber is recommended and must be combined with adequate amounts of fluid. Insufficient amounts of fiber in the diet and insufficient fluids contribute to constipation. Fiber is the indigestible material that gives plants their structure. It is abundant in raw fruits and vegetables and in unrefined grains and cereals.

Vitamins and Minerals

Older adults who consume five servings of fruits and vegetables daily will obtain adequate intake of vitamins A, C, and E and also potassium. However, Americans of all ages eat less than half of the recommended amounts of fruits and vegetables. Vitamin B12 plays a key role in anti-aging, but 50% of adults over the age of 50 years are deficient. Vitamin B12 deficiency is a common and underrecognized condition (Hooshmand et al., 2016). After the age of 50 years, the stomach produces less gastric acid, which makes vitamin B12 absorption less efficient. Older adults should increase their intake of the crystalline form of vitamin B12 from fortified foods such as whole-grain breakfast cereals. Other food sources include salmon, tuna, grass-fed beef, sardines, eggs, and cottage cheese. Individuals who take proton pump inhibitors (e.g., Prilosec, Prevacid) show increased risk of vitamin B12 deficiency when these medications are taken for 2 years. Individuals consuming a vegetarian diet and those with some form of weight-loss surgery are also more likely to be low in the vitamin. Calcium and vitamin D are essential for bone health and may prevent osteoporosis and decrease the risk of fracture (Chapter 21).

OBESITY (OVERNUTRITION)

Most of the world's population live in countries where overweight and obesity kills more people than underweight. Since the 1990s, the prevalence of older adults who are obese has doubled. Every country, except for those in sub-Saharan Africa, faces alarming obesity rates that have risen 82% since 2000. In the United States, approximately 35% of adults over 60 years are obese, with a higher prevalence in women (38%) than men (32%) (Gretebeck et al., 2017). By 2030, nearly one in two adults will be obese (Ward et al., 2019). Overweight and obesity are associated with increased health care costs, functional impairments, disability, chronic disease, and nursing home admission. Obesity is a major risk factor for the most common disabling conditions—osteoarthritis, atherosclerosis, diabetes, and stroke (Kritchevsky, 2017).

The World Health Organization (WHO) (2020) defines overweight and obesity as follows: overweight is a body mass index (BMI) greater than or equal to 25; obesity is a BMI greater than or equal to 30. However, there is no consensus about the best way to measure obesity in the older population. Normal changes in body composition may make BMI less accurate. Fat mass increases with age and lean mass decreases, and BMI underestimates total adiposity. Additionally, most older adults also decline in height, resulting in overall overestimation of obesity.

Although there is strong evidence that obesity in younger people decreases life expectancy and has a negative effect on functionality and morbidity, less is known about the benefits and risks of obesity in older adults compared with children and adults. Older adults who are overweight or obese do not have the same risk of morbidity and mortality as do younger individuals, particularly if obesity develops late in life. In what has been termed the *obesity paradox*, some research has found that for people who have survived to 70 years of age, mortality risk is lowest in those with a BMI classified as overweight (Kalish, 2016).

Higher BMI is associated with an increased risk of osteoarthritis, diabetes, and disability, but when weight gain occurs in late life, there is less time to impose metabolic and cardiovascular health risks. Obesity may protect against bone density loss and hip fracture, and for frail older adults with severely decreased functional status, obesity may be regarded as a protective factor with regard to functionality and mortality.

Further research is needed to understand how long-term intentional weight loss and associated shifts in body composition affect the onset of chronic disease (Bowman et al., 2017). Weight loss recommendations for older adults should be carefully considered on an individualized basis with attention to the weight history and medical conditions. A critical goal is to maintain or increase quality of life and physical function. Because weight loss is accompanied by a decline in free fat mass, activities to maintain muscle strength, such as progressive resistance training, should be included in all weight loss plans for older adults. Maintaining a healthy weight throughout life can prevent many illnesses and functional limitations as a person grows older.

MALNUTRITION (UNDERNUTRITION)

Malnutrition is a recognized geriatric syndrome. The most common definition of malnutrition is too little or too much energy, protein, and nutrients, which can cause adverse effects on a person's body and its function and clinical outcomes. Malnutrition happens when a person has an imbalance between the nutrients they need and those that they receive and can result from overnutrition and undernutrition. The rising incidence of malnutrition among older adults has been documented in acute care, long-term care, and the community.

Malnutrition among hospitalized patients is estimated to affect as many as one in two patients at admission, while many others develop malnutrition throughout hospitalization (Avelino-Silva & Jaluul, 2017). Up to 50% of older adult patients are malnourished when discharged from the hospital. Malnutrition is estimated to occur in up to 15% of community-dwelling older adults, 20% to 60% of hospitalized older adults, and 30% to 85% of those living in nursing facilities. These figures are expected to rise dramatically in the next 30 years with the aging of the population. Those at greatest risk are older women, minorities, and people who are poor or live in rural areas. Being 75 years of age and older is an independent risk factor for poor nutrition (Crogan, 2017; Tilly, 2017). Malnutrition among older adults is clearly a serious challenge for health professionals in all settings.

Characteristics

The understanding of malnutrition is evolving and research is ongoing. No single marker has been identified to diagnose adult malnutrition of any etiology. Characteristics have been identified to determine malnutrition (Mueller, 2015) (Box 10.3). Malnutrition is a complex syndrome that can develop following two primary trajectories. It can occur when the individual does not consume sufficient amounts of micronutrients (i.e., vitamins, minerals, phytochemicals) and macronutrients (i.e., protein, carbohydrates, fat, water) required to maintain organ function and healthy tissues. This type of malnutrition can occur from prolonged undernutrition or overnutrition. In contrast, inflammation-related malnutrition develops as a consequence of injury, surgery, or disease states that trigger inflammatory mediators that contribute to increased metabolic rate and impaired nutrient utilization (Cederholm & Jensen, 2017; Mogensen & DiMaria-Ghalili, 2015).

Inflammation is increasingly identified as an important underlying factor that increases risk of malnutrition and a contributing factor to suboptimal responses to nutritional intervention and increased risk of mortality. Weight loss frequently occurs in both trajectories but weight alone is not an indicator of nutritional status. Individuals also experience malnutrition when they take in enough calories but miss important nutrients that affect their nutritional status (Tilly, 2017).

BOX 10.3   Characteristics of Malnutrition

For a diagnosis of malnutrition, two or more of the following characteristics must be present:
- Insufficient energy intake
- Weight loss
- Loss of muscle mass
- Loss of subcutaneous fat
- Localized or generalized fluid accumulation that may mask weight loss
- Diminished functional status as measured by handgrip strength

Consequences

Malnutrition is a precursor to frailty and has serious consequences, including infections, pressure injuries, anemia, hypotension, impaired cognition, sarcopenia (low muscle mass associated with aging), hip fractures, prolonged hospital stay, institutionalization, increased dependence, reduced quality of life, and increased morbidity and mortality (Tilly, 2017). Malnourished patients are twice as likely to develop pressure injuries and three times as likely to have infections. Almost half of the patients who fall during hospitalization are reported to be malnourished. Finally, older adults who are admitted to the hospital with malnutrition are more likely to have longer hospital stays and die before discharge (Avelino-Silva & Jaluul, 2017). Many factors contribute to the occurrence of malnutrition in older adults (Box 10.4).

BOX 10.4   Risk Factors for Malnutrition

- Chronic diseases
- Acute illness/trauma
- Polypharmacy
- Overly restrictive diets
- Poor dentition
- Dysphagia
- Poor functional status; inability to prepare food
- Depression
- Altered mental status/dementia
- Social isolation and limited social supports
- Lack of transportation to purchase food
- Socioeconomic deprivation

FACTORS AFFECTING FULFILLMENT OF NUTRITIONAL NEEDS

Lifelong Eating Habits

The nutritional state of a person reflects the individual's dietary history and present food practices. "Foodways are defined as the eating habits and culinary practices of a people, region, or historical period" (Furman, 2014, p. 80). This includes unique eating patterns of various cultural and religious groups. Foodways influence food preferences, meal expectation, and nutritional intake. Eating habits do not always coincide with fulfillment of nutritional needs and may especially affect the ability and desire to consume food that is not consistent with individual foodways. The meaning of food and mealtimes, often established in childhood, "become[s] more poignant with age" (Furman, 2014, p. 83). The Joint Commission and Centers for Medicare and Medicaid

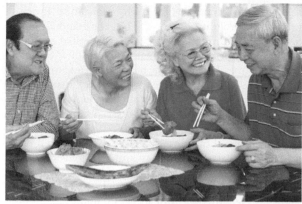

Older adults enjoying a meal together. (© iStock.com/monkey-businessimages.)

Services (CMS) (2014) specify assessment of dietary needs, restrictions, and cultural considerations in a patient safety tool (Box 10.5).

Lifelong habits of dieting or eating fad foods also echo through the later years. Individuals may fall prey to advertisements that claim specific foods can reverse aging or rid one of chronic conditions. Following the MyPlate for Older Adults (Fig. 10.1) is best for an ideal diet, with changes based on particular problems, such as hypercholesteremia. Individuals should be counseled to base their dietary decisions on valid research and consultation with their primary care provider. For the healthy individual, essential nutrients should be obtained from food sources rather than relying on dietary supplements.

Socialization

The fundamentally social aspect of eating has to do with sharing and the feeling of belonging that it provides. All of us use food as a means of giving and receiving love, friendship, or belonging. The presence of others during meals is a significant predictor of caloric intake. The meaning and enjoyment of eating can often be challenged as a person ages, requires hospitalization or nursing home residence, or experiences chronic illnesses, loneliness, depression, isolation, and functional limitations. Disinterest in food may also result from the effects of medication or disease processes. Misuse and abuse of alcohol are prevalent among older adults and are growing public health concerns. Excessive drinking interferes with nutrition. Drinking alcohol depletes the body of necessary nutrients and often replaces meals, thus making an individual susceptible to malnutrition (Chapter 24).

The elderly nutrition program, authorized under Title III of the Older Americans Act (OAA), is the largest national food and nutrition program specifically for older adults. Programs and services include congregate nutrition programs, home-delivered nutrition services (Meals-on-Wheels), and nutrition screening and education. The program is not means tested, and participants may make voluntary confidential contributions for meals. The OAA does require targeting services to those in greatest social and economic need. A large percentage of program participants are likely to be socioeconomically deprived, minorities, living alone, and have disability or poor health. A recent study reported that facilitators of good nutrition in these types of programs included adherence to traditional (culturally appropriate diet) and peer networks (Sadarangani et al., 2019). Home-delivered meals have been shown to be most effective in improving nutrition and other outcomes for older adults (Tilly, 2017). Increased attention should be given to providing meals that include traditional foods and evaluating the effectiveness of these kinds of programs on nutritional health.

Socioeconomic Deprivation

There is a strong relationship between poor nutrition and socioeconomic deprivation. Older adults are the fastest-growing food-insecure population in the United States, which means they are not sure where or how they will get their next meal. Older adults are likely to be food insecure if they live in a southern state, have a disability, are younger than 69 years, live with a grandchild, and/or are Black or Hispanic (National Council on Aging, 2018). Individuals with low incomes may need to choose between fulfilling needs such as food, heat, telephone bills, medications, and health care visits. Some older adults eat only once per day in an attempt to make their income last through the month.

The Supplemental Nutrition Assistance Program (SNAP), a program of the USDA, Food and Nutrition Services, offers nutrition assistance to eligible, socioeconomically deprived individuals and families, but older adults are less likely than any other age group to use food assistance programs. Three out of five older adults who qualify for SNAP do not participate. Some individuals may not see the benefit, and others, especially those who lived through the Great Depression, are very reluctant to accept welfare. Low participation rates are also a result of barriers related to mobility and technology required to apply for benefits. Additionally, recent restrictions on eligibility for SNAP have been introduced in the United States and will further limit access for many older adults.

Free food programs, such as donated commodities, are also available at distribution centers (food banks) for those with limited incomes. Although this is another valuable option, use of such programs is not always feasible. One takes a chance on the types of food available on any particular day or week; quantities distributed are frequently too large for the single older adult or the older couple to use or even carry from the distribution site; the site may be too far away or difficult to reach; and the time of food distribution may be inconvenient.

There are cafeterias and restaurants that provide special meal prices for older adults, but costs have risen with increases in food costs. The previous advantages of eating out have diminished. Yet many single older adults eat out for most meals. More older adults are eating at fast food restaurants that typically do not offer low-fat/low-salt menu items. Providing education about the nutritional content of fast food and other convenient ways to enhance healthy nutritional intake is important (Box 10.2).

Transportation

Available and easily accessible transportation may be limited for older adults. Many small, long-standing neighborhood food stores have been closed in the wake of the expansion of larger supermarkets, which are located in areas that serve a greater segment of the population. Small convenience stores may not have a selection of healthy foods. Functional impairments may make it difficult to walk to the market, to reach it by public transportation, or to carry a bag of groceries while using a cane or walker. Fear is apparent in older adults' consideration of transportation. They may fear walking in the street and being mugged, not being able to cross the street in the time it takes the traffic light to change, or being knocked down or falling as they walk in crowded streets. Despite reduced senior citizen bus fares, many older adults remain very fearful of attack when using public transportation.

Transportation by taxicab or other transportation services may be unrealistic for an individual on a limited income. Senior citizen organizations in many parts of the United States have been helpful in providing older adults with van service to shopping areas. In housing complexes, it may be possible to schedule group trips to the supermarket. Resources in rural areas are more limited. It is important for nurses to be knowledgeable about transportation resources in the community. In addition, many older adults, particularly widowed men, may have never learned to shop and prepare food. Often, individuals have to rely on others to shop for them, and this may be a cause of concern depending on the availability of support and the reluctance to be dependent on someone else, particularly family. For those who own a computer, shopping over the Internet and having groceries delivered offers advantages, although prices may be higher than those in the stores.

CHRONIC DISEASES AND CONDITIONS AFFECTING NUTRITION

Many chronic diseases and their sequelae pose nutritional challenges for older adults. Heart failure and chronic obstructive pulmonary disease (COPD) are associated with fatigue, increased energy expenditure, and decreased appetite. Dietary interventions for diabetes are essential but may also affect customary eating patterns and require lifestyle changes. Conditions of the teeth and dental problems also affect nutrition (Chapter 11). Functional and cognitive impairments associated with chronic disease interfere with the individual's ability to shop, cook, and eat independently. More detailed information on chronic illness can be found in Chapters 20 to 23.

The side effects of medications prescribed for chronic conditions may further impair nutritional status. There are clinically significant drug-nutrient interactions that result in nutrient loss, and evidence is accumulating that shows the use of nutritional supplements may counteract these possible drug-induced nutrient depletions. A thorough medication review is an essential component of nutritional evaluation, and individuals should receive education about the effects of prescription medications, herbals, and supplements on nutritional status (Chapter 9).

Chronic Conditions That Affect Nutrition

Although there are several physiological and functional changes in the gut associated with aging (Chapter 4), the majority of the problems are the result of extrinsic factors. Polypharmacy, high-fat, high-volume meals, inactivity, and comorbid conditions are all aggravating factors. Some conditions that often affect nutritional intake, gastroesophageal reflux disease (GERD), diverticular disease, and dysphagia are discussed here.

Gastroesophageal Reflux Disease

GERD is a syndrome defined as mucosal damage from the movement of gastric contents backward from the stomach into the esophagus. It is the most common GI disorder affecting older adults. GERD is diagnosed empirically based on history and response to treatment. When the symptoms do not resolve with standard treatment, an endoscopy is indicated (Iannetti, 2017).

Etiology. The majority of GERD cases are caused by abnormalities of the lower esophageal sphincter (LES). When this muscle relaxes and allows reflux or is generally weak, GERD may occur. Risk factors include hiatal hernia, obesity, pregnancy, cigarette smoking, or inhaling secondhand smoke. People of all ages can develop GERD; some for unknown reasons.

Signs and symptoms. Although complaints of simple "heartburn" are often from dyspepsia, when other signs and symptoms are added, it is a greater concern. The classic complaints indicative of GERD are heartburn plus regurgitation—a sensation of burning in the throat as partially digested food and stomach acid inappropriately return to the posterior oropharynx. Older adults more commonly have more atypical symptoms of persistent cough, exacerbations of asthma, laryngitis, and intermittent chest pain. Abdominal pain may occur within 1 hour of eating, and symptoms are worse when lying down with the added pressure of gravity on the LES. Consumption of alcohol before or during eating exacerbates the reflux.

Complications. Persistent symptoms may lead to esophagitis, peptic strictures, esophageal ulcers (with bleeding), and, most importantly, Barrett's esophagus, a precursor to cancer. The most serious complication is the development of pneumonia from the aspiration of stomach contents. Dental caries may be caused by chronic exposure to gastric acids.

Treatment. The management of GERD combines lifestyle changes with pharmacological preparations, used in a stepwise fashion. Lifestyle modifications include eating smaller meals; stopping eating 3 to 4 hours before bed; avoiding high-fat foods, alcohol, caffeine, and nicotine; and sleeping with the head of the bed elevated. Weight reduction and smoking cessation are helpful. These strategies alone may control the majority of symptoms when complications are not present. Pharmacological preparations begin with over-the-counter antacids, such as Tums and Rolaids, and progress to H_2 blockers, such as ranitidine (Zantac), and then proton pump inhibitors, such as lansoprazole (Prevacid). In severe cases of GERD, surgical tightening of the LES may be necessary.

A nurse will work with the older adult to identify situations that aggravate GERD symptoms (e.g., overeating, consuming alcohol at mealtime) and develop the best strategies to deal with them.

Diverticular Disease

Diverticula are small herniations or sac-like outpouchings of mucosa that extend through the muscle layers of the colon wall, almost exclusive of the sigmoid colon. They form at weak points in the colon wall, usually where arteries penetrate and provide nutrients to the mucosal layer. Usually less than 1 cm in diameter, diverticula have thin, compressible walls if empty or firm walls if full of fecal matter. The prevalence of diverticular disease increases with age. The risk factors for diverticular disease can be found in Box 10.6. Diverticulitis is an acute inflammatory complication of diverticulosis.

> ## BOX 10.6   Risk Factors for Diverticular Disease
>
> - Family history
> - Personal history of gallbladder disease
> - Low dietary intake of fiber
> - Use of medications that slow fecal transit time
> - Chronic constipation
> - Obesity

Etiology. Although the exact etiology of diverticular disease is unknown, it is thought to be the result of a low-fiber diet, especially one accompanied by increased intra-abdominal pressure and chronic constipation. Smoking and obesity have been linked to diverticulitis and physical activity is associated with a decreased risk.

Signs and symptoms. The majority of persons with diverticulosis are completely asymptomatic, and the condition is found only when a barium enema, colonoscopy, or computed tomography (CT) scan is performed for some other reason. Persons with uncomplicated diverticulitis complain of abdominal pain, especially in the left-lower quadrant, and may have a fever and elevated white blood cell count, although the latter symptoms may be delayed or absent in older adults. The physical evaluation may be completely negative. Rectal bleeding is typically acute in onset, is painless, and stops spontaneously.

Complications. The complications of diverticulitis are rupture, abscess, stricture, or fistula. With any perforation, peritonitis is likely. Individuals with these complications may have an elevated pulse rate or are hypotensive; however, in older adults, unexplained lethargy or confusion may be seen. A lower-left quadrant mass may be palpated. Complicated diverticulitis is always considered an emergency and requires hospitalization for treatment and possible surgical repair.

Treatment. For persons with diverticulosis, the goal is prevention of diverticulitis. High-fiber diets (25 to 30 g/day) have been cited in American, European, and Asian studies as protective against diverticulosis. In addition, persons should strive for intake of six to eight glasses of fluid per day, preferably with little caffeine. Acute diverticulitis can be quite painful. The nurse works with the individual to find effective and safe comfort strategies that include pain medication and creative nonpharmacological approaches such as massage, hot or cold packs, stretching exercises, relaxation, music, or meditation techniques. Uncomplicated diverticulitis is treated with antibiotics and a clear liquid diet and is usually managed in the outpatient setting.

Dysphagia

Dysphagia, or difficulty swallowing, is a prevalent and growing concern in the older adult population. Swallowing is a complex process with some 50 pairs of muscles and many nerves working together to receive food into the mouth, prepare it, and move it from mouth to stomach. Normally, swallowing is a rapid and seamless act but involves several phases, and dysphagia can occur secondary to deficits in any of the phases of swallowing. Any condition that weakens or damages the muscles and nerves used for swallowing may cause dysphagia. Examples include individuals with diseases of the nervous system, such as amyotrophic lateral sclerosis (ALS) and Parkinson's disease (Chapter 23). Stroke or head injury may weaken or affect coordination of the swallowing muscles or limit sensation in the mouth and throat. Cerebrovascular accidents are the leading cause of neurological dysphagia and occur in 51% to 73% of patients with stroke (Paik & Moberg-Wolff, 2017) (Chapter 22). In addition, cancer of the head, neck, or esophagus may cause swallowing problems. Memory loss and cognitive deficits may also make it difficult to chew or swallow (Box 10.7) (Chapter 25).

The most common type of dysphagia is oropharyngeal dysphagia (OD). OD is a highly prevalent but largely unrecognized health issue. Prevalence is highest in older adults with neurological conditions and increases with advancing age and frailty. Up to 47% of frail older adults hospitalized for acute illness suffer from OD and it affects more than 50% of nursing home residents.

Dysphagia is a serious problem and has negative consequences, including severe distress during meals, aspiration with the consequence of chronic bronchial inflammation and aspiration pneumonia, weight loss, reduced food and fluid intake with the consequence of malnutrition and dehydration, and increased risk of

---

BOX 10.7   Risk Factors for Dysphagia

- Cerebrovascular accident
- Parkinson's disease
- Neuromuscular disorders (ALS, MS, myasthenia gravis)
- Dementia
- Head and neck cancer
- Traumatic brain injury
- Aspiration pneumonia
- Inadequate feeding technique
- Poor dentition

ALS, Amyotrophic lateral sclerosis; *MS,* multiple sclerosis.

---

death. Aspiration is the most profound and dangerous problem for older adults experiencing dysphagia. The 30-day mortality from health care–associated aspiration pneumonia is 30% (Wirth et al., 2016).

Recognizing and Analyzing Cues: Dysphagia

Screening and identification of cues is important and serves to identify those patients with the greatest risk of dysphagia. It is important to obtain a careful history of the older adult's response to dysphagia and to observe the person during mealtime. Symptoms that alert the nurse to possible swallowing problems are presented in Box 10.8. If dysphagia is suspected, a comprehensive

---

BOX 10.8   Symptoms of Dysphagia or Possible Aspiration

- Difficult, labored swallowing
- Drooling
- Copious oral secretions
- Coughing, choking at meals
- Holding or pocketing food/medications in the mouth
- Difficulty moving food or liquid from mouth to throat
- Difficulty chewing
- Nasal voice or hoarseness
- Wet or gurgling voice
- Excessive throat clearing
- Food or liquid leaking from the nose
- Prolonged eating time
- Pain with swallowing
- Unusual head or neck posturing while swallowing
- Sensation of something stuck in the throat during swallowing; sensation of a lump in the throat
- Heartburn
- Chest pain
- Hiccups
- Weight loss
- Frequent respiratory tract infections, pneumonia

clinical examination of swallowing and referral to a speech-language pathologist (SLP) is essential. A comprehensive examination includes a clinical swallowing evaluation, comprehensive medical history, physical examination of oral and motor function, and evaluation of food intake. Instrumental assessment includes video fluoroscopy swallowing study (VFSS) and fiberoptic endoscopic evaluation of swallowing (FEES). Nothing-by-mouth (NPO) status should be maintained until the swallowing evaluation is completed.

Nursing Actions: Dysphagia

After the swallowing evaluation, a decision must be made about the person's potential for functional improvement of the swallowing disorder and the person's safety in swallowing liquid and solid food. The main goal of dysphagia therapy is to reduce morbidity and mortality associated with chest infections and poor nutritional status. Nurses work closely with speech therapists and dietitians to implement interventions to prevent aspiration. Interventions include postural changes, such as chin tucks or head turns while swallowing, and modification of bolus volume, consistency, temperature, and rate of presentation. Diets may be modified in texture from pudding-like to nearly normal-textured solids. Liquids may range from spoon thick to honey-like, nectar-like, and thin. Commercial thickeners and thickened products are also available. The evidence is not strong that texture-modified food and thickened liquids reduce the impact of dysphagia. Additionally, patients often do not prefer this kind of food, which may reduce nutritional intake.

Neuromuscular electrical stimulation has received clearance by the US Food and Drug Administration for treatment of dysphagia. This therapy involves the administration of small electrical impulses to the swallowing muscles in the throat and is used in combination with traditional swallowing exercises. Research on the appropriate management of swallowing disorders in older adults, particularly during acute illness and in long-term care facilities, is very limited, and additional study is essential (Wirth et al., 2016). A protocol for preventing aspiration in older adults with dysphagia, and directions to access a video presentation of dysphagia, can be found in Box 10.2. Suggested interventions that nurses can utilize to prevent aspiration during hand feeding are presented in Box 10.9.

A comprehensive analysis of swallowing problems and other factors that influence intake must be conducted before initiating severely restricted diet modifications or considering the use of feeding tubes, particularly in older adults with end-stage dementia or those at the end of life. There is little evidence of a reduction in the risk of aspiration pneumonia with tube feeding in any

---

> **BOX 10.9 Tips for Best Practice**
> ### Preventing Aspiration in Patients With Dysphagia: Hand Feeding
>
> - Provide a 30-minute rest period before meal consumption; a rested person will likely have less difficulty swallowing.
> - The person should sit at 90 degrees during all oral intake and maintain 90-degree positioning for at least 1 hour after intake.
> - Adjust rate of feeding and size of bites to the person's tolerance; avoid rushed or forced feeding.
> - Alternate solid and liquid boluses.
> - Have the person swallow twice before the next mouthful.
> - Stroke under chin downward to initiate swallowing.
> - Follow speech therapist's recommendation for safe swallowing techniques and modified food consistency (may need thickened liquids, pureed foods).
> - If facial weakness is present, place food on the nonimpaired side of the mouth.
> - Avoid sedatives and hypnotics that may impair cough reflex and swallowing ability.
> - Keep suction equipment ready at all times.
> - Supervise all meals.
> - Monitor temperature.
> - Observe color of phlegm.
> - Visually check the mouth for pocketing of food in cheeks.
> - Check for food under dentures.
> - Provide mouth care every 4 hours and before and after meals, including denture cleaning.

---

group of adult patients, and in fact, enteral nutrition is generally cited as a risk factor for aspiration pneumonia (Finucane, 2017). However, there may be certain circumstances when providing temporary short-term tube feeding may be appropriate (e.g., individuals with stroke and resulting dysphagia and other conditions when it may be possible to resume oral nutrition at some point). Chapter 10 discusses concerns related to the use of feeding tubes for individuals with dementia.

❖ USING CLINICAL JUDGMENT TO PROMOTE HEALTHY AGING: NUTRITIONAL HEALTH

Nurses are often the first to identify patients in need of nutrition intervention and are integral to encouraging nutritional intake from admission to discharge. Evaluation of nutritional health in older adults can be difficult in the absence of severe malnutrition. Similar to other illness presentations, cues to nutritional problems present more subtly, and older adults are less likely than younger people to show signs of malnutrition and nutrient malabsorption.

◆ Recognizing and Analyzing Cues: Nutritional Health

Nutritional screening is the first step in identifying individuals who are at risk of malnutrition or have undetected malnutrition. Based on findings of a preliminary screening, a more comprehensive analysis may be indicated. Because of the high incidence of malnutrition and often nonspecific symptoms, nutrition risk screening should be performed routinely and can be incorporated into annual health checks for those aged 75 years and older. If the individual is hospitalized or in a long-term care facility, screening and identification of concerns should be conducted within 24 hours of admission and periodically reassessed throughout the stay (Avelino-Silva & Jaluul, 2017).

There are several screening tools specific to older individuals, and screening can be completed in any setting. The Nutrition Screening Initiative Checklist (Fig. 10.2) can be self-administered or completed by a family member or any member of the health care team. The MNA-SF (Box 10.2) provides a simple, quick, and valid method of identifying older adults who are at risk of malnutrition. The Self-MNA is a simple tool designed to help older adults determine whether they are getting the nutrition they need. The tool is available in English, Bulgarian, Danish, Finnish, German, Greek, Italian, Portuguese, Spanish, and Swedish. Further information on how to access the MNA and a video demonstrating a nurse administering the tool can be found in Box 10.2.

The Minimum Data Set 3.0 (MDS 3.0) (Chapter 8), used in long-term care facilities, is also a useful screening tool for nutritional risk. The MDS does not establish malnutrition, but rather is a tool to generate a care plan (Mueller, 2015). The MDS includes the range of cues that can be used to identify potential nutritional problems, risk factors, and the potential for improved function. Triggers for a more thorough investigation of problems include weight loss, alterations in taste, medical therapies, prescription medications, hunger, parenteral or intravenous feedings, mechanically altered or therapeutic diets, percentage of food left uneaten, pressure injuries, and edema.

When malnutrition or risk of it is detected, a comprehensive analysis of presenting cues (physical, psychosocial) is indicated and will provide the most conclusive data about a person's actual nutritional state. Interprofessional approaches are key to further investigation and determination of needed actions and should involve medicine, nursing, dietary, physical, occupational and speech therapy, and social work. The collective results provide the data needed to identify the immediate and the potential nutritional problems so that plans for supervision, assistance, and education in the attainment of adequate nutrition can be implemented. Components of a comprehensive analysis include interview, history, physical examination, anthropometric data, laboratory data, food/nutrient intake, and functional status. A summary is presented in Box 10.10. Explanations of several components are discussed in the following sections.

◆ Food/Nutrient Intake

Frequently, a 24-hour diet recall compared with the MyPlate for Older Adults (Fig. 10.1) can provide an estimate of nutritional adequacy. When the individual

---

Read the statements below. Circle the number in the Yes column for those that apply to you or someone you know. For each "yes" answer, score the number listed. Total your nutritional score.

	YES
I have an illness or condition that made me change the kind or amount of food I eat.	2
I eat fewer than two meals per day.	3
I eat few fruits, vegetables, or milk products.	2
I have three or more drinks of beer, liquor, or wine almost every day.	2
I have tooth or mouth problems that make it hard for me to eat.	2
I don't always have enough money to buy the food I need.	4
I eat alone most of the time.	1
I take three or more different prescriptions or over-the-counter drugs each day.	1
Without wanting to, I have lost or gained 10 pounds in the past 6 months.	2
I am not always physically able to shop, cook, and/or feed myself.	2

Total Nutritional Score _____

0-2 indicates good nutrition
3-5 moderate risk
6+ high nutritional risk

FIG. 10.2 Nutrition Screening Initiative. (Courtesy The Nutrition Screening Initiative, Washington, DC.)

BOX 10.10 Recognizing and Analyzing Cues to Nutritional Health

Dietary History and Current Intake
- Food preferences and habits; meaning and significance of food to the individual; do they eat alone?
- Cultural or religious food habits
- Ability to obtain and prepare food including adequate finances to obtain nutritious food
- Social activities and normal patterns; meal frequency
- Control over food selection and choices
- Fluid intake
- Alcohol intake
- Special diet
- Vitamins/minerals/supplement use
- Chewing/swallowing problems
- Functional limitations that impair independence in eating
- Cognitive changes affecting appetite/ability to feed self
- Depression screen if indicated

History/Physical
- Chief complaint, medical history, chronic conditions, presence or absence of inflammation (fever, hypothermia, signs of systemic inflammatory response), usual weight and any loss or gain, fluid retention, loss of muscle/fat, oral health and dentition, medication use

Anthropometric Measurements
- Body mass index
- Height
- Current weight and usual adult weight
- Recent weight changes
- Skinfold measurements

Biochemical Analysis
- Complete blood count
- Protein status
- Lipid profile
- Electrolytes
- Blood urea nitrogen (BUN)/creatinine ratio

Food/Nutrient Intake
- Periods of inadequate intake (nothing-by-mouth [NPO] status)
- 24-hour or 3-day diet record

Functional Assessment
- Hand-grip strength
- Standard functional assessment (Chapter 8)

Adapted from Mathew, M., & Jacobs, M. (2014). Malnutrition and feeding problems. In R. Ham, P. Sloane, G. Warshaw, et al. (Eds.), *Primary care geriatrics: a case-based approach* (6th ed, p. 318). Philadelphia: Elsevier Saunders.

cannot supply all of the requested information, it may be possible to obtain data from a family member or another source such as a shopping receipt. There will be times, however, when information will not be as complete as one would like, or the individual, too proud to admit that he or she is not eating, will furnish erroneous information. Other areas of the comprehensive analysis will provide additional data from other sources. Keeping a dietary record for 3 days is another tool. This can be completed by the individual, family, or caregivers. The diet recall includes what foods were eaten, when food was eaten, and the amounts eaten. Computer analysis of the dietary records provides information on energy and vitamin and mineral intake. Printouts can provide the individual and the health care provider with a visual graph of the intake.

Accurate completion of 3-day dietary records in hospitals and long-term care facilities can be problematic, and intake may be either underestimated or overestimated. Standardized observational protocols should be developed to ensure accuracy of oral intake documentation and the adequacy and quality of feeding assistance during mealtimes. Nurses should ensure that direct caregivers are educated on the proper observation and documentation of intake and should closely monitor performance in this area.

◆ Weight/Height Considerations

Weight change (from usual) offers the most useful information on nutritional status, and a detailed weight history should be obtained along with current weight. History should include a history of weight loss, if the weight loss was intentional or unintentional, and during which period it occurred. A history of anorexia is also important and many older adults, especially women, have limited their weight throughout life. Debate continues in the quest to determine the appropriate weight charts for an older adult. Although weight alone does not indicate the adequacy of diet, unplanned fluctuations in weight are significant and should be evaluated.

Accurate weight patterns are sometimes difficult to obtain in long-term care settings. Procedures for weighing people should be established and followed consistently to obtain an accurate representation of weight changes. Weighing procedure should be supervised by licensed personnel, and changes should be reported immediately to the provider. Correct weight values might be met for height, but weight changes may be the result of fluid retention, edema, or ascites and merit investigation. A weight loss of 5% of usual body weight in 6 to 12 months is the most widely accepted definition for clinically important weight loss in older adults. In long-term care facilities, a loss of more than 5% of body weight in 1 month, more than 7.5% in 3 months, or more than 10% in 6 months is considered a significant indicator of poor nutrition and an MDS trigger.

Height should always be measured and never estimated or given by self-report. If the person cannot stand, an alternative way of measuring standing height is knee-height using special calipers. An alternative to knee-height measurements is a demi-span measurement, which is half the total arm span. Measurement of BMI in older adults can be unreliable and does not provide the same clues to health status in older adults as it does in younger people. A BMI of less than 23 classifies an older adult (older than age 65 years) as underweight and may require nutrition intervention. Health risks associated with a BMI of 18.5 to 25 in younger populations may not apply to those older than 65 years of age (Chernoff, 2014; Sauer et al., 2016).

◆ Biochemical Analysis/Measures of Visceral Protein

The relevance of laboratory tests of serum albumin, prealbumin, and transferrin, as indicators of malnutrition, is limited. These acute-phase proteins do not consistently or predictability change with weight loss, calorie restriction, or negative nitrogen balance. They appear to be a better indication of the severity of inflammatory response rather than poor nutritional status. Further investigation of the significance of low protein levels is needed (Avelino-Silva and Jaluul, 2017).

◆ Nursing Actions: Nutritional Health

Causes of poor nutrition are complex, and all of the factors emphasized in this chapter are important to evaluate when planning individualized interventions to ensure adequate nutrition for older adults. For the community-dwelling older adult, nutrition education and problem solving with the individual and family members or caregivers on the best way to resolve the potential or actual nutritional deficit is important. Referrals to community-based nutrition programs, if indicated, can assist in enhancing nutrition. Older adults in hospitals and long-term care facilities are more likely to be admitted with malnutrition, be at high risk of malnutrition, and have disease conditions that contribute to malnutrition. Severely restricted diets, long periods of NPO status, and insufficient time and staff for feeding assistance also contribute to inadequate nutrition. Older adults with dementia are particularly at risk of weight loss and inadequate nutrition (Chapter 25).

An important nursing role to enhance nutritional health is assisting with meal intake and supervising other staff and family members in hospitals and nursing facilities. Inherent in the role are (1) identification of issues related to performance at mealtimes (ability to eat independently, quality of assistance if needed, adequate intake); (2) modification of the environment to be pleasurable for eating; (3) supervision of eating; (4) provision of guidance and support to staff on feeding techniques that enhance intake and preserve dignity and independence; and (5) evaluation of outcomes.

The incidence of eating disability in long-term care is high, with estimates that 50% of all residents cannot eat independently. Inadequate staffing in long-term care facilities is associated with poor nutrition and hydration, and research has shown that it can be an impossible task to feed the number of people who need assistance (Kayser-Jones, 1997). In response to concerns about the lack of adequate assistance during mealtime in long-term care facilities, the CMS implemented a rule that allows feeding assistants with 8 hours of approved training to help residents with eating. Feeding assistants must be supervised by a registered nurse (RN) or licensed practical-vocational nurse (LPN-LVN). Family members may also be willing and able to assist at mealtimes and also provide a familiar social context for the patient.

Assistance with meals in hospitals is also a concern and programs to address the unique needs of hospitalized patients have been implemented in some hospitals. Further research is needed on the effectiveness of feeding assistance programs in hospital settings. Boxes 10.11 and 10.12 present best-practice tips to improve nutritional intake in hospitals and long-term care facilities. Chapter 25 discusses nutritional concerns for individuals with neurocognitive disorders and interventions to enhance nutrition. Prevention of undernutrition and malnutrition and the maintenance of dietary needs and food intake are also ethical responsibilities. No older adult should be hungry or thirsty because he or she cannot shop, cook, buy and prepare food, or eat independently. Nor should any older adult have to suffer because of a lack of assistance with these activities in whatever setting the person may reside.

◆ Restrictive Diets and Caloric Supplements

The use of restrictive therapeutic diets for frail older adults in long-term care (low cholesterol, low salt, no concentrated sweets) often reduces food intake without significantly helping the clinical status of the individual (Pioneer Network and Rothschild Foundation, 2011). Dispensing a small amount of calorically dense oral nutritional supplement (2 calories/mL) during the routine medication pass may have a greater effect on weight gain than a traditional supplement (1.06 calories/mL) with or between meals. Small volumes of nutrient-dense supplement may have less of an effect on appetite and will enhance food intake during meals and snacks. This delivery method allows nurses to observe and document

---

BOX 10.11   Tips for Best Practice
Improving Nutritional Intake in Hospitals

- Evaluate nutritional and oral health status, including ability to eat and amount of assistance needed.
- Ensure proper fit and cleanliness of dentures and denture use.
- Provide oral hygiene, and allow the person to wash his or her hands before meals.
- Ensure environment is conducive to eating (remove objects such as urinals and bed pans; clear bedside tables). Ask yourself whether you would want to eat the food in the environment in which it is presented.
- Position patient for safe eating (head of bed elevated or sit in a chair if possible).
- Stop nonessential clinical activity during meals (e.g., procedures, rounds, medication administration).
- Ensure that all nursing staff are aware of the patients who need assistance with eating and that adequate help is provided.
- Ensure that all necessary items are on the tray; prepare all food on the tray if needed; butter bread, open containers, provide straws, provide adaptive equipment as needed.
- Consider volunteers or family members to assist with eating and train and supervise.
- Administer medication for pain or nausea on a schedule that provides comfort at mealtime.
- Determine food preferences; provide for choices in food; include foods appropriate to cultural and religious customs.
- Accurately evaluate dietary intake using a validated method.
- Make dietary changes/referrals readily.
- Make food available 24 hours/day—provide snacks between meals and at night.
- Limit periods of nothing-by-mouth NPO status and provide food as soon as patient is able to eat.
- Consider liberalizing therapeutic diet if intake is inadequate; offer diet options/alternatives as indicated, including flavor enhancement.

From Furman E. (2014). The Theory of Compromised Eating Behavior. Research in Gerontological Nursing. 7(2):78–86. doi:10.3928/19404921-20130930-01. Reprinted with permission from SLACK Incorporated.

BOX 10.12   Tips for Best Practice
Improving Nutritional Intake in Long-Term Care

- Evaluate nutritional and oral health status.
- Evaluate ability to eat and amount of assistance needed.
- Serve meals with the person in a chair rather than in bed when possible.
- Provide analgesics and antiemetics on a schedule that provides comfort at mealtime.
- Determine food preferences; provide for choices in food; include foods appropriate to cultural and religious customs.
- Consider buffet-style dining, use of steam tables rather than meal delivery service from trays, café or bistro-type dining.
- Make food available 24 hours/day—provide snacks between meals and at night.
- Do not interrupt meals to administer medication if possible.
- Limit staff breaks to before and after mealtimes to ensure adequate staff are available to assist with meals.
- Walk around the dining area or the rooms at mealtime to determine if food is being eaten or if assistance is needed.
- Encourage family members to share the mealtimes for a heightened social situation.
- If caloric supplements are used, offer them between meals or with the medication pass.
- Ensure proper fit of dentures and denture use.
- Provide oral hygiene, and allow the person to wash his or her hands before meals.
- Have the person wear his or her glasses during meals.
- Sit while feeding the person who needs assistance, use touch, and carry on a social conversation.
- Provide soft music during the meal.
- Use small, round tables seating six to eight people. Consider using tablecloths and centerpieces.
- Seat people with similar interests and abilities together and encourage socialization.
- Involve in restorative dining programs.
- Make diets as liberal as possible depending on health status, especially for frail elders who are not consuming adequate amounts of food.
- Consider a referral to occupational therapist for individuals experiencing difficulties with eating.

---

consumption. A growing body of evidence suggests that supplementation might improve outcomes of hospitalized patients, including length of stay, costs, and readmissions (Avelino-Silva & Jaluul, 2017).

Further studies and randomized clinical trials are needed to evaluate the effectiveness of nutritional supplementation. The American Geriatrics Society (2014) recommends avoiding high-calorie supplements for treatment of anorexia in older adults. Instead, recommendations are to optimize social supports, provide feeding assistance, and clarify patient goals and expectations. Unintentional weight loss is a common problem for medically ill or frail older adults. Although high-calorie supplements increase weight in older adults, there is no evidence that they affect other important clinical outcomes, such as quality of life, mood, functional status, or survival.

◆ Pharmacological Therapy

The American Geriatrics Society (2014) does not recommend drugs that stimulate appetite (orexigenic drugs) to treat anorexia or malnutrition in older adults.

Use of drugs such as megestrol acetate results in minimum improvement in appetite and weight gain, no improvement in quality of life or survival, and increased risk of thrombotic events, fluid retention, and death. Systematic reviews of cannabinoids, dietary polyunsaturated fatty acids (DHA and EPA), thalidomide, and anabolic steroids have not identified adequate evidence for the efficacy and safety of these agents for weight gain.

◆ Patient Education

Education should be provided on nutritional requirements for health, special diet modifications for chronic illness management, the effect of age-associated changes and medication on nutrition, effective feeding techniques, and community resources to assist in maintaining adequate nutrition. Medicare covers nutrition therapy for select diseases, such as diabetes and kidney disease.

KEY CONCEPTS

- Diet can affect longevity and, when combined with lifestyle changes, reduce disease risk.
- Clinical judgment begins with the recognition and analysis of clinical cues through observation of physical data and integration of the range of complex factors that may affect nutritional health, including lifelong eating habits, income, chronic illness, dentition, mood disorders, capacity for food preparation, and cognitive and functional limitations. An interprofessional approach is the most effective in developing solutions and taking action.
- Overweight and obesity are major public health concerns around the globe. The proportion of older adults who are obese has doubled in the past 30 years.
- A rising incidence of malnutrition among older adults has been documented in acute care, long-term care, and the community and is expected to rise dramatically in the next 30 years.
- Malnutrition is a precursor to frailty and has serious consequences, including infections, pressure injuries, anemia, hypotension, impaired cognition, hip fractures, prolonged hospital stay, institutionalization, and increased morbidity and mortality.
- Making mealtime pleasant for older adults who are unable to eat unassisted is a nursing challenge; mealtime must be made enjoyable, and adequate assistance must be provided.
- Dysphagia is a serious problem and contributes to weight loss, malnutrition, dehydration, aspiration pneumonia, and death. Careful assessment of risk factors, observation for signs and symptoms, and collaboration with speech-language pathologists on interventions are essential.

ACTIVITIES AND DISCUSSION QUESTIONS

1. Which factors affect the nutrition of the older adult?
2. Give specific examples of nursing actions to provide better nutrition for older adults in the community, in acute care, and in long-term care settings.
3. Choose one of the contributing factors to malnutrition and nursing actions to reduce risk.
4. Assess your nutrition using the Nutrition Screening Initiative and discuss your score and risk.
5. How is dysphagia evaluated and which actions may be helpful in preventing aspiration?

NEXT-GENERATION NCLEX® EXAMINATION-STYLE QUESTIONS

The nurse is completing the monthly nursing assessment of Mr. Dawson. Mr. Dawson is a 92-year-old male. He has been at the long-term care facility for the past 5 years. His weight this month is 300 pounds (BMI 26.6 kg/m²). His blood pressure is 145/82 mmHg, heart rate 90 beats per minute, respirations 18 breaths per minute and temperature 97.4°F. He responds to questions appropriately. During the physical examination at 0900 hours, the nurse notes Mr. Dawson is drooling and coughing intermittently. His upper dentures fall when he opens his mouth for evaluation. His lungs are clear on examination and his heart has regular rhythm.

Choose the most likely options for the information missing from the statements below by selecting from the lists of options provided.

The nurse recognizes that _____1_____, ___2_____, and ____3_____ put Mr. Dawson at increased risk of _____4_____ and he should be ___5_____ until the _____ 6_____ is completed.

Options
Overnutrition
Swallowing evaluation
Depression
Coughing after eating
NPO
Dry mouth
Dysphagia
Copious secretions
Difficulty chewing
Occupational therapy

REFERENCES

American Geriatrics Society. *Choosing wisely: five things physicians and patients should question,* 2014. http://www.choosingwisely.org/american-geriatrics-society-releases-second-choosing-wisely-list-identifies-5-more-tests-and-treatments-that-older-patients-and-providers-should-question/.

Avelino-Silva, T. J., & Jaluul, O. (2017). Malnutrition in hospitalized older patients: management strategies to improve patient care and clinical outcomes. *Int J Geront, 11*(2), 56–61.

Baugreet, S., Hamill, R. M., Kerry, J. P., & McCarthy, S. N. (2017). Mitigating nutrition and health deficiencies in older adults: a role for food innovation? *J Food Sci, 82*(4), 848–855.

Bowman, K., Delgado, J., Henley, W. E., et al. (2017). Obesity in older people with and without conditions associated with weight loss: follow-up of 955,000 primary care patients. *J Gerontol A Biol Sci Med Sci, 72*(2), 203–209.

Buys, D. R., Flood, K. L., Real, K., Chang, M., & Locher, J. L. (2013). Mealtime assistance for hospitalized older adults: a report on the SPOONS volunteer program. *J Gerontol Nur, 39*(9), 18–22.

Cederholm, T., & Jensen, G. L. (2017). To create a consensus on malnutrition diagnostic criteria: a report from the Global Leadership Initiative on Malnutrition (GLIM) meeting at the ESPEN Congress 2016. *Clin Nutr, 36*, 7–10.

Chernoff, R. (2014). *Geriatric nutrition: the health professionals handbook,* ed. 4. Burlington, MA: Jones and Bartlett Learning.

Crogan, N. L. (2017). Nutritional problems affecting older adults. *Nurs Clin North Am, 52*, 433–445.

Finucane, T. E. (2017). Questioning feeding tubes to treat dysphagia. *JAMA Intern Med, 177*(3), 443.

Furman, E. (2014). The theory of compromised eating behavior. *Res Gerontol Nurs, 7*(2), 78–86.

Gretebeck, K. A., Sabatini, L. M., Black, D. R., & Gretebeck, R. J. (2017). Physical activity, functional ability, and obesity in older adults: a gender difference. *J Gerontol Nurs, 43*(9), 38–46.

Gropper, S. S., Tappen, R. M., & Vieira, E. R. (2019). Differences in nutritional and physical health indicators among older African Americans, European Americans, and Hispanic Americans. *J Nutr Gerontol Geriatr, 38*(3), 205–217.

Hooshmand, B., Mangialasche, F., Kalpouzos, G., et al. (2016). Association of vitamin B12, folate, and sulfur amino acids with brain magnetic resonance imaging measures in older adults: a longitudinal population-based study. *JAMA Psychiatry, 73*(6), 606–613.

Iannetti, A. (2017). Updates on the management of GERD disease. *J Gastrointest Dig Syst, 7*, 523.

Kalish, V. B. (2016). Obesity in older adults. *Prim Care, 43*(1), 137–144.

Kayser-Jones, J. (1997). Inadequate staffing at mealtime: implications for nursing and health policy. *J Gerontol Nurs, 23*, 14–21.

Kritchevsky, S. B. (2017). Taking obesity in older adults seriously. *J Gerontol A Biol Sci Med Sci, 73*(1), 57–58.

Lustbader, W. (1999). Thoughts on the meaning of frailty. *Generations, 13*, 21.

McEvoy, C. T., Guyer, H., Langa, K. M., & Yaffe, K. (2017). Neuroprotective diets are associated with better cognitive function: the Health and Retirement Study. *J Am Geriatr Soc, 65*, 1857–1862.

Mogensen, K. M., & DiMaria-Ghalili, R. A. (2015). Malnutrition in older adults. *Today's Dietician, 17*(9), 56.

Mueller, C. M. (2015). Nutrition assessment and older adults. *Top Clin Nutr, 30*(1), 94–102.

National Council on Aging. *SNAP and senior hunger facts,* 2018. https://www.ncoa.org/news/resources-for-reporters/get-the-facts/senior-hunger-facts/.

Paik, N. J., & Moberg-Wolff, A. (2017). Dysphagia. *Medscape.* https://emedicine.medscape.com/article/2212409-overview.

Sadarangani, T. R., Johnson, J. J., Chong, S. K., et al. (2019). Using the social ecological model to identify drivers of nutrition risk in adult day settings serving East Asian older adults. *Res Gerontol Nurs, 12*, 1–12.

Sauer, A. C., Alish, C. J., Strausbaugh, K., West, K., & Quatrara, B. (2016). Nurses needed: identifying malnutrition in hospitalized older adults. *NursingPlus Open, 2*, 21–25.

Simmons, S. F., Osterweil, D., & Schnelle, J. F. (2001). Improving food intake in nursing home residents with feeding assistance: a staffing analysis. *J Gerontol A Biol Sci Med Sci, 56*(12), M790–M794.

The Joint Commission. (2014). *Patient Safety Tool: Advancing effective communication, cultural competence and patient- and family-centered care: a roadmap for hospitals.* OakbrookTerrace, IL: The Joint Commission.

Tilly, J. (2017). White Paper: Opportunities to improve nutrition for older adults and reduce risk of poor health outcomes. *National Resource Center on Nutrition and Aging.* http://nutritionandaging.org/opportunities-to-improve-nutrition-for-older-adults-and-reduce-risk-of-poor-health-outcomes/.

Tufts University. *MyPlate for Older Adults,* 2016. http://hnrca.tufts.edu/myplate/.

US Department of Health and Human Services and US Department of Agriculture: *2015—2020 Dietary Guidelines for Americans,* ed. 8, 2015–2020. https://health.gov/dietaryguidelines/2015/guidelines/.

Ward, Z., Bleich, S., Cardock, AL., et al. (2019). Projected state-level prevalence of adult obesity and severe obesity. *NEJM, 381*, 2440–2450.

Wirth, R., Dziewas, R., Beck, A. M., et al. (2016). Oropharyngeal dysphagia in older adults—from pathophysiology to adequate intervention: a review and summary of an international expert meeting. *Clin Interv Aging, 11*, 189–208.

World Health Organization. Obesity and overweight. 2020. https://www.who.int/news-room/fact-sheets/detail/obesity-and-overweight.

11

Clinical Judgment to Promote Hydration and Oral Health

Theris A. Touhy

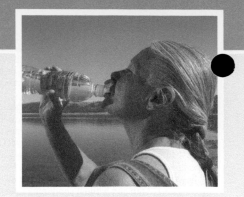

http://evolve.elsevier.com/Touhy/gerontological/

LEARNING OBJECTIVES

Upon completion of this chapter, the reader will be able to:
- Identify factors that influence hydration management in older adults.
- Describe nursing actions for prevention and treatment of dehydration.
- Demonstrate understanding of the relationship between oral health and disease.
- Utilize clinical judgment to identify and evaluate nursing actions to maintain hydration and oral health in a variety of settings.

THE LIVED EXPERIENCE

I know I don't drink enough water—coffee, yes; water, no. It's hard when you are in a wheelchair and only have one arm that works. This smart little student nurse really fixed me up. She gave me a plastic water bottle and attached it to my chair on my good side. Now wherever I go, the water goes.

Jack, age 84

HYDRATION MANAGEMENT

Hydration management is the promotion of an adequate fluid balance, which prevents complications resulting from abnormal or undesirable fluid levels. Water, an accessible and available commodity to almost all people, is often overlooked as an essential part of nutritional requirements. Water's function in the body includes thermoregulation, dilution of water-soluble medications, facilitation of renal and bowel function, and creation of requisite conditions for and maintenance of metabolic processes.

Daily needs for water can usually be met by functionally independent older adults through intake of fluids with meals and social drinks. However, a significant number of older adults (up to 85% of those 85 years of age and older) drink less than 1 liter of fluid per day. Older adults, with the exception of those requiring fluid restrictions, should consume at least 1500 mL of fluid per day. Maintenance of fluid balance (fluid intake equals fluid output) is essential to health, regardless of a person's age.

Age-related changes (Chapter 4), medication use, functional impairments, and comorbid medical and emotional illnesses place some older adults at risk of changes in fluid balance, especially dehydration. Hydration habits, as described by Mentes (2012), also influence how and why individuals consume liquids. Each group has different hydration habits that can guide evaluation and design of nursing actions. Providing targeted nursing actions to those at greatest risk may decrease the prevalence of dehydration (Box 11.1).

BOX 11.1   Typology of Hydration Problems

CAN DRINK: Capable of accessing and consuming fluids but may not know what adequate intake is or may forget to drink as a result of cognitive impairment. May need education about daily fluid needs and the importance of reporting any changes; verbal encouragement and prompting; easy access to fluids.

CAN'T DRINK: Physically incapable of accessing or safely consuming fluids related to physical dependence or swallowing disorders. May need dysphagia prevention interventions; physical aids to assist with drinking (e.g., sports bottle, sippy cup); swallowing evaluation and safe swallowing techniques; oral care; foods rich in fluid (smoothies); adequate assistance.

WON'T DRINK: Highest risk of dehydration. Capable of consuming fluids safely but do not because of fear of being incontinent; or have lower cognitive abilities and consume limited amounts of fluid at a time (sippers). Interventions may include offering frequent small amounts of fluid at each contact (preferred beverages); providing fluid with activities; implementing toileting programs; promoting education about maintaining fluid intake.

END OF LIFE: Terminally ill individuals who may have hydration patterns described in other categories. Hydration will be dependent on resident and family preference, advance directives.

From Mentes J. (2006). A Typology of Oral Hydration: Problems Exhibited by Frail Nursing Home Residents. *J Gerontol Nurs.* 32(1) 13–19. doi:10.3928/0098-9134-20060101-09. Reprinted with permission from SLACK Incorporated.

DEHYDRATION

Dehydration is a complex condition resulting in a reduction of total body water. In older adults, dehydration most often develops as a result of disease, age-related changes, and/or the effects of medication. Dehydration is not primarily a result of lack of access to water. Dehydration is considered a geriatric syndrome that is frequently associated with common diseases (e.g., diabetes, respiratory illness, heart failure) and frailty. It is often an unappreciated comorbid condition that exacerbates an underlying condition such as a urinary tract infection, respiratory tract infection, or worsening depression.

Dehydration is a significant risk factor for delirium, thromboembolic complications, infections, kidney stones, constipation and obstipation, falls, medication toxicity, renal failure, seizure, electrolyte imbalance, hyperthermia, and delayed wound healing (McCrow et al., 2016; Mentes & Aronow, 2016). In community-dwelling older adults, physical performance and cognitive processing are both affected by mild dehydration (Mentes & Gaspar, 2020).

Adults older than 65 years have the highest rates of acute care admissions for dehydration as a primary diagnosis. Dehydration is estimated to be present in half of long-term care residents. In the long-term care setting, difficulties in communication, mobility, cognitive function, and eating prevent many from accessing fluid independently, and a recent study reported that the majority of residents are not even consuming 1500 mL of fluids per day (Namasivayam-MacDonald et al., 2018).

⚡ SAFETY ALERT

Dehydration is a problem prevalent among older adults in all settings. If not treated adequately, mortality from dehydration can be as high as 50% (Faes et al., 2007).

Risk Factors for Dehydration

The presence of physical or emotional illness, surgery, trauma, frailty, or conditions of higher physiological demands increases the risk of dehydration. Older adults are particularly at risk of dehydration because their kidneys are less able to concentrate urine and some medications (diuretics) increase fluid excretion. However, the main reason for dehydration is reduced fluid intake (Namasivayam-MacDonald et al., 2018). When the fluid balance of older adults is at risk, the limited capacity of homeostatic mechanisms becomes significant. With age, daily fluid intake tends to decrease, and adults aged 85 years and older, on average, drink the least amount of fluid at 850 cc per day. Even simple disruptions in food and fluid intake can precipitate an episode of dehydration. Careful monitoring of intake is important during hospitalization and long-term care placement because several missed meals can contribute to hydration problems (Mentes & Gaspar, 2020).

❖ USING CLINICAL JUDGMENT TO PROMOTE HEALTHY AGING: DEHYDRATION

◆ Recognizing and Analyzing Cues: Dehydration

Prevention of dehydration is essential, but evaluation is complex in older adults. Cues present differently, and clinical signs may not appear until dehydration is advanced. Attention to risk factors for dehydration is very important (Box 11.2). In addition, the Minimum Data Set (MDS) 3.0 (Chapter 8) provides guidelines for the evaluation of dehydration and fluid maintenance in nursing home residents. Education should be provided to older adults and their caregivers on the need for fluids and the signs and symptoms of dehydration. Acute situations such as vomiting, diarrhea, or febrile episodes should be identified quickly and treated. Evaluation of

BOX 11.2   Risk Factors for Dehydration in Older Adults

- Age-related changes
- Medications: diuretics, laxatives, angiotensin-converting enzyme (ACE) inhibitors, psychotropics
- Use of four or more medications
- Functional deficits
- Communication and comprehension problems
- Oral problems
- Dysphagia
- Delirium
- Dementia
- Hospitalization
- Low body weight
- Diagnostic procedures requiring fasting
- Inadequate assistance with fluid/food intake
- Diarrhea
- Fever
- Vomiting
- Infections
- Bleeding
- Draining wounds
- Artificial ventilation
- Fluid restrictions
- High environmental temperatures
- Multiple comorbidities

hydration status must be conducted on admission to the hospital or nursing facility, particularly for those who are frail, and must be regularly monitored throughout their stay and at discharge (McCrow et al., 2016).

Signs/Symptoms of Dehydration

Typical signs of dehydration may not always be present in older adults, and symptoms are often atypical. Skin turgor at the sternum, commonly included in the evauation of dehydration, is an unreliable marker in older adults because of the loss of subcutaneous tissue with aging. Dry mucous membranes in the mouth and nose, longitudinal furrows on the tongue, orthostasis, speech incoherence, rapid pulse rate, extremity weakness, dry axilla, and sunken eyes may indicate dehydration. However, the diagnosis of dehydration must be biochemically proven.

Laboratory Tests

Serum osmolarity readings ≥ 300 mOsmol/L are indicative of dehydration in older adults (Hooper et al., 2016). Although most cases of dehydration have an elevated blood urea nitrogen (BUN) measurement, there are many other causes of an elevated BUN/creatinine ratio,

therefore this test cannot be used alone to diagnose dehydration in older adults. Recent research reports that urinary measures reflecting hydration status in older adults (urine color, osmolarity, volume) should not be used because these measures are not sensitive or specific enough (Hooper et al., 2016). However, urine patterns and color should be observed for changes.

◆ Nursing Actions: Dehydration

Nursing actions are derived from a comprehensive analysis of cues and consist of risk identification and hydration management (Box 11.3). Any older adult who has functional or cognitive impairments and is dependent on others for fluid intake is particularly at risk. Those who develop fever, diarrhea, vomiting, or a nonfebrile infection should be monitored closely by implementing intake and output records and providing additional fluids. NPO (nothing-by-mouth) requirements for diagnostic tests and surgical procedures should be as short as possible for older adults, and adequate fluids should be given once tests and procedures are completed. A 2-hour suspension of fluid intake is recommended for many procedures. Fluid intake needs to be monitored throughout a hospital stay and adequate assistance provided to maintain fluid intake.

BOX 11.3   Simple Screen for Dehydration

Drugs (e.g., diuretics)	**T**achycardia
End of life	**I**ncontinence (fear of)
High fever	**O**ral problems/sippers
Yellow urine turns dark	**N**eurological impairment
Dizziness (orthostasis)	(confusion)
Reduced oral intake	**S**unken eyes
Axilla dry	

From Thomas, D., Cote, T., Lawhorne, L., et al. (2008). Understanding clinical dehydration and its treatment, *J Am Med Dir Assoc* 9(5), 292–301.

Hydration management involves both acute and ongoing management of oral intake (Box 11.4). Oral rehydration therapy is the first treatment approach for dehydration. Individuals with mild to moderate dehydration who can drink and do not have significant mental or physical compromise resulting from fluid loss may be able to replenish fluids orally. Water is considered the best fluid to offer, but other clear fluids may also be useful depending on the person's preference. Box 11.4 presents tips to maintain hydration.

BOX 11.4   Tips for Best Practice

Maintaining Hydration

1. Calculate a daily fluid goal.
   - All older adults should have an individualized fluid goal determined by a documented standard for daily fluid intake. At least 1500 mL of fluid/day should be provided.
2. Compare current intake to fluid goal to evaluate hydration status.
3. Provide fluids consistently throughout the day.
   - Provide 75% to 80% of fluids at mealtimes and the remainder at other times such as medication times.
   - Offer a variety of fluids and fluids that the person prefers.
   - Standardize the amount of fluid that is offered with medication administration (e.g., at least 6 oz).
4. Plan for at-risk individuals.
   - Have fluid rounds midmorning and midafternoon.
   - Provide two 8-oz glasses of fluid in the morning and evening.
   - Provide modified fluid containers based on resident's abilities— for example, lighter cups and glasses, weighted cups and glasses, plastic water bottles with straws (attach to wheelchairs, deliver with meals).

- Make fluids accessible at all times and be sure individuals can access them—for example, filled water pitchers, fluid stations, or beverage carts in congregate areas.
- Allow adequate time and staff for eating or feeding. Meals can provide two-thirds of daily fluids.
- Encourage family members to participate in feeding and offering fluids.
5. Perform fluid regulation and documentation.
   - Document complete intake including hydration habits.
   - Know volumes of fluid containers to accurately calculate fluid consumption.
   - For individuals who are not continent, teach caregivers to observe incontinent pads or briefs for amount and frequency of urine, color changes, and odor, and report variations from individual's normal pattern.

Adapted from Mentes, J. C. (2012). Managing oral hydration. In M. Boltz, E. Capezuti, T. Fulmer, et al, (Eds), *Evidence-based geriatric nursing protocols for best practice* (4th ed, pp. 419–438). New York: Springer.

◆ Rehydration Methods

Rehydration methods depend on the severity and type of dehydration and may include intravenous or hypodermoclysis (HDC). A general rule is to replace 50% of the loss within the first 12 hours (or 1 L/day in afebrile individuals) or sufficient quantity to relieve tachycardia and hypotension. Further fluid replacement can be administered more slowly over a longer period of time. It is important to monitor for symptoms of overhydration (unexplained weight gain, pedal edema, neck vein distention, shortness of breath), especially in individuals with heart failure or renal disease. Individuals taking selective serotonin reuptake inhibitors (SSRIs) should have serum sodium levels and hydration status closely monitored because of a risk of hyponatremia (Chapter 9). Increasing fluid intake may aggravate an evolving hyponatremia.

◆ Hypodermoclysis

HDC (also known as clysis) is an infusion of isotonic fluids into the subcutaneous space. HDC is safe, easy to administer, and a useful alternative to intravenous administration for persons with mild to moderate dehydration, particularly those patients with altered mental status. HDC cannot be used in severe dehydration or for any situation requiring more than 3 L over 24 hours. Common sites of infusion are the lateral abdominal wall; the anterior or lateral aspects of the thighs; the

infraclavicular region; and the back, usually the interscapular or subscapular regions with a fat fold at least 1 inch thick. Normal saline (0.9%), half-normal saline (0.45%), 5% glucose in water infusion (D5W), or lactated Ringer's solution can be used.

HDC offers a wider range of infusion sites than traditional intravenous (IV) therapy and can be far less painful, especially when veins are difficult to find because of dehydration. IV access can also be difficult when older adults have mental status changes. HDC is considered a simple, safe, well-tolerated, and low-cost procedure that can be administered in almost any setting. It can also be administered in the home setting to provide hydration for individuals at the end of life (Coelho et al., 2020). Nurses have little knowledge of HDC as a fluid replacement therapy and there is need for more clinical studies to promote decision-making and guide clinical practice (Gomes et al., 2017). Other resources on hydration can be found in Box 11.5.

ORAL HEALTH

Orodental health is integral to general health. Orodental health is a basic need that is increasingly neglected with advanced age, debilitation, and limited mobility. Age-related changes in the oral cavity (Chapter 4), medical conditions, poor dental hygiene, and lack of dental

BOX 11.5   Resources for Best Practice

Hydration and Oral Care

The Hartford Institute for Geriatric Nursing (Consultgeri.org): Nursing Standard of Practice Protocols: Oral health care in aging, hydration management. Oral health assessment, The Kayser-Jones Brief Oral Health Status Examination (BOHSE). https://consultgeri.org/try-this/general-assessment/issue-18.

Oral Cancer Foundation: Check Your Mouth (www.checkyourmouth.org)—interactive website to assist individuals in self-screening for oral cancer/oral changes.

Oral Health America: Tooth Wisdom: Oral Health for Older Adults. https://www.toothwisdom.org/tag/oha/.

Smiles for Life: http://www.smilesforlifeoralhealth.org/buildcontent.aspx?tut=555&pagekey=62948&cbreceipt=0: National curriculum to help primary care clinicians integrate oral health care into care of patients.

BOX 11.7   Tips for Best Practice

Promoting Oral Health

- Encourage annual dental exams, including individuals with dentures.
- Brush and floss twice daily; use a fluoride dentifrice and mouthwash.
- Ensure dentures fit well and are cleaned regularly.
- Maintain adequate daily fluid intake (1500 mL).
- Avoid tobacco.
- Limit alcohol.
- Eat a well-balanced diet.
- Use an ultrasonic toothbrush (more effective in removing plaque).
- Use a commercial floss handle for easier flossing.
- Adapt toothbrush if manual dexterity is impaired. Use a child's toothbrush or enlarge the handle of an adult-sized toothbrush by adding a foam grip or wrapping it with gauze or rubber bands to increase handle size.

care contribute to poor oral health. Older adults who are dependent on caregivers for bodily care assistance exhibit worse oral hygiene than those who are self-sufficient. Poor oral health is recognized as a risk factor for dehydration, malnutrition, and a number of systemic diseases, including pneumonia, joint infections, cardiovascular disease, and poor glycemic control in type 1 and type 2 diabetes. Poor oral health is an important public health issue and a growing burden to countries worldwide. Health disparities are evident across and within regions and result from living conditions and availability of oral health services. *Healthy People 2020*

 ## BOX 11.6   Healthy People 2020

Dental Health Goals for Older Adults

- Prevent and control oral and craniofacial diseases, conditions, and injuries, and improve access to preventive services and dental care.
- Reduce the proportion of adults with untreated dental decay.
- Reduce the proportion of older adults with untreated caries.
- Reduce the proportion of adults who have ever had a permanent tooth extracted because of dental caries or periodontal disease.
- Reduce the proportion of older adults 65 to 74 years of age who have lost all of their natural teeth.
- Reduce the proportion of adults 45 to 74 years of age with moderate or severe periodontitis.
- Increase the proportion of oral and pharyngeal cancers detected at the earliest stages.

Data from US Department of Health and Human Services, Office of Disease Prevention and Health Promotion (2012). *Healthy People 2020*. http://www.healthypeople.gov/2020.

addresses oral health (US Department of Health and Human Services, 2020) (Box 11.6). Tips for promotion of oral health are presented in Box 11.7.

Common Oral Problems

Xerostomia (Mouth Dryness)

Xerostomia and hyposalivation are present in approximately 30% of older adults and can affect eating, swallowing, and speaking and contribute to dental caries and periodontal disease. Adequate saliva is necessary for the beginning stage of digestion, helping to break down starches and fats. It also functions to clear the mouth of food debris and prevent overgrowth of oral microbes. The flow of saliva does not decrease with age, but medical conditions and medications affect salivary flow (Becerra, 2017). More than 400 medications have a side effect of hyposalivation, including antihypertensives, antidepressants, antihistamines, antipsychotics, diuretics, and anti-Parkinson agents.

Treatment of xerostomia. A review of all medications is important, and if medication side effects are contributing to dry mouth, medications may be changed or altered. Affected individuals should practice good oral hygiene practices and have regular dental care to screen for decay. Consumption of adequate water intake and avoidance of alcohol and caffeine are recommended. Over-the-counter saliva substitutes (Oral Balance Gel, MouthKote) and salivary stimulants such as Biotene, Xylitol gum, and sugarless candy can be helpful.

Oral Cancer

Oral cancers occur more with age. The median age at diagnosis is 61 years; men are affected twice as often as women. It is much more common in Hungary and France than in the United States and much less common in Mexico and Japan. The 5-year survival rate is 60% and has not changed significantly since the late 1960s. This is largely the result of late identification of the disease. There are several types of oral cancer, but around 90% are squamous cell carcinomas. Historically, the majority of individuals are over the age of 40 years at the time of discovery; however, the incidence is increasing in those under this age. Exact causes are becoming clearer and include the human papilloma virus 16 and the use of "smokeless" chewing or spit tobacco. In a younger age group, including those who have never used any tobacco products, human papilloma virus may be replacing tobacco as the primary causative agent. This virus is sexually transmitted between partners and is also responsible for more than 90% of all cervical cancers. Risk factors are listed in Box 11.8.

> ### BOX 11.8   Risk Factors for Oral Cancer
>
> Tobacco, including smokeless tobacco
> Alcohol
> Oncogenic viruses (especially human papillomavirus)
> Genetic susceptibility

From Stein, P., Miller, C., Fowler, C. (2014). Oral disorders. In R. Ham, P. Sloane, G. Warshaw, et al, (Eds.), *Primary care geriatrics: A case-based approach* (6th ed.). Philadelphia: Elsevier.

Early detection is essential, but more than 60% of oral cancers are not diagnosed until an advanced stage. Early signs and symptoms may be subtle and not recognized by the individual or health care provider. Common areas for oral cancer to develop are the tongue, tonsils, oropharynx, the gums, and the floor of the mouth. Oral examinations can assist in early identification and treatment. All persons, especially those older than 50 years of age, with or without dentures, should have oral examinations on a regular basis. A new initiative from the Oral Cancer Foundation *Check Your Mouth* (www.checkyourmouth.org) is built around an interactive website designed to help individuals learn to self-discover suspicious tissue changes in their own mouths. Box 11.9 lists common signs and symptoms of oral cancer.

Once diagnosed, therapy options are based on diagnosis and staging and include surgery, radiation, and chemotherapy. If detected early, these cancers can almost always be treated successfully. Individuals with treated oral cancer will need to have follow-up examinations for the rest of their lives, because another cancer can develop later in the mouth, lung, throat, or other areas (Oral Cancer Foundation, 2018).

> ### BOX 11.9   Signs and Symptoms of Oral and Throat Cancer
>
> - Swelling or thickening, lumps or bumps, or rough spots or eroded areas on the lips, gums, or other areas inside the mouth
> - Velvety white, red, or speckled patches in the mouth
> - Persistent sores on the face, neck, or mouth that bleed easily
> - Unexplained bleeding in the mouth
> - Unexplained numbness or pain or tenderness in any area of the face, mouth, neck, or tongue
> - Soreness in the back of the throat; a persistent feeling that something is caught in the throat
> - Difficulty chewing or swallowing, speaking, or moving the jaw or tongue
> - Hoarseness, chronic sore throat, or changes in the voice
> - Dramatic weight loss
> - Lump or swelling in the neck
> - Severe pain in one ear—with a normal eardrum
> - Pain around the teeth; loosening of the teeth
> - Swelling or pain in the jaw; difficulty moving the jaw

Oral Care

Nearly one-third of individuals older than 65 years of age have untreated tooth decay. Nearly one in five adults 65 years and older have lost all of their teeth (edentulous), primarily as a result of periodontitis, which occurs in about 68% of those in this age group (CDC, 2016). There has been a dramatic reduction in the prevalence of tooth loss as knowledge increases and more people use fluorides, improve nutrition, engage in new oral hygiene practices, and take advantage of improved dental health care. However, many individuals may not have had the advantages of new preventive treatment, and those with functional and cognitive limitations may be unable to perform oral hygiene.

Access to dental care for older adults may be limited and cost prohibitive. In the existing health care system, dental care is a low priority. Medicare does not provide any coverage for oral health care services, and few Americans 75 years of age or older have private dental insurance. Medicaid coverage for dental treatment varies from state to state, but funding has decreased and coverage can be limited. Older adults have fewer dentist visits than any other age group. Those with the poorest oral health are those who are economically disadvantaged and lack insurance. Being disabled, homebound, or institutionalized increases the risk of poor oral health. Access to dentists in long-term care facilities is very limited, and many are unwilling to provide care in these facilities (Jablonski et al., 2017). If a long-term care resident needs dental care, transportation to a dentist's office is required, which is not only costly but often not possible because of the individual's condition. In many undeveloped countries, there is a shortage of trained dental professionals and dental care is nonexistent except that provided by groups such as medical and dental ministries from other countries.

❖ USING CLINICAL JUDGMENT TO PROMOTE HEALTHY AGING: ORAL HEALTH

◆ Recognizing and Analyzing Cues: Oral Health

Good oral hygiene and timely evaluation of oral health are nursing responsibilities. Oral care is "oral infection control" (Jablonski-Jaudon et al., 2016, p. 15). The relationship between poor oral health and systemic infections, such as pneumonia, is well documented (Jablonski et al., 2017). In addition, examination of the mouth can serve as an early warning system for some diseases and lead to early diagnosis and treatment. Evaluation of the mouth, teeth, and oral cavity is an essential part of the health examination (Chapter 8) and especially important when an individual is hospitalized or in a long-term care facility.

An oral examination should be included as part of a general medical examination in primary care (Becerra, 2017). The MDS 3.0 requires information obtained from an oral health evaluation. Federal regulations mandate an annual examination for residents of long-term care facilities. Although the oral examination is best performed by a dentist, nurses in health care settings can provide oral health screenings using an instrument such as the Kayser-Jones Brief Oral Health Status Examination (BOHSE) (Box 11.5).

◆ Nursing Actions: Oral Health

Nurses may be involved in promoting oral health through teaching individuals or caregivers recommended interventions, screening for oral disease, and making dental referrals, or by providing, supervising, and evaluating oral care in hospitals and long-term care facilities. Box 11.10 presents information on providing oral hygiene.

Older adults and those who may care for them should be taught proper care of dentures and oral tissue to prevent odor, stain, plaque buildup, and oral infections. All nursing staff should be knowledgeable about care of dentures (Box 11.11). Dentures are very personal and expensive possessions, and utmost care should be taken when handling, cleaning, and storing dentures, especially in hospitals and long-term care facilities. It is not uncommon to hear that dentures were lost, broken, or mixed up with those of others, or not removed and cleaned during a hospital or nursing home stay. Dentures should be marked, and many states require all newly made dentures to contain the client's identification. Denture marking kits are easily available and provide a simple, efficient, and permanent means of marking dentures.

Broken or damaged dentures and dentures that no longer fit because of weight loss or changes in the oral cavity are a common problem for older adults. Many older adults believe that there is no longer a need for oral care once they have dentures, but regular professional attention is important. Rebasing of dentures is a technique to improve the fit of dentures. Ill-fitting dentures or dentures that are not cleaned contribute to oral problems (lesions, stomatitis) and to poor nutrition and reduced enjoyment of food.

BOX 11.10 Tips for Best Practice

Provision of Oral Care

1. Explain all actions to the individual; use gestures and demonstration as needed; cue and prompt to encourage as much self-care performance as possible.
2. If the individual is in bed, elevate their head by raising the bed or propping the head with pillows, and have the individual turn their head to face you. Place a clean towel across the chest and under the chin, and place a basin under the chin.
3. If the individual is sitting in a stationary chair or wheelchair, stand behind the individual and stabilize their head by placing one hand under the chin and resting the head against your body. Place a towel across the chest and over the shoulders.
4. The basin can be kept handy in the individual's lap or on a table placed in front of or at the side of the patient. A wheelchair may be positioned in front of the sink.
5. If the individual's lips are dry or cracked, apply a light coating of petroleum jelly or use lip balm.
6. Inspect the oral cavity to identify teeth in ill repair, pain, lesions, or inflammation.
7. Brush and floss the individual's teeth (use an electric toothbrush if possible, with sulcular brushing (around and below the gumline). It may be helpful to retract the lips and cheek with a tongue blade or fingers in order to see the area that is being cleaned. Use a mouth prop as needed if the individual cannot hold their mouth open. If manual flossing is too difficult, use a floss holder or interproximal brush to clean the proximal surfaces between the teeth. Use a dentifrice containing fluoride.
8. Provide the conscious individual with fluoride rinses or other rinses as indicated by the dentist or hygienist.

BOX 11.11 Tips for Best Practice

Providing Denture Care

1. Remove dentures or ask individual to remove dentures. Observe ability to remove dentures.
2. Inspect oral cavity.
3. Rinse denture or dentures after each meal to remove soft debris. Do not use toothpaste on dentures because it abrades denture surfaces.
4. Once each day, preferably before retiring, remove denture and brush thoroughly.
   a. Although an ordinary soft toothbrush is adequate, a specially designed denture brush may clean more effectively. (CAUTION: Acrylic denture material is softer than natural teeth and may be damaged by being brushed with very firm bristles.)
   b. Brush denture over a sink lined with a facecloth and half-filled with water. This will prevent breakage if the denture is dropped.
   c. Hold the denture securely in one hand, but do not squeeze. Hold the brush in the other hand. Never use a commercial tooth powder because it is abrasive and may damage the denture materials. Plain water, mild soap, or sodium bicarbonate may be used.
   d. When cleaning a removable partial denture, great care must be taken to remove plaque from the curved metal clasps that hook around the teeth. This can be done with a regular toothbrush or with a specially designed clasp brush.
5. After brushing, rinse denture thoroughly; then place it in a denture-cleaning solution and allow it to soak overnight or for at least a few hours. (Note: Acrylic denture material must be kept wet at all times to prevent cracking or warping.) In the morning, remove denture from the cleaning solution and rinse it thoroughly before inserting it into the person's mouth. Use denture paste if necessary to secure dentures.
6. Dentures should be worn constantly except at night (to allow relief of compression on the gums) and replaced in the mouth in the morning.

◆ Oral Hygiene in Hospitals and Long-Term Care

Oral care is an often neglected part of daily nursing care and should receive the same priority as other kinds of care. Illness, acute care situations, and functional and cognitive impairments make the provision of oral care difficult. When the person is unable to carry out their dental/oral regimen, it is the responsibility of the caregiver to provide oral care. Factors contributing to less than adequate oral care include inadequate knowledge of how to provide care, lack of appropriate supplies, inadequate training and staffing, and lack of oral care protocols. Most nursing curricula offer limited training and education in oral care practices, and graduates may therefore be unprepared to implement nursing actions to promote oral health (Red and O'Neal, 2020).

In the acute care setting, good oral care is crucial to the prevention of ventilator-associated pneumonia (VAP), one of the most common hospital-acquired infections and a leading cause of morbidity and mortality in intensive care units (ICUs). Attention to oral care is essential in all settings but often not consistently implemented. In an observational study of oral hygiene care interventions provided by nurses to older adults in post-acute hospital settings, oral hygiene care was supported in just over one-third of encounters. Denture care was inconsistently performed; also, nurses did not encourage adequate self-care of natural teeth by patients and infrequently moisturized tissues (Coker et al., 2017). Mouth care may be perceived as a comfort measure rather than a critical component of infection control.

Individuals residing in long-term care facilities are particularly vulnerable to problems with oral care as a result of functional and cognitive impairments. A large number are dependent on staff for the provision of oral hygiene. Older adults with dementia often resist caregiving activities associated with mouth care. Care-resistant behavior (CRB) is one of the primary reasons for the omission of mouth care (Hoben et al., 2017; Jablonski-Jaudon et al., 2016). Long-term care residents with dementia who exhibit CRBs are three times more likely to have more tooth decay than those who allow mouth care.

Use of the research-based intervention, the MOUTh (Managing Oral Hygiene Using Threat reduction strategies), has been shown to prevent and minimize CRBs when providing oral care to individuals with dementia. Components include (1) an evidence-based mouth care protocol; (2) recognition of CRBs; and (3) strategies designed to lower the perception of mouth care as a threatening, scary, or assaultive activity. Strategies include approach, establishing rapport, avoiding speaking down to the individual (elderspeak), gestures/pantomime, cueing, and chaining (initiating the action with the expectation that the individual will take over). For a link to a video demonstrating techniques, see Box 11.5. Techniques may have applicability to other activities that trigger CRB, such as bathing (Chapter 25) (Jablonski-Jaudon et al., 2016).

The use of therapeutic rinses (e.g., chlorhexidine) that are broad-spectrum antimicrobial agents has been shown to help control plaque and reduce VAP by 40% (Erickson, 2016). These can be used in conjunction with brushing or instead of brushing in those unable to tolerate brushing. A correlation between tongue coating and aspiration pneumonia risk points to the benefit of including tongue cleaning as part of mouth care (Erickson, 2016). Many long-term care institutions have implemented programs, such as special training of nursing assistants for dental care teams, dental care champions, providing visits from mobile dentistry units on a routine basis, or using dental students to perform oral screening and cleaning of teeth (Kohli et al., 2017).

◆ Other Considerations in Oral Hygiene Provision

Tube feeding is associated with significant pathologic colonization of the mouth, greater than that observed in people who received oral feeding. Individuals with dysphagia (Chapter 10) often receive inadequate mouth care and experience poor oral health (Jablonski et al., 2017). Recommendations are that individuals receiving tube feeding should have their teeth brushed twice a day, but techniques and safety have not been determined (Huang et al., 2017). In hospitals, nurses routinely provide mouth care to patients unable to swallow using toothbrushes connected to wall suction. In a pilot study, Jablonski et al. (2017) examined the effectiveness of using soft toothbrushes dipped in alcohol-free mouthwash for individuals with dysphagia in long-term care settings without access to suction equipment. The protocol resulted in improved oral hygiene without aspiration. Foam swabs are available to provide oral hygiene but do not remove plaque as well as toothbrushes. Foam swabs may be used to clean the oral mucosa of an edentulous older adult. Research into the oral hygiene status of non-oral feeding patients and optimal and safe oral care interventions for individuals with dysphagia and tube feeding is needed, especially in long-term care and home settings (Ohno et al., 2017).

⚡ SAFETY ALERT

Lemon glycerin swabs should never be used for oral care. In combination with decreased salivary flow and xerostomia, they inhibit salivary production, causing dry mouth and promoting bacterial growth (Booker et al., 2013).

KEY CONCEPTS

- Age-related changes, medication use, functional impairments, and comorbid medical and emotional illnesses place some older adults at risk of changes in fluid balance, especially dehydration.
- Dehydration is considered a geriatric syndrome that is frequently associated with common diseases (e.g., diabetes, respiratory illness, heart failure) and declining health in frail older adults.

- In older adults, dehydration most often develops as a result of disease, age-related changes, and/or the effects of medication; dehydration is not primarily caused by lack of access to water.
- Prevention and early detection of dehydration is essential, but recognizing and analyzing cues are complex in older adults. Cues present differently than in younger individuals, and clinical signs may not appear until dehydration is advanced.
- Age-related changes in the oral cavity, the presence of medical conditions, the practice of poor dental hygiene, and lack of dental care contribute to poor oral health. Poor oral health is a risk factor for dehydration and malnutrition, as well as a number of systemic diseases, including pneumonia, joint infections, cardiovascular disease, and poor glycemic control in type 1 and type 2 diabetes.
- Good oral hygiene and timely evaluation of oral health are essentials of nursing care.
- Nurses may be involved in promoting oral health by teaching individuals or caregivers recommended interventions, by screening for oral disease and making dental referrals, or by providing, supervising, and evaluating oral care in hospitals and long-term care facilities.

ACTIVITIES AND DISCUSSION QUESTIONS

1. What are some of the risk factors for dehydration in an older adult who is hospitalized for pneumonia?
2. What are your suggestions for enhancing fluid intake for individuals with dementia residing in skilled nursing facilities?
3. Which factors influence adequate dental care among older adults?
4. What are suggestions to encourage better oral care in hospitalized older adults and residents of long-term care facilities?

NEXT-GENERATION NCLEX® EXAMINATION-STYLE QUESTIONS

Mr. Rosenthal, 86 years old, resides in assisted living and requires assistance with dressing each day. He has a history of Type 2 diabetes, heart failure, hypertension, and mild cognitive impairment. His medications include glipizide 10 mg twice daily, metformin 850 mg twice daily, lisinopril 40 mg daily, metolazone 20 mg daily, and donepezil 10 mg at bedtime. Mr. Rosenthal eats his meals in the common dining area; he states he likes the companionship. He is 6′ tall and last week his weight was 135 pounds (BMI 18.31 kg/m^2). He ambulates with a rolling walker and enjoys spending time in the gardens, pruning the rose bushes and planting; when he is in the gardens, he wears a straw hat and always has his water bottle at his side. Mr. Rosenthal saw his health care provider last week and a urinalysis was obtained. The results:

- Urine is straw color and clear, pH 4.5, urine specific gravity 1.003, nitrite negative and leukocyte esterase trace, blood negative, WBC 2/hpf, and bacteria occasional.

Use an X to indicate which client factors listed in the left column may place this client at risk of dehydration.

Client Factors	Risk of Dehydration
86 years old	
Metolazone 20 mg daily	
Results of urinalysis	
Lisinopril 40 mg daily	
Eats in common dining area	
BMI 18.31 kg/m^2	

REFERENCES

Becerra, K. (2017). Oral health in older patients: a job for primary care. *Medscape.* https://www.medscape.com/viewarticle/881460.

Centers for Disease Control and Prevention. *Facts about older adult oral health,* 2016. https://www.cdc.gov/oralhealth/basics/adult-oral-health/adult_older.htm.

Coelho, T., Wainstein, A., Drummond-Lage, A. (January 6, 2020). Hypodermoclysis as a strategy for patients with end-of-life cancer in home care settings. *American J Hospice and Palliative Medicine.* https://doi.org/10.1177/1049909119897401.

Coker, E, Ploeg, J., Kaasalainen, S., & Carter, N. (2017). Observations of oral hygiene care interventions provided by nurses to hospitalized older people. *Geriatr Nurs, 38*(1), 17–21.

Erickson, L. E. (2016). The mouth-body connection. *Generations, 40*(3), https://www.asaging.org/blog/mouth%E2%88%92body-connection.

Faes, M. C., Spift, M. G., Olde, M. G., et al. (2007). Dehydration in geriatrics. *Geriatr Aging, 10,* 590.

Gomes, N. S., DaSilva, A., & Zago, L. (2017). Nursing knowledge and practices regarding subcutaneous fluid administration. *Rev Bras Enferm, 70*(5). http://www.scielo.br/scielo.php?pid=S0034-71672017000501096&script=sci_arttext.

Hoben, M., Kent, A., Kogagi, N., et al. (2017). Effective strategies to motivate nursing home residents in oral care and to prevent or reduce responsive behaviors to oral care: a systematic review. *PLoS One, 12*(6), e0178913.

Hooper, L., Bunn, D. K., Abdelhamid, A., et al. (2016). Water-loss (intracellular) dehydration assessed using urinary tests: how well do they work? Diagnostic accuracy in older people. *Am J Clin Nutr, 104,* 121–131.

Huang, S., Chiou, C., & Liu, H. (2017). Risk factors for aspiration pneumonia related to improper oral hygiene behavior in community dysphagia persons with nasogastric tube feeding. *J Dent Sci, 12*(4), 375–381.

Jablonski, R. A., Winstead, V., Azuero, A., et al. (2017). Feasibility of providing safe mouth care and collecting oral and fecal microbiome samples from nursing home residents with dysphagia: proof of concept study. *J Gerontol Nurs, 43*(9), 9–15.

Jablonski-Jaudon, R. A., Kolanowski, A. M., Winstead, V, Jones-Townsend, C., & Azuero, A. (2016). Maturation of the MOUTh intervention: from reducing threat to relationship-centered care. *J Gerontol Nurs, 42*(3), 15–23.

Kohli, R., Nelson, S., Ulrich, S., Finch, T., Hall, K., & Schwarz, E. (2017). Dental care practices and oral health training for professional caregivers in long-term care facilities: an interdisciplinary approach to address oral health disparities. *Geriatr Nurs, 38*(4), 296–301.

McCrow, J., Morton, M., Travers, C., Harvey, K., & Eeles, E. (2016). Associations between dehydration, cognitive impairment, and frailty in older hospitalized patients: an exploratory study. *J Gerontol Nurs, 42*(5), 19–27.

Mentes, J., & Gaspar, P. (2020). Hydration management. *Jour Gerontol Nurs, 46*(2), 19–28.

Mentes, J. C., & Aronow, H. (2016). Comparing older adults presenting with dehydration as a primary diagnosis versus a secondary diagnosis in the emergency department. *J Aging Res Clin Pract, 5*(4), 181–186.

Mentes, J. C. (2012). Managing oral hydration. In M. Boltz, E. Capezuti, & T. Fulmer (Eds.), *Evidence-based geriatric nursing protocols for best practice* (ed. 4, pp. 419–438). New York, NY: Springer.

Namasivayam-MacDonald, A. M., Slaughter, S. E., Morrison, J., et al. (2018). Inadequate fluid intake in long term care residents: prevalence and determinants. *Geriatr Nurs, 39,* 330–335.

Ohno, T., Heshiki, Y., Kogure, M., Sumi, Y., & Miura, H (2017). Comparison of oral assessment results between non-oral and oral feeding patients: a preliminary study. *J Gerontol Nurs, 43*(4), 23–28.

Oral Cancer Foundation: Screening, 2019. https://oralcancerfoundation.org/screening.

Red, A., & O'Neal, P. (2020). Implementation of an evidence-based oral care protocol to improve the delivery of mouth care in nursing home residents. *J Gerontol Nurs, 46*(5), 33–38.

US Department of Health and Human Services, Office of Disease Prevention and Health Promotion: *Healthy People 2020,* 2012. Available at http://www.healthypeople.gov/2020.

12

Clinical Judgment to Promote Bladder and Bowel Health

Theris A. Touhy

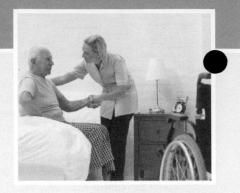

http://evolve.elsevier.com/Touhy/gerontological/

LEARNING OBJECTIVES

Upon completion of this chapter, the reader will be able to:
- Explain the types of urinary incontinence (UI) and their causes.
- Identify risk factors for UI and accidental bowel leakage and describe appropriate nursing actions.
- Utilize clinical judgment skills to recognize and analyze cues and determine nursing actions to promote bowel and bladder health.

THE LIVED EXPERIENCE

"UI (urinary incontinence) is like being a bad kid or a big baby."

"There's nothing that can be done. Well, I don't think there is anything else but a diaper."

"Sometimes I have to wet my bed before they get here, you know, and they are all busy and I have to wait for somebody, then I can't control it."

"I do something that is very wrong. I try not to drink too much but that's so wrong. So how can you drink a lot, you would be soaked all the time."

Comments from participants in a study of living with urinary incontinence in long-term care (MacDonald & Butler, 2007).

UI is a preventable and treatable condition and yet, "continence remains undervalued and UI remains underassessed. Even though UI is a basic nursing issue, nurses are not claiming it as one."

Comment from expert continence care nurses (Mason et al., 2003, p. 3).

The body must remove waste products of metabolism to sustain healthy function, but bladder activity and bowel activity are fraught with social implications. Bladder and bowel function in later life, although normally only slightly altered by the physiological changes of aging (Chapter 4), can contribute to problems severe enough to interfere with the ability to continue independent living and can seriously threaten the body's capacity to function and to survive. The effects of uncontrolled bladder and bowel action are a threat to the person's independence and well-being. Elimination is a private matter, not publicized socially. In most cultures, children are taught early to deal with their own body waste. Deviations from this are socially unacceptable and can lead to chastisement, ostracism, and social withdrawal. Nurses are in a key position to generate solutions and take actions to enhance continence and improve function, independence, and quality of life for older adults. Additionally, providing education about bladder health is an important nursing action for individuals of all ages (Box 12.1).

BOX 12.1 Promotion of a Healthy Bladder

- Drink 8 to 10 glasses of water a day before 8 p.m.
- Eliminate or reduce the use of coffee, tea, brown cola, and alcohol, particularly before bedtime.
- Empty bladder completely before and after meals and at bedtime.
- Urinate whenever the urge arises; never ignore the urge.
- Limit the use of sleeping pills, sedatives, and alcohol because they decrease sensation of needing to urinate.
- Make sure toilet is nearby with a clear path to it and good lighting, especially at night. Consider a grab bar or a raised toilet seat if there is difficulty getting on and off the toilet.
- Maintain ideal body weight.
- Get regular physical exercise.
- Avoid smoking.
- Seek professional treatment for complaints of burning, urgency, pain, blood in urine, or difficulties maintaining continence.

❖ USING CLINICAL JUDGMENT TO PROMOTE HEALTHY AGING: BLADDER HEALTH

◆ Urinary Incontinence

Urinary incontinence (UI) is the involuntary loss of urine sufficient to be a problem. UI is an important yet neglected geriatric syndrome. UI is a stigmatized, underreported, underdiagnosed, undertreated condition that is erroneously thought to be part of normal aging. Similar to other conditions experienced by older adults, many observed and reported cues of UI are ascribed to normal aging and accepted rather than being identified as indicators of the treatable condition of UI. Less than half of older adults with UI mention this problem to their health care provider (Hsu et al., 2016). On average, women wait 6.5 years from the first time they experience symptoms until they obtain a diagnosis for their bladder control problems. Instead, they try to cope with the condition on their own, with variable success. Older individuals are less likely to receive evidence-based care for UI complaints than younger people (Gibson & Wagg, 2014; Wilde et al., 2014).

Individuals may not seek treatment for UI because they are embarrassed to talk about the problem or think that it is a normal part of aging. They may be unaware that successful treatments are available. Men may be unlikely to report UI to their primary care provider because they feel it is a woman's disease. Older adults want more information about bladder control, and nurses must take the lead in implementing approaches to continence promotion and public health education about UI. Nurses are intimately involved in providing personal hygiene care and are often the ones to identify UI. It is essential that they assume a leading role in improving outcomes for individuals with UI. However, nursing staff tend to view UI as an inconvenience rather than a condition requiring assessment and treatment.

Research has identified nurses' negative attitudes toward the older adult population, lack of knowledge about UI, inadequate assessment, diagnosis, or proper documentation of the condition, and limited use of evidence-based protocols for UI. In a recent study in the acute care setting, nurses were often unaware of UI assessment tools, designed their own assessment tools, or used assessment tools that were not validated for use with older adults. Evaluation of urine control problems was infrequently performed, and the most common nursing actions to manage UI were adult incontinence pads and adult briefs (Colborne and Dahlke, 2017).

Without an adequate knowledge base of continence care and use of evidence-based practice protocols, nursing care will continue to consist of only containment strategies, such as the use of pads and briefs, to manage UI. Often, these are used out of convenience, nursing habit, and patient preference, or due to lack of time (Colborne & Dahlke, 2017). Nurses in all practice settings who care for older adults should be prepared to identify and analyze cues and utilize clinical judgment to implement nursing actions that promote continence. There is a growing role for nurses in continence care, and advanced training and certification are available through specialty organizations such as the Society of Urologic Nurses and Associates and the Wound, Ostomy and Continence Nurses Society (Holtzer-Goor et al., 2015; Spencer et al., 2017).

◆ UI Facts and Figures

Because of the high prevalence and chronic but preventable nature of UI, it is most appropriately considered a public health problem. UI is more common in women than men by a ratio of two to one. More than 50% of women and 25% of men aged 65 years and older, not residing in health care facilities or institutions, reported symptoms of UI of varying severities. Approximately 50% of men and women over the age of 65 years living in residential care facilities reported UI and another 50% reported both fecal incontinence and UI (Searcy, 2017). UI is more prevalent than diabetes, Alzheimer's disease, and many other chronic conditions that have prompted more attention and treatment. The direct medical costs of UI are similar to those of coronary heart disease and higher than the costs of diabetes (Holtzer-Goor et al., 2015).

◆ Risk Factors for UI

UI is often the result of multiple risk factors (Box 12.2). Age-related changes in the renal and urological systems (Chapter 4) and other physiological, pathological, and

BOX 12.2 Risk Factors for UI

- Age
- Immobility, functional limitations
- Diminished cognitive capacity (dementia, delirium)
- Medications (those with anticholinergic properties, diuretics)
- Smoking
- High caffeine intake
- Low fluid intake
- Obesity
- Constipation, fecal impaction
- Pregnancy, vaginal delivery, episiotomy, forceps birth, large baby
- Environmental barriers
- Diabetes, stroke, Parkinson's disease, multiple sclerosis, spinal cord injury
- Hysterectomy
- Pelvic muscle weakness, pelvic organ prolapse
- Childhood nocturnal enuresis
- Prostate surgery
- Estrogen deficiency
- Arthritis and/or back problems
- Depression
- Benign prostatic hypertrophy (BPH)

functional changes can result in a loss of continence. However, UI should never be considered a normal part of aging and requires evaluation and treatment. "The maintenance of continence is complex requires a functional lower urinary tract and pelvic floor, sufficient cognition to interpret the desire to void and locate a toilet, adequate mobility and dexterity to manipulate clothing and allow safe walking to the toilet, and an appropriate environment in which to allow this" (Gibson & Wagg, 2014). All of these factors need to be considered when recognizing and analyzing the range of cues contributing to UI symptoms.

For older men, risk factors include diabetes mellitus (DM), hypertension, problems with memory, stroke, functional impairment, and benign prostatic hyperplasia (BPH). BPH is a common condition that can cause problems with urine storage and voiding, and the severity of the symptoms may be unrelated to the size of the prostate. BPH should not be considered a strictly prostatic disease because it has been demonstrated that the entire lower urinary tract is involved in a complex pathophysiology (Albisinni et al., 2016; Jiwraika et al., 2018).

Older adults with dementia are at high risk of UI. Dementia does not cause UI but affects the ability of the individual to recognize the urge to void and to find a bathroom. Mobility problems and dependency in transfers are better predictors of continence status than dementia, suggesting that individuals with dementia may have the

potential to remain continent as long as they are mobile. Drugs that increase urinary output and sedatives, tranquilizers, and hypnotics, which produce drowsiness, confusion, or limited mobility, promote incontinence by dulling the transmission of the desire to urinate.

◆ Consequences of UI

UI affects quality of life and has physical, psychosocial, and economic consequences. UI is identified as a marker of frailty in community-dwelling older adults. UI is more common and more severe in older adults and associated with sequelae not seen in younger people, such as increased risk of falls, fractures, hospitalization, and admission to long-term care. Cues to be examined will differ in older adults. UI affects self-esteem and increases the risk of depression, anxiety, loss of dignity and autonomy, social isolation, falls, skin breakdown, and avoidance of sexual activity (Ostaszkiewicz, 2017).

Older adults with UI experience a loss of independence and self-confidence and feelings of shame and embarrassment. In a survey of hospitalized older adults, 67% considered bladder and bowel incontinence to be a state the same as, or worse than, death. "Despite the value individuals place on being continent, many nurses do not consider incontinence to be a clinically important issue" (Ostaszkiewicz, 2017, p. 11).

The psychosocial impact of UI affects the individual and family and professional caregivers. An important nursing role is to provide education to caregivers about UI and strategies to assist in practical and effective management. The provision of continence care to a dependent individual or an individual with cognitive impairment can be challenging and cause significant distress for both caregivers and care recipients. Continence care is frequently a trigger for agitation or aggression in individuals with cognitive impairment who may perceive intimate personal care interventions as frightening (Chapter 25).

◆ Types of UI

Incontinence is classified as either *transient* (acute) or *established* (chronic). *Transient* incontinence has a sudden onset, is present for 6 months or less, and is usually caused by treatable factors such as urinary tract infections (UTIs), delirium, constipation and stool impaction, and increased urine production caused by metabolic conditions such as hyperglycemia and hypercalcemia. Hospitalized older adults are at risk of developing transient UI and may also be at risk of being discharged without resolution of the condition. Use of medications such as diuretics, anticholinergic agents, antidepressants, sedatives, hypnotics, calcium channel blockers, and α-adrenergic agonists and blockers can also lead to

TABLE 12.1	Types and Symptoms of UI
Type	**Symptoms**
Stress	Loss of small amount of urine with activities that increase intra-abdominal pressure (coughing, sneezing, exercising, lifting, bending); More common in women but can occur in men after prostate surgery/treatment; Postvoid residual (PVR) low.
Urge	Loss of moderate to large amount of urine before getting to toilet; inability to suppress need to urinate; Frequency and nocturia may be present; PVR low; May be associated with overactive bladder (OAB) characterized by urinary frequency (>8 voids/24 h), nocturia, urgency, with or without urinary incontinence (UI). About half of individuals with OAB have urge UI.
Overflow	Nearly constant urine loss (dribbling), hesitancy in starting urine, slow urine stream, passing small volumes of urine, feeling of incomplete bladder emptying; may be urge, stress, or mixed UI with high residuals; PVR high.
Functional	Lower urinary tract intact but individual unable to reach toilet because of environmental barriers, physical limitations, cognitive impairment, lack of assistance, difficulty managing belts, zippers, getting a dress up and undergarments down, or sitting on a toilet; May occur with other types of UI; more common in individuals who are institutionalized.
Mixed	Combination of more than one UI problem; usually stress and urge.

transient UI. *Established* UI may have either a sudden or a gradual onset and is categorized into the following types: (1) stress, (2) urge, (3) overflow, (4) functional UI, and (5) mixed UI (Table 12.1).

❖ USING CLINICAL JUDGMENT TO PROMOTE HEALTHY AGING: UI

◆ Recognizing and Analyzing Cues: UI

A case-finding question about bladder and bowel problems (e.g. "Have you ever leaked urine/water?) is recommended as part of all interactions between older adults and clinicians (Shaw & Wagg, 2016). Health care personnel must begin to change their thinking about incontinence and acknowledge that incontinence can be cured in about 80% of individuals (National Association for Continence, 2017). If it cannot be cured, it can be treated to minimize its detrimental effects. In frail older adults, interventions will improve UI in most cases, but complete continence may not be a realistic goal (Enberg & Li, 2017).

Recognizing and analyzing cues related to UI represent a multidimensional process targeted to identify continence patterns, alterations in continence, and contributing factors. If the individual is being admitted to a hospital, home care agency, or skilled nursing facility, it is important to document the presence or absence of UI, past continence patterns, the presence or absence of an indwelling urinary catheter, and the reasons for

the catheter if present. In the long-term care setting, the Minimum Data Set (MDS) 3.0 (Chapter 8) provides an evidence-based overview of the important and relevant information to evaluate bladder continence based on the Medicare guidelines.

Individuals in long-term care facilities should have an evaluation of continence on admission and whenever there is a change in cognition, physical ability, or urinary tract function. An environmental evaluation including the accessibility of bathrooms, the adequacy of room lighting, the availability of assistance, and the use of aids such as raised toilet seats or commodes is also important.

For individuals with UI, the nurse collaborates with the interprofessional team (1) to determine whether UI is transient or established (or both); (2) to determine the type of UI; and (3) to identify and document possible etiologies of the UI, including a review of risk factors (Spencer et al., 2017). Additional evaluation is presented in Box 12.3. Box 12.4 provides information on a video of a nurse conducting an evaluation for transient UI. More extensive examinations are considered after the initial findings are evaluated. Individuals who do not fit a simple pattern for UI should be referred promptly for urodynamic assessment.

◆ Nursing Actions: UI

Nursing actions focus primarily on the appropriate evaluation of continence, teaching about treatments, and implementation and evaluation of supportive and therapeutic modalities to promote and restore continence

BOX 12.3 Tips for Best Practice
Recognizing and Analyzing Cues in Evaluation of Bladder Function

Screening Questions

"Have you ever leaked urine/water? If yes, how much does it bother you?"

"Do you ever leak urine/water on the way to the bathroom?"

"Do you ever use pads, tissue, or cloth in your underwear to catch urine/water?"

"Do you dribble urine/water most of the time?"

"Do you have any burning, hesitancy, or pain with urination?"

Screening Instruments

Urogenital Distress Inventory—6

Incontinence Impact Questionnaire Male Urinary Distress Inventory

Bladder (Voiding) Diary (Fig. 12.1)

Kept for 3 to 7 days by the individual or caregiver

Voiding record for even 1 day can be helpful

Patterns of Fluid Intake

Usual fluid intake over 24 hours

Types of fluids and time consumed

Decreased or increased urine output

Bowel Patterns

Frequency, consistency, straining

Use of laxatives

Exploration of Symptoms of Urinary Incontinence (UI)

When did UI start?

What have you done to manage the problem?

How often does it occur?

What things make it better or worse?

How severe is it?

Presence of voiding symptoms: hesitancy, straining, slow stream, intermittency, spraying

RED FLAGS: Hematuria, pain on urination

Focused History (Medical, Neurological, Gynecological, Genitourinary)

Review past health history: possible contributing factors to UI, pertinent diagnoses (heart failure, stroke, diabetes mellitus, multiple sclerosis, Parkinson's disease)

Medication Review

Review all medications including over-the-counter with focus on diuretics, anticholinergics, psychotropics, α-adrenergic blockers, α-adrenergic agonists, calcium channel blockers

Review use of alcohol

Focused Evaluation

Screen for depression

Cognitive, functional

Observe Individual Using the Toilet

Ability to reach a toilet and use it, time it takes to reach the toilet, finger dexterity for clothing manipulation; character of the urine (color, odor, sediment); difficulty starting or stopping urinary stream.

Physical Examination

Abdominal, rectal, genital: Assess for suprapubic distention indicative of urinary retention.

Observe for signs of perineal irritation, itching, burning, lesions, discharge, tenderness, thin and pale genital tissues (atrophic vaginitis), dyspareunia, pelvic organ prolapse.

Check for fecal impaction, tenderness

Other Tests That May Be Ordered

Urinalysis; culture and sensitivity if clinically significant systemic or urinary symptoms.

If indicated, postvoid residual (bladder sonography or catheterization) 16 minutes or less postvoid.

Adapted from Shaw, C., & Wagg, A. (2016). Urinary incontinence in older adults, *Med Older Adults 45*, 1.

and to prevent incontinence-related complications, such as skin breakdown. The nurse should share appropriate resources and explain clinical information and differences in treatment choices (Box 12.5). Supportive and therapeutic modalities to promote and restore continence are discussed in the following section.

◆ Lifestyle Modifications

Several lifestyle factors have been associated with either the development or the exacerbation of UI. These include increased fluid intake, weight reduction, smoking cessation, bowel management, avoiding caffeine and alcohol

(if identified as causative factors), and physical activity. Research has shown that women with stress UI who undergo a 5% to 10% weight loss experience a positive impact on UI symptoms. This is most likely due to the effects of reduced abdominal weight, intraabdominal pressure, and intravesicular pressure. The benefits of weight loss in frail older adults is more complex (Chapter 10).

◆ Promotion of Continence-Friendly Environment

An evaluation of environmental, functional, and cognitive cues is important to determine factors that may affect the individual's ability to use the toilet in public

Bladder Diary ("Uro-Log")

Complete one form for each day for 4 days before your appointment with a health care provider. In order to keep the most accurate diary possible, you'll want to keep it with you at all times and write down the events as they happen. Complete the record from 6 am to 9 pm. Take the completed forms with you to your appointment.

Your Name: _____

Date: _____

Time	Fluids		Foods		Did you urinate?		Accidents		
							Leakage	Did you feel an urge to urinate?	What were you doing at the time?
	What kind?	How much?	What kind?	How much?	How many times?	How much? (sm, med, lg)	How much? (sm, med, lg)		Sneezing, exercising, etc.
Sample	Coffee	1 cup	Toast	1 slice	✓✓	med	sm	Yes	(No)	Running
6-7 a.m.								Yes	No	
7-8 a.m.								Yes	No	
8-9 a.m.								Yes	No	
9-10 a.m.								Yes	No	
10-11 a.m.								Yes	No	
11-12 noon								Yes	No	
12-1 p.m.								Yes	No	

FIG. 12.1 Bladder diary.

BOX 12.4   Resources for Best Practice

Catheter Out (https://www.catheterout.org/): Protocols, Educational tools, Toolkit

Continence Product Advisor (https://www.continenceproducta-dvisor.org/): Impartial advice for continence product users and health care professionals

Hartford Institute for Geriatric Nursing (consultgeri.org): Try This Series: Urinary incontinence assessment in older adults. Part 1: Transient Incontinence (includes link to video of assessment), Part 2: Persistent Incontinence; Prevention of catheter-associated urinary tract infection

International Continence Society: Educational materials, product guide, research, advocacy

National Association for Continence (NAC): Comprehensive site for information for caregivers, professional clinicians, and individuals on UI and FI. Includes educational materials, product guide, advocacy, bowel and bladder diaries, OAB treatment tracker.

National Institute of Diabetes and Digestive and Kidney Disease (NIDDK): The NIDDK Bowel Control Awareness Campaign

Safe Care Campaign: Preventing health care and community associated infections: urinary tract infections

Simon Foundation for Continence: Educational materials, resources and products. Stool diary and Bristol Form Stool Scale

FI, Fecal incontinence; *OAB*, overactive bladder; *UI*, urinary incontinence.

BOX 12.5   Tips for Best Practice
Teaching About Nursing Actions for UI

- Use therapeutic communication skills and a positive and supportive attitude to help individuals overcome any embarrassment about UI.
- Teach about the range of interventions available for management of UI.
- Share helpful resources for continence management.
- Share techniques found useful by others.
- Collaborate with the individual to help him or her choose the most appropriate and acceptable intervention based on needs.
- Assist individual to develop a detailed, realistic action plan and set goals.
- Determine an evaluation plan to assess the effectiveness of interventions.
- Review progress, identify any barriers to implementation, set alternative goals, or select alternate treatments if indicated.
- Reinforce effort and persistence.

From Wilde, M., Bliss, D., Booth, J., et al. (2014). Self-management of urinary and fecal incontinence, *Am J Nurs, 114*(2), 38–45.

settings, at home, and in the hospital and institutional settings. Observing the individual using the toilet should be included in any evaluation of UI. If the individual is in a hospital or institution, occupational therapists can be helpful in these assessments and provide suggestions and equipment for improved abilities (e.g., elevated toilet seat, grab bars).

Accessibility to toilets and the availability of toileting assistance in a timely manner are identified risk factors for UI in older adults who are frail, particularly those who are institutionalized. Toileting aids such as grab bars, raised toilet seats, toilet visibility, signage, and images may be effective in older adults with cognitive impairment or visual-perceptual deficits. For those who are not able to go to the toilet independently, the availability of timely toileting assistance is critical to all other interventions for UI. In all settings, nurses play a key role in arranging the environment to facilitate toilet use and assist the individual to maintain or return to continence.

◆ Behavioral Techniques

Behavioral techniques, such as scheduled (timed) voiding, prompted voiding (PV), habit retraining, bladder retraining, and pelvic floor muscle exercises (PFMEs), are recommended as first-line treatment of UI. Because UI in older adults can have multiple precipitating factors, a single intervention may not be adequate, and more complex, multicomponent interventions may be required (Gibson & Wagg, 2014). Behavioral interventions have a good basis in research and can be implemented by nurses without extensive and expensive evaluation. Selection of a modality and interventions will depend on a comprehensive evaluation, the type of incontinence and its underlying cause, and whether the outcome is to cure or to minimize the extent and complications of the incontinence.

◆ *Scheduled (timed) voiding.* Scheduled (timed) voiding is used to treat urge and functional UI in both cognitively intact and cognitively impaired older adults. The individual uses the toilet at fixed intervals, such as every 4 hours. The schedule or timing of voiding can be based on common voiding patterns (voiding on arising, before and after meals, midmorning, midafternoon, and bedtime).

◆ *Pelvic floor muscle exercises.* PFMEs, also called Kegel exercises, involve repeated voluntary pelvic floor muscle contraction. The targeted muscle is the pubococcygeal muscle, which forms the support for the pelvis and surrounds the vagina, the urethra, and the rectum. The goal of the repetitive contractions is to strengthen the muscle and decrease UI episodes. PFMEs are recommended for stress, urge, and mixed UI in older women and have also been shown to be helpful for men who have undergone prostatectomy. PFMEs can also be used to avoid an incontinence episode associated with urge UI.

Biofeedback may improve PFME teaching and outcomes, but further research is needed. Medicare covers biofeedback for individuals who do not improve after 4 weeks of a trial of PFMEs.

Reports of a study evaluating an app with instructions for PFMEs for treating stress UI suggest that it may be a feasible way to deliver high-quality care in a cost-effective manner to large groups of individuals (Sjöström et al., 2017). Box 12.6 presents a protocol for PFMEs.

◆ *Habit retraining.* The individual's voiding pattern is identified, usually by means of a voiding diary (Fig. 12.1). A schedule is then devised so that the individual uses the toilet to avoid UI episodes identified from the diary.

◆ *Bladder retraining.* Bladder retraining aims to increase the time interval between the urge to void and voiding. This method is appropriate for individuals with urge UI who are cognitively intact and independent in toileting or after removal of an indwelling catheter. Bladder retraining involves frequent voluntary voiding to keep bladder volume low and suppression of the urge to void using PFMEs, distraction, or relaxation techniques. When the individual feels the urge to urinate, they use the urge control techniques. After the urge subsides, the individual walks at a normal pace to the toilet. The initial toileting frequency is every 2 hours and is progressively lengthened to 4 hours over the course of days or weeks, depending on tolerance.

◆ *Prompted voiding (PV).* PV is a technique that combines scheduled voiding with monitoring, prompting, and verbal reinforcement. The objective of PV is to increase self-initiated voiding and decrease the number of episodes of UI. The person is assisted to the toilet at predetermined times during waking hours if they request it and receives positive feedback for voiding successfully. PV is associated with modest short-term improvement in daytime UI in individuals residing in long-term care settings (Lai & Wan, 2017).

Newly admitted individuals to long-term care facilities who are incontinent (and able to use the toilet) should receive a 3- to 5-day trial of PV or other toileting programs. The trial can be helpful in demonstrating responsiveness to toileting and determining patterns of and symptoms associated with the incontinence. PV is also combined with functional intervention training in which direct care givers incorporate strengthening exercises into toileting routines (Shaw & Wagg, 2016).

◆ Use of Urinary Catheters

Intermittent catheterization is a technique used in people with urinary retention related to a weak detrusor muscle (e.g., diabetic neuropathy), those with a blockage of the

BOX 12.6   Pelvic Floor Muscle Training Exercises

Purpose

Prevent the involuntary loss of urine by strengthening the muscles under the uterus, bladder, and bowel.

Who Should Perform These Exercises?

Men and women who have problems with urine leakage or bowel control.

Identifying Pelvic Floor Muscles

When urinating, start to go and then stop. Feel the muscles in your vagina, bladder, or anus get tight and move up. These are the pelvic floor muscles. If you feel them tighten, you have done the exercise right.

If you are still not sure you are tightening the right muscle, keep in mind that all the muscles of the pelvic floor relax and contract at the same time. Because these muscles control the bladder, rectum, and vagina, the following tips may help:

Women: Inset a finger into your vagina. Tighten the muscles as if you are holding your urine; then let go. You should feel the muscles tighten and move up or down. These are the same muscles you would tighten if you were trying to prevent yourself from passing gas.

Men: Insert a finger into your rectum. Tighten the muscles as if you were holding your urine; then let go. You should feel the muscles tighten and move up and down. These are the same muscles you would tighten if you were trying to prevent yourself from passing gas.

Note: Nurses can teach correct muscle identification when performing a rectal or vaginal examination.

Pelvic Floor Muscle Exercises (PFME) Routine

1. Begin by emptying your bladder.
2. You can lie down, stand up, or sit in a chair.
3. Tighten the pelvic floor muscles and hold for a count of 10.
4. Relax the muscles completely for a count of 10.
5. Do 10 repetitions, 3 to 5 times a day.
6. Breathe deeply and relax your body when doing the exercises.
7. It is very important to keep the abdomen, buttocks, and thigh muscles relaxed when doing PFME.
8. After 4 to 6 weeks, most people see some improvement but it may take as long as 3 months. The regimen should be continued for 12 weeks.
9. After a few weeks, you can also try doing a single PFME contraction at times when you are likely to leak.

From US National Library of Medicine, NIH National Institutes of Health (2018). Pelvic floor muscle training exercises, *Medline Plus*. http://www.nlm.nih.gov/medlineplus/ency/article/003975.htm.

BOX 12.7   Indications for Indwelling Urinary Catheter Use

- Presence of acute urinary retention or bladder outlet obstruction
- Need for accurate measurements of urinary output in critically ill patients
- Perioperative use for selected surgical procedures: urological or other surgery on contiguous structures of the genitourinary tract; anticipated prolonged surgery duration (should be removed in post-anesthesia unit); patients expected to receive large-volume infusions or diuretics during surgery; need for intraoperative monitoring of urinary output
- Assistance in healing of open sacral or perineal wounds in individuals with UI
- Requirement for prolonged patient immobilization (e.g., potentially unstable thoracic or lumbar spine, multiple traumatic injuries such as pelvic fractures)
- Improvement in comfort for end-of-life care if needed

urethra (e.g., benign prostatic hypertrophy [BPH]), or those with reflux incontinence related to a spinal cord injury. The goal is to maintain 300 mL or less of urine in the bladder. Most of the research on intermittent catheterization has been conducted with children or young adults with spinal cord injuries, but it may be useful for older adults who are able to self-catheterize. It provides an important alternative to indwelling catheterization.

Indwelling catheter use is not appropriate in any setting for long-term management (more than 30 days) (Box 12.7). Regulatory standards in nursing homes follow these same guidelines, and the use of indwelling catheters must be justified on the basis of medical conditions and failure of other efforts to maintain continence. In hospitals, the use of indwelling catheters is often unjustified and they are used inappropriately or left in place too long. Hospitalized older adults are more likely to have urinary catheters placed without indication, of which 50% have been shown to have been improperly used.

Those with more care needs, cognitive impairment, and pressure injuries are at higher risk of catheter placement (Hu et al., 2017). Reasons for this include (1) convenience to manage UI; (2) lack of knowledge of risks associated with use and alternative treatments; (3) providers not tracking continued use; and (4) lack of valid continence assessment tools for older adults. Misuse of catheterization should be considered a medical error.

External catheters (condom catheters) are sometimes used in males who are incontinent and cannot use the toilet. Long-term use of external catheters can lead to fungal skin infections, penile skin maceration, edema, fissures, contact burns from urea, UTIs, and septicemia. The catheter should be removed and replaced daily and the penis cleaned, dried, and aired to prevent irritation, maceration, and the development of skin breakdown. If the catheter is not sized appropriately and not applied and monitored correctly, strangulation of the penile shaft can occur.

There is also a external female urinary collection device that is a feasible alternative to an indwelling urinary catheter or intervention for urinary incontinence and minimizes the risk for skin injury and infection. The collection device conforms to the perineal area between the labia and the urethra. The device is connected to low continuous suction providing a sump mechanism to collect and measure urine output. In addition, there is a continuous air flow promoting a microclimate environment to the perineum region (Beeson and Davis, 2018).

◆ Use of Absorbent Products

Some individuals prefer to use absorbent products in addition to toileting interventions to maintain "social continence" and a wide variety of products are available (Box 12.4). Disposable types are available in several sizes, determined by hip and waist measurements, or as one size made to fit all. Many of these undergarments now look like regular underwear, and you even see them in stylish television commercials. Nurses should avoid the use of the word "diaper," since it is infantilizing and demeaning to older adults—the word "brief" is preferred. It is important that individuals are counseled to purchase proper continence products that will wick moisture away from the skin. These products are costly but they protect skin integrity. Women may tend to use menstrual pads, but these do not absorb significant amounts of fluid.

◆ Pharmacological Approaches

Medications are not considered first-line treatment but can be considered in combination with behavioral strategies in some cases. Behavioral therapy, alone or in combination with other interventions, is generally more effective than pharmacologic treatments alone in treating both stress and urge UI and should be the primary intervention (Balk et al., 2019). Pharmacological treatment (anticholinergic, antimuscarinic agents) may be indicated for urge UI and overactive bladder (OAB). These include oxybutynin (Oxytrol, Ditropan, Ditropan XL), tolterodine (Detrol, Detrol LA), trospium chloride (Sanctura), darifenacin (Enablex), fesoterodine (Toviaz), and solifenacin (VESIcare).

All of these medications have similar efficacy in reducing urge UI frequency, and the choice of medication depends on avoidance of adverse drug effects, drug-drug and drug-disease interactions, dosing frequency, titration range, and cost. β_3-Agonists (mirabegron) are a new class of medications for urge UI and OAB. They should not be used in individuals with severe uncontrolled hypertension, hepatic insufficiency, or bladder obstruction from BPH, or in those taking antimuscarinic agents. These medications can also raise digoxin levels.

Dosages of medications for urge UI and OAB should be started low and titrated with careful attention to side effects and drug interactions. A trial of 4 to 8 weeks is adequate and recommended. If one medication is not effective, another may be tried. Undesirable side effects of anticholinergic medications such as dry mouth and eyes, constipation, and cognitive impairment are problematic. People with narrow-angle glaucoma cannot use these medications, and they should not be combined with cholinesterase inhibitors. These medications can be especially problematic for those with cognitive impairment.

None of these medications have been evaluated in older adults who are frail and should only be considered after all potentially remediable comorbid conditions/factors are evaluated and addressed and there has been an appropriate trial of behavioral and lifestyle interventions. With cautious use, there may be some benefit in pharmacological management of symptom control. Drug treatment should generally be avoided in individuals who make no attempt to use the toilet when assisted, become agitated when toileted, or are so cognitively and functionally impaired that there is no prospect for meaningful benefit (Enberg & Li, 2017).

◆ Surgical Treatment and Nonsurgical Devices

There are numerous surgical treatments for urge and stress UI available for individuals when they are referred to a specialist. These include in-office urethral bulking agents, surgical placements of urethral slings and bladder neck suspensions for stress UI, and intradetrusor botulinum toxin injection. For individuals with urge UI associated with OAB who have not responded to conservative or pharmacological therapies, sacral neuromodulation (SNM) may be recommended. SNM stimulates the sacral nerve root to control urination and can be an office-based 12-week treatment or a surgical implantation of a sacral neuromodulator system. Surgical SNM includes implantation of the Medtronic Interstim Therapy device, FDA-approved for bladder dysfunction, including UI and fecal incontinence, and has shown efficacy for decreasing symptoms of UI (El-Azab & Siegel, 2019). There is limited evidence on surgical treatments for UI in older adults who are frail; however, age alone is not a contraindication to surgical treatment (Enberg & Li, 2017; Searcy, 2017; Shaw & Wagg, 2016).

There are a variety of intravaginal or intraurethral devices to relieve stress UI. These include intravaginal support devices, pessaries, external occlusive devices, and urethral plugs for women. For men, there are foam penile clamps. The pessary, used primarily to prevent uterine prolapse, is a device that is fitted into the vagina and exerts pressure to elevate the urethrovesical junction of the pelvic floor. The individual is taught to insert and remove the pessary, much like inserting and removing a diaphragm used for contraception. The pessary is removed weekly or monthly for cleaning with soap and water and then reinserted. Adverse effects include vaginal infection, low back pain, and vaginal mucosal erosion. Another concern is the danger of forgetting to remove the pessary. An evaluation of the stress UI by the health care provider should be conducted to determine whether these devices would be helpful.

URINARY TRACT INFECTIONS (UTIs)

UTIs are the most common cause of bacterial sepsis in older adults and are 10 times more common in women than in men. The clinical spectrum of UTIs ranges from asymptomatic and recurrent UTIs to sepsis associated with UTI requiring hospitalization. There is significant disagreement in clinical practice as to what constitutes a UTI, and overdiagnosis of UTI is a significant problem in the older adult population. Recognizing and analyzing cues to UTIs in older adults is complex because signs and symptoms present differently, particularly in nursing home residents.

Cognitively impaired individuals may not be able to report symptoms, and nurses often rely on nonspecific signs and symptoms (lack of appetite, change in behavior) as indicators of UTI. It is widely believed that UTI in older adults can manifest atypically, but there is little evidence that nonspecific symptoms, when present in isolation, are reliable indicators of UTI (Crnich et al., 2017; Kitsler et al., 2017). The presence of nonspecific signs/symptoms in the absence of fever or urinary tract symptoms should trigger consideration of noninfectious conditions rather than a UTI.

Asymptomatic bacteriuria is transient and considered benign in older women. Significant bacteriuria and urinary symptoms are common, often occur together, and generally resolve spontaneously in noncatheterized, medically stable adults without structural or functional urinary tract abnormalities. Neither is linked strongly to serious urinary tract disease or to a likelihood of benefit from antibiotic treatment (Finucane, 2017). The American Geriatrics Society recommends that antimicrobials should not be used to treat bacteriuria in older adults unless specific urinary tract symptoms are present (American Geriatrics Society, 2014). However, antibiotic treatment is common even though more than half of the antibiotics initiated for suspected UTIs are unnecessary or inappropriate (Crnich et al., 2017).

Screening urine cultures should also not be performed in individuals who are asymptomatic. As many as half of all positive urine cultures should be considered false positives for the presence of a UTI (Kistler et al., 2017). The diagnosis of symptomatic UTI is made when the patient has both clinical features (painful urination, lower abdominal pain/tenderness, blood in urine, new or worsening urinary urgency or frequency, incontinence, and fever) and laboratory evidence of a UTI. Treatment is with antibiotics selected by identifying the pathogen, knowing local resistance rates, and considering adverse effects.

Catheter-Associated Urinary Tract Infections

Catheter-associated urinary tract infections (CAUTIs) are UTIs that occur in a patient with an indwelling catheter or within 48 hours of catheter removal. CAUTIs are one of the most common health care–associated infections (HAI) (CDC, 2018). CAUTIs are the leading cause of secondary bloodstream infections and were among the first hospital-acquired conditions (HACs) targeted for nonpayment by Medicare in 2008 (Timmons et al., 2017). One of the goals of *Healthy People 2020* is to prevent, reduce, and ultimately eliminate HAIs.

Too often, catheters are inserted inappropriately and not removed in a timely manner. Continence evaluation and interventions are often lacking in acute care settings. Recommendations to improve practice and decrease CAUTIs include standardized catheter removal protocols; catheter reminders, stop orders, nurse-initiated removal protocols; use of evidence-based guidelines to prevent CAUTIs; education of staff, patients, and families about CAUTI; and use of a urinary catheter bundle (Mody et al., 2017; Quinn et al., 2020). Box 12.8 presents Tips for Best Practice for prevention of CAUTI.

⚡ SAFETY ALERT

Long-term catheter use increases the risk of recurrent urinary tract infections leading to urosepsis, urethral damage in men, urethritis, or fistula formation. Catheter-associated urinary tract infection is one of the most common health care–associated infection in the United States, and Medicare no longer reimburses hospitals for this infection. Indwelling catheters should be inserted only for appropriate conditions and must be removed as soon as possible, and alternatives should be investigated (e.g., condom catheters, intermittent catheterization, toileting programs).

BOX 12.8   **Tips for Best Practice**

Prevention of CAUTI: ABCDE

A	Adherence to general infection control principles (hand hygiene, surveillance, aseptic catheter insertion, proper maintenance of a sterile, closed, unobstructed drainage system, and education).
B	Be sure to use protocol in place to avoid unnecessary catheterizations.
C	Condom catheters or other alternatives to an indwelling catheter such as intermittent catheterization should be considered in appropriate patients.
D	Do not use the indwelling catheter unless you must. Do not use antimicrobial catheters. Do not irrigate catheters unless obstruction is anticipated (e.g., as might occur with bleeding after prostatic or bladder surgery). Do not clean the periurethral area with antiseptics (cleansing of the meatal surface during daily bathing or showering is appropriate).
E	Early removal of the catheter using a reminder or nurse-initiated removal protocol.

CAUTI, Catheter-associated urinary tract infection.
From Centers for Disease Control and Prevention (CDC). *National and State Healthcare-associated infections (HAI) progress report,* 2018. https://www.cdc.gov/hai/data/portal/progress-report.html.

BOWEL ELIMINATION

Bowel function of older adults, although normally only slightly altered by the physiological changes of age (Chapter 4), can be a source of concern and a potentially serious problem, especially for older adults who are functionally impaired. Normal elimination should be an easy passage of feces, without undue straining or a feeling of incomplete evacuation or defecation.

Constipation

Constipation is defined as a reduction in the frequency of stool or difficulty in formation or passage of stool. The Rome Criteria outline the operational definitions of constipation and should be used as a guide to diagnosis as well as a tool for teaching individuals about constipation (Box 12.9). Constipation is one of the most common gastrointestinal complaints encountered in clinical practice in all settings. Many individuals, both the lay public and health care professionals, may view constipation as a minor problem or nuisance. However, it is associated with impaired quality of life, significant health care costs, and a large economic burden. Constipation can also have very serious consequences including fecal impaction, bowel obstruction, cognitive dysfunction, delirium, falls, and increased morbidity and mortality. Individuals with chronic constipation are also at greater risk of developing colorectal cancer and benign colorectal neoplasms (Guérin et al., 2014).

BOX 12.9   **Rome III Criteria for Defining Chronic Functional Constipation in Adults**

Two or more of the following for at least 12 weeks in the preceding 12 months:
- Straining with defecation more than 25% of the time
- Lumpy or hard stools more than 25% of the time
- Sensation of incomplete emptying more than 25% of the time
- Manual maneuvers used to facilitate emptying in more than 25% of defecations (digital evacuation or support of the pelvic floor)
- Fewer than three bowel movements per week

From Lacy, B., Mearin, F., Chang, L., Chey, W. et al. (2016). Bowel Disorders. *Gastroenterology, 150,* 1393–1407.

Constipation is a symptom, not a disease. It is a reflection of poor habits, delayed response to the colonic reflex, and many chronic illnesses—both physical and psychological—and a common side effect of medication. Diet and activity level play a significant role in constipation. Constipation and other changes in bowel habits can also signal more serious underlying problems, such as colonic dysmotility or colon cancer. Thorough evaluation is important, and these complaints should not be blamed on age alone. It is important to note that alterations in cognitive status, incontinence, increased temperature, poor appetite, or unexplained falls may be the only clinical symptoms of constipation in cognitively impaired or frail older adults.

Fecal Impaction

Fecal impaction is a major complication of constipation. It is especially common in older adults who are incapacitated and institutionalized and those who require narcotic medications (e.g., end-of-life care). Symptoms of fecal impaction include malaise; loss of appetite; abdominal bloating/pain; nausea; vomiting; urinary retention; elevated temperature; incontinence of bladder or bowel; leaking of stool; alterations in cognitive status; fissures; hemorrhoids; and intestinal obstruction. Unrecognized, unattended, or neglected constipation eventually leads to fecal impaction. Digital rectal examination for impacted stool and abdominal x-rays will confirm the presence of impacted stool. Continued obstruction by a fecal mass may eventually impair sensation, leading to the need for larger stool volume to stimulate the urge to defecate, which contributes to megacolon.

Paradoxical diarrhea, caused by leakage of fecal material around the impacted mass, may occur. Reports of diarrhea in older adults must be thoroughly evaluated before the use of antidiarrheal medications, which further complicate the problem of fecal impaction. Stool analysis for *Clostridium difficile* toxin should be ordered in patients who develop new-onset diarrhea, especially for those who live in a communal setting or have been recently hospitalized.

Removal of a fecal impaction is at times worse than the misery of the condition. Management of fecal impaction requires the digital removal of the hard, compacted stool from the rectum with use of lubrication containing lidocaine jelly. In general, this is preceded by an oil-retention enema to soften the feces in preparation for manual removal. Use of suppositories is not effective because their action is blocked by the amount and size of the stool in the rectum. Several sessions or days may be necessary to cleanse the sigmoid colon and rectum totally of impacted feces. Once this is achieved, attention should be directed to planning a regimen that includes adequate fluid intake, increased dietary fiber, administration of medications if needed, and many of the suggestions presented later in the chapter for prevention of constipation. Protocols and policies for removal of a fecal impaction should be in place in all facilities.

For patients who are hospitalized or residing in long-term care settings, accurate bowel records are essential; unfortunately, they are often overlooked or inaccurately completed. Education about the importance of bowel function and the accurate reporting of size, consistency, and frequency of bowel movements should be provided to all direct care providers as well as families caring for older adults in the home. This is especially important for frail or cognitively impaired older adults to prevent fecal impaction, a serious and often dangerous condition.

❖ USING CLINICAL JUDGMENT TO PROMOTE HEALTHY AGING: BOWEL FUNCTION

◆ Recognizing and Analyzing Cues: Bowel Function

Identification of cues to altered bowel function and implementing nursing actions to promote bowel health represent an important nursing responsibility. The precipitants and causes of constipation must be included in the evaluation of bowel function. A review of these factors will also determine whether the individual is at risk of altered bowel function and if any of the known risks are modifiable. Constipation has different meanings to different people. The recognition and analysis of cues begin with clarification of what the person means by constipation and discussion of the criteria for the diagnosis (Box 12.9).

It is important to obtain a bowel history including usual patterns, frequency of bowel movements, size, consistency, any changes, and occurrence of straining and hard stools. However, recall of bowel frequency has been shown to be unreliable in establishing the presence of constipation. Having the individual keep a bowel diary (Box 12.4) and using the Bristol Stool Form Scale (Lewis & Heaton, 1997), which provides a visual description of stool appearance, will be more accurate. Other important data to be obtained are presented in Box 12.10.

BOX 12.10   Tips for Best Practice
Evaluation of Constipation

Sample Questions
- What is your usual bowel pattern?
- How many minutes did you sit on the bedpan or toilet before you had your bowel movement?
- How much did you have to strain before you had your bowel movement?
- Do you think you are constipated? If yes, why do you think so?
- Have you had any abdominal pain, nausea, vomiting, weight loss, blood in your bowel movement, or rectal pain?
- Have you had any bowel or rectal surgery?
- What type of physical activity do you engage in and how often?

Review of Food and Fluid Intake
Medication Review
- Include over-the-counter (OTC), herbal preparations, supplements

Psychosocial History
- With attention to depression, anxiety, and stress management

Review of Concurrent Medical Conditions
Other Measures
- Bowel diary
- Bristol Stool Form Survey

Focused Physical Examination
- Abdominal exam to detect masses, distention, tenderness, high-pitched or absent bowel sounds
- If these abnormalities are present, primary care provider should be contacted
- Rectal exam, following institutional policy, to identify painful anal disorders such as hemorrhoids or fissures, rectal prolapse, stool presence in the vault, strictures, masses, anal reflex

Other Tests as Indicated
- Complete blood count, fasting glucose, chemistry panel, thyroid studies
- Flexible sigmoidoscopy, colonoscopy, computed tomography scan, abdominal x-ray

From McKay, S., Fravel, M., Scanlon, C. (2014). Management of constipation, *J Gerontol Nurs, 38*(7):9–16.

◆ Nursing Actions: Bowel Function

◆ Nonpharmacological Treatment

The first action is to examine the medications the person is taking and to eliminate those that can cause constipation, preferably changing to medications that do not carry that side effect. Medications are the leading cause of constipation, and almost any drug can cause constipation. Nonpharmacological interventions for constipation that have been implemented and evaluated are as follows: (1) fluid and diet related, (2) physical activity, (3) environmental manipulation, (4) toileting regimen, and (5) a combination of these. Fluid intake of at least 1.5 L per day, unless contraindicated, is the cornerstone of constipation therapy, with fluids coming mainly from water.

A gradual increase in fiber intake, either as supplements or incorporated into the diet, is generally recommended. Fiber helps stools become bulkier and softer and move through the body more quickly. This will produce easier and more regular bowel movements. High fiber intake is not recommended for individuals who are immobile or do not consume at least 1.5 L of fluid per day.

◆ *Physical activity.* Physical activity is important as an intervention to stimulate colon motility and bowel evacuation. Daily walking for 20 to 30 minutes, if tolerated, is helpful, especially after a meal. Pelvic tilt exercises and range-of-motion (passive or active) exercises are beneficial for those who are less mobile or who are bedridden. Exercise and physical activity are discussed in Chapter 13.

◆ *Positioning.* The squatting or sitting position, if the individual is able to assume it, facilitates bowel function. A similar position may be obtained by leaning forward and applying firm pressure to the lower abdomen or by placing the feet on a stool. Rocking back and forth while sitting solidly on the toilet may facilitate stool movement. Massaging the abdomen or rectum may also help stimulate the bowel.

◆ *Toileting regimen.* Establishing a routine for toileting promotes or normalizes bowel function (bowel retraining). The gastrocolic reflex occurs after breakfast or supper and may be enhanced by a warm drink. Given privacy and ample time (a minimum of 10 minutes), many will have a daily bowel movement. However, any urge to defecate should be followed by a trip to the bathroom. Older adults dependent on others to meet toileting needs should be assisted to maintain normal routines and provided opportunities for routine toilet use. Box 12.11 presents a bowel training program.

◆ Pharmacological Treatment

When changes in diet and lifestyle are not effective, the use of laxatives is considered. Use of these medications, both prescribed and OTC, is high. The extensive use of laxatives among older adults in the United States can be considered a cultural habit. In the past, weekly doses of rhubarb, cascara, castor oil, and other types of laxatives

---

BOX 12.11   Tips for Best Practice

Bowel Training Program

1. Obtain a bowel history and establish a schedule for the bowel training program that is normal and comfortable for the patient and conforms to their lifestyle.

2. Ensure adequate fiber and fluid intake (normalize stool consistency).
   a. Fiber
      i. Add high-fiber foods to diet (dried fruit, dried beans, vegetables, and wheat products).
      ii. Suggest adding one to three tablespoons of bran or Metamucil to the diet once or twice each day. (Titrate dosage on the basis of response.)
   b. Fluid
      i. Consume 2 to 3 L daily (unless contraindicated).
      ii. Four ounces of prune, fig, or pear juice (or a warm fluid) may be given daily as a stimulus (e.g., 30 to 60 min before the established time for defecation).

3. Encourage an exercise program.
   a. Pelvic tilt, modified sit-ups for abdominal strength
   b. Walking for general muscle tone and cardiovascular system
   c. More vigorous program if appropriate

4. Establish a regular time for the bowel movement.
   a. Established time depends on patient's schedule.
   b. Best times are 20 to 40 minutes after regularly scheduled meals, when the gastrocolic reflex is active.
   c. Attempts at evacuation should be made daily within 15 minutes of the established time and whenever the patient senses rectal distention.
   d. Instruct patient about normal posture for defecation. (The patient normally sits on the toilet or bedside commode; for the patient who is unable to get out of bed, the left side–lying position is best.)
   e. Instruct the patient to contract the abdominal muscles and "bear down."
   f. Have the patient lean forward to increase the intra-abdominal pressure by use of compression against the thighs.
   g. Stimulate the anorectal reflex and rectal emptying if necessary.

5. Insert a rectal suppository or mini-enema into the rectum 15 to 30 minutes before the scheduled bowel movement, placing the suppository against the bowel wall; or insert a gloved, lubricated finger into the anal canal and gently dilate the anal sphincter.

---

were consumed and believed by many to promote health. The belief that cleaning out the colon and having a daily bowel movement is paramount to maintaining good health still persists in some groups. Providing information about normal bowel function, definition of constipation, and lifestyle modifications can assist in promoting healthy bowel habits without the use of laxatives.

Older adults receiving opiates need to have a constipation prevention program in place because these drugs delay gastric emptying and decrease peristalsis. Correction of constipation associated with opiate use requires senna or an osmotic laxative to overcome the strong opioid effect. Stool softeners and bulking agents alone are inadequate.

Enemas. Enemas of any type should be reserved for situations in which other methods produce no response or when it is known that there is an impaction. Enemas should not be used on a regular basis. A normal saline or tap water enema (500 to 1000 mL) at a temperature of 105°F is the best choice. Sodium citrate enemas are another safe choice. Soapsuds and phosphate enemas irritate the rectal mucosa and should not be used. Oil retention enemas are used for refractory constipation and in the treatment of fecal impaction.

> ### ⚡ SAFETY ALERT
>
> Sodium phosphate enemas (e.g., Fleets) should not be used in older adults because they may lead to severe metabolic disorders associated with high mortality and morbidity.

◆ Alternative Treatments

Combinations of natural fiber, fruit juices, and natural laxative mixtures are often recommended in clinical practice, and some studies have found an increase in bowel frequency and a decrease in laxative use when these mixtures are used (Box 12.12). Although research is still limited, many modalities of complementary and alternative medicine, such as probiotic bacteria, traditional herbal medicines, biofeedback, and massage, are also used to treat constipation.

> ### BOX 12.12 Natural Laxative Recipe
>
> **Power Pudding**
> *Ingredients*
> 1 cup wheat bran
> 1 cup applesauce
> 1 cup prune juice
>
> *Directions*
> Mix and store in refrigerator. Start with administration of 1 tablespoon/day. Increase slowly until desired effect is achieved and no disagreeable symptoms occur.

ACCIDENTAL BOWEL LEAKAGE/FECAL INCONTINENCE

Fecal incontinence (FI) is defined by the International Continence Society as the involuntary loss of liquid or solid stool that is a social and hygienic problem (Markland, 2014). Although fecal incontinence is the most common terminology used, results of a large study of female patients, the term "accidental bowel leakage" was preferred over FI (Brown et al., 2012; Paquette et al., 2015). Both terms will be used in this chapter but "accidental bowel leakage" may be the preferred term for nurses to use when caring for individuals with this health concern.

Prevalence of FI varies with the study population: 2% to 17% in community-dwelling older adults; 50% to 65% in older adults in nursing homes; and 33% in hospitalized older adults. Higher prevalence rates are found among patients with diabetes, irritable bowel syndrome, stroke (new onset, 30%; 16% at 3 years poststroke), multiple sclerosis, and spinal cord injury (Grover et al., 2010). A lack of consistency in the definitions used for FI and differences in populations studied and methodology affect statistics. Additionally, accurate estimates are difficult to obtain because many people are reluctant to discuss this disorder and many primary care providers do not ask about it.

Often FI is associated with urinary incontinence, and up to 50% to 70% of patients with UI also carry the diagnosis of FI. FI can be transient (episodes of diarrhea, acute illness, fecal impaction) or persistent. Fecal incontinence, like urinary incontinence, has devastating social ramifications for the individuals and families who experience it. UI and FI share similar contributing factors, including damage to the pelvic floor as a result of surgery or trauma, neurological disorders, functional impairment, immobility, and dementia.

Bowel continence and defecation depend on coordination of sensory and motor innervation of the rectum and anal sphincters. Impairment of the anorectal unit, such as weakness from prolonged straining secondary to constipation, or overt anal tears seen after vaginal delivery in women (35%) are common causes of FI. Injury from obstetrical trauma is often delayed in onset and many women do not manifest symptoms until after the age of 50 years.

❖ USING CLINICAL JUDGMENT TO PROMOTE HEALTHY AGING: ACCIDENTAL BOWEL LEAKAGE (FI)

◆ Recognizing and Analyzing Cues: Accidental Bowel Leakage (FI)

Recognition and analysis of cues begin with a complete client history as in UI (Box 12.3) and investigation into stool consistency and frequency, use of laxatives or enemas, surgical and obstetrical history, medications, effect of bowel leakage on quality of life, focused physical examination with attention to the gastrointestinal system, and a bowel record. A digital rectal examination should be performed to identify any presence of a mass, impaction, or occult blood.

◆ Nursing Actions: Accidental Bowel Leakage (FI)

Nursing actions are implemented to assist the individual in managing and/or restoring bowel continence. Dietary and medical management are recommended as first-line management. Therapies similar to those used to treat UI such as environmental manipulation (access to toilet); dietary alterations; habit training schedules; PFMEs; improving transfer and ambulation ability; sphincter training exercises; biofeedback; medications; and/or surgery to correct underlying defects are effective. Studies have shown that 22% to 54% of individuals can have improvement in accidental bowel leakage with formal counseling from a specialist regarding dietary habits, fluid management, bowel routines, and changes to medications (Paquette et al., 2015). Providing resources and educational information is important and will help in self-management (see Box 12.4). Other interventions are presented in Box 12.13.

BOX 12.13 Tips for Best Practice
Nursing Actions for Accidental Bowel Leakage

- Use therapeutic communication skills and a positive and supportive attitude to help individuals overcome any embarrassment.
- Use the term accidental bowel leakage rather than fecal incontinence.
- Emphasize the importance of thorough evaluation.
- Teach about the range of interventions available for management.
- Share helpful resources for continence management.
- Have individual keep a bowel diary and identify triggers. For example, if eating a meal or drinking a cup of coffee stimulates defecation, use the toilet at a given time after the trigger event. Have a regular toileting routine.
- Encourage being prepared. Schedule outings, appointments, exercise routines around anticipated bowel patterns; suggest keeping a change of underwear, clothing, and toileting supplies when out; use an absorbent pad and have bags to dispose of pad if soiled; deodorant sprays for odor; wear darker clothing when away from home so that if soiling occurs, it will be less noticeable; when out, scan environment for toilet locations.
- Avoid greasy and flatus-producing foods, dairy products, fruits with edible seeds, acidic citrus fruits, nuts, spicy foods, and other foods that trigger leakage. Bake or broil foods instead of frying; eat meals at regular times; eat after public events to reduce likelihood of leakage.

From Wilde, M., Bliss, D., Booth, J., et al. (2014). Self-management of urinary and fecal incontinence, *Am J Nurs 114*(2), 38–45.

Pharmacological interventions may include the use of antidiarrheal medications and fiber therapy. Biofeedback may also be recommended, and there are some surgical options that can be considered if conservative interventions are not successful. SNM may also be considered as a first-line surgical option and has been shown to reduce the frequency of episodes. Injection of bulking agents into the anal canal has been reported to reduce accidental bowel leakage, but guidelines suggest a weak recommendation for this treatment based on moderate-quality evidence (Paquette et al., 2015). Further study is needed on these types of treatments.

The effectiveness of interventions in fecal incontinence will be self-evident but will take time. As in the treatment of UI, goals must be realistic. It cannot be stated too often or too strongly that nurses must always provide immaculate skin care to persons with incontinence, because self-esteem and skin integrity depend on it.

▌ KEY CONCEPTS

- Urinary incontinence is not a part of normal aging. UI is a symptom of an underlying problem and requires thorough recognition and analysis of cues to design nursing actions to promote bladder health.
- Urinary incontinence can be minimized or cured, and there are many therapeutic modalities available for treatment of UI that nurses can implement. Behavioral and lifestyle approaches are first-line interventions.
- Health promotion teaching, identification of risk factors, comprehensive evaluation of UI, education of informal and formal caregivers, and use of evidence-based interventions are basic continence competencies for nurses.
- A number of interventions for urinary incontinence are applicable to the management of bowel incontinence.
- Evaluation and management of bowel function are important nursing responsibilities. The precipitants and causes of constipation must be included in the evaluation of bowel function. Increased fluid intake, changes in diet, physical activity, bowel training programs, and review of medications with constipation side effects are important nonpharmacological interventions.

▌ ACTIVITIES AND DISCUSSION QUESTIONS

1. Discuss risk factors for UI in older adults.
2. What health teaching would you provide to a 70-year-old woman who asks you if it is normal to leak urine

when coughing or sneezing? What suggestions could you give her to deal with this concern?

3. When you are at your clinical site, ask the nurses what concerns they have with the bowel elimination of their patients.

NEXT-GENERATION NCLEX® EXAMINATION-STYLE QUESTIONS

Case Study 1

The assistive personnel report that Ms. Miller, an 87-year-old resident, has a change in her response level. Ms. Miller has late-stage Alzheimer's disease, hypertension, and osteoporosis. On regular days, she will attempt to speak to the staff even though her speech is garbled. She enjoys sitting up in bed or in a chair next to someone and listening to music. Upon evaluation, Ms. Miller opens her eyes when her name is called, but otherwise does not respond to verbal stimuli. Her blood pressure is 140/60 mmHg, heart rate is 74 beats/min, rhythm is regular, respiratory rate is even with 18 breaths/min, temperature 98.9°F, with oxygen saturation of 95% on room air. Lung sounds are clear to auscultation throughout lung fields, bowel sounds are hypoactive, abdomen is slightly distended, and Ms. Miller grunts with abdominal palpation. Ms. Miller has no peripheral edema and her skin is warm, dry, and intact. Intake and output records from yesterday show a small bowel movement with each void and 50% meal intake. Laboratory results include:

- BUN/Creatinine is 22 mg/dL and 1.6 mg/dL,
- Na/Cl is 145 mmol/L and 105 mmol/L,
- Glucose is 105 mg/dL.
- Urine is amber and clear, pH 5.0, nitrite negative and leukocyte esterase trace, blood negative, WBC 2/hpf, and bacteria occasional.

Highlight the evaluation data that require follow-up by the nurse.

Case Study 2

Ms. Franklin, 68 years old, is seen in the clinic for urinary incontinence. Her history includes hypertension, Type 2 diabetes, and osteoarthritis, treated with lisinopril/hydrochlorothiazide 20 mg/25 mg daily, glipizide/metformin 2.5 mg/500 mg twice a day, and celecoxib 200 mg daily. She states she delayed seeking care as she felt uncomfortable talking to her health care provider about the issue and thought all women experienced incontinence. The problem has worsened; she leaks through her incontinence liner pads at times. Two of her daughters convinced her to come to the clinic for treatment.

Upon further questioning by the nurse, it is revealed that Ms. Franklin has reduced her caffeine intake to one cup of coffee per day but has also decreased her overall fluid intake to reduce her incontinence. When asked to describe her incontinence, she states that she loses urine before she can make it to the bathroom and she needs to urinate frequently. She also gets up to use the bathroom several times each night. She states her last bowel movement was this morning after breakfast; she normally has a soft bowel movement each day. Ms. Franklin's vital signs are blood pressure 125/82 mmHg, heart rate 88 beats per minute, respirations 14 breaths per minute, temperature 97.9°F. She is 5'4' and weighs 200 pounds. Her lab results include:

- BUN/Creatinine is 22 mg/dL and 1.6 mg/dL,
- Na/Cl is 145 mmol/L and 105 mmol/L,
- Glucose is 115 mg/dL.
- Urine is amber and clear, pH 5.0, nitrite negative and leukocyte esterase negative, RBC 2/hpf, WBC 2/hpf, and bacteria negative.

Use an X to indicate which actions listed in the left column would be included in the plan of care.

Actions	Plan of Care
Ask client to complete a 3-day bladder diary	
Teach client to lengthen toileting frequency progressively to every 4 hours	
Use a 3-day trial of prompted voiding combined with the use of absorbent products	
Teach client pelvic floor muscle exercises	
Encourage intake of 2 liters of fluid per day	
Reduce weight by 10%	
Encourage client to use over-the-counter laxatives to maintain routine bowel movements	

REFERENCES

Albisinni, S., Biaou, I., Marcelis, Q., et al. (2016). New medical treatments for lower urinary tract symptoms due to benign prostatic hyperplasia and future perspectives. *BMC Urology, 16*(1), 58.

American Geriatrics Society Choosing Wisely Workgroup. (2014). American Geriatrics Society identifies another five things that healthcare providers and patients should question. *J Am Geriatr Soc, 62*(5), 950–960.

Balk, E., Rofeberg, V., Adam, G., et al. (2019). Pharmacological and nonpharmacological treatments for urinary incontinence in women. *Annals of Int Med, 170*(7), 465–476.

Beeson, T., & Davis, C. (2018). Urinary management with an external female collection device. *J Wound Ostomy Continence Nurs, 45*(2), 187–189.

Brown, H. W., Wexner, S. D., Segall, M. M., Brezoczky, K. L., & Lukacz, E. S. (2012). Accidental bowel leakage in the mature women's health study. *Int J Clin Pract, 66*(11), 1101–1108.

Centers for Disease Control and Prevention (CDC). *National and State Healthcare-associated infections (HAI) progress report,* 2018. https://www.cdc.gov/hai/data/portal/progress-report.html.

Colborne, M., & Dahlke, S. (2017). Nurses' perceptions and management of urinary incontinence in hospitalized older adults. *An Integr Rev J Gerontol Nurs, 43*(10), 46–55.

Crnich, C. J., Jump, R. L., & Nace, D. A. (2017). Improving management of urinary tract infections in older adults: a paradigm shift or therapeutic nihilism? *J Am Geriatr Soc, 65*, 1661–1663.

El-Azab, A. S., & Siegel, S. W. (2019). Sacral neuromodulation for female pelvic floor disorders. *Arab J Urol, 17*(1), 14–22.

Enberg, S., & Li, H. (2017). Urinary incontinence in frail older adults. *Urologic Nurs, 37*(3), 119–124.

Finucane, T. E. (2017). Urinary tract infection"—requiem for a heavyweight. *J Am Geriatr Soc, 65*, 1650–1655.

Gibson, W., & Wagg, A. (2014). New horizons: urinary incontinence in older adults. *Age Ageing, 43*, 157–163.

Grover, M., Busby-Whitehead, J., Palmer, M. H., et al. (2010). Survey of geriatricians on the effect of fecal incontinence on nursing home referral. *J Am Geriatr Soc, 58*, 1058.

Guérin, A., Mody, R., Fok, B., et al. (2014). Risk of developing colorectal cancer and benign colorectal neoplasm in patients with chronic constipation. *Aliment Pharmacol Ther, 40*(1), 83–92.

Holtzer-Goor, K. M., Gaultney, J. G., van Houten, P., et al. (2015). Cost-effectiveness of including a nurse specialist in the treatment of urinary incontinence in primary care in the Netherlands. *PLoS One, 10*(10), e0138225.

Hsu, A., Suskind, A., & Huang, A. J. (2016). Urinary incontinence among older adults. In L. Lindquist (Ed.), *New directions in geriatric medicine* (pp. 49–69). New York: Springer.

Hu, F., Chuan-Hsiu, T., Huey-Shyan, L., et al. (2017). Inappropriate urinary catheter reinsertion in hospitalized older patients. *American J Inf Control, 45*(1), 8–12.

Jiwrajka, M., Yaxley, W., Ranasinghe, S., et al. (2018). Drugs for benign prostatic hypertrophy. *Aust Prescr, 41*(5), 150–153.

Kitsler, C. E., Zimmerman, S., Scales, K., et al. (2017). The antibiotic prescribing pathway for presumed urinary tract infections in nursing home residents. *J Am Geriatr Soc, 65*, 1719–1725.

Lacy, B., Mearin, F., Chang, L., Chey, W. et al. (2016). Bowel Disorders. *Gastroenterology, 150*, 1393–1407.

Lai, C. K. Y., & Wan, X (2017). Using prompted voiding to manage urinary incontinence in nursing homes: can it be sustained? *J Am Med Dir Assoc, 18*(6), 509–514.

Lewis, S. J., & Heaton, K. W. (1997). Stool form scale as a useful guide to intestinal transit time. *Scand J Gastroenterol, 32*, 920–924.

MacDonald, D. G., & Butler, L. (2007). Silent no more: elderly women's stories of living with urinary incontinence in long-term care. *J Gerontol Nurs, 33*, 14–20.

Markland, A., et al. (2014). Constipation and fecal incontinence. In R. Ham, R. Sloane, & G. Warshaw et al. (Eds.), *Primary care geriatrics* (6th ed., pp. 281–291). Philadelphia: Elsevier.

Mason, D. J., Newman, D. K., & Palmer, M. H. (2003). Changing UI practice. *Am J Nurs, 103*, 129.

Mody, L., Greene, M. T., Meddings, J., et al. (2017). A national implementation program to prevent catheter-associated urinary tract infection in nursing home residents. *JAMA Intern Med, 177*(8), 1154–1162.

National Association for Continence. *Urinary incontinence overview, facts and statistics,* 2017. https://www.nafc.org/urinary-incontinence/.

Ostaszkiewicz, J. (2017). A conceptual model of the risk of elder abuse posed by incontinence and care dependence. *Int J Older People Nurs, 13*(2), e12182.

Paquette, I. M., Varma, M. G., Kaiser, A. M., Steele, S. R., & Rafferty, J. F. (2015). The American Society of Colon and Rectal Surgeons clinical practice guideline for the treatment of fecal incontinence. *Dis Colon Rectum, 58*, 623–636.

Quinn, M., Ameling, J. M., Forman, J., et al. (2020). Persistent barriers to timely catheter removal identified from clinical observation and interviews. *Jt Comm J Qual Patient Saf, 46*(2), 99–108.

Searcy, J. A. R (2017). Geriatric urinary incontinence. *Nurs Clin North Am, 52*, 447–455.

Shaw, C., & Wagg, A. (2016). Urinary incontinence in older adults. *Med Older Adults, 45*(1).

Sjöström, M., Lindholm, L., & Samuelsson, E. (2017). Mobile app for treatment of stress urinary incontinence: a cost-effectiveness analysis. *J Med Int Res, 19*(5), e154.

Spencer, M., McManus, K., & Sabourin, J. (2017). Incontinence in older adults: the role of the geriatric multidisciplinary team. *BC Med J, 59*(2), 99–105.

Staller, K., et al: Abstract Sa1711. Presented at Digestive Disease Week, May 2-5, 2020; Chicago [meeting cancelled].

Timmons, B., Vess, J., & Conner, B. (2017). Nurse-driven protocol to reduce indwelling catheter time: a health care improvement initiative. *J Nurs Care Qual, 32*(2), 104–107.

Wilde, M. H., Bliss, D. Z., Booth, J., Cheater, F. M., & Tannenbaum, C. (2014). Self-management of urinary and fecal incontinence. *Am J Nurs, 114*(2), 38–45.

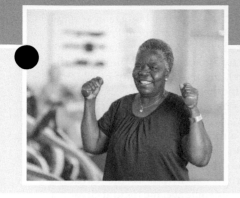

Clinical Judgment to Promote Healthy Rest, Sleep, and Activity

Theris A. Touhy

LEARNING OBJECTIVES

Upon completion of this chapter, the reader will be able to:
- Identify factors that affect rest, sleep, and activity as we age.
- Discuss the importance of sleep and activity to the health and well-being of older adults.
- Describe the beneficial effects of exercise and appropriate exercise regimens for older adults.
- Utilize clinical judgment to identify and evaluate nursing actions for rest, sleep, and promotion of activity

THE LIVED EXPERIENCE

You know, I never get a decent night's sleep. I wake up at least four times every night, and I just know I won't get back to sleep. I really don't want to keep taking pills for sleep, but when I lie there awake, I just think of all the difficult times and situations I can't manage. After a while, I'm really in a stew about everything.

Richard, a 67-year-old recent retiree

This is really beginning to tire me out. Richard keeps waking me at night because he can't sleep. I try to tell him to get up and read or something. I really need my sleep if I'm going to get to work on time. I wonder if Richard needs to see a doctor. Maybe he is depressed about being retired and alone while I'm at work. I'll talk to him about it.

Clara, Richard's wife

Rest, sleep, and activity depend on one another. Inadequacy of rest and sleep affects any activity, whether it is considered strenuous exertion or performance of activities of daily living (ADLs). Activity, in turn, is necessary to maintain physical and physiological integrity (e.g., cardiopulmonary endurance and function; musculoskeletal strength, agility, and structure), and it helps a person obtain adequate sleep. Rest, sleep, and activity contribute greatly to overall physical and mental well-being.

REST AND SLEEP

The human organism needs rest and sleep to conserve energy, prevent fatigue, provide organ respite, and relieve tension. Sleep is an extension of rest, and both are physiological and mental necessities for survival. Sleep is a basic need. Rest occurs with sleep in sustained unbroken periods. Sleep occupies one-third of our lives and is a vital function that affects cognition and performance. Research into the physiology of sleep suggests that the restorative function of sleep may be a consequence of the enhanced removal of potentially neurotoxic waste products that accumulate in the awake central nervous system.

Sleep is a barometer of health, and attention to sleep and actions to address sleep concerns and actions to address sleep concerns should receive as much attention as other vital signs. There is increasing awareness of the relationship between sleep problems and health outcomes, including premature mortality, osteoporosis, cardiovascular disease, diabetes, metabolic disease, impaired cognition and physical function, anxiety and depression, pain, and decreased quality of life (Jike et al., 2018; Silva et al., 2016). Impaired sleep has been associated with Alzheimer's disease. Studies show that sleep plays a role in clearing beta-amyloid out of the brain. A build-up of beta-amyloid is linked to impaired brain function and Alzheimer's disease (Chapter 23). A recent small study demonstrated that beta-amyloid increased about 5% in the brains of the participants after losing just one night of sleep (Shokri-Kojori et al., 2018).

Insufficient sleep is a public health epidemic, and the Centers for Disease Control and Prevention (CDC, 2018) has called for continued public health surveillance of sleep quality, duration, behaviors, and disorders to monitor for sleep difficulties and their health impact. Sleep problems also constitute a global epidemic, affecting up to 45% of the world's population. Because of the public health burden of chronic sleep loss and sleep disorders, and the low awareness of poor sleep health, *Healthy People 2020* includes sleep health as a special topic area (Box 13.1).

Biorhythm and Sleep

Our lives proceed in a series of rhythms that influence and regulate physiological function, chemical concentrations, performance, behavioral responses, moods, and the ability to adapt. It is clear that body temperature, pulse rate, blood pressure, and hormonal levels change significantly and predictably in a circadian rhythm. Circadian rhythms are linked to the 24-hour day by time cues (zeitgebers), the most important of which is the light-dark cycle. Biorhythms vary between individuals, and age-related changes in biorhythms (circadian rhythms) are relevant to health and the process of aging. With aging, there is a reduction in the amplitude of all circadian endogenous responses (e.g., body temperature, pulse rate, blood pressure, hormonal levels).

The most important biorhythm is the circadian sleep–wake rhythm. As people age, the natural circadian rhythm may become less responsive to external stimuli, such as changes in light during the course of the day. In addition, the endogenous changes in the production of melatonin are diminished, resulting in less sleep efficacy and further disruption of restorative sleep (Saccomano, 2014). Genetic research is investigating pathways linking sleep, circadian rhythm, metabolism, functioning, and disease, and genome-wide determinants of sleep duration (Mukherjee et al., 2018).

Sleep and Aging

The predictable pattern of normal sleep is called **sleep architecture**. The body progresses through stages of sleep consisting of **rapid eye movement (REM)** sleep and **non-rapid eye movement (NREM)** sleep. Most of the changes in sleep architecture in healthy adults begin between the ages of 40 and 60 years. The age-related changes include less time spent in N3 sleep (formerly called Stages 3 and 4) (slow wave sleep) and more time spent awake or in N1 (formerly called Stage 1) sleep. The changes contribute to fragmented sleep and early awakening (Suzuki et al., 2017).

Time spent in REM sleep also declines with age, and transitions between N1 and N2 (stages 1 and 2) are more common. REM sleep is seen as important for older adults, since it is a time for the brain to replenish neurotransmitters essential for remembering, learning, and problem solving. Declines in N3 and N4 sleep begin between 20 and 30 years of age and are nearly complete by the age of 50 to 60 years. In adults over 90 years, N3 sleep may disappear completely (Xiong and Hategan, 2019).

Research suggests that the deterioration of a cluster of neurons associated with regulating sleep patterns, the ventrolateral preoptic nucleus, may be responsible for sleep decline in aging. The more neurons that are lost, the more difficult it is for the person to sleep. For individuals with dementia, the link between the loss of neurons is greater and causes more problems with sleep (Petrovsky et al., 2018). The changes that occur in sleep with aging are summarized in Box 13.2.

 BOX 13.1 Healthy People 2020

Sleep Health

Goals
- Increase public knowledge of how adequate sleep and treatment of sleep disorders improve health, productivity, wellness, quality of life, and safety on roads and in the workplace.
- Increase the proportion of persons with symptoms of obstructive sleep apnea who seek medical evaluation.
- Increase the proportion of adults who get sufficient sleep.

From US Department of Health and Human Services, Office of Disease Prevention and Health Promotion: *Healthy People 2020,* 2012. http://www.healthypeople.gov/2020.

BOX 13.2 Changes in Sleep With Age

- More time spent in bed awake before falling asleep
- Total sleep time and sleep efficiency are reduced
- Periods awake are frequent, increasing after age 50 years (>30 min of wakefulness after sleep onset in >50% of older subjects)
- Daytime napping
- Changes in circadian rhythm (early to bed, early to rise)
- Sleep is subjectively and objectively lighter (more stage 1, little stage 4, more disruptions)
- Rapid eye movement (REM) sleep is short, less intense, and more evenly distributed
- Frequency of abnormal breathing events is increased
- Frequency of leg movements during sleep is increased

Adapted from Saccomano, S. (2014). Sleep disorders in older adults, *J Gerontol Nurs 40*(3), 38–45.

⚡ SAFETY ALERT

Poor sleep is not an inevitable consequence of aging, but rather an indicator of health status and calls for investigation. Older adults with good general health, positive moods, and engagement in more active lifestyles and meaningful activities report better sleep and fewer sleep complaints.

Sleep Disorders

Insomnia

Insomnia is the most common sleep disorder worldwide (Bhaskar et al., 2016). The American Academy of Sleep Medicine defines insomnia as the subjective perception of difficulty with sleep initiation, duration, consolidation, or quality that results in some form of daytime impairment (Matheson & Hainer, 2017). The diagnosis of insomnia requires that the person has difficulty falling asleep for at least 1 month and that impairment in daytime functioning results from difficulty sleeping. Insomnia is classified as either primary or comorbid.

Primary insomnia implies that no other cause of sleep disturbance has been identified. Comorbid insomnia is more common and is associated with psychiatric and medical disorders, medications, and primary sleep disorders, such as obstructive sleep apnea (OSA) or restless legs syndrome (RLS). Comorbid insomnia does not suggest that these conditions cause insomnia but that insomnia and the other conditions co-occur and each may require attention and treatment (Winkelman, 2015).

More than half of older adults suffer from insomnia and sleep complaints are generally higher in women than in men (Theorell-Haglöw et al. 2018; World Association of Sleep Medicine, 2018). Chronic insomnia is a significant risk factor for cognitive decline in men. Insomnia

is also associated with an increased risk of cardiovascular-related and all-cause mortality as well as a predictor of long-term care placement (Suzuki et al., 2017). The number of insomnia symptoms is associated with an increased risk of falls in older adults, and the use of sleeping medications, irrespective of insomnia symptoms, further increases fall risk (Chen et al., 2017) (Chapter 15).

There are many influencing factors for insomnia, including physiological, psychological, and environmental (Box 13.3). Prescription and nonprescription medications and alcohol create sleep disturbances (Box 13.4). The times of day that medications are given can also contribute to sleep problems—for example, a diuretic given before bedtime or a sedating medication given in the morning.

Insomnia and Alzheimer's disease sleep disruption affects approximately 60% to 70% of older adults with

---

BOX 13.3 Risk Factors for Sleep Disturbances in Older Adults

Physical Health
- Age-related changes in sleep architecture
- Comorbidities (cardiovascular disease, diabetes, pulmonary disease, musculoskeletal disorders); CNS disorders (Parkinson's disease, seizure disorder, dementia); GI disorders (hiatal hernia, GERD, PUD); urinary disorders (incontinence, BPH)
- Pain
- Polypharmacy
- Lack of exercise
- Excessive napping
- Sleep disorders (apnea, restless legs syndrome, periodic leg movement, rapid eye movement behavior disorder, alcohol, smoking)

Psychological Condition
- Depression, anxiety, delirium, psychosis
- Life stressors/response to stress
- Sleep-related beliefs
- Sleep habits (daily sleep/activity cycle, napping)
- Loneliness
- Loss of partner
- Poor sleep hygiene

Physical Environment
- Environmental noises, institutional routines
- Caregiving for a dependent older adult
- Limited exposure to sunlight
- New environment

BPH, Benign prostatic hyperplasia; *CNS,* central nervous system; *GERD,* gastroesophageal reflux disease; *GI,* gastrointestinal; *PUD,* peptic ulcer disease.
Adapted from Teodorescu, M. (2014). Sleep disruptions and insomnia in older adults, *Consultant 54*(3), 166–173.

BOX 13.4   Medications Affecting Sleep

Selective serotonin reuptake inhibitors (SSRIs)
Antihypertensives (clonidine, beta blockers, reserpine, methyldopa)
Anticholinergics
Sympathomimetic amines
Diuretics
Opiates
Cough and cold medications
Thyroid preparations
Phenytoin
Cortisone
Levodopa

BOX 13.5   Sleep Diary

Instructions: Record the following for 2 to 4 weeks. Should be completed by the person or the caregiver if the person is unable. Record when you:

- Go to bed
- Go to sleep
- Wake up
- Get out of bed
- Take naps
- Exercise
- Consume alcohol
- Consume caffeinated beverages

From Centers for Disease Control and Prevention (2013). *What should I do if I can't sleep?* https://www.cdc.gov/sleep/about_sleep/cant_sleep.html.

---

dementia and varies by dementia subtype. Individuals with Lewy body dementia and Parkinson's dementia have the highest prevalence of sleep disruption (90%), and 25% to 60% of individuals with Alzheimer's disease have sleep disruptions or abnormal circadian rhythms. Multiple factors contribute to sleep disruption in dementia, including degenerative changes in the suprachiasmatic nuclei (SCN) of the hypothalamus, which generates the circadian rhythm, psychiatric, and medical comorbidities, and physiological changes associated with aging (Scales et al., 2018).

Additionally, decreased exposure to daytime light and increased exposure to nighttime noise and light contributes to disrupted sleep (Figueiro et al., 2019). A recent study (Evans and Kovach, 2020) reported that discomfort from musculoskeletal pain, respiratory distress, gastrointestinal discomfort, and urinary retention affected quality of sleep in persons with dementia. Evaluation of pain and other sources of discomfort affecting sleep in persons with dementia is important in improving sleep quality. Sleep disruption is associated with increased neuropsychiatric symptoms, functional decline, morbidity, and mortality. Sleep disruption is a major predictor of institutionalization and caregiver burden. Caregivers of individuals with dementia also experience poor sleep quality, and this influences caregiver stress and health problems (Leggett et al., 2018; Petrovsky et al., 2018).

❖ USING CLINICAL JUDGMENT TO PROMOTE HEALTHY AGING: SLEEP

◆ Recognizing and Analyzing Cues: Sleep

Sleep habits should be reviewed with older adults in all settings. Many people do not seek treatment for insomnia and may blame poor sleep on the aging process. Nurses are in an excellent position to evaluate sleep and suggest actions to improve the quality of the sleep of older adults.

"No other group of health care providers watch more people sleep than nurses" (Dean et al., 2016, p. 438).

Evaluation of sleep disturbances and awareness of contributing factors to poor sleep (pain, chronic illness, medications, alcohol use, depression, anxiety) are important. Nurses should learn how well the person sleeps at home, how many times the person is awakened at night, what time the person retires, level of physical activity during the day, and which rituals occur at bedtime. Rituals include bedtime snacks, watching television, listening to music, or reading—activities whose execution is crucial to the individual's ability to fall asleep. The sleep diary or log is also an important part of evaluation (Box 13.5). This information will provide an accurate account of the person's sleep problem and help identify the sleep disturbance. A period of 2 to 4 weeks is needed to obtain a clear picture of the sleep problem. A self-rating scale, the Pittsburgh Sleep Quality Index (PSQI), can be used to measure the quality and patterns of sleep in the older adult, and daytime sleepiness can be evaluated with the Epworth Sleepiness Scale, both recommended by the Hartford Institute for Geriatric Nursing (Box 13.6).

BOX 13.6   Resources for Best Practice

Sleep

Hartford Institute for Geriatric Nursing: Try This: General Assessment Series: Epworth Sleepiness Scale and Pittsburg Sleep Quality Index; Want to know more: Sleep: Nursing Standard Practice Protocol, Excessive Sleepiness.

National Heart Lung and Blood Institute: Sleep apnea. https://www.nhlbi.nih.gov/health-topics/sleep-apnea.

Willis-Ekbom Foundation: RLS/WED symptom diary. http://www.willis-ekbom.org/about-rls-wed/publications?

Nursing Actions: Sleep Promotion

Nonpharmacological Treatment

Treatment actions begin after a thorough sleep history has been recorded and, if possible, a sleep log obtained. Nonpharmacological interventions are considered first-line treatment for insomnia. Education should be provided on changes in sleep architecture with aging and the importance of attention to sleep hygiene principles to promote good sleep habits.

Cognitive behavioral therapy for insomnia is a multidimensional approach combining psychological and behavioral therapies that include healthy sleep habits, relaxation techniques, circadian rhythm interventions, and cognitive therapy (Box 13.7). A combination of approaches is most effective, and these interventions have been reported to be an effective and practical treatment for chronic insomnia in older adults (Anderson, 2018; Haynes et al., 2018). Cognitive training programs (Chapter 5) may improve sleep quality and cognitive performance. Tai Chi Qigong (TCQ), a less complex form of tai chi movements, can be considered a useful nonpharmacological approach for sleep complaints for individuals with cognitive impairment (Chan et al., 2016).

Sleep in hospitals and nursing homes. In hospital and institutional settings, promotion of a good sleep environment is important. Studies have shown that as many as 22% to 61% of hospitalized patients experience impaired sleep (Dean et al., 2016). A multidisciplinary approach to identify sources of noise and light, such as equipment and staff interactions, could result in modification without compromising safety and quality of patient care. Sleep deprivation because of noise can potentially exacerbate delirium. Noise from monitoring equipment alarms and infusion devices and the ringing from telephones cause an elevation of heart rate (Grossman et al., 2017; McGough et al., 2018). Nursing staff should ensure that patients complete a full sleep cycle of 90 minutes before waking for nonemergency reasons such as checking for incontinence or doing routine tasks.

Individuals experiencing dementia often have severe dysfunctions of their sleep–wake and rest–activity patterns (sundowning, excessive daytime sleepiness, nocturnal wandering, agitation, irritability, day–night reversal, decreased cognitive functioning). Daytime light exposure is a major synchronizer of circadian rhythms. When individuals with dementia are in controlled environments (hospitals, long-term care facilities), daytime light exposure may be limited, exacerbating their symptoms. Tailored light interventions designed to maximally affect the circadian system have been reported to improve sleep in individuals with moderate to late-stage dementia (Figueiro et al., 2019).

Pharmacological Treatment

The use of over-the-counter (OTC) sleep aids, as well as the use of prescription sedative and hypnotic medications, is increasing in the United States. Individuals over the age of 60 years receive 33% of all hypnotic prescriptions, although they constitute only 14% of the population. The American Geriatrics Society (AGS) Beers Criteria (2015)

BOX 13.7 Interventions for Insomnia

Healthy Sleep Habits
- Keep a consistent sleep schedule. Get up at the same time every day, even on weekends or during vacations.
- Set a bedtime that is early enough to get at least 7 hours of sleep.
- Don't go to bed unless sleepy.
- If you don't fall asleep after 20 minutes, get out of bed.
- Establish a relaxing bedtime routine.
- Use bed only for sleep and sex.
- Make bedroom quiet and relaxing. Keep the room at a comfortable, cool temperature.
- Limit exposure to bright light in the evenings.
- Turn off electronic devices at least 30 minutes before bedtime.
- Don't eat a large meal before bedtime. If hungry at night, eat a light, healthy snack.
- Exercise regularly and maintain a healthy diet.
- Avoid caffeine, alcohol, and tobacco in the late afternoon or evening.

- Reduce fluid intake before bedtime.
- Limit or avoid daytime napping.

Relaxation Techniques
- Diaphragmatic breathing
- Progressive relaxation
- White noise or music
- Guided imagery
- Stretching
- Yoga or tai chi

Circadian Rhythm Interventions
- Cue circadian rhythm by connecting with environmental signals (light exposure, meals, activity, medications).
- Maintain stable daytime routines with meals, activity, and medications.
- Increase duration and intensity of bright light or sunlight exposure during the day.
- Melatonin 1 to 2 hours before bedtime may be helpful.

Adapted from American Academy of Sleep Medicine (2017). *Healthy sleep habits.* http://www.sleepeducation.org/essentials-in-sleep/healthy-sleep-habits.

strongly suggests avoiding any type of benzodiazepine for the treatment of insomnia because these medications are associated with adverse outcomes including motor vehicle accidents, impaired cognition, and falls (Markota et al., 2016; Maust et al., 2016; Schroeck et al., 2016). Adverse reactions to these medications are also increasing. Use of narcotic pain medications and sedatives, and the use of alcohol in combination with these medications and other prescribed medications, is a growing concern (Chapter 28).

Individuals should be educated on the proper use of medications, their side effects, and their interactions with alcohol and other prescription drugs. Pharmacological treatments for sleep disorders may be used in combination with behavioral interventions but must be managed with caution in older adults (Albert et al., 2017). In long-term care settings, there are specific regulatory guidelines on the use of hypnotics, including appropriate prescribing and tapering and discontinuation of use.

> ⚡ **SAFETY ALERT**
>
> Benzodiazepines or other sedative-hypnotics should not be used in older adults as a first choice of treatment for insomnia (American Geriatrics Society, 2015).

OTC drugs such as diphenhydramine, found in many OTC sleep products such as Tylenol PM, are often thought to be relatively harmless but should be avoided because of antihistaminic and anticholinergic side effects. Other OTC sleep aid preparations contain ingredients such as kava kava, valerian root, melatonin, chamomile, and tryptophan. Because these ingredients are not regulated, information and outcomes of efficacy may not be known. Endogenous nocturnal melatonin, a major loop for circadian rhythm, may have decreased levels in older adults. Melatonin, taken 1 to 2 hours before bedtime, may replicate the natural secretion pattern of melatonin and lead to improvements in the circadian regulation of the sleep–wake cycle. Routine use of OTC medications for sleep may delay appropriate evaluation and treatment of contributing medical or psychological conditions, identification of sleep disorders, and appropriate counseling and treatment. The individual should report use of all OTC drugs to their health care provider since they may interact with other medications.

Benzodiazepine receptor agonists, such as zolpidem (Ambien), eszopiclone (Lunesta), and zaleplon (Sonata), are considered benzodiazepine-like in their action because they induce sleep easily. They can have detrimental effects, causing changes in mental status (delirium), memory loss, falls and fractures, daytime drowsiness, and increased risk of motor vehicle accidents, with only minimal improvement in sleep latency and duration (American Geriatrics Society, 2014). Zolpidem is the medication most often implicated in emergency department visits for adverse drug events in adults (Hampton et al., 2014). The US Food and Drug Administration (FDA, 2019) has added a black box warning on patient medication guides and prescription information for insomnia drugs such as zolpidem, zaleplon, and eszopiclone, calling attention to side effects that can lead to serious injury or death. Rare but serious incidents have occurred when users of these medications experienced complex sleep behaviors: sleepwalking, sleep driving, and engaging in other activities when not fully awake.

> ⚡ **SAFETY ALERT**
>
> Thorough evaluation of sleep problems should be conducted before medication use. Nonpharmacological interventions are first-line treatment. If sleeping medications are used, they should be taken immediately before bedtime because of their rapid action. Short-term use (2 to 3 weeks, never more than 90 days) is recommended.

Sleep Disordered Breathing and Sleep Apnea

Sleep disordered breathing (SDB) affects approximately 25% of older individuals (more men than women), and the most common form is obstructive sleep apnea (OSA). Untreated obstructive sleep apnea (OSA) is related to heart failure, cardiac dysrhythmias, stroke, type 2 diabetes, cognitive decline, osteoporosis, and even death (Kapur et al., 2017; Leng et al., 2017). The diagnosis of OSA is often delayed in older adults and symptoms are blamed on age (McMillan & Morrell, 2016). Severe OSA is also related to increased blood glucose in Black individuals. Developing interventions to promote regular sleep schedules may prove useful in improving blood glucose controls and preventing type 2 diabetes among Black patients (Yano et al., 2020).

Age-related decline in the activity of the upper airway muscles, resulting in compromised pharyngeal patency, predisposes older adults to OSA. A high body mass index (BMI) and large neck circumference have been identified as risk factors for OSA. Losing weight is an effective treatment for OSA, and recent studies have shown that increased tongue fat may explain the relationship between obesity and OSA. Results of a recent study reported that a reduction in tongue fat volume was the primary link between weight loss and sleep apnea improvement (Wang et al., 2020). Other risk factors for OSA are presented in Box 13.8.

BOX 13.8   Risk Factors for Obstructive Sleep Apnea

- Increasing age
- Increased neck circumference (not as significant in older adults)
- Male gender
- Anatomical abnormalities of the upper airway
- Upper airway resistance and/or obstruction
- Family history
- Excess weight
- Use of alcohol, sedatives, or tranquilizers
- Smoking
- Hypertension

Recognizing and Analyzing Cues: SDB

The diagnosis of OSA is often delayed in older adults and symptoms blamed on age (McMillan and Morrell, 2016). If the person has a sleeping partner, it is often the partner who reports the nighttime symptoms. If there is a sleeping partner, they may move to another room to sleep because of the disturbance to their own rest.

The individual with SDB may present with complaints of insomnia or daytime sleepiness and insomnia should be evaluated as discussed previously, including the use of screening instruments such as the Epworth Sleepiness Scale (Box 13.6). Symptoms of OSA and information from the sleeping partner, if present, are obtained. Recognition of OSA in older adults may be more difficult because there may not be a sleeping partner to report symptoms. If presenting symptoms suggest the disorder, a tape recorder can be placed at the bedside to record snoring and breathing sounds during the night. A medication review is always indicated when investigating sleep complaints. The upper airway, including the nasal and pharyngeal airways, should be examined for anatomical obstruction, tumors, or cysts. Comorbid conditions such as heart failure and diabetes should be evaluated and managed appropriately.

Nursing Actions: SDB and OSA

If OSA is suspected, a referral for a sleep study should be conducted. A sleep study or polysomnogram is a multiple-component test that electronically transmits and records specific physical activities during a full night of sleep. Sleep studies can be done in a special center or at home with a portable diagnostic device. If done at a sleep center, you will sleep in a bed at the center for the duration of the study. Removable sensors are placed on the scalp, face, eyelids, chest, limbs, and a finger. The sensors record brain waves, heart rate, breathing effort and rate, oxygen levels, and muscle movements before, during, and after sleep. Mild, moderate, or severe sleep apnea can be diagnosed based on the number of sleep apnea events that occur in an hour during the sleep study (National Heart Lung and Blood Institute, 2018).

Therapy will depend on the severity and type of sleep apnea and the presence of comorbid illnesses. Treatment of sleep apnea may involve avoidance of alcohol and sedative-hypnotic medications, cessation of smoking, avoidance of supine sleep positions, increased physical activity, development of healthy sleep habits, and weight loss. There should be risk counseling about impaired judgment from sleeplessness and the possibility of accidents when driving.

Continuous positive airway pressure (CPAP) is the most commonly recommended treatment for OSA and generally can reverse this condition quickly with the appropriate titration of devices (Downey et al., 2018). The CPAP device delivers pressurized air through tubing to a nasal mask or nasal pillows, which are fitted around the head. The pressurized air acts as an airway splint and gently opens the individual's throat and breathing passages, allowing the individual to breathe normally, but only through the nose (Fig. 13.1). Teaching should be provided about the effects of untreated OSA and the need for treatment emphasized.

A stepwise approach during the initiation of therapy and continued monitoring can foster better use of CPAP or prevent discontinuation of therapy. CPAP nonadherence is a major challenge with estimates indicating about half of individuals either discontinue the therapy or are not adherent (use for less than 4 hours per night) (Jacobsen et al., 2017; Nadal et al., 2018). If the individual requires surgery or pain management, precautions should be taken to make sure the airway stays open during surgery or when selecting pain medications.

Mandibular repositioning mouthpieces are devices that cover the lower and upper teeth and hold the jaw in a position that prevents it from blocking the upper

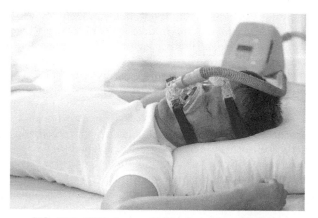

FIG. 13.1 CPAP device. (© iStock.com/cherrybeans.)

airway. These devices may be recommended as an alternative treatment for individuals who prefer this type of device, experience adverse effects with CPAP, and have mild sleep apnea that occurs only while lying on their back. These devices are custom fit by a dentist who specializes in correcting tooth or jaw problems. These appliances also require a stable dentition and may be problematic for individuals with dentures or extensive tooth loss (Dean et al., 2016). Implants that are surgically implanted can benefit some people with sleep apnea. The device senses breathing patterns and delivers mild stimulation to certain muscles that open the airways during sleep. The FDA has approved one implant as a treatment for sleep apnea. Further research is needed to determine how effective the implant is in treating sleep apnea.

Restless Legs Syndrome/Willis-Ekbom Disease

Restless legs syndrome/Willis-Ekbom disease (RLS/WED) is a neurological movement disorder of the limbs that is often associated with a sleep complaint. Individuals with RLS/WED have an uncontrollable need to move the legs, often accompanied by discomfort in the legs. Other symptoms include paresthesia; creeping sensations; crawling sensations; tingling, cramping, and burning sensations; pain; or even indescribable sensations. RLS/WED has a circadian rhythm, with the intensity of the symptoms becoming worse at night and improving toward the morning. Symptoms may be temporarily relieved by movement.

An estimated 7% to 10% of adults in North America and Europe have the disease. The disorder is familial in about 50% of individuals, and several predisposing genes have been identified through genome-wide association studies (Suzuki et al., 2017). RLS/WED is less common in Asian populations. Incidence is about twice as high in women, and although the disease may begin at any age (including childhood), many individuals who are severely affected are middle-aged or older. RLS/WED may be a contributing factor to nighttime agitation in persons with Alzheimer's disease (Richards et al., 2020). Symptoms become more frequent and last longer with age (National Institute of Neurological Disorders and Stroke [NINDS], 2017).

In most cases, RLS/WED is a primary idiopathic disorder, but it can also be associated with underlying medical disorders including iron deficiency, end-stage renal disease (especially in individuals requiring dialysis), diabetes, and pregnancy. Antidepressants, antihypertensives, and neuroleptic medications can aggravate RLS/WED symptoms. Increased BMI, caffeine use, alcohol or tobacco use, sleep deprivation, and sedentary lifestyle may also be contributing factors. Other contributing factors being studied include iron metabolism and neurotransmitter dysfunctions involving dopamine and glutamate (NINDS, 2017).

Diagnosis of RLS/WED is based on symptoms, and a sleep study may be indicated. Possible contributing conditions should be evaluated, and all individuals with symptoms should be tested for iron deficiency with a complete iron panel. If iron stores are low, iron replacement is needed. Medication treatment should only start when symptoms have a significant impact on quality of life in terms of frequency and severity; intermittent treatment might be considered in intermediate cases. Medications used include levodopa, benzodiazepines, or low-potency opioids. The chronic persistent form of the disorder may be treated with nonergot dopamine agonists (pramipexole, ropinirole, rotigotine patch) or with gabapentin, gabapentin enacarbil, and pregabalin (Garcia-Borreguero et al., 2016).

Nonpharmacological therapy includes stretching of the lower extremities, mild to moderate physical activity, hot baths, massage, acupressure, relaxation techniques, and avoidance of caffeine, alcohol, and tobacco. Individuals should be encouraged to keep a symptom diary for 7 to 14 days to identify triggers and aid in diagnosis. The Restless Legs Syndrome Foundation (2018) provides a symptom diary on their website (Box 13.6).

Rapid Eye Movement Sleep Behavior Disorder

REM sleep behavior disorder (RBD) is characterized by loss of voluntary muscle atonia during REM sleep associated with complex behavior while dreaming. Individuals report elaborate enactment of their dreams, often with violent content, during sleep. This may include violent behaviors, such as punching and kicking, with the potential for injury of both the individual and the bed partner. The mean age at emergence of RBD is 60 years and it is more common in males (National Sleep Foundation, 2018; Suzuki et al., 2017).

The chronic form is usually idiopathic or associated with Parkinson's disease and dementia with Lewy bodies and 80% to 90% of individuals with RBD eventually develop a neurodegenerative disorder. The acute form of the disorder can be caused by toxic-metabolic abnormalities, drug or alcohol withdrawal, and medications (tricyclic antidepressants, monoamine oxidase inhibitors, cholinergic agents, and selective serotonin reuptake inhibitors [SSRIs]). Diagnosis is based on history, symptoms, and a sleep study to test for the key features of the disorder. Clonazepam curtails or eliminates the disorder about 90% of the time, but side effects of daytime sleepiness and dizziness are of concern in older adults. If clonazepam is not effective, some antidepressants or melatonin may reduce the behaviors. A safe environment in the bedroom should be provided (Suzuki et al., 2017).

Circadian Rhythm Sleep Disorders

In circadian rhythm sleep disorders (CRSDs), relatively normal sleep occurs at abnormal times. Two clinical presentations are seen: advanced sleep phase disorder (ASPD) and irregular sleep-wake disorder (ISWD). In ASPD, the individual begins and ends sleep at unusually early times (e.g., going to bed as early as 6 or 7 p.m. and waking up between 2 and 5 a.m.). Not all individuals with an advanced sleep phase have ASPD. If they are not bothered by their sleep phases and have no functional impairment, we may just consider them "morning" people. In ISWD, sleep is dispersed across the 24-hour day in bouts of irregular length. Factors contributing to these disorders are age-related changes in sleep and circadian rhythm regulation combined with decreased levels of light exposure and activity.

A combination of good sleep hygiene practices and methods to delay the timing of sleep and wake times is recommended as treatment for ASPD. Bright light therapy is designed to promote the synchronization of circadian rhythms with environmental light–dark cycles through stimulation of the suprachiasmatic nucleus or nuclei (SCN) area of the brain in the hypothalamus responsible for controlling circadian rhythms (Scales et al., 2018) (Box 13.7). Bright light therapy is a reasonably low-cost treatment that, unlike medication usage, does not generally result in residual effects and tolerance. It should be noted that older adults may be less sensitive to light because of age-related changes that may influence the effectiveness of light therapy (Kim & Duffy, 2018).

In ISWD, the individual may obtain enough sleep over the 24-hour period, but time asleep is broken into at least three different periods of variable length. Erratic napping occurs during the day, and nighttime sleep is severely fragmented and shortened. Chronic insomnia and/or daytime sleepiness are present. ISWD is most commonly encountered in individuals with dementia, particularly those who are institutionalized.

ACTIVITY

Few factors contribute as much to health in aging as being physically active. The adage "use it or lose it" certainly applies to muscles and physical fitness. Regular physical activity throughout life is essential for healthy aging. Physical activity enhances health and functional status while also decreasing the number of chronic illnesses and functional limitations

---

> **BOX 13.9   Health Benefits of Physical Activity**
>
> - Reduced risk of hypertension, coronary artery disease, heart attack, stroke, diabetes, colon and breast cancers, metabolic syndrome, depression
> - Reduced adverse blood lipid profile
> - Prevention of weight gain
> - Improved cardiorespiratory and muscular fitness
> - Reduced risk of falls and hip fracture
> - Improved sleep quality
> - Improved bone and functional health
> - Decreased risk of early death (life expectancy increased even in persons who do not begin exercising regularly until the age of 75 years)
> - Improved functional independence
> - Improvement in walking speed, strength, functional ability of frail nursing home residents with diagnoses ranging from arthritis to lung disease and dementia

often assumed to be a part of growing older (Lee et al., 2017). Moderate physical activity may be beneficial for neurometabolic function and assist in combating Alzheimer's-related changes in midlife (Dougherty et al., 2017) (Box 13.9). The frail health and loss of function we associate with aging are, in large part, a result of physical inactivity. "Reduced physical mobility and immobility contribute to the development of geriatric syndromes (pressure injuries, urinary incontinence, falls, functional decline, and delirium)" (Gray-Miceli, 2017, p. 471) (Chapter 8).

Physical Activity and Aging

Despite a large body of evidence about the benefits of physical activity to maintain and improve function, only 16% of older adults meet the national guideline recommendations for physical activity. With advancing age (75 years and older), participation is even lower with only 9% of men and 6% of women meeting the recommended guidelines (U.S. Department of Health & Human Services, 2017). For women, patterns of physical activity have been reported to decline between the ages of 55 and 64 years and again at the age of 75 years and older. These may be prime times to enhance education on the benefits of physical activity for women as they age. The levels of physical activity among older adults have not improved over the past decade in the United States (Du et al., 2019). Increasing physical activity for people of all ages is a global concern in both developed and developing countries. Physical inactivity is identified as a leading risk factor for global mortality (hypertension, smoking, high blood glucose level, physical

BOX 13.10 Healthy People 2020

Physical Activity

- Reduce the proportion of adults who engage in no leisure-time physical activity.
- Increase the proportion of adults who engage in aerobic physical activity or at least moderate intensity for at least 150 minutes/week, or 75 minutes/week of vigorous intensity, or an equivalent combination.

From US Department of Health and Human Services, Office of Disease Prevention and Health Promotion (2012). *Healthy People 2020*. http://www .healthypeople.gov/2020.

inactivity, obesity). *Healthy People 2020* goals for physical activity can be found in Box 13.10.

Physical activity is important for all older adults, not just active healthy older adults. Even a small amount (at least 30 minutes) of moderate activity several days a week can improve health. Studies have found that increasing physical activity improves health outcomes in individuals with chronic illnesses (regardless of severity) and in those with functional impairment. Increasing evidence suggests that high-quality exercise programs are central to older adults who are either frail or sarcopenic (Morley, 2016). Exercise training appears to improve brain health or lower the risk of dementia and may also improve the ability to perform activities of daily living (ADLs) in individuals with dementia and consequently reduce caregiver burden (Ding et al., 2018; Lee et al., 2017). Regardless of age or situation, older adults can find some activity suitable for their condition. Reducing sedentary time, independent of physical activity, has cardiovascular, metabolic, and functional benefits in older adults. Any amount of exercise is better than being sedentary, and even a little activity is better than none (Jefferis et al., 2018).

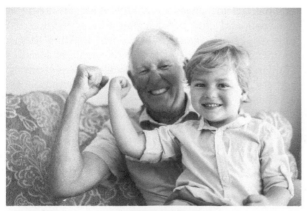

Physical activity is important for all older adults. (© iStock.com /Squaredpixels.)

❖ USING CLINICAL JUDGMENT TO PROMOTE HEALTHY AGING: PHYSICAL ACTIVITY

◆ Recognizing and Analyzing Cues: Physical Activity

Functional abilities and mobility are essential components of evaluation of activity abilities in older adults. For individuals 65 years of age and older, if they are relatively fit and have no limiting health conditions, initiation of a moderate-intensity exercise program is safe and does not require any type of cardiac screening (Lee et al., 2017). The consensus is that there is minimal cardiovascular risk to engaging in physical activity and a much greater risk in maintaining a sedentary lifestyle. Individuals with specific health conditions, such as cardiovascular disease and diabetes, may need to take extra precautions and seek medical advice before beginning an exercise program. Frail individuals will need more comprehensive evaluation to adapt exercise recommendations to their abilities and ensure benefit without compromising safety.

◆ Nursing Actions: Physical Activity

The Centers for Disease Control and Prevention (CDC) "Growing Stronger" program materials are very useful to help determine a safe exercise program and provide detailed information about appropriate exercises and precautions (Box 13.11). Nurses should be knowledgeable about recommended physical activity guidelines, educate individuals about the importance of exercise and physical activity, and provide exercise counseling on ways to incorporate exercise into daily routines. Many older adults mistakenly believe that they are

BOX 13.11   Resources for Best Practice

Physical Activity

Alzheimer's Society: Exercise and physical activity for individuals with dementia: https://www.alzheimers.org.uk/info/20029 /daily_living/15/exercise_and_physical_activity/2.

Centers for Disease Control and Prevention: Making physical activity a part of an older adult's life. Includes exercise program information, videos, success stories, ways to overcome barriers (Growing Stronger program and resources for strength training including pictures/videos).

National Center on Health, Physical Activity and Disability: 14 Weeks to a healthier you: http://www.ncpad.org /14weeks.

National Institute on Aging: Exercise and physical activity: your everyday guide from the National Institute on Aging.

BOX 13.12   Exercise Guidelines

Older Adults Need at Least

- 2 hours and 30 minutes (150 minutes) of moderate-intensity aerobic activity (e.g., brisk walking, swimming, bicycling) every week *and*
- Muscle-strengthening activities on two or more days that work all major muscle groups (legs, hips, abdomen, chest, shoulders, and arms)

  Additionally: Stretching (flexibility) and balance exercises (particularly for older adults who are at risk of falls) are also recommended. Yoga and tai chi exercises have been shown to be of benefit to older adults in terms of improving flexibility and balance and reducing pain and enhancing psychological well-being (Miller & Taylor-Piliae, 2014). Tai chi can be adapted for level of function and mobility status. Home-based balance-training exercise programs are also available.

From Centers for Disease Control and Prevention (2015). *How much physical activity do older adults need?* https://www.cdc.gov/physicalactivity/basics/adults/index.htm.

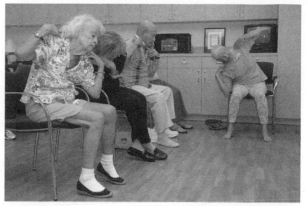

Age is not a barrier to fitness and exercise. 95-year-old Vera Paley leads yoga class. (Courtesy Louis and Anne Green Memory and Wellness Center of the Christine E. Lynn College of Nursing at Florida Atlantic University.)

too old to begin a fitness program. Older adults are less likely to receive exercise counseling from their primary care providers than younger individuals are. Research has noted that health care providers value the benefits of physical activity but have inadequate knowledge of specific recommendations. Giving specific advice about the type and frequency of exercise is important (CDC, 2015; Lee et al., 2017). Nurses can also design and lead exercise and physical activity programs for groups of older adults in the community or in long-term care.

Physical Activity Guidelines

Guidelines for physical activity for adults 65 years of age or older who are generally fit and have no limiting health conditions are presented in Box 13.12. Recommendations for all adults include participation in 30 minutes of exercise of moderate intensity for 5 or more days of the week. People do not have to be active for 30 minutes at a time but can accumulate 30 minutes over 24 hours. As little as 10 minutes of exercise has health benefits, and three 10-minute bouts of activity have the same fitness effects as one 30-minute bout. All four types of exercise should be practiced for the most benefits (Fig. 13.2).

Chair yoga, a gentle form of yoga practiced sitting in a chair or standing while holding on to the chair for support, is well suited for older adults who cannot participate in traditional yoga or standing exercises and can improve flexibility (Park et al., 2017).

Muscle-strengthening exercises without weight bearing also provide more joint stability for individuals with lower extremity OA. Swimming is a low-risk activity that provides aerobic benefit, and water-based exercises are particularly beneficial for individuals with arthritis or other mobility limitations.

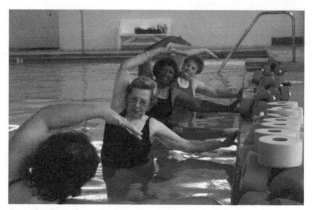

Aquatic Exercise. Aquatic programs are beneficial for older adults with mobility and joint problems. They improve circulation, muscle strength, and endurance and provide socialization and relaxation. (© iStock.com/ftwitty.)

Incorporating Physical Activity Into Lifestyle

One does not have to invest in expensive gym equipment or gym memberships to incorporate the recommended physical activity guidelines into their daily routine. Hand weights (or use cans of food as weights), a chair, and an exercise mat can easily get the individual started. Individuals may also be able to integrate

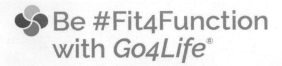
Be #Fit4Function with *Go4Life*®

Exercise and be active every day so you can keep doing what's most important to you.

Practice all 4 types of exercise for the most benefits.

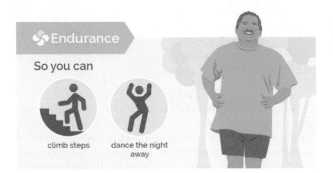

Endurance

So you can

climb steps

dance the night away

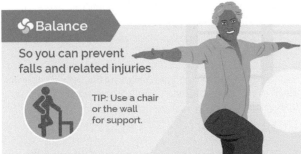

Balance

So you can prevent falls and related injuries

TIP: Use a chair or the wall for support.

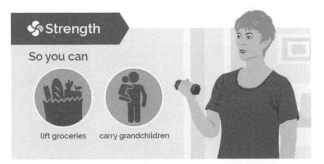

Strength

So you can

lift groceries

carry grandchildren

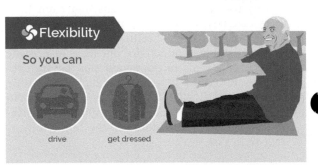

Flexibility

So you can

drive

get dressed

Visit go4life.nia.nih.gov and be #Fit4Function.

Get exercise ideas, motivational tips, and more from *Go4Life*®, an exercise and physical activity campaign for older adults from the National Institute on Aging at NIH.

Go4Life®

FIG. 13.2 Practice All Four Types of Exercises for the Most Benefits. (Image courtesy of the National Institute on Aging/National Institutes of Health.)

activity into daily life rather than doing a specific exercise. Examples include walking, golfing, tennis, biking, raking leaves, yard work/gardening, dancing, washing windows or floors, washing and waxing the car, and swimming and water-based exercises. The Wii game system offers other possibilities for exercise at all levels and is increasingly used by older adults in their own homes and in senior living facilities to encourage physical activity, improve balance, and provide enjoyable entertainment. Dancing is another enjoyable activity to promote physical and cognitive function and socialization. In a study comparing dancing to endurance training, dancing improved reaction time and working memory. Only dancing led to improvement in posture and balance (Rehfeld et al., 2017).

Many assisted living facilities and SNFs provide gym equipment. The SilverSneakers program, the nation's leading exercise program for active community-dwelling older adults, is a membership benefit through some of the Medicare health plans. Local community centers often provide exercise programs for older adults, and many gyms in the United States have reduced-cost memberships for individuals older than 65 years of age. Some have trainers on staff with expertise in exercises appropriate for older individuals. Nurses can share resources in the community, and communities should be encouraged to provide accessible and affordable options for physical activity.

Special Considerations

The benefits of physical activity extend to more physically frail older adults, those who are nonambulatory or experience cognitive impairment, and those residing in assisted living facilities (ALFs) or SNFs. In fact, these individuals may benefit most from an exercise program in terms of function and quality of life. Nursing home residents should be involved in an exercise program two to three times per week (Morley, 2016). There are many creative and enjoyable ideas for enhancing physical activity, such as using lower extremity cycling equipment, marching in place, tossing a ball, stretching, using resistive bands (Chen et al., 2016), group exercises (Kocic et al., 2018), and chair yoga.

Individuals with cognitive impairment are often not included in physical activity programs. Results of research suggest that older adults with cognitive impairment who participate in exercise programs may improve strength and endurance, mood and behavior, cognitive function, and ability to perform ADLs. Elements of successful exercise interventions with individuals with dementia include individualized approaches, caregiver involvement, strength-training interventions, one-component exercises, and enjoyable activities (Forbes et al., 2015; Rodriguez-Larrad et al., 2017; Schwenk et al., 2014). Although further research is needed to understand the level and intensity of exercise that is beneficial for each type of dementia, exercise should be a component of the plan of care (Li et al., 2019) (Box 13.11).

KEY CONCEPTS

- Sleep is a barometer of health and can be considered one of the vital signs.
- Complaints of sleep difficulties should be thoroughly investigated and not attributed to age. An important nursing role is recognition and analysis of cues suggesting sleep disturbances and identification and evaluation of nursing actions to improve sleep health.
- Nonpharmacological interventions are first-line treatments for sleep problems. Benzodiazepines or other sedative-hypnotics should not be used in older adults. If sleeping medications are prescribed, benzodiazepine receptor agonists are preferred and used only short term (2 to 3 weeks, never more than 90 days).
- All sleeping medications, including OTC, have adverse effects that include daytime drowsiness, changes in mental status, and increased likelihood of falls.
- Few factors contribute to health in aging as much as being physically active.
- Physical activity enhances health and functional status while also decreasing the number of chronic illnesses and functional limitations often assumed to be part of growing older.
- The physical activity levels of older adults remain low and have not improved over the past decade.
- Nursing actions to assist older adults to improve physical activity include evaluation of functional abilities, mobility, level of activity, education, and exercise counseling.
- Individuals who are nonambulatory or experience cognitive impairment and those residing in assisted living facilities (ALFs) or skilled nursing facilities (SNFs) may benefit most from an exercise program in terms of function and quality of life.

ACTIVITIES AND DISCUSSION QUESTIONS

1. Which age-related changes affect rest, sleep, and activity in older adults?
2. How would you evaluate an older adult for adequacy or inadequacy of rest, sleep, and activity?
3. Which interventions would be helpful to promote adequate sleep in acute care? In long-term care?
4. Develop an exercise prescription for an older adult residing in the community.

REFERENCES

Albert, S. M., Roth, T., Toscani, M., Vitiello, M. V., & Zee, P. (2017). Sleep health and appropriate use of OTC sleep aids in older adults-recommendations of a Gerontological Society of America workgroup. *Gerontologist, 57*(2), 163–170.

American Geriatrics Society Choosing Wisely Group. (2014). American Geriatrics Society identifies another five things that healthcare providers and patients should question. *J Am Geriatr Soc, 62*(5), 950–960.

American Geriatrics Society. (2015). 2015 Beers Criteria Update Expert Panel: American Geriatrics Society 2015 updated Beers criteria for potentially inappropriate medication use in older adults. *J Am Geriatr Soc, 63*(11), 2227–2246.

Anderson, K. N. (2018). Insomnia and cognitive behavioural therapy—how to assess your patient and why it should be a standard part of care. *J Thorac Dis, 10*(Suppl 1), S94–S102.

Bhaskar, S., Hemavathy, D., & Prascad, S. (2016). Prevalence of chronic insomnia in adult patients and its correlation with medical comorbidities. *J Family Med Prim Care, 5*(4), 780–784.

Centers for Disease Control and Prevention (CDC). *CDC declares sleep disorders a public health epidemic,* 2018. https://www.sleepdr .com/the-sleep-blog/cdc-declares-sleep-disorders-a-public -health-epidemic/.

Centers for Disease Control and Prevention. *How much physical activity do older adults need?* 2015. https://www.cdc.gov /physicalactivity/basics/adults/index.htm.

Chan, A. W., Yu, D. D., Choi, K. C., Lee, D. T., Sit, J. W., & Chan, H. Y. (2016). Tai chi qigong as a means to improve night-time sleep quality among older adults with cognitive impairment: a pilot randomized controlled trial. *Clin Interv Aging, 11*, 1277–1286.

Chen, T. Y., Lee, S., & Buxton, O. M. (2017). A greater extent of insomnia symptoms and physician-recommended sleep medication use predict fall risk in community-dwelling older adults. *Sleep, 40*(11). https://academic.oup.com/sleep/article/40/11 /zsx142/4159943.

Dean, G., Klimpt, M., Morris, J., et al. (2016). Excessive sleepiness. In M. Boltz, E. Capezuti, T. Fulmer, & D. Zwicker (Eds.), *Evidence-based geriatric nursing protocols for best practice* (ed. 5, pp. 431–441). New York: Springer.

Ding, K., Tarumi, T., Zhu, D. C., et al. (2018). Cardiorespiratory fitness and white matter neuronal fiber integrity in mild cognitive impairment. *J Alzheimers Dis, 61*(2), 729–739.

Dougherty, R. J., Schultz, S. A., Kirby, T. K., et al. (2017). Moderate physical activity is associated with cerebral glucose metabolism in adults at risk for Alzheimer's disease. *J Alzheimers Dis, 58*(4), 1089–1097.

Downey, R., Mosenifar, Z., Gold, P., et al. (2018). Obstructive sleep apnea (OSA) treatment and management. *Medscape.* January 9. https://emedicine.medscape.com/article/295807-treatment.

Du, Y., Lu, B., Sun, Y., et al. (2019). Trends in adherence to the physical activity guidelines for Americans for aerobic activity and time spent on sedentary behavior among US adults, 2007-2016. *JAMA Network Open, 2*(7), e197597.

Evans, C., & Kovach, C. (2020). The association between physiological sources of pain and sleep quality in older adults with and without dementia. *Res Gerontol Nurs, 13*(6), 297–306.

Figueiro, M., Plitnick, B., Roohan, C., et al. (2019). Effects of a tailored lighting intervention on sleep quality, rest-activity, mood, and behavior in older adults with Alzheimer disease and related dementias: a randomized clinical trial. *Journal of Clinical Sleep Medicine, 15*(12). https://jcsm.aasm.org/doi/full/10.5664/jcsm.8078.

Forbes, D., Forbes, S. C., Blake, C. M., Thiessen, E. J., & Forbes, S. (2015). Exercise programs for people with dementia. *Cochrane Database Syst Rev,* (4), CD006489.

Garcia-Borreguero, D., Silber, M. H., Winkelman, J. W., et al. (2016). Guidelines for the first-line treatment of restless legs syndrome/ Willis-Ekbom disease, prevention and treatment of dopaminergic augmentation: a combined task force of the IRLSSG, EURLSSG, and the RLS-foundation. *Sleep Med, 21*, 1–11.

Gray-Miceli, D. (2017). Impaired mobility and functional decline in older adults: evidence to facilitate a practice change. *Nurs Clin North Am, 52*, 469–487.

Grossman, M. N., Anderson, S. L., Worku, A., et al. (2017). Awakenings? Patient and hospital staff perceptions of nighttime disruptions and their effect on patient sleep. *J Clin Sleep Med, 13*(2), 301–306.

Hampton, L. M., Daubresse, M., Chang, H. Y., Alexander, G. C., & Budnitz, D. S. (2014). Emergency department visits by adults for psychiatric medication adverse effects. *JAMA Psychiatry, 79*(9), 1006–1014.

Haynes, J., Talbert, M., Fox, S., & Close, E. (2018). Cognitive behavioral therapy in the treatment of insomnia. *South Med J, 111*(2), 75–80.

Jacobsen, A. R., Eriksen, F., Hansen, R. W., et al. (2017). Determinants for adherence to continuous positive airway pressure therapy in obstructive sleep apnea. *PLoS One, 12*(12), e0189614.

Jefferis, B. J., Parsons, T. J., Sartini, C., et al. (2018). Objectively measured physical activity, sedentary behavior and all-cause mortality in older men: does volume of activity matter more than pattern of accumulation? *Br J Sports Med, 53*(16), bjsports-2017-098733.

Jike, M., Itani, O., Watanabe, N., Buysse, D. J., & Kaneita, Y. (2018). Long sleep duration and health outcomes: a systematic review, meta-analysis and meta-regression. *Sleep Med Rev, 39*, 25–36.

Kapur, V. K., Auckley, D. H., Chowdhuri, S., et al. (2017). Clinical practice guideline for diagnostic testing for adult obstructive sleep apnea: an American Academy of sleep medicine clinical practice guideline. *J Clin Sleep Med, 13*(3), 479–504.

Kim, J. H., & Duffy, J. F. (2018). Circadian rhythm sleep-wake disorders in older adults. *Sleep Med Clin, 13*(1), 39–50.

Lee, P. G., Jackson, E. A., & Richardson, C. R. (2017). Exercise prescription in older adults. *Am Fam Physician, 95*(7), 425–432.

Leggett, A., Polenick, C. A., Maust, D. T., et al. (2018). "What hath night to do with sleep?" The caregiving context and dementia caregivers' nighttime awakenings. *Clin Gerontol, 41*(2), 158–166.

Leng, Y., McEvoy, C. T., Allen, I. E., & Yaffe, K. (2017). Association of sleep-disordered breathing with cognitive function and risk of cognitive impairment: a systematic review and meta-analysis. *JAMA Neurol, 74*(10), 1237–1245.

Li, B., Liu, C., Wan, Q., & Yu, F. (2019). An integrative review of exercise interventions among community-dwelling adults with Alzheimer's disease. *Int J Older People Nursing,* November. https://doi.org/10.1111/opn.12287.

Markota, M., Rummans, T. A., Bostwick, J. M., & Lapid, M. I. (2016). Benzodiazepine use in older adults: dangers, management, and alternative therapies. *Mayo Clin Proc, 91*(11), 1632–1639.

Matheson, E., & Hainer, B. L., (2017). Insomnia: Pharmacologic therapy, *Am Fam Physician, 96*(1), 29–35.

Maust, D. T., Kales, H. C., Wiechers, I. R., Blow, F. C., & Olfson, M. (2016). No end in sight: benzodiazepine use among older adults in the United States. *J Am Geriatr Soc, 64*(12), 2546–2553.

McGough, N. N. H., Keane, T., Uppal, A., et al. (2018). Noise reduction in progressive care units. *J Nurs Care Qual, 33*(2), 166–172.

McMillan, A., & Morrell, M. J. (2016). Sleep disordered breathing at the extremes of age: the elderly. *Breathe (Sheff), 12*(1), 50–60.

Morley, J. E. (2016). High-quality exercise programs are an essential component of nursing home care. *J Am Med Dir Assoc, 17*, 373–375.

Mukherjee, S., Saxena, R., & Palmer, L. J. (2018). The genetics of obstructive sleep apnoea. *Respirology, 23*, 18–27.

Nadal, N., de Batlle, J., Barbé, F., et al. (2018). Predictors of CPAP compliance in different clinical settings: primary care versus sleep unit. *Sleep & Breath, 22*(1), 157–163.

National Heart Lung and Blood Institute. Sleep apnea. https://www.nhlbi.nih.gov/health-topics/sleep-apnea.

National Institute of Neurological Disorders and Stroke. *Restless legs syndrome fact sheet*, 2017. https://www.ninds.nih.gov/Disorders/Patient-Caregiver-Education/Fact-Sheets/Restless-Legs-Syndrome-Fact-Sheet.

National Sleep Foundation. *REM behavior disorder and sleep*, 2018. https://sleepfoundation.org/sleep-disorders-problems/rem-behavior-disorder.

Park, J., McCaffrey, R., Newman, D., Liehr, P., & Ouslander, J. G. (2017). A pilot randomized controlled trial of the effects of chair yoga on pain and physical function among community-dwelling older adults with lower extremity osteoarthritis. *J Am Geriatr Soc, 65*, 592–597.

Petrovsky, D. V., McPhillips, M. V., Li, J., Brody, A., Caffeé, L., & Hodgson, N. A. (2018). Sleep disruption and quality of life in persons with dementia: a state-of-the-art review. *Geriatr Nurs, 39*(6), 640–645.

Rehfeld, K., Müller, P., Aye, N., et al. (2017). Dancing or fitness sport? The effects of two training programs on hippocampal plasticity and balance abilities in healthy seniors. *Front Hum Neurosci, 11*, 305.

Restless Legs Syndrome Foundation. *RLS symptom diary*, 2018. https://www.rls.org/file/symptom-diary.pdf.

Richards, K., Morrison, J., Rangel, A. et al. (2020). Nighttime agitation and restless leg syndrome in persons with Alzheimer's Disease. *Res in Gerontol Nurs, 13*(6), 280–288.

Rodriguez-Larrad, A., Arrieta, H., Rezola, C., et al. (2017). Effectiveness of a multicomponent exercise program in the attenuation of frailty in long-term nursing home residents: study protocol for a randomized clinical controlled trial. *BMC Geriatr, 17*, 60.

Saccomano, S. (2014). Sleep disorders in older adults. *J Gerontol Nurs, 40*(3), 38–45.

Scales, K., Zimmerman, S., & Miller, S. J. (2018). Evidence-based non-pharmacological practice to address behavioral and psychological symptoms of dementia. *Gerontologist, 58*(Suppl 1), S88–S102.

Schroeck, J. L., Ford, J., Conway, E. L., et al. (2016). Review of safety and efficacy of sleep medicines in older adults. *Clin Ther, 38*(11), 2340–2372.

Schwenk, M., Dutzi, I., Englert, S., et al. (2014). An intensive exercise program improves motor performance in patients with dementia:

translational model of geriatric rehabilitation. *J Alzheimers Dis, 39*(3), 487–498.

Shokri-Kojori, E., Wang, G. J., Wiers, C. E., et al. (2018). β-Amyloid accumulation in the human brain after one night of sleep deprivation. *Proc Natl Acad Sci USA, 115*(17), 4483–4488.

Silva, A. A., de Mello, R. G., Schaan, C. W., Fuchs, F. D., Redline, S., & Fuchs, S. C. (2016). Sleep duration and mortality in the elderly: a systematic review with meta-analysis. *BMJ Open, 6*, Article e008119.

Suzuki, K., Miyamoto, M., & Hirata, K. (2017). Sleep disorders in the elderly: diagnosis and management. *J Gen Fam Med, 18*(2), 61–71.

Theorell-Haglöw, J., Miller, C. B., Bartlett, D. J., Yee, B. J., Openshaw, H. D., & Grunstein, R. R. (2018). Gender differences in obstructive sleep apnoea, insomnia and restless legs syndrome in adults — what do we know? A clinical update. *Sleep Med Rev, 38*, 28–38.

US Food and Drug Administration. *FDA adds boxed warning for risk of serious injuries caused by sleepwalking with certain prescription insomnia medications*. https://www.fda.gov/drugs/drug-safety-and-availability/fda-adds-boxed-warning-risk-serious-injuries-caused-sleepwalking-certain-prescription-insomnia.

U.S. Department of Health & Human Services: Facts and Statistics Physical Activity (2017). https://www.hhs.gov/fitness/resource-center/facts-and-statistics/index.html#:~:text=Less%20than%205%25%20of%20adults,of%20physical%20activity%20each%20week.&text=Only%2035%20%E2%80%93%2044%25%20of%20adults,65%2D74%20are%20physically%20active.

Wang, S., Keenan, B., Wiemken, A., et al. (2020). Effect of weight loss on upper airway anatomy and the apnea hypopnea index: the importance of tongue fat. *Am J Respiratory and Critical Care.* https://doi.org/10.1164/rccm.201903-0692OC.

Winkelman, J. W. (2015). Clinical Practice. Insomnia disorder. *N Engl J Med, 373*(15), 1437–1444.

World Association of Sleep Medicine. *World Sleep Day*, 2018. http://worldsleepday.org.

Xiong, G., & Hategan, A. (2019). Geriatric sleep disorder, *Medscape*, December 21. https://emedicine.medscape.com/article/292498-overview?pa=FoKIu4vX0dMcRVgVjSVTmYLaTejRnqVqku9xeP7q1BqUA5zw3fPxKTv30G3JQT0e8SIvl8zjYv73GUyW5rsbWA%3D%3D. Accessed December 2020.

Yano, Y., Gao, Y., & Johnson, D. A., et al. (2020). Sleep characteristics and measures of glucose metabolism in Blacks: the Jackson heart study. *J Am Heart Assoc, 28* April.

14

Clinical Judgment to Promote Healthy Skin

Theris A. Touhy

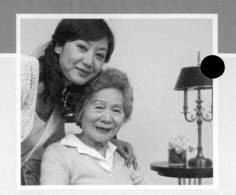

http://evolve.elsevier.com/Touhy/gerontological/

LEARNING OBJECTIVES

Upon completion of this chapter, the reader will be able to:

- Identify skin conditions commonly found in later life.
- Identify preventive, maintenance, and restorative measures for skin health.
- Identify risk factors for pressure injuries and describe nursing actions for prevention and treatment.
- Use clinical judgment to recognize and analyze cues of skin problems in older adults.
- Identify and evaluate nursing actions to promote skin health.

THE LIVED EXPERIENCE

An elderly woman and her little grandson, whose face was sprinkled with bright freckles, spent the day at the zoo. Lots of children were waiting in line to get their cheeks painted by a local artist who was decorating them with tiger paws.

"You've got so many freckles, there's no place to paint!" a girl in the line said to the little fellow.

Embarrassed, the little boy dropped his head. His grandmother knelt down next to him.

"I love your freckles. When I was a little girl, I always wanted freckles," she said, while tracing her finger across the child's cheek. "Freckles are beautiful."

The boy looked up, "Really?"

"Of course," said the grandmother. "Why just name me one thing that's prettier than freckles?"

The little boy thought for a moment, peered intensely into his grandma's face, and softly whispered, "Wrinkles."

Anonymous

Gerontological nurses have an instrumental role in promoting the health of the skin of individuals who seek their care. Skin care may be often overlooked when the focus is on management of chronic illness or acute problems. However, skin conditions can be challenging concerns, affecting health and compromising quality of life. Thorough assessment and intervention based on age-related evidence-based protocols is important to healthy aging and best-practice gerontological nursing.

SKIN

The skin is the largest organ of the body. Exposure to heat, cold, water, trauma, friction, and pressure notwithstanding, the skin's function is to maintain a homeostatic environment. Healthy skin is durable, pliable, and strong enough to protect the body by absorbing, reflecting, cushioning, and restricting various substances and forces that might enter and alter its function; yet it is sensitive enough to relay subtle messages to the brain. When the integument malfunctions or is overwhelmed, discomfort, disfigurement, or death may ensue. However, nurses can promptly recognize and help to prevent many of the sources of danger to a person's skin in the promotion of the best possible health.

Many age-related changes in the skin are visible; similar changes in other organs of the body are not so readily observed. Although there are some changes related to the aging process (Chapter 4), genetics and environmental factors (ultraviolet [UV] radiation, tobacco smoke, inflammatory responses, and gravity) contribute to these changes (McCance & Huether, 2014). The most common skin problems of aging are xerosis (dry skin), pruritus, seborrheic keratosis, herpes zoster, and cancer. Those who are immobilized or medically fragile are at risk of fungal infections and pressure injuries, both major threats to wellness.

COMMON SKIN PROBLEMS

Xerosis

Xerosis is extremely dry, cracked, and itchy skin. Xerosis is the most common skin problem experienced and may be linked to a dramatic age-associated decrease in the amount of epidermal filaggrin, a protein required for binding keratin filaments into macrofibrils. This leads to separation of dermal and epidermal surfaces, which compromises the nutrient transfer between the two layers of the skin. Xerosis occurs primarily in the extremities, especially the legs, but can also affect the face and the trunk. The thinner epidermis of older skin makes it less efficient, allowing more moisture to escape. Inadequate fluid intake worsens xerosis because the body will pull moisture from the skin in an attempt to combat systemic dehydration. Box 14.1 presents Tips for Best Practice in prevention and treatment of xerosis.

Pruritus

One of the consequences of xerosis is *pruritus*, that is, itchy skin. It is a symptom, not a diagnosis or disease, and is a threat to skin integrity because of the attempts to relieve it by scratching. It is aggravated by perfumed

---

BOX 14.1   Tips for Best Practice

Prevention and Treatment of Xerosis

Assessment

- Evaluate for dehydration, nutritional deficiencies, systemic diseases (diabetes mellitus, hypothyroidism, renal disease), and open lesions
- Determine precipitating and alleviating factors
- Evaluate current treatment and effectiveness

Interventions

- Maintain environment of 60% humidity
- Promote adequate fluid intake; skin can only be rehydrated with water
- Creams, lubricants, emollients should be applied to towel-patted dry, damp skin immediately after a bath; water-laden emulsions without perfumes or alcohol should be used
- Mineral oil or Vaseline is effective and more economical than commercial lotions and oils
- Use only tepid water for bathing; avoid long-duration baths; daily baths and showers may not be needed; advise sponge bathing
- Use super-fatted soaps or skin cleansers (Cetaphil, Dove, Caress soaps; Neutrogena and Oil of Olay bath washes); avoid deodorant soaps except in places such as axilla and groin
- In cases of extreme dryness, petroleum jelly can be applied to affected area before bed (can use cotton gloves and socks to cover hands/feet)

---

detergents, fabric softeners, heat, sudden temperature changes, pressure, vibration, electrical stimuli, sweating, restrictive clothing, fatigue, exercise, and anxiety. Medication side effects are another common cause of pruritus. Pruritus may also accompany systemic disorders such as chronic renal failure and biliary or hepatic disease. Subacute to chronic generalized pruritus that awakens the individual is an indication to look for secondary causes (especially lymphoma or hematological conditions) (Endo & Norman, 2014).

A gerontological nurse should always listen carefully to the patient's ideas of why the pruritus is occurring and the patient's description of aggravating and relieving factors. If rehydration of the stratum corneum (outer layer of the skin) and other measures to prevent and treat xerosis are not sufficient to control itching, cool compresses, oatmeal, or Epsom salt baths may be helpful. Failure to control the itching increases the risk of eczema, excoriations, cracks in the skin, inflammation, and infection arising from the usually linear excoriations resulting from scratching. Nurses should be alert to signs of infection.

Scabies

Scabies is a skin condition that causes intense itching, particularly at night. Scabies is caused by a tiny burrowing mite called *Sarcoptes scabiei*. Scabies is contagious and can be passed easily by an infested person to household members, caregivers, or sexual partners. Scabies can spread easily through close physical contact in a family, childcare group, or school class. Scabies outbreaks have occurred among patients, visitors, and staff in institutions such as nursing homes and hospitals. These types of outbreaks are frequently the result of delayed diagnosis and treatment of crusted (Norwegian) scabies. Some immunocompromised, disabled, or debilitated persons are at risk for this form of scabies.

Individuals with crusted scabies have thick crusts of skin that contain large numbers of scabies mites and eggs. In addition to spreading through skin-to-skin contact, crusted scabies can transmit indirectly through contamination of clothing, linen, and furniture. Because the characteristic itching and rash of scabies can be absent in crusted scabies, there may be misdiagnosis and delayed or treated inadequately, resulting in continued transmission. To diagnose scabies, a close skin examination is conducted to look for signs of mites, including their characteristic burrows. A scraping may be taken from an area of skin for microscopic examination to determine the presence of mites or their eggs.

Scabies treatment involves eliminating the infestation with prescribed lotions and creams. Two or more applications, about a week apart, may be necessary, especially for crusted scabies. Treatment is usually provided to family members and other close contacts even if they show no signs of scabies infestation. Medication kills the mites, but itching may not stop for several weeks. Oral medications may be prescribed for individuals with altered immune systems, for those with crusted scabies, or for those who do not respond to prescription lotions and creams. All clothes and linen used at least three times before treatment should be washed in hot, soapy water and dried with high heat. Rooms used by the person with crusted scabies should be thoroughly cleaned and vacuumed (Centers for Disease Control and Prevention [CDC], 2020a).

Purpura

Thinning of the dermis leads to increased fragility of the dermal capillaries and to easy rupture of blood vessels with minimal trauma. Extravasation of the blood into the surrounding tissue, commonly seen on the dorsal forearm and hands, is called *purpura*. Most cases are not related to a pathological condition. The incidence of purpura increases with age as a result of the normal changes in the skin. Persons who take blood thinners are especially prone to acquiring purpura. For those who find that they are prone to purpura, it is advisable to use protective garments such as long-sleeved pants and shirts. Health care personnel must be advised to be gentle while providing care to persons with sensitive or easily traumatized skin.

Skin Tears

Skin tears (STs) are painful, acute, accidental wounds, perhaps more prevalent than PIs, and are largely preventable. STs are frequently caused by trauma, are slow to heal, and may become chronic wounds. If not managed properly, they can be susceptible to secondary wound infections. STs occur in individuals in all settings from long-term care to active individuals in the community, but older adults are at highest risk. Physiological changes in the skin such as dermal and subcutaneous tissue loss and xerosis contribute to risk factors for STs in older adults. Older adults who are dependent on others for total care are at greatest risk of STs, and independent ambulatory older adults are at second highest risk. The top causes of STs include equipment injury, patient transfers, falls, activities of daily living, and treatment and dressing removal. The literature pertaining to the prevalence and incidence of STs and risk factors is very limited.

Management of STs includes proper assessment of ST category, control of bleeding, cleansing with nontoxic solutions (normal saline or nonionic surfactant cleaners), use of appropriate dressings that provide moist wound healing, protection of periwound skin, management of exudate, prevention of infection, implementation of prevention protocols, and education. Skin flaps, if present, should not be removed but instead rolled back over the open, cleaned area. Steri-Strips can be very useful; suturing is not recommended. A Skin Tear Tool Kit (LeBlanc & Baranoski, 2017), dressing recommendations, and comprehensive information on assessment and prevention can be found on the International Skin Tear Advisory Panel website provided in Box 14.2.

Keratoses

There are two types of keratosis: seborrheic and actinic. *Actinic keratosis* is a precancerous lesion and *seborrheic keratosis* is a benign growth that appears mainly on the trunk, the face, the neck, and the scalp as single or multiple lesions. One or more lesions are present on nearly all adults older than 65 years and are more common in men. An individual may have dozens of these benign lesions. Seborrheic keratosis is a waxy, raised lesion, flesh colored or pigmented in various sizes. The lesions have a "stuck-on" appearance, as if they could be scraped off. Seborrheic keratoses may be removed by a

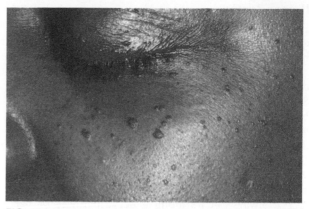

FIG. 14.2 Dermatosis papulosa nigra. (From Neville, B., Damm, D. D., Allen, C. M., et al. (2009). *Oral and maxillofacial pathology* (3rd ed.). St Louis: Saunders.)

dermatologist for cosmetic reasons (Fig. 14.1). A variant seen in darkly pigmented persons occurs mostly on the face and appears as numerous small, dark, possibly tag-like lesions (Fig. 14.2).

Actinic keratosis is a precancerous lesion that is thought to be in the middle of the spectrum between photoaging changes and squamous cell carcinoma. It is directly related to years of overexposure to UV light. Risk factors are older age and fair complexion. It is found on faces, lips, and hands and forearms—areas of chronic sun exposure in everyday life. Actinic keratosis is characterized by rough, scaly, sandpaper-like patches, pink to reddish-brown on an erythematous base (Fig. 14.3). Lesions may be single or multiple; they may be painless or mildly tender. The person with actinic keratoses should be monitored by a dermatologist every 6 to 12 months for any change in appearance of the lesions. Early recognition, treatment, and removal of these lesions are easy and important and may be combined with topical field therapy (Endo & Norman, 2014).

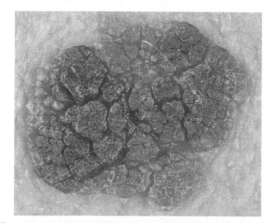

FIG. 14.1 Seborrheic keratosis in older adults. (From Habif, T. P. (2010). *Clinical dermatology: A color guide to diagnosis and therapy* (5th ed.). St Louis: Mosby.)

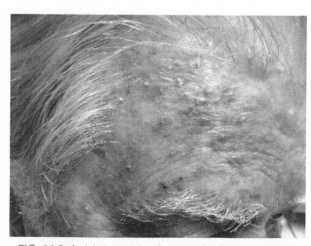

FIG. 14.3 Actinic keratosis. (Courtesy Dr. Robert Norman.)

Herpes Zoster

Herpes Zoster (HZ), or shingles, is a viral infection frequently seen in adults over 50 years of age, those who have medical conditions that compromise the immune system, or people who receive immunosuppressive drugs. About one of every three people in the United States will develop HZ in their lifetime. HZ is caused by reactivation of latent varicella-zoster virus (VZV) within the sensory neurons of the dorsal root ganglion decades after initial VZV infection is established. More than 90% of the world's population is infected with this virus, and about half of all cases occur in individuals 60 years of age or older (CDC, 2020b).

HZ always occurs along a nerve pathway or *dermatome* (Fig. 14.4). The more dermatomes involved, the more serious the infection, especially if it involves the head. When eyes are affected, it is always a medical emergency. Most HZ occurs in the thoracic region, but it can also occur in the trigeminal area and cervical, lumbar, and sacral areas. HZ vesicles never cross the midline. In most cases, the severity of the infection increases with age. It is important to differentiate HZ from herpes simplex. Herpes simplex does not occur in a dermatome pattern and is recurrent.

The onset of HZ may be preceded by itching, tingling, or pain in the affected dermatome several days before the outbreak of the rash. During the healing process, clusters of papulovesicles develop along a nerve pathway. The lesions themselves eventually rupture, crust over, and resolve. Scarring may result, especially if scratching or poor hygiene leads to a secondary bacterial infection. HZ is infectious until it becomes crusty. Prompt treatment with the oral antiviral agents

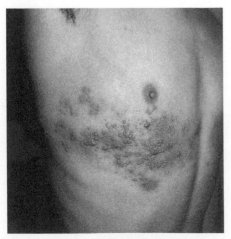

FIG. 14.4 Herpes zoster. (From Harding, M. M., Kwong, J., Roberts, D., Hagler, D., Reinisch, C. (2020). *Lewis's medical-surgical nursing* (11th ed.). St Louis: Mosby.)

acyclovir, valacyclovir, and famciclovir may shorten the length and severity of the illness; however, to be effective, the medications must be started as soon as possible after the rash appears. Analgesics may help relieve pain. Wet compresses, calamine lotion, and colloidal oatmeal baths may help relieve itching.

Two shingles vaccines are licensed and recommended in the United States. Zoster vaccine live (ZVL, Zostavax) has been used since 2006 and recombinant zoster vaccine (RZV, Shingrix), has been used since 2017. Shingrix is recommended as the preferred shingles vaccine. It is recommended that individuals get the Shingrix vaccine even if they have had previous vaccination with Zostavax. Two doses of Shingrix are required with the second dose given 2–6 months after the first dose. Shingrix should not be given within 2 months of receiving Zostavax.

Vaccination is recommended for all individuals aged 50 years and older who have no contraindications, including those who report a previous episode of zoster or who have chronic medical conditions (CDC, 2020b). Shingrix induces a strong and persistent immune response in older adults and is more than 90% effective at preventing shingles and long-term nerve pain (Bastidas et al., 2019). *Healthy People 2020* includes a goal of increasing the percentage of adults who are vaccinated against zoster (shingles) in the overall goal of reducing or eliminating cases of vaccine-preventable diseases.

Postherpetic neuralgia (PHN) is a common complication of HZ that is minimized for those who are immunized. PHN is a chronic, often debilitating painful condition that can last months or even years. Older adults are more likely to have PHN and to have longer-lasting and more severe pain. Another complication of HZ is eye involvement, which occurs in 10% to 25% of zoster episodes and can result in prolonged or permanent pain, facial scarring, and loss of vision.

The pain of PHN has been difficult to control and can significantly affect quality of life. Treatment should include medical, psychological, complementary and alternative medicine options, and rehabilitation. The best evidence studies for medications indicate that the most effective are the tricyclic antidepressants, gabapentin and pregabalin, carbamazepine (for trigeminal neuralgia), opioids, tramadol, topical lidocaine patch, and duloxetine or venlafaxine. Assessment and management of pain is discussed in Chapter 18.

Candidiasis *(Candida albicans)*

The fungus *Candida albicans* (referred to as yeast) is present on the skin of healthy individuals of any age. However, under certain circumstances and in the right environment, a fungal infection can develop. Persons who are obese or malnourished, are receiving antibiotic or steroid therapy, or have diabetes are at increased risk. *Candida* grows especially well in areas that are moist, warm, and dark, such as in skinfolds, in the axilla, in the groin area, and under pendulous breasts. It can also be found in the corners of the mouth associated with the chronic moisture of angular cheilitis. In the vagina it is also called a "yeast infection." If this is found in an older woman, it may mean that she has undiagnosed or poorly controlled diabetes.

Inside the mouth a *Candida* infection is referred to as "thrush" and is associated with poor hygiene and immunocompromised individuals, such as those who have long-term steroid use, who are receiving chemotherapy, or test positive for or are infected with human immunodeficiency virus (HIV), or have acquired immunodeficiency syndrome (AIDS). In the mouth, candidiasis appears as irregular, white, flat to slightly raised patches on an erythematous base that cannot be removed by scraping. The infection can extend into the throat and cause swallowing to be painful. In severely immunocompromised persons, the infection can extend down the entire gastrointestinal tract.

On skin, *Candida* is usually maculopapular, glazed, and dark pink in persons with less pigmentation and grayish in persons with more pigmentation. If it is advanced, the central area may be completely red and/or dark and weeping with characteristic bright red and/or dark satellite lesions (distinct lesions a short distance from the center). At this point the skin may be edematous, itching, and burning. The best approach to managing fungal infections is to prevent them, and the key to prevention is limiting the conditions that encourage fungal growth. Prevention is prioritized for persons who are obese, bedridden, incontinent, or diaphoretic.

Photo Damage of the Skin

Although exposure to sunlight is necessary for the production of vitamin D, the sun is also the most common cause of skin damage and skin cancer. More than 90% of the visible changes commonly attributed to skin aging are caused by the sun (Skin Cancer Foundation, 2020). With aging, years of sun exposure are accumulated and the epidermis is thinner, significantly increasing the risk for older adults. The damage (photo or solar damage) comes from prolonged exposure to UV light from the environment or in tanning booths. Although the amount of sun-induced damage varies with skin type, genetics, and geographical location, much of the associated damage is preventable. Ideally, preventive measures begin in childhood, but clinical evidence has shown that some improvement can be achieved at any time by limiting sun exposure and using sunscreens regularly regardless of skin tones.

SKIN CANCERS

Facts and Figures

Skin cancer (including melanoma and nonmelanoma skin cancer) is the most common of all cancers. Skin cancer is a major public health problem, and skin cancers in the United States, unlike many other cancers, continue to rise. One in five Americans will develop skin cancer in the course of a lifetime (Skin Cancer Foundation, 2020). Caucasian populations generally have a much higher risk of getting nonmelanoma or melanoma skin cancers than dark-skinned populations, but individuals of all skin colors should minimize sun exposure. Individuals with pale or freckled skin, fair or red hair, and blue eyes belong to the highest-risk group. About 90% of nonmelanoma skin cancers are associated with exposure to UV radiation from the sun.

Basal Cell Carcinoma

Basal cell carcinoma is the most common malignant skin cancer. It occurs mainly in older age groups but is increasingly occurring in younger persons. It is slow growing, and metastasis is rare. A basal cell lesion can be triggered by extensive sun exposure, especially burns, chronic irritation, and chronic ulceration of the skin. It is more prevalent in light-skinned persons. It usually begins as a pearly papule with prominent telangiectasias (blood vessels) or as a scar-like area with no history of trauma (Fig. 14.5). Basal cell carcinoma is also known to ulcerate. It may be indistinguishable from squamous cell carcinoma and is diagnosed by biopsy. Early detection and treatment are necessary to minimize disfigurement. Treatment is usually surgical with either simple excision or Mohs micrographic surgery.

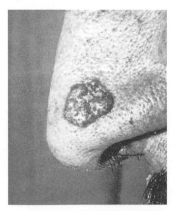

FIG. 14.5 Basal cell carcinoma. (Courtesy Gary Monheit, MD, University of Alabama at Birmingham School of Medicine.)

Squamous Cell Carcinoma

Squamous cell carcinoma is the second most common skin cancer. However, it is aggressive and has a high incidence of metastasis if not identified and treated promptly. Major risk factors include sun exposure, fair skin, and immunosuppression. Individuals in their mid-60s who have been or are chronically exposed to the sun (e.g., persons who work outdoors or are athletes) are prime candidates for this type of cancer. Less common causes include chronic stasis ulcers, scars from injury, and exposure to chemical carcinogens, such as topical hydrocarbons, arsenic, and radiation (especially for individuals who received treatments for acne in the mid-twentieth century) (Endo & Norman, 2014).

The lesion begins as a firm, irregular, fleshy, pink-colored nodule that becomes reddened and scaly, much like actinic keratosis, but it may increase rapidly in size. It may also be hard and wart-like with a gray top and horny texture, or it may be ulcerated and indurated with raised, defined borders (Fig. 14.6). Because it can appear so differently, it is often overlooked or thought to be insignificant. All persons, especially those who live in sunny climates, should be regularly screened by a dermatologist. Treatment depends on the size, histologic features, and patient preference and may include electrodesiccation and curettage, Mohs micrographic surgery, aggressive cryotherapy, or topical 5-fluorouracil. Once a person has been diagnosed with a squamous cell carcinoma, they need to be routinely followed because the majority of recurrences are within the first few years.

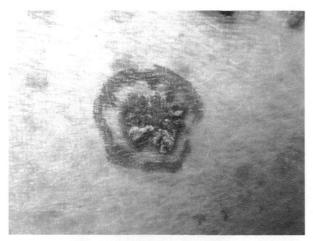

FIG. 14.6 Squamous cell carcinoma. (From Ham, R. J., Sloane, P. D., Warshaw, G. A., et al. (2014). *Primary care geriatrics* (6th ed.). Philadelphia: Saunders. Used with permission, University of Utah Department of Dermatology.)

Melanoma

Melanoma, a neoplasm of the melanocytes, affects the skin or, less commonly, the retina. Melanoma has a classic multicolor, raised appearance with an asymmetrical, irregular border. It may appear to be of any size, but the surface diameter is not necessarily reflective of the size beneath the surface, similar in concept to an iceberg. It is treatable if diagnosed early, before it has a chance to invade surrounding tissue. Melanoma accounts for less than 2% of skin cancer cases, but it causes most skin cancer deaths. Melanoma is highly curable if the cancer is detected in its earliest stages and treated promptly (Skin Cancer Foundation, 2020).

Incidence and Prevalence

The number of new cases of melanoma in the United States has been increasing for at least 30 years. Overall, the lifetime risk of developing melanoma is about 1 in 50 for the White population, 1 in 1000 for Black individuals, and 1 in 200 for the Hispanic population. Melanoma rates among middle-aged adults, especially women, have increased in the past four decades. Men have a higher rate of melanoma than women, and an individual who has already had a melanoma has a higher risk of developing another one.

Risk Factors

Risk factors for melanoma include a personal history of melanoma; the presence of atypical, large, or numerous (more than 50) moles; sun sensitivity; history of excessive sun exposure and severe sunburns; use of tanning booths; natural blond or red hair color; diseases or treatments that suppress the immune system; and a history of skin cancer. Increasing age along with a history of sun exposure increases a person's risk even further. The legs and backs of women and the backs of men are the most common sites of melanoma. Many studies have linked melanoma on the trunk, legs, and arms to frequent sunburns, especially in childhood. Blistering sunburns before the age of 18 years are thought to damage Langerhans cells, which affect the immune response of the skin and increase the risk of a later melanoma. Two-thirds of melanomas develop from preexisting moles; only one-third arise alone.

Although melanoma occurs more often in older adults, it is one of the most common cancers in people younger than 30 years. Exposure to indoor tanning, common in developed countries, is thought to be contributing to the increasing rates of melanoma and other skin cancers among younger individuals. Indoor tanning increases the risk of melanoma by 75% when use is started before the age of 35 years. Worldwide, there are more skin cancer cases as a result of indoor tanning than there are lung cancer cases caused by smoking

(Skin Cancer Foundation, 2020). This is considered a major public health issue, with many states limiting minors' access to tanning salons.

Tanning devices have been reclassified by the Federal Drug Administration to Class II (moderate risk devices) and all sunlamp products, which include tanning beds and booths, must now carry the FDAs strictest "Black Box" warning stating that the product should not be used by people under the age of 18 years. *Healthy People 2020* includes objectives to reduce the proportion of adolescents and adults using indoor tanning devices (USDHSS, 2012).

Age-related skin changes, such as thinning and diminished numbers of melanocytes, significantly increase the risk for solar damage and subsequent skin cancer. Nurses have an active role in the prevention and early recognition of skin cancers. This role may include working with community awareness and education programs and screening clinics and providing direct care. By far the most important preventive nursing action is to provide education regarding skin cancer risk factors and adequate lifelong protective measures (Box 14.3).

Careful skin inspection is essential, and nurses should be vigilant in observing skin for changes that require further evaluation. Patient education also includes teaching individuals how to examine their skin once a month to look for warning signs or any suspicious lesions. If the individual has a partner, partners can perform regular checks of each other's skin, watching for signs of change and the need to contact a primary care provider or dermatologist promptly. For a person with keratosis and multiple freckles (nevi), photographing the body parts may be a useful reference. The adage "when in doubt, get it checked" is an important one, and regular screenings should be a part of the health care of all older adults. The "ABCDE" approach to assessing such potential lesions is used (Box 14.4).

BOX 14.3 Promoting Healthy Skin

- Seek the shade, especially between 10 a.m. and 4 p.m.
- Don't get sunburned
- Avoid tanning and never use UV tanning beds
- Cover up with clothing, including a broad-brimmed hat and UV blocking sunglasses
- Use a broad-spectrum (UVA/UVB) sunscreen to your entire body 30 minutes before going outside. Reapply every 2 hours after swimming or excessive sweating.
- Keep newborns out of the sun
- Examine your skin head-to-toe every month
- See a dermatologist at least once a year for a professional skin exam

From: Skin Care Foundation (2020). Skin cancer prevention. https://www.skincancer.org/skin-cancer-prevention/sun-protection/.

BOX 14.4 Danger Signs: Remember ABCDE

A Asymmetry of a mole (one that is not regularly round or oval)
B Border is irregular
C Color variation (areas of black, brown, tan, blue, red, white, or a combination)
D Diameter greater than the size of a pencil eraser (although early stages may be smaller)
E Elevation and enlargement[a]

[a]Lesions that change, itch, bleed, or do not heal are also alarm signals.
From Skin Cancer Foundation (2018). *Do you know your ABCDEs?* https://www.skincancer.org/skin-cancer-information/melanoma/mclanoma-warning-signs-and-images/do-you-know-your-abcdes.

PRESSURE INJURIES (PIs)

Aging carries a high risk of the development of PIs; 70% of PIs occur in older adults. PIs are recognized as one of the geriatric syndromes (Chapter 8), and *Healthy People 2020* has addressed this issue with a goal of reducing the rate of PI-related hospitalizations among older adults. Although prevention and treatment of PIs require an interprofessional approach, PIs are considered specifically a nurse-sensitive indicator by the US National Database of Nursing Quality Indicators (Ayello et al., 2017) and a nurse-sensitive indicator for hospital-acquired pressure injuries (HAPIs) (Al-Majid et al., 2017). Nurses play a key role in the prevention of PIs and selection of evidence-based treatment strategies.

Definition

The National Pressure Injury Advisory Panel (NPIAP) and the European Pressure Ulcer Advisory Panel (EPUAP) constitute an international collaboration convened to develop evidence-based recommendations to be used throughout the world to prevent and treat pressure-related injuries. In 2016, the NPIAP began using the term pressure injury to replace pressure ulcer to describe more accurately PIs to both intact and ulcerated skin. In addition to the change in terminology, Arabic numbers are now used in the names of the stages instead of Roman numerals. Stages have been more fully described and two additional PI definitions have been added. In 2019, the third edition of the guidelines were released (https://npiap.com/). The National Pressure Ulcer Advisory Panel (NPUAP) changed its name to The National Pressure Injury Advisory Panel (NPIAP) as well.

A PI is defined as "localized damage to the skin and/or underlying soft tissue usually over a bony prominence or related to a medical or other device." The injury can present as intact skin or an open ulcer and may be painful. The injury occurs as a result of intense pressure and/or prolonged pressure or pressure in combination with shear. The tolerance of soft tissue for pressure and shear may also be affected by microclimate, nutrition, perfusion, comorbidities, and condition of the soft tissue.

Scope of the Problem

PIs cause pain, loss of function, extended length of hospitalization and long-term care stays, and increase in related costs. Reported prevalence rates of hospital acquired pressure injuries (HAPIs) are as high as 38% in the acute care setting, 42% in critical care patients, 17% in home care, and 23% in long-term care. PIs are a major challenge worldwide and a major cause of morbidity, mortality, and health care burden globally (Ramundo et al., 2018). The epidemiology of PIs varies appreciably by clinical setting. Critically ill patients in the intensive care unit (ICU) are considered to be at the greatest risk of PI development as a result of high acuity and the multiple interventions and therapies they receive (Alderden et al., 2017).

HAPI rates have decreased across the United States. However, despite growing resources invested into the development and implementation of evidence-based prevention protocols, the rates of facility-acquired PIs are still much higher in many clinical areas across the globe, especially in high-risk populations such as older adults and critically ill patients (Rondinelli et al., 2018). Concern over the global problem of PIs had led the NPIAP to establish a Pressure Ulcer/Injury Registry, the first database of its type to allow clinicians to input cases of PIs in an effort to provide statistically significant rigorous analysis of the variables associated with the development of unavoidable PIs.

Cost and Regulatory Requirements

Treatment of PIs is costly in terms of both health care expenditure and patient suffering. The development of a stage/category 3 or 4 PI is considered a "never event" (preventable serious medical errors or adverse events that should never happen to a patient). Hospitals no longer receive additional reimbursement to care for a patient who has acquired PIs under the hospital's care, which has the potential to increase the financial strain greatly for facilities that fail to rise to this challenge. In long-term care facilities, when PIs develop after admission and are identified as avoidable, civil monetary penalties can be assessed.

Characteristics

PIs can develop anywhere on the body but are seen most frequently on the posterior aspects, especially the sacrum, the heels, and the greater trochanters. Secondary areas of breakdown include the lateral condyles of knees and ankles. The pinna of the ears, occiput, elbows, and scapulae are other areas subject to breakdown. The heel is particularly prone to the development of PIs because of its anatomy. It consists of skin overlying a cup-like shell of connective tissue that essentially forms a sealed compartment, creating a compartment of fat with comparatively low vascularity that is prone to ischemia. The shell of connective tissue and sealed compartment structure inhibit distribution of external pressure. Additionally, the small surface area of contact and little subcutaneous tissue lead to PI when pressure is exerted directly on bone (Ramundo et al., 2018).

> ### ⚡ SAFETY ALERT
>
> Approximately 25% to 35% of pressure injuries are on heels. Those with peripheral vascular disease (PVD) are at high risk. Keep heels elevated off the bed with a pillow under calf or use heel suspension boots. Prophylactic multilayer foam dressings, in conjunction with a pressure injury prevention program, are recommended for prevention of pressure injuries on the heel (Ramundo et al., 2018).

Classification

The EPUAP and NPIAP classification of PIs is presented in Box 14.5. The following two additional PI definitions have also been added:

Medical Device–Related Pressure Injury: Medical device–related pressure injuries (MDRPIs) result from the use of devices designed and applied for diagnostic or therapeutic purposes. The resultant PI generally conforms to the pattern or shape of the device. The injury should not be staged using the staging system.

Mucosal Membrane Pressure Injury: A mucosal membrane PI is found on mucous membranes with a history of a medical device in use at the location of the injury. Because of the anatomy of the tissue, these injuries cannot be classified.

PIs are always classified by the highest stage "achieved" and reverse staging is never used. This means that the wound is documented as the stage representing the maximal damage and depth that has occurred. As the wound heals, it fills with granulation tissue composed of endothelial cells, fibroblasts, collagen, and an extracellular matrix. Muscle, subcutaneous fat, and dermis are not replaced. A stage 4 PI that is healing does not revert to stage 3 and then stage 2. It remains defined as a healing stage 4 PI.

Risk Factors

Many factors increase the risk of pressure injuries, including changes in the skin, comorbid illnesses,

BOX 14.5 Pressure Injury Stages

Deep Tissue Pressure Injury (DTPI): Persistent Nonblanchable Deep Red, Maroon, or Purple Discoloration

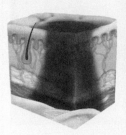

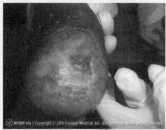

Heel, ethnic skin

Intact or nonintact skin with localized area of persistent non-blanchable deep red, maroon, or purple discoloration or epidermal separation revealing a dark wound bed or blood-filled blister. Pain and temperature change often precede skin color changes. Discoloration may appear differently in darkly pigmented skin. This injury results from intense and/or prolonged pressure and shear forces at the bone–muscle interface. The wound may evolve rapidly to reveal the actual extent of tissue injury or may resolve without tissue loss. If necrotic tissue, subcutaneous tissue, granulation tissue, fascia, muscle, or other underlying structures are visible, this indicates a full-thickness pressure injury (Unstageable, Stage 3, or Stage 4). Do not use DTPI to describe vascular, traumatic, neuropathic, or dermatological conditions.

Stage 1 Pressure Injury: Nonblanchable Erythema of Intact Skin

Intact skin with a localized area of nonblanchable erythema, which may appear differently in darkly pigmented skin. Presence of blanchable erythema or changes in sensation, temperature, or firmness may precede visual changes. Color changes do not include purple or maroon discoloration; these may indicate deep tissue pressure injury.

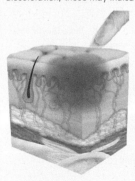

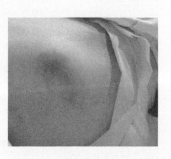

Stage 2 Pressure Injury: Partial-Thickness Skin Loss With Exposed Dermis

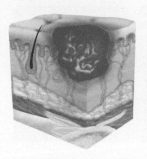

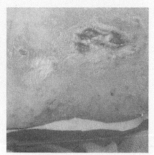

Partial-thickness loss of skin with exposed dermis. The wound bed is viable, pink or red, and moist, and may also present as an intact or ruptured serum-filled blister. Adipose (fat) is not visible and deeper tissues are not visible. Granulation tissue, slough, and eschar are not present. These injuries commonly result from adverse microclimate and shear in the skin over the pelvis and shear in the heels. This stage should not be used to describe moisture-associated skin damage (MASD) including incontinence-associated dermatitis (IAD), intertriginous dermatitis (ITD), medical adhesive–related skin injury (MARS), or traumatic wounds (skin tears, burns, abrasions).

Stage 3 Pressure Injury: Full-Thickness Skin Loss

Full-thickness loss of skin, in which adipose (fat) is visible in the ulcer and granulation tissue and epibole (rolled wound edges) are often present. Slough and/or eschar may be visible. Undermining and tunneling may occur. Fascia, muscle, tendon, ligament, cartilage, and/or bone are not exposed. If slough or eschar obscures the extent of tissue loss this is an Unstageable Pressure Injury.

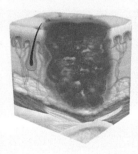

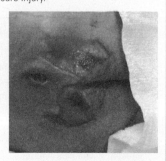

Continued

BOX 14.5   Pressure Injury Stages—cont'd

Stage 4 Pressure Injury: Full-Thickness Skin and Tissue Loss

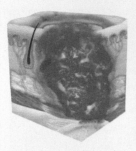
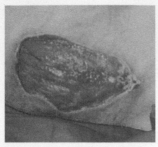

Full-thickness skin and tissue loss with exposed or directly palpable fascia, muscle, tendon, ligament, cartilage, or bone in the ulcer. Slough and/or eschar may be visible. Epibole (rolled edges), undermining, and/or tunneling often occur. Depth varies by anatomical location. If slough or eschar obscures the extent of tissue loss, this is an Unstageable Pressure Injury.

Unstageable Pressure Injury: Obscured Full-Thickness Skin and Tissue Loss

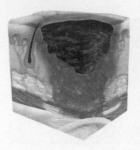
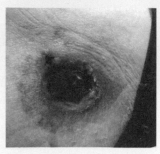

Full-thickness skin and tissue loss in which the extent of tissue damage within the ulcer cannot be confirmed because it is obscured by slough or eschar. If slough or eschar is removed, a Stage 3 or Stage 4 pressure injury will be revealed. Stable eschar (e.g., dry, adherent, intact without erythema or fluctuance) on an ischemic limb or the heels should not be removed.

From the National Pressure Ulcer Advisory Panel (NPUAP) (2016). National Pressure Ulcer Advisory Panel (NPUAP) announces a change in terminology from pressure ulcer to pressure injury and updates the stages of pressure injury. Reprinted with permission of the NPUAP, 2016.
DTPI photo: From NPUAP. Stages 1–4 photos: From Cameron, M. H., & Monroe, L. (Eds.) (2011). *Physical rehabilitation for the physical therapist assistant*. St Louis: Saunders.
Unstageable photo: From Ham, R. J., Sloane, P. D., Warshaw, G. A., et al, (Eds.) (2014). *Primary care geriatrics* (6th ed.). Philadelphia: Elsevier.

nutritional status, frailty, surgical procedures (especially orthopedic/cardiac), cognitive deficits, incontinence, and reduced mobility (Box 14.6). A major risk factor is the combination of intensity and duration of pressure and tissue tolerance. Individuals confined to a bed or chair and who are unable to shift weight or reposition themselves at regular intervals are at high risk. Tissue tolerance, in addition to unrelieved pressure, contributes to the risk of a PI. Tissue tolerance is related to the ability of the tissue to distribute and compensate for pressure exerted over bony prominences. Factors that affect tissue tolerance include moisture, friction, shear

BOX 14.6   Pressure Injury Risk Factors

Prolonged Pressure/Immobilization

Lying in bed or sitting in a chair or wheelchair without changing position or relieving pressure over an extended period
Lying for hours on hard x-ray and operating tables
Neurological disorders (coma, spinal cord injuries, cognitive impairment, or cerebrovascular disease)
Fractures or contractures
Debilitation: older adults in hospitals and nursing homes
Pain
Sedation
Shearing forces (moving by dragging on coarse bed sheets)

Disease/Tissue Factors

Impaired perfusion; ischemia
Fecal or urinary incontinence; prolonged exposure to moisture

Malnutrition, dehydration
Chronic diseases accompanied by anemia, edema, renal failure, malnutrition, peripheral vascular disease, or sepsis
Previous history of pressure injuries

Additional Risk Factors for the Critically Ill

Norepinephrine infusion
Acute Physiology and Chronic Health Evaluation (APACHE II) score
Anemia
Age older than 40 years
Multiple organ system disease or comorbid complications
Length of hospital stay

From McCance, K. L., & Huether, S. E. (2014). *Pathophysiology* (7th ed.). St Louis: Elsevier.

force, nutritional status, age, sensory perception, and arterial pressure.

In darker-pigmented persons, redness and blanching may not be observed as early signs of skin damage. In dark skin, early signs of skin damage can manifest as a purplish color or appear like a bruise. It is important to observe for induration, darkening, change in color from surrounding skin, or a shadowed appearance of the skin. The affected skin area, when compared with adjacent tissues, may be firm, warmer, cooler, or painful. Many pressure injuries in dark skin are missed because presentation is different than in other skin types. Recognizing this early cue and taking action during hospital and nursing home stays are important.

Prevention of Pressure Injuries

The importance of prevention of PIs has been frequently emphasized and is the key to treatment. Key elements of PI prevention are presented in Box 14.7. A comprehensive PI program that includes multiple interventions (care bundle) appears to be related to better outcomes. A bundle is composed of a set of evidence-based practices that, when performed collectively and reliably, have been shown to improve patient outcomes. Involvement of the patient and family may enhance the effectiveness of care bundles (Roberts et al., 2017).

Core preventive strategies include recognizing and analyzing risk, evaluation of skin, nutritional status, repositioning, and appropriate support surfaces. Interventions that address limited mobility, compromised skin integrity, and nutritional support have been associated with improvements in PI rates. A recent quality improvement study reported that nurse practitioners assuming a leadership role as wound care consultants in acute care may be instrumental in decreasing HAPI rates (Irvin et al., 2017).

> ### BOX 14.7   Key Elements of a Pressure Injury Prevention Program
>
> - Skin evaluation for all patients looking for pressure injury
> - Daily risk evaluation
> - Daily skin inspection
> - Moisture management
> - Optimizing nutrition and hydration
> - Minimizing pressure (posture changes)
> - Pressure injury nursing care education
> - Establishment of a wound care team
> - Interprofessional cooperation
>
> From Jin, Y., Jin, T., Lee, S. (2017). Automated pressure injury risk assessment system incorporated into an electronic record system, *Nurs Res 66*(6), 462–472.

Systematic prevention programs have been shown to decrease HAPIs. The On-Time Pressure Injury Prevention Program (AHRQ, 2014) has been shown to reduce the incidence of PIs in long-term care. Tools to document PI healing and treatments and reports to monitor the healing process are available (Box 14.2). Despite recognition of its importance, PI prevention strategies are not consistently implemented and PIs continue to have a negative impact on patient outcomes and health care costs in a variety of care settings.

Education programs on PI, both for practicing nurses and student nurses, are essential and should be a part of institutional and educational curricula. Innovative approaches to education are important and may include "just in time" interactive educational methods, including mobile phone apps. The Department of Veterans Affairs (VA) has developed an innovative mobile app for veterans and caregivers working to prevent and treat PIs—the VA Pressure Ulcer/Injury Resource app (VA PUR) (Box 14.2). Continuing professional development for PI prevention and management needs to be interprofessional and include evidence-based educational material and strategies. Professional nursing checklists for competence and performance evaluations need to be implemented at all levels (novice to expert).

Consequences of Pressure Injuries

PIs are costly to treat and prolong recovery and extend rehabilitation. Complications include the need for grafting or amputation, sepsis, or even death and may lead to legal action by the individual or their representative against the caregiver. The personal impact of a PI on health and quality of life is also significant and not well understood or researched. Findings from a study exploring patients' perceptions of the impact of a PI and its treatment on health and quality of life suggest that PIs cause suffering, pain, discomfort, and distress that are not always recognized or adequately treated by nursing staff. PIs have a profound impact on the patients' lives—physically, socially, emotionally, and mentally (Spilsbury et al., 2007). The link to several patient's stories, presented in video format, can be found in Box 14.2.

Are Pressure Injuries Always Preventable?

PI development is a multicausal event. In the vast majority of cases, appropriate actions for prevention and treatment can prevent or minimize PI development. Both the NPIAP (Edsberg et al., 2014) and the Wound, Ostomy, and Continence Nurses Society (WOCN Society) (Schmitt et al., 2017) have published statements on avoidable and unavoidable PIs. Clinical situations can severely impair efforts to prevent PIs. Some of these are preexisting deep tissue injury (DTI) (but no visible ulceration); immobility; hemodynamic instability; medical devices; compromised nutrition; and the patient who is nearing the end of life (Edsberg et al., 2014).

Skin failure is an emerging concept, particularly in the palliative care setting. "Skin is the largest organ of the body, and it fails like any other organ system" (Levine, 2017a, p. 201). Skin failure has been defined as "the state in which tissue tolerance is so compromised that cells can no longer survive in zones of physiological impairment that include hypoxia, local mechanical stress, impaired delivery of nutrients, and buildup of metabolic byproducts. This includes PIs, wounds that occur at life's end, and in the setting of multisystem organ failure" (Levine, 2017a). Skin failure can occur in the course of acute and chronic illness and at the end of life when the body is shutting down.

Skin failure at the end of life is not the same as PIs. Preventing wound deterioration or healing may not be realistic goals for individuals at the end of life. The focus of wound management at the end of life is comfort and involves symptom control, stabilization of existing wounds, and prevention of additional wounds and infectious complications. If opportunity for wound healing is limited, maintenance of the wound in the present state may be the outcome. In some situations, palliative wounds may benefit from interventions such as surgical debridement or support surfaces even if the goal is not to heal the wound. The plan of care must be consistent with the patient and family goals and wishes. Further research is needed to fully understand the development of unavoidable PI in situations of high risk such as at the end of life (Levine, 2017a).

❖ USING CLINICAL JUDGMENT TO PROMOTE HEALTHY AGING: PRESSURE INJURIES

Nursing staff, as direct caregivers, are key team members who monitor and evaluate the skin, identify risk factors, and implement numerous preventive nursing actions. The nurse alerts the health care provider to the need for prescribed treatments, recommends treatments, and administers and evaluates the changing status of the wound(s) and adequacy of treatments.

◆ Recognizing and Analyzing Cues: Risk of Pressure Injury

Careful inspection of the skin and use of instruments to evaluate risk are performed on admission and whenever there is a change in the status of the patient (Box 14.8). In long-term care facilities, the MDS 3.0 provides guidelines for the evaluation of skin integrity and PIs with accompanying care guidelines (Chapter 8). Evaluation begins with a history, detailed head-to-toe skin examination,

---

> **BOX 14.8   Guidelines for Evaluation of Skin**
>
> **Acute care:** On admission, reassess at least every 24 hours or sooner if patient's condition changes
> **Long-term care:** On admission, weekly for 4 weeks, then quarterly and whenever resident's condition changes
> **Home care:** On admission and at every nurse visit

Data from NPUAP (2007). *Pressure ulcer prevention points.* http://www.npuap.org/wp-content/uploads/2012/03/PU_Prev_Points.pdf.

nutritional evaluation, and analysis of laboratory findings. Laboratory values that have been correlated with risk of the development and the poor healing of PIs include those that reflect anemia and poor nutritional status. Visual and tactile inspection of the entire skin surface with special attention to bony prominences is essential. Nurses should look for any interruption of skin integrity or other changes, including redness or *hyperemia*. Special attention must be given to the observation of dark skin because tissue injury will appear differently in lighter skin. Assessment of pain related to the PI (dressing changes, turning) is important so that appropriate treatment can be given to relieve pain (Chapter 18).

If pressure is present, it should be relieved and the area evaluated in 1 hour. Pressure areas and surrounding tissue should be palpated for changes in temperature and tissue resilience. Blisters or pimples with or without hyperemia and scabs over weight-bearing areas in the absence of trauma should be considered suspect. Inspection is best accomplished in nonglare daylight or, if that is not possible, with focused lighting. Special attention should be directed to affected areas when an individual uses orthotic devices such as corsets, braces, prostheses, postural supports, splints, slings, or casts and to areas of skin around other devices such as endotracheal and tracheostomy tubes.

Early identification of risk status is critical so that timely interventions can be designed to address specific risk factors. The Braden Scale for Predicting Pressure Sore Risk, developed by nurses Barbara Braden and Nancy Bergstrom, is widely used and clinically validated. The Braden Scale is available online and used in most health care institutions (Murphree, 2017) (Box 14.2). This scale evaluates the risk of PIs on the basis of a numerical scoring system of six risk factors: sensory perception, moisture, activity, mobility, nutrition, and friction/shear. Because the Braden Scale does not include all of the risk factors for PIs, it is recommended that it be used as an adjunct rather than in place of clinical judgment. A thorough patient history to evaluate other risk factors such as age, medications, comorbidities (diabetes, peripheral vascular disease), history of PIs, and other factors, is important to address fully the risk of PI development so that appropriate preventive actions can be developed.

◆ Nursing Actions: PI

The goal of prevention is to help maintain skin integrity against the various environmental, mechanical, and chemical assaults that are potential causes of breakdown. Nursing actions include (1) eliminating friction and irritation to the skin, such as from shearing, and reducing moisture so that tissues do not macerate; (2) managing incontinence and enhancing mobility; and (3) displacing body weight from prominent areas to facilitate circulation to the skin. Nurses should be familiar with the types of supportive surfaces so that the most effective products are used. The Support Surface Algorithm (SSA) is an evidence-based tool that helps determine a strong protocol for addressing PIs (Box 14.2). Use lifting devices to move the person rather than dragging the person during transfers and position changes. Use pillows or foam wedges so that skin surfaces do not touch, and use devices that eliminate pressure on heels.

Repositioning is generally regarded as one of the most important and effective measures for preventing PI, but there is no consensus on the frequency or type of repositioning most effective for individual patients. For some, 4-hour repositioning may be adequate while for others, even hourly repositioning would not prevent PI. Historically, 2-hour turning has been recommended regardless of the individual need. Hampton (2017) argues that this recommendation originated from Florence Nightingale who recognized the importance of repositioning when caring for soldiers in the Crimean War. She did not stipulate the timing, but it took 2 hours to work round the large ward from bed one and back to bed one. Hence the myth of 2-hourly turns was born.

Techniques for proper positioning are directed at offloading pressure and individualized for each individual. These techniques include a change in body position, head of bed adjustment, micro-shifting, and utilization of the appropriate pillows, wedges, and sleep surfaces. Continuous bedside pressure mapping (CBPM) devices (Fig. 14.7) enable caregivers and patients to visualize, evaluate, and monitor pressure points between the patient and the support surface (beds or wheelchairs) and to undertake the necessary actions to successfully offload pressure.

The pressure sensing mat measures pressure from thousands of discrete points and converts pressure (measured in mmHg) into color with red/orange/yellow corresponding to higher pressures and blue/green corresponding to lower pressures. Based on systematic review and meta-analysis, the current literature demonstrates that PI-monitoring devices are associated with a

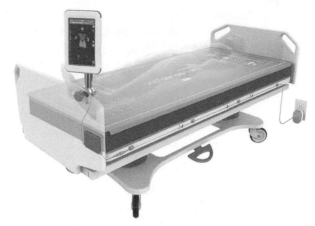

FIG. 14.7 Continuous Bedside Pressure Mapping (CBPM) Devices. (Used with permission from Wellsense, Inc.)

strong reduction in the risk of developing PIs in acute and skilled nursing settings (Lucchini et al., 2020; Walia et al., 2017) These devices provide critical, real-time information to clinicians and patients to implement prevention guidelines.

> ### ⚡ SAFETY ALERT
>
> Individuals placed on pressure redistribution mattresses continue to need turning and repositioning according to an individualized schedule.

Consultation with the nutritional team is important. Nutritional intake should be monitored, along with the serum albumin, hematocrit, and hemoglobin levels. Caloric, protein, vitamin, and/or mineral supplementation can be considered if there is evidence of deficiencies of these nutrients. Routine use of higher than the recommended daily allowance of vitamin C and zinc for the prevention and/or treatment of PIs is not supported by evidence (Jamshed & Schneider, 2010). Nurses promote nutritional health by ensuring that the person receives adequate assistance with eating and that dining time is a pleasant experience for the person (Chapter 10). PI prevention education programs need to be provided to all levels of health care providers, patients, families, and caregivers.

PIs are evaluated with each dressing change and repeated on a weekly, biweekly, and as-needed basis. The purpose is to evaluate specifically and carefully the effectiveness of treatment. The PUSH tool (Pressure Ulcer Scale for Healing) (National Pressure Ulcer Advisory Panel, 2014) provides a detailed form that covers all aspects of PI evaluation and takes a short time to complete (Fig. 14.8). Photographic documentation is highly

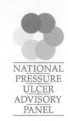

NATIONAL
PRESSURE
ULCER
ADVISORY
PANEL

Pressure Ulcer Scale for Healing (PUSH)
PUSH Tool 3.0

Patient Name_____ Patient ID# _____

Ulcer Location _____ Date _____

Directions:

Observe and measure the pressure ulcer. Categorize the ulcer with respect to surface area, exudate, and type of wound tissue. Record a sub-score for each of these ulcer characteristics. Add the sub-scores to obtain the total score. A comparison of total scores measured over time provides an indication of the improvement or deterioration in pressure ulcer healing.

LENGTH X WIDTH (in cm²)	0	1	2	3	4	5	Sub-score
	0	< 0.3	0.3 – 0.6	0.7 – 1.0	1.1 – 2.0	2.1 – 3.0	
	6	7	8	9	10		
	3.1 – 4.0	4.1 – 8.0	8.1 – 12.0	12.1 – 24.0	> 24.0		
EXUDATE AMOUNT	0 None	1 Light	2 Moderate	3 Heavy			Sub-score
TISSUE TYPE	0 Closed	1 Epithelial Tissue	2 Granulation Tissue	3 Slough	4 Necrotic Tissue		Sub-score
							TOTAL SCORE

Length x Width: Measure the greatest length (head to toe) and the greatest width (side to side) using a centimeter ruler. Multiply these two measurements (length x width) to obtain an estimate of surface area in square centimeters (cm²). Caveat: Do not guess! Always use a centimeter ruler and always use the same method each time the ulcer is measured.

Exudate Amount: Estimate the amount of exudate (drainage) present after removal of the dressing and before applying any topical agent to the ulcer. Estimate the exudate (drainage) as none, light, moderate, or heavy.

Tissue Type: This refers to the types of tissue that are present in the wound (ulcer) bed. Score as a "4" if there is any necrotic tissue present. Score as a "3" if there is any amount of slough present and necrotic tissue is absent. Score as a "2" if the wound is clean and contains granulation tissue. A superficial wound that is reepithelializing is scored as a "1". When the wound is closed, score as a "0".

   4 – **Necrotic Tissue (Eschar):** black, brown, or tan tissue that adheres firmly to the wound bed or ulcer edges and may be either firmer or softer than surrounding skin.

   3 – **Slough:** yellow or white tissue that adheres to the ulcer bed in strings or thick clumps, or is mucinous.

   2 – **Granulation Tissue:** pink or beefy red tissue with a shiny, moist, granular appearance.

   1 – **Epithelial Tissue:** for superficial ulcers, new pink or shiny tissue (skin) that grows in from the edges or as islands on the ulcer surface.

   0 – **Closed/Resurfaced:** the wound is completely covered with epithelium (new skin).

www.npuap.org
11F

PUSH Tool Version 3.0: 9/15/98
©National Pressure Ulcer Advisory Panel

FIG. 14.8 Push Tool. (Used with permission from National Pressure Injury Advisory Panel [NPIAP].)

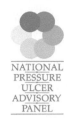

NATIONAL
PRESSURE
ULCER
ADVISORY
PANEL

Pressure Ulcer Healing Chart
To monitor trends in PUSH Scores over time
(Use a separate page for each pressure ulcer)

Patient Name_____ Patient ID# _____

Ulcer Location _____ Date _____

Directions:
Observe and measure pressure ulcers at regular intervals using the PUSH Tool.
Date and record PUSH Sub-scores and Total Scores on the Pressure Ulcer Healing Record below.

Pressure Ulcer Healing Record													
Date													
Length x Width													
Exudate Amount													
Tissue Type													
PUSH Total Score													

Graph the PUSH Total Scores on the Pressure Ulcer Healing Graph below.

PUSH Total Score	Pressure Ulcer Healing Graph												
17													
16													
15													
14													
13													
12													
11													
10													
9													
8													
7													
6													
5													
4													
3													
2													
1													
Healed = 0													
Date													

www.npuap.org
11F

PUSH Tool Version 3.0: 9/15/98
©National Pressure Ulcer Advisory Panel

FIG. 14.8 (continued)

recommended both at the onset of the problem and at intervals during treatment.

If there are no signs of healing from week to week or worsening of the wound is seen, then either the treatment is insufficient or the wound has become infected; in both cases, treatment must be changed. Determining the cause of the PI is important so that appropriate preventive measures can be implemented. The care team, in consultation with the individual and family, reviews the evaluation and care plan and determines, if possible, if the underlying cause is reversible so that appropriate treatment decisions can be made to ensure patient comfort. Consultation with a wound care specialist is advisable for wounds that are extensive or nonhealing. Specialized nurses such as enterostomal therapists or nurse practitioners, who may work with wound centers or surgeons, provide consultation in nursing homes, offices, or clinics.

◆ Pressure Injury Dressings

The type of dressing selected is based on careful evaluation of the condition of the PI; the presence of granulation, necrotic tissue, and slough; the amount of drainage; the microbial status; and the quality of the surrounding skin. If the wound has necrotic tissue, it must be debrided. Debridement methods include mechanical (whirlpool, wet-to-dry); sharp (scalpel, scissors); enzymatic (collagenase); and autolytic (hydrocolloid, hydrogel). Wound cleansing should be done with nontoxic preparations; normal saline is recommended. Other principles are presented in Box 14.9. Box 14.10 presents general guidelines for PI dressings.

There are many PI products and devices available but little research evidence regarding whether particular wound dressings or topical treatments and devices have a beneficial impact on wound healing, even compared with basic dressings (Westby et al., 2017). Quality research is needed on the effectiveness of the most widely used dressings and should include time to healing and whether healing occurs. Cost-effectiveness should also be considered.

BOX 14.9 Mnemonic for Pressure Injury Treatment: DIPAMOPI

Debride
Identify and treat infection
Pack dead space lightly
Absorb excess exudate
Maintain moist wound surface
Open or excise closed wound edges
Protect healing wound from infection/trauma
Insulate to maintain normal temperature

BOX 14.10 Factors to Consider in Selecting Pressure Injury Dressing

- Shallow, dry wounds with no/minimal exudate need hydrating dressings that add or trap moisture; very shallow wounds require cover dressing only (gels/transparent adhesive dressings, thin hydrocolloid, thin polyurethane foam).
- Shallow wounds with moderate to large exudate need dressings that absorb exudate, maintain moist surface, support autolysis if necrotic tissue is present, protect and insulate, and protect surrounding tissue (hydrocolloids, semipermeable polyurethane foam, calcium alginates, gauze). Cover with an absorptive cover dressing.
- Deep wounds with moderate to large exudate require filling of dead space, absorption of exudate, maintenance of moist environment, support of autolysis if necrotic tissue present, protection, and insulation (copolymer starch, dextranomer beads, calcium alginates, foam cavity). Cover with gauze pad, ABD, transparent thin film, or polyurethane foam.

Although further research is needed, the use of prophylactic multilayer silicone foam dressings, particularly on the heel and sacrum, can help in the prevention of PIs and shear and friction injuries and improve the microclimate of the skin. Prophylactic dressings must be considered an adjunct treatment to be used alongside standard pressure relieving measures (Ramundo et al., 2018).

Other general categories of wound care–related devices include compression therapy devices; off-weighting devices (off-loading); adjunctive therapies such as electrical stimulation and ultrasound and hyperbaric oxygen therapy (HBOT); negative pressure wound therapy (NPWT); and pressure redistribution surfaces (specialty beds, support surfaces). An evidence-based approach is recommended in the selection and prescription of equipment to prevent and manage wounds. Levine (2017b) comments that NPWT is an expensive cure-oriented treatment that is frequently overused in situations where treatment is hopeless. Health professionals need to consult reviews such as the Cochrane Review and clinical practice guidelines such as those from NPIAP when determining the most appropriate device or treatment. Specific product information can also be found in Box 14.2.

Provision of education to patients, families, and professional staff must also be included in any skin care program. Patient and family needs must be integrated into the plan of care. Teach the individual and their family about the normal healing process and keep them informed about progress (or lack of progress) toward healing, including signs and symptoms that should be brought to the professional's attention and education about any devices used.

KEY CONCEPTS

- The skin is the largest and most visible organ of the body; it has multiple roles in maintaining a person's health.
- Maintaining adequate oral hydration and skin lubrication will reduce the incidence of xerosis and other skin problems.
- The best way to minimize the risk of skin cancer is to avoid prolonged sun exposure.
- The primary risk factors for PI development are immobility and reduced activity.
- Changes in the skin with age, comorbid illnesses, nutritional status, low body mass, shear, and friction also increase PI risk. Individuals at greatest risk include those who are confined to a bed or chair and unable to shift weight or reposition themselves.
- Structured protocols and prevention bundles should be present in all facilities and have been shown to reduce PI development.
- A PI is documented by stage, which reflects the greatest degree of tissue damage, and as it heals, reverse staging is not appropriate.
- A PI covered in dead tissue (eschar or slough) cannot be staged until it is debrided.
- Darkly pigmented skin will not display the "typical" erythema of a stage 1 PI or early DTI; therefore, early recognition and analysis of cues in dark skinned individuals and closer vigilance is necessary.

ACTIVITIES AND DISCUSSION QUESTIONS

1. Describe the common skin conditions an older adult is likely to experience.
2. What is the nurse's responsibility in health promotion related to skin integrity?
3. How would you counsel an older adult about getting the Shingrix vaccine even if they have had previous vaccination with Zostavax?
4. What are early cues to deep pressure tissue injury in dark-skinned individuals?
5. Which evidence-based protocols can the nurse utilize for prevention of pressure injuries?

NEXT-GENERATION NCLEX® EXAMINATION-STYLE QUESTIONS

Ms. Patel, a 76-year-old female, is being admitted to skilled services following hospitalization for heart failure. She has a history of diabetes type 2, hypertension, osteoporosis, and peripheral vascular disease. She had a stroke 5 years ago and has left-sided hemiparesis. However, she can transfer herself from bed to wheelchair and propel herself around the facility. She is 5'6" and laughs when she says she has shrunk a couple of inches over the past decade. Her weight is 225 pounds and her BMI is 36.31 kg/m². Ms. Patel is oriented to person, place, and time. She denies any pain, although she says she takes acetaminophen at bedtime, because her left side aches after a day of activity. Her blood pressure is 138/86 mmHg, temperature 97.2°F, heart rate 96 beats per minute, respiratory rate 14 breaths per minute, oxygen saturation 96% on room air.

On examination, there is a dark pink, maculopapular rash under her left breast; it has a scalloped border with a white rim. Her left lateral olecranon process has a half-moon shaped wound with separation of the layers of skin with the edges rolled, the base of the wound is red and moist; the sacrum has a shallow wound measuring $2.6 \text{ mm} \times 2 \text{ mm} \times 2 \text{ mm}$; the wound bed is viable, red, and moist. On her left ischial tuberosity, there is a wound measuring $5 \text{ mm} \times 4.5 \text{ mm} \times 4 \text{ mm}$. Slough covers 25% of the wound bed; undermining that measures 3 mm is present from the 9 o'clock position to the 2 o'clock position. The wound has a moderate amount of serosanguinous drainage. Ms. Patel's left lateral malleolus has an area the size of a dime that is non-blanchable and tender. On her left heel, there is an intact, fluid-filled blister.

Choose the most likely options for the information missing from the statement below by selecting from the list of options provided.

The assessment findings indicate the client has a _____1_____ on her left lateral olecranon process; a _____2_____ on her sacrum; a _____3_____ on her left ischial tuberosity; a _____4_____ on her left lateral malleolus; and a _____5_____ on her left heel.

Options
Stage I pressure injury
Stage II pressure injury
Stage III pressure injury
Stave IV pressure injury
Unstageable Injury
Suspected deep tissue injury
Medical device related injury
Skin tear
Maceration

REFERENCES

Alderden, J., Cummins, M. R., Pepper, G. A., et al. (2017). Midrange Braden subscale scores are associated with increased risk for pressure injury development among critical care patients. *J Wound Ostomy Continence Nurs, 44*(5), 420–428.

Agency for Healthcare Research and Quality (AHQR) Safety Program for Nursing Homes. (2014). *On-time pressure ulcer prevention*. Rockville, MD: Agency for Healthcare Research and Quality. Content last reviewed November 2014. http://www.ahrq.gov/professionals/systems/long-term-care/resources/ontime/pruprev/pruprev-intro.html.

Ayello, E. A., Zulkowski, K., Capezuti, E., Jicman, W. H., & Sibbald, R. G. (2017). Educating nurses in the United States about pressure injuries. *Advance in Skin Wound Care, 30*(2), 83–94.

Bastidas, A., de la Sema, J., El Idrissi, M., et al. (2019). Effect of recombinant zoster vaccine on incidence of herpes zoster after autologous stem cell transplantation: a randomized clinical trial. *JAMA, 322*(2), 123–133.

Centers for Disease Control and Prevention: *Scabies*, 2020a. https://www.cdc.gov/parasites/scabies/index.html.

Centers for Disease Control and Prevention: *Shingles (herpes zoster)*, 2020b. https://www.cdc.gov/shingles/index.html.

Edsberg, L. E., Langemo, D., Baharestani, M. M., et al. (2014). Unavoidable pressure injury: state of the science and consensus outcomes. *Journal of Wound Ostomy Continence Nursing, 41*(4), 313–314.

Endo, J., Norman, R. (2014). Skin problems. In R. Ham, P. Sloane, G. Warshaw, J. Potter, & E. Flaherty (Eds.), *Ham's primary care geriatrics* (ed. 6, pp. 573–587). Philadelphia, PA, Elsevier Saunders.

Hampton, S. (2017). Could lateral tilt mattresses be the answer to pressure ulcer prevention and management? *Br Journal of Community Nursing, 22*(Suppl 3), S6–S12.

Irvin, C., Sedlak, E., Walton, C., Collier, S., & Bernhofer, E. I. (2017). Hospital-acquired pressure injuries: the significance of the advanced practice registered nurse's role in a community hospital. *Journal of American Association Nursing Practice, 29*(4), 203–208.

Jamshed, N., & Schneider, E. (2010). Is the use of supplemental vitamin C and zinc for the prevention and treatment of pressure ulcers evidence-based? *Annals Longterm Care, 18*, 28–32.

LeBlanc, K., & Baranoski, S. (2017). Skin tears: finally recognized. *Adv Skin Wound Care, 30*(2), 62–63.

LeBlanc, K., Baranoski, S., Christensen, D., et al. (2016). The art of dressing selection: a consensus statement on skin tears and best practice. *Advance in Skin Wound Care, 29*(1), 32–46.

Levine, J. M. (2017a). Skin failure: a new paradigm. *GeriPal*. http://www.geripal.org/2017/10/skin-failure-new-paradigm.html.

Levine, J. M. (2017b). Palliative wound care: a new frontier. *GeriPal*. http://www.geripal.org/2017/09/palliative-wound-care-new-frontier.html Last accessed March 2020.

Lucchini, A, Bambi, S, Elli, S, Tuccio, S, et al. (2020). Continuous monitoring of contact pressures in a general ICU: a prospective observational study. *Assist Inferm Ric, 39*(1), 5–12.

McCance, K. L., & Huether, S. E. (2014). Structure, function, and disorders of the integument. In K. L. McCance, & S. E. Huether (Eds.), *Pathophysiology* (ed. 7, pp. 1616–1651). St Louis, MO: Elsevier.

Murphree, R. W. (2017). Impairments in skin integrity. *Nursing Clinic North American, 52*, 405–417.

National Pressure Ulcer Advisory Panel: *PUSH tool,* 2014. https://npiap.com/page/Resources.

Ramundo, J., Pike, C., & Pittman, J. (2018). Do prophylactic foam dressings reduce heel pressure injuries?. *Journal of Wound Ostomy Continence Nursing, 45*(1), 75–82.

Roberts, S., Wallis, M., McInnes, E., et al. (2017). Patients' perceptions of a pressure ulcer prevention care bundle in hospital: a qualitative descriptive study to guide evidence-based practice. *Worldviews Evidence Based Nursing, 14*(5), 385–393.

Rondinelli, J., Zuniga, S., Kipnis, P., Kawar, L. N., Liu, V., & Escobar, G. J. (2018). Hospital-acquired pressure injury: risk-adjusted comparisons in an integrated healthcare delivery system. *Nursing Research, 67*(1), 16–25.

Schmitt, S., Andries, M. K., Ashmore, P. M., et al. (2017). WOCN Society position paper: Avoidable versus unavoidable pressure ulcers/injuries. *Journal of Wound Ostomy Continence Nursing, 44*(5), 458–468.

Scott, R. G., & Thurman, K. M. (2014). Visual feedback of continuous bedside pressure mapping to optimize effective patient repositioning. *Advance Wound Care, 3*(5), 376–382.

Skin Cancer Foundation: What you need to know about skin cancer 2020. Accessed February 2020. https://www.skincancer.org/.

Spilsbury, K., Nelson, A., Cullum, N., Iglesias, C., Nixon, J., & Mason, S. (2007). Pressure ulcers and their treatment and effects on quality of life: hospital inpatient perspectives. *Journal of Advance Nursing, 57*, 494–504.

United States Department of Health and Human Services, Office of Disease Prevention and Health Promotion (2012). *Healthy People 2020, 2012.*

Walia, G, Wong, A, Lo, A, Mackert, G, et al. (2016). Efficacy of monitoring devices in support of prevention of pressure injuries: systematic review and meta-analysis. *Advances in Skin & Wound Care, 29*, 568–574.

Westby, M. J., Dumville, J. C., Soares, M. O., Stubbs, N., & Norman, G. (2017). Dressings and topical agents for treating pressure ulcers. *Cochrane Database of System Review*. http://www.cochrane.org/CD011947/WOUNDS_which-dressings-or-topical-agents-are-most-effective-healing-pressure-ulcers.

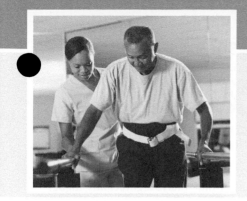

Clinical Judgment to Reduce Fall Risk and Injuries

Theris A. Touhy

http://evolve.elsevier.com/Touhy/gerontological/

LEARNING OBJECTIVES

Upon completion of this chapter, the reader will be able to:
- Identify factors that increase vulnerability to falls.
- Recognize and analyze the cues that indicate fall risk.
- List several actions to reduce fall risks and identify those at high risk.
- Describe the effects of physical restraints and identify alternative safety interventions.
- Utilize clinical judgment to identify and evaluate nursing actions to reduce falls and injury.

THE LIVED EXPERIENCE

After that fall last year when I slipped on the urine in the bathroom, I feel so insecure. I find myself taking small, shuffling steps to avoid falling again, but it makes me feel awkward and clumsy. When I was younger, I never worried about falling, but now I'm so afraid I will break a bone or something.

Betty, aged 75 years

FALLS

Falls are defined as any sudden drop from one surface to a lower surface with or without injury. Falls are one of the most important geriatric syndromes (Chapter 8) and the leading cause of morbidity and mortality for older adults. Falls are the most common adverse event in health care facilities and the leading cause of injury-related emergency department (ED) visits and injury-related deaths in older adults. Of particular concern, rates of fall-related ED visits and hospitalizations are increasing (de Vries et al., 2018) (Fig. 15.1). Each year, about one-third of adults aged 65 years or older and half of those aged 80 years and older will fall. More than half of those will fall more than once (Taylor-Piliae et al., 2017). Nearly half of all falls result in injury, of which 10% are serious.

About 3% to 20% of hospital inpatients fall at least once during their hospitalization (Quigley et al., 2016). Between 50% and 75% of nursing home residents fall

annually, twice the rate of community-dwelling older adults, and these falls result in more serious complications than other falls (Centers for Disease Control and Prevention [CDC], 2017). Nearly 50% of hospital admissions and most nursing home placements are a direct result of fall-related injuries such as hip fractures, upper limb injuries, and traumatic brain injuries (Taylor-Piliae et al., 2017). Estimates are that up to two-thirds of falls may be preventable (Gray-Miceli et al., 2016).

Falls are a significant public health problem and are considered a nursing-sensitive quality indicator. Falls with resultant fractures, dislocations, and crushing injuries are considered one of the ten hospital-acquired conditions (HAC) that are not covered under Medicare. All falls in long-term care facilities are considered sentinel events and must be reported to Centers for Medicare and Medicaid Services (CMS) with penalties of fines. *Healthy People 2020* includes several goals related to falls (Box 15.1).

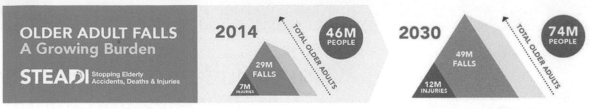

FIG. 15.1 Older Adult Falls: A Growing Burden. (From Centers for Disease Control and Prevention (2017). *STEADI Stopping Elderly Accidents, Deaths & Injuries*. https://www.cdc.gov/steadi/materials.html.)

⚡ SAFETY ALERT

The Quality and Safety Education for Nurses (QSEN) project has developed quality and safety measures for nursing and proposed targets for the knowledge, skills, and attitudes to be developed in nursing prelicensure and graduate programs. Education on falls and fall risk reduction is an important consideration in the QSEN safety competency, which addresses the need to minimize risk of harm to patients and providers through both system effectiveness and individual performance. Safe and effective transfer techniques are an important component of safety measures.

♥ BOX 15.1 Healthy People 2020

Falls, Fall Prevention, Injury

- Reduce the rate of emergency department visits due to falls among older adults.
- Reduce fatal and nonfatal injuries.
- Reduce hospitalizations for nonfatal injuries.
- Reduce emergency department visits for nonfatal injuries.
- Reduce fatal and nonfatal traumatic brain injuries.

From US Department of Health and Human Services, Office of Disease Prevention and Health Promotion (2012). *Healthy People 2020.* http://www.healthypeople.gov/2020.

Consequences of Falls

Hip Fractures

More than 95% of hip fractures among older adults are caused by falling, usually by falling sideways. Hip fractures are associated with considerable morbidity and mortality. The likelihood of recovery to prefracture level of function is less than 50% regardless of the individual's previous level of function. Returning to a high level of function is particularly low in those older than 85 years of age, with multiple comorbid conditions, or dementia. Morbidity and mortality are high, with approximately 10% of patients dying within 1 month, 30% at 1 year, and 80% at 8 years following hip fracture. This excess mortality persists for 10 years after the fracture and is higher in men. White women have significantly higher hip fracture rates than Black women as a result of a higher incidence of osteoporotic changes (CDC, 2017).

Traumatic Brain Injury

Traumatic brain injury (TBI) is associated with almost half of all admissions for major trauma in older adults. Older adults (75 years of age and older) have the highest rates of TBI-related hospitalization and death. Advancing age negatively affects the outcome after TBI, even with relatively minor head injuries. Factors that place the older adult at greater risk of TBI include the presence of comorbid conditions, use of antiplatelet and anticoagulant medications, and changes in the brain with age. Preinjury use of antiplatelet and anticoagulant medications is especially problematic with head trauma and increases the risk of traumatic intracranial hemorrhage and premature disability and death (Nishijima et al., 2017).

Brain changes with age, although clinically insignificant, do increase the risk of TBIs and especially subdural hematomas, which are much more common in older adults. There is a decreased adherence of the dura mater to the skull, increased fragility of bridging cerebral veins, and increases in the subarachnoid space and atrophy of the brain, which create more space within the cranial vault for blood to accumulate before symptoms appear.

Falls are the leading cause of TBI, but older adults may experience TBI with seemingly more minor incidents (e.g., sharp turns or jarring movement of the head). Some patients may not even remember the incident. TBIs have been associated with an earlier age of dementia onset and increasing the risk of Parkinson's disease (Gardner et al., 2018; Schaffert et al., 2018). In cases of moderate to severe TBI, there will be cognitive and physical sequelae obvious at the time of injury or shortly afterward that will require emergency treatment. However, older adults who experience a minor incident with seemingly lesser trauma to the head often present with more insidious and delayed symptom onset. Because of changes in the aging brain, there is an increased risk of slowly expanding subdural hematomas.

TBIs are often missed or misdiagnosed among older adults. If clinicians do not have information on the usual cognitive status of an older adult, manifestations of TBI are often misinterpreted as signs of dementia, which can lead to inaccurate prognoses and limit implementation of appropriate treatment. Health professionals should have a high suspicion of TBI in an older adult who falls and strikes their head or experiences even a minor event, such as sudden twisting of the head. For older adults who are receiving warfarin and experience minor head injury with a negative computed tomography (CT) scan, a protocol of 24-hour observation followed by a second CT scan is recommended. Box 15.2 presents signs and symptoms of TBI.

BOX 15.2 Signs and Symptoms of Traumatic Brain Injury in Older Adults[a]

Symptoms of Mild TBI
- Low-grade headache that will not dissipate
- Slowness in thinking, speaking, acting, or reading
- Getting lost or easily confused
- Feeling tired all the time, lack of energy or motivation
- Change in sleep pattern
- Loss of balance, feeling light-headed or dizzy
- Increased sensitivity to sounds, lights, distractions
- Blurred vision or eyes that tire easily
- Loss of sense of taste or smell
- Ringing in the ears
- Change in sex drive
- Mood changes

Symptoms of Moderate to Severe TBI
- Severe headache that gets worse or does not disappear
- Repeated vomiting or nausea
- Seizures
- Inability to wake from sleep
- Dilation of one or both pupils
- Slurred speech
- Weakness or numbness in the arms or legs
- Loss of coordination
- Increased confusion, restlessness, or agitation

[a]Older adults taking blood thinners should be seen immediately by a health care provider if they have a bump or blow to the head, even if they do not have any of the symptoms listed here.

Fear of Falling (Fallophobia)

Even if a fall does not result in injury, falls contribute to a loss of confidence that leads to reduced physical activity, increased dependency, and social withdrawal. Fear of falling (fallophobia) may restrict an individual's life space (area in which an individual performs activities). Fear of falling is an important predictor of general functional decline and a risk factor for future falls. Fallophobia is a significant cue to identifying risk of falls and implementing nursing actions for prevention. Nursing staff may also contribute to fear of falling in their patients by telling them not to get up by themselves or by using restrictive devices to keep them from independently moving. This further decreases mobility, safety, and function and increases fall risk. Mobility loss is common in older adults who are hospitalized for acute illness and is associated with poor outcomes, including loss of muscle mass and strength, long hospital stays, falls, and declines in ADL abilities post discharge. "Mobility loss is critical in the cascade to dependency" (Wald et al., 2019, p. 67).

Recommendations from a White Paper Report include mobility assessments, prescribed exercise programs, and changing the emphasis from the focus on falls to a focus on safe mobility (Martinez-Velilla et al., 2019). It is important to listen to the story of the individual's experience related to falling and the personal impact the fall experience has had on their life. In collaboration with the older adult, the nurse can more effectively design individualized actions to enhance independence, mobility, safety, and reduce fall risk. It is important to explore the personal accounts of older adults in research about falls and other experiences, but there exists little research in this area (Gray-Miceli, 2017).

Fall Risk Factors

Falls are a symptom of a problem and are rarely benign in older adults. The etiology of falls is multifactorial and the result of a convergence of risk factors across biological and behavioral aspects of the individual and factors in their environment. Episodes of acute illness or exacerbations of chronic illness are times of high fall risk and falls may indicate impending illness (Taylor-Piliae et al., 2017). New-onset delirium is a common cause of falls (Morley, 2017). Gray-Miceli and colleagues (2010, 2016) developed seven types of fall classifications based on research in nursing homes (Box 15.3). Several important risk factors are discussed below with implications for nursing actions.

⚡ SAFETY ALERT

A history of falls is a significant risk factor, and individuals who have fallen have three times the risk of falling again and being injured compared with persons who did not fall in the past year. Recurrent falls are often the result of the same underlying cause but can also be an indication of disease progression (e.g., heart failure, Parkinson's disease) or a new acute problem (e.g., infection, dehydration) (Taylor-Piliae et al., 2017).

BOX 15.3 Fall Classifications

- Falls resulting from acute events such as orthostatic hypotension, loss of balance, syncope
- Falls resulting from chronic events such as chronic dizziness or lower extremity weakness
- Falls resulting from medications
- Falls resulting from environmental mishaps
- Falls resulting from equipment malfunction
- Falls resulting from poor safety awareness
- Falls resulting from poor patient judgment

From Gray-Miceli, D., deCordova, P., Crane, G., Quigley P., Ratcliffe, S. (2016). Nursing home registered nurses' and licensed practical nurses' knowledge of causes of falls, *J Nurs Care Qual 31*(2),153–160.

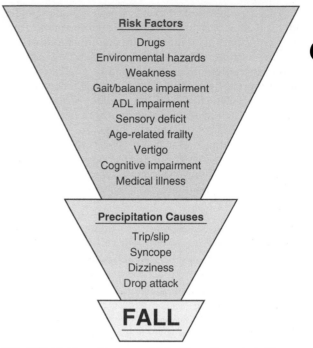

FIG. 15.2 Multifactorial nature of falls. (From Ham, R. J., Sloane, P. D., Warshaw, G. A., et al. (2014). *Primary care geriatrics* (6th ed.). Philadelphia: Elsevier.)

Individual risk factors can be categorized as either intrinsic or extrinsic. Intrinsic risk factors are unique to each individual and are associated with factors such as reduced vision and hearing, unsteady gait, cognitive impairment, acute and chronic illnesses, and effects of medications. Extrinsic risk factors are external to the individual and related to the physical environment and include lack of support equipment for bathtubs and toilets, height of beds, condition of floors, poor lighting, inappropriate footwear, and improper use of assistive devices (Fig. 15.2). Falls in the young–old and the healthier old occur more frequently because of external reasons; however, with increasing age and comorbid conditions, internal and locomotor reasons become increasingly prevalent as factors contributing to falls. The risk of falling increases as the number of risk factors increases.

Most falls occur from a combination of intrinsic and extrinsic factors that combine at a certain point in time. Community-dwelling older adults may fall for different reasons than individuals living in long-term care. Environmental factors (indoors and outdoors) may bring a higher risk of falls when combined with current health conditions. Falls in health care settings are more often related to the health status of the individual and the change in their environment (Kruschke & Butcher, 2017).

Inadequate staffing in health care settings is also a factor that may increase fall risk if patients attempt to get up for bathroom use or get out of bed because help is not readily available. Other factors may also influence risk for falls, including stressful life events such as illness, accidents, death of spouse/partner or close relatives or friends, loss of pet, financial trouble, a move or change in residence, or giving up an important hobby. Recognition and analysis of these cues associated with falls are important in determining actions for prevention.

Gait Disturbances

More than 60% in community-dwelling individuals over the age of 80 years experience gait disorders. Gait disorders are associated with a threefold increase in fall risk. Marked gait disorders are not normally a consequence of aging alone but are more likely indicative of an underlying pathological condition. Arthritis of the knee may result in ligamentous weakness and instability, causing the legs to give way or collapse. Diabetes, dementia, Parkinson's disease, stroke, alcoholism, and vitamin B deficiencies may cause neurological damage and resultant gait problems (Pirker & Katzenschlager, 2017). Gait deformities affect walking and balance. Fall assessments need to include assessment of gait using tools such as the Timed Up and Go (TUG) test (Fig. 15.3) and 30-Second Chair Stand.

Foot Deformities

Foot deformities and ill-fitting footwear also contribute to gait problems and potential for falls. Care of the feet is an important aspect of mobility, comfort, and a stable gait and is often neglected. Little attention is given to a person's feet until they interfere with walking and moving and ultimately the ability to remain independent. Foot problems are often unrecognized and untreated,

ASSESSMENT

Timed Up & Go (TUG)

Patient _____

Date _____

Time _____ ☐ AM ☐ PM

Purpose: To assess mobility

Equipment: A stopwatch

Directions: Patients wear their regular footwear and can use a walking aid, if needed. Begin by having the patient sit back in a standard arm chair and identify a line 3 meters, or 10 feet away, on the floor.

OBSERVATIONS

Observe the patient's postural stability, gait, stride length, and sway.

Check all that apply:

① **Instruct the patient:**

NOTE: Always stay by the patient for safety.

When I say **"Go,"** I want you to:

1. Stand up from the chair.
2. Walk to the line on the floor at your normal pace.
3. Turn.
4. Walk back to the chair at your normal pace.
5. Sit down again.

② **On the word "Go," begin timing.**
③ **Stop timing after patient sits back down.**
④ **Record time.**

☐ Slow tentative pace
☐ Loss of balance
☐ Short strides
☐ Little or no arm swing
☐ Steadying self on walls
☐ Shuffling
☐ En bloc turning
☐ Not using assistive device properly

These changes may signify neurological problems that require further evaluation.

Time in Seconds: _____

An older adult who takes ≥12 seconds to complete the TUG is at risk for falling.

CDC's STEADI tools and resources can help you screen, assess, and intervene to reduce your patient's fall risk. For more information, visit www.cdc.gov/steadi

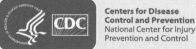

Centers for Disease Control and Prevention
National Center for Injury Prevention and Control

2017

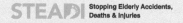

STEADI Stopping Elderly Accidents, Deaths & Injuries

FIG. 15.3 Timed Up and Go (TUG). (From Centers for Disease Control and Prevention. https://www.cdc.gov /steadi/pdf/TUG_Test-print.pdf.)

leading to considerable dysfunction. Older adults may consider foot problems and foot pain to be part of aging rather than a treatable medical condition (Menz, 2016).

As we age, feet are subjected to a lifetime of stress and may not be able to continue to adapt and inflammatory changes in bone and soft tissue can occur. Foot problems are present in a large number of older adults and may include foot pain, nail fungus, dry skin, corns and calluses, bunions, and neuropathy. Some older adults are unable to walk comfortably, or at all, because of neglect of corns, bunions, and overgrown nails. Other causes of problems may be traced to loss of fat cushioning and resilience with aging, diabetes, ill-fitting shoes, poor arch support, excessively repetitive weight-bearing activities, obesity, or uneven distribution of weight on the feet.

Foot health and function may reflect systemic disease or give early clues to physical illness. Sudden or gradual changes in the condition of nails or skin of the feet or the appearance of recurring infections may be precursors of more serious health problems. Rheumatological disorders such as the various forms of arthritis can also affect the feet. Gout occurs most often in the joint of the great toe but is a systemic disease. Both diabetes and peripheral vascular disease (PVD) commonly cause problems in the lower extremities that can quickly become life-threatening (Chapter 20).

Care of the foot takes a team approach, including the individual, the nurse, the podiatrist, and the primary health care provider. Nursing care of an individual with foot problems should be directed toward providing optimal comfort and function, removing possible mechanical irritants, and decreasing the likelihood of infection. The nurse has the important function of assessing the feet for clues of functional ability and their owner's well-being (Box 15.4). Difficulty cutting toenails is common in older adults, since it requires joint flexibility, manual dexterity, and visual acuity, and nurses often care for toenails. Appropriate cutting of toenails is important, and safety precautions are essential. Nurses can identify potential and actual problems and make referral to or seek assistance as needed from the primary care provider or podiatrist for any changes in the feet. Regular podiatry treatment can maintain or improve foot health in older adults.

Orthostatic and Postprandial Hypotension

Declines in depth perception, proprioception, and normotensive response to postural changes are important factors that contribute to falls (Finucane et al., 2017). Clinically significant orthostatic hypotension (OH) is a common clinical finding in older adults who are frail and has been reported to be present in up to 50% of older adults in nursing homes. OH is considered a decrease of

---

BOX 15.4   Tips for Best Practice

Recognizing and Analyzing Cues to Care of the Foot

Observation of Mobility
- Gait
- Use of assistive devices
- Footwear type and pattern of wear

Past Medical History
- Neuropathies
- Musculoskeletal limitations
- Peripheral vascular disease (PVD)
- Vision problems
- History of falls
- Pain affecting movement

Bilateral Assessment
- Color
- Circulation and warmth
- Pulses
- Structural deformities
- Skin lesions
- Lower-extremity edema
- Evidence of scratching
- Abrasions and other lesions
- Rash or excessive dryness
- Condition and color of toenails

---

20 mmHg (or more) in systolic pressure and/or a decrease of 10 mmHg (or more) in diastolic pressure with position change from lying or sitting to standing. Measurement of OH in everyday nursing practice is often overlooked or assessed inaccurately and needs to be included as a competency in nursing education and practice (Box 15.5). However, there is considerable variability in the recommendations by clinical experts regarding the timing and position of blood pressure measurements, and further research is needed (Lipsitz, 2017). The detection of OH is of clinical importance to fall prevention because OH is treatable.

Postprandial hypotension (PPH) is associated with increased risk of syncope and falls. PPH occurs after ingestion of a carbohydrate meal and may be related to the release of a vasodilatory peptide, but research is needed on the epidemiology and pathophysiology of PPH. PPH is usually asymptomatic and may be overlooked. Patients with neurological disease and diabetes have a higher frequency of PPH. Lifestyle interventions such as increasing water intake before eating or eating smaller, more frequent meals may be important, but further research is needed. Older individuals with

BOX 15.5 Measuring Orthostatic Blood Pressure

- Orthostatic hypotension is more common in the morning, and therefore assessment should occur then.
- Ask the individual to lie down for 5 minutes.
- Measure blood pressure and pulse rate in both arms. Use the arm with the higher blood pressure for measurements following position change.
- Ask the individual to stand (use safety precautions as needed). If unable to stand, measure blood pressure sitting with feet hanging.
- Take the blood pressure immediately after standing and ask about dizziness.
- Repeat blood pressure and pulse rate measurements after standing for 3 minutes and ask about dizziness.
- A drop in BP of ≥20 mmHg or in diastolic BP of ≥10 mmHg or experiencing light-headedness, dizziness, or loss of balance is considered abnormal.

From Momeyer M. (2014). Orthostatic Hypotension in Older Adults with Dementia. *J Gerontol Nurs.* 40(6) 22-29. doi:10.3928/00989134-20140421-01. Reprinted with permission from SLACK Incorporated.

risk factors should be cautioned against sudden rising from sitting or supine positions, particularly after eating. Measurement of OH should be conducted after a fall, particularly if related to a meal (Krbot Skoric et al., 2017).

Cognitive Impairment

Older adults with cognitive impairment are at double the risk of falling compared with age-matched individuals, with reports of 60% to 80% falling within a year of diagnosis of dementia. A twofold increased fall risk is present even in mild impairment (Peach et al., 2017). Cognition plays a crucial role in control of gait and individuals with cognitive impairment may have an altered gait pattern. Other factors such as medications (neuroleptics), visual acuity, functional impairments, falls history, insight, memory, and behavior contribute to the complex mix of risk factors for falls in this population.

There is little research on fall prevention programs for individuals with cognitive impairment, but combined cognitive and physical interventions have been reported to improve balance, functional mobility, and gait speed in individuals with mild cognitive impairment. Further research is needed to determine the most appropriate fall risk-reduction programs for the different stages of dementia (Lach et al., 2017). Fall risk evaluation should include more specific cognitive risk factors, and cognitive assessment measures need to be conducted more frequently with individuals at risk of falls (Booth et al., 2015, 2016).

Vision and Hearing

Vision and hearing impairment have been associated with falls and should be assessed in older adults and corrected as much as possible (Chapter 19). Poor visual acuity, reduced contrast sensitivity, decreased visual field, cataracts, and use of nonmiotic glaucoma medications have all been associated with falls. There is little research on interventions for either vision or hearing problems and falls and fractures (Gopinath et al., 2016; Gupta et al., 2017).

Medications

Medications implicated in increasing fall risk include those causing potentially dangerous side effects including drowsiness, mental confusion, problems with balance, loss of urinary control, and sudden drops in blood pressure with standing. These include antidepressants, antihypertensives, diuretics, some analgesics, sedative-hypnotics, and psychotropic medications. The association between psychotropic medications and falls is well established (de Vries et al., 2018). Antidepressant use is also associated with an increased risk of hip fracture among older adults (Torvinen-Kiiskinen et al., 2017).

The literature on cardiovascular medications as potential fall-risk–increasing drugs is conflicting and needs further research. In a systematic meta-analysis (de Vries et al., 2018), loop diuretics and digitalis were consistently associated with increased fall risk. Additionally, the initiation of cardiovascular drugs showed an association with increased risk of falling. When cardiovascular drugs are prescribed, beginning with a smaller dose, increasing the dose slowly, monitoring response, and fall prevention teaching are important.

Medication review is an evidence-based strategy for reducing falls among older adults. Attention to medications should become a key focus of public health educational efforts and fall prevention in all settings (Phelan et al., 2017). All medications, including over-the-counter (OTC) and herbal medications, should be reviewed and limited to those that are absolutely essential. The addition of any new medication should trigger a fall risk evaluation (Musich et al., 2017). Psychotropic prescribing should be carefully considered, initiated at low doses, and monitored closely. If these medications are being used, patient teaching should be provided related to fall risk, fall prevention interventions, appropriate dosing, and use of other medications, such as benzodiazepines, and alcohol (Chapter 24). Chapter 9 discusses geropharmacology and Chapter 25 discusses the use of these medications and alternative approaches for behavioral symptoms that may occur in individuals with dementia.

❖ USING CLINICAL JUDGMENT TO PROMOTE HEALTHY AGING: FALL PREVENTION

◆ Recognizing and Analyzing Cues: Fall Risk

The American Geriatrics Society/British Geriatrics Society *Clinical Practice Guideline: Prevention of Falls in Older Persons* (2010) recommends that fall risk analysis be an integral part of primary health care for the older adult. All older adults should be asked whether they have fallen in the past year and whether they experience difficulties with walking or balance. In addition, ask about falls that did not result in an injury and the circumstances of a near-fall, mishap, or misstep because this may provide important information for prevention of future falls. Older adults may be reluctant to share information about falls for fear of losing independence, therefore the nurse must use judgment and empathy in eliciting information about falls, assuring the individual that there are many modifiable factors to increase safety and to help maintain independence.

The risk analysis varies with the target population. General guidelines are as follows:

- Low-risk community-dwelling individuals should be asked at least once a year about fall occurrence and circumstances.
- Individuals who report a single fall should be evaluated for mobility impairment and unsteadiness using a simple observational test (Fig 15.3), and those who demonstrate mobility problems or unsteadiness should be referred for further assessment.
- High-risk populations (individuals who have had multiple falls in the past year, have abnormalities of gait and/or balance, have received medical attention related to a fall, or reside in a nursing home) should undergo a more comprehensive risk analysis.

◆ Considerations in Hospital/Long-Term Care

Individuals admitted to acute or long-term care settings should have an initial analysis of fall risk on admission, after any change in condition, and at regular intervals during their stay. This is an ongoing process that includes multiple and continual types of fall risk analysis and evaluation following a fall or intervention to reduce the risk of a fall. An interprofessional team (physician or nurse practitioner, nurse, risk manager, physical and occupational therapists, and other designated staff) should be involved in planning care on the basis of findings from the evaluations. Nurses bring expert knowledge of patient activities, abilities, and needs from a 24-hours-per-day, 7-days-per-week perspective to help the team implement the most appropriate actions and evaluate outcomes.

Identifying Fall Risk

A single screening question, "Have you fallen in the past year?" is highly effective (Tatum et al., 2018). Other key questions that can be asked to alert clinicians to fall risk and the need for more follow-up include: (1) Have you fallen in the past year? (2) Do you feel unsteady when standing or walking? (3) Are you worried about falling? Red flag risk factors such as osteoporosis, mobility problems, or anticoagulant therapy also alert the clinician of the need for further assessment. A screening tool that can be completed by the individual is available from the STEADI (*Stopping Elderly Accidents, Deaths, and Injuries*) program (CDC, 2017) (Box 15.6).

Fall risk instruments are still commonly included in fall prevention interventions; instruments that are utilized need to be reliable and valid and nurses need to use them judiciously. Often, these instruments are completed in a

---

BOX 15.6 Resources for Best Practice

Fall Prevention and Restraint Alternatives

- **Agency for Healthcare Research and Quality (AHRQ):** Preventing falls in hospitals: a toolkit for improving quality of care. https://www.ahrq.gov/professionals/systems/hospital/fallpxtoolkit/index.html.
- **Centers for Disease Control and Prevention (CDC):** STEADI (Stopping Elderly Accidents, Deaths and Injuries): Educational materials for patients and providers; Check for safety: a home fall prevention checklist for older adults; Safe patient handling for schools of nursing (curricular materials). https://www.cdc.gov/steadi/materials.html.
- **Gericareonline:** Story of Your Falls. http://www.gericareonline.net/tools/eng/falls/index.html
- **HELP (Hospital Elder Life) Program:** http://www.hospitalelderlifeprogram.org/public/public-main.php.
- **Hartford Institute for Geriatric Nursing (consultgeri.org):** Fall prevention: assessment, diagnosis, intervention strategies, Hendrich II Fall Risk Model; Avoiding restraints in hospitalized older adults with dementia; Dementia series, therapeutic activity kits.
- **National Council on Aging:** National Falls Prevention Resource Center.https://www.ncoa.org/center-for-healthy-aging/falls-resource-center/.
- **The GROW Program:** Getting residents out of wheelchairs. http://www.thegrowprogram.net/.
- **The Joint Commission: Targeted Solutions Tool for Preventing Falls (TST):** Provides in-depth support to help hospitals in fall prevention efforts. https://www.centerfortransforminghealthcare.org/tst_pfi.aspx.
- **Veterans Affairs (VA) National Center for Patient Safety:** Falls Toolkit. https://www.patientsafety.va.gov/professionals/onthejob/falls.asp.

routine manner and risk factors are not identified or may not be known because of lack of assessment and knowledge of the individual's history. A fall risk score is not an adequate predictor of falls. To be able to prevent a fall, it is important to know why someone is at risk of falling, identification of the individual's actual fall and injury risk factors, factors that are modifiable and those that are not, treatment of modifiable factors, and helping patients compensate for those that are not modifiable. This information is obtained from comprehensive fall risk analysis. Additional research is needed to develop valid, reliable instruments to differentiate levels of fall risk in various settings.

The National Center for Patient Safety recommends the Morse Falls Scale, but not for use in long-term care. The Hendrich II Fall Risk Model, which also includes a modified Get Up and Go test, is recommended by the Hartford Foundation for Geriatric Nursing (Box 15.6). This instrument has been validated with skilled nursing and rehabilitation populations and is also easy to use in the outpatient setting. In the skilled nursing facility, the Minimum Data Set (MDS 3.0) includes information about history of falls and hip fractures, observation of balance during transitions and walking (moving from seated to standing, walking, turning around, moving on and off toilet, and transfers between bed and chair or wheelchair) (Chapter 8).

Postfall Assessment (PFA)

A comprehensive analysis of a fall is an integral component of fall prevention programs in institutional settings. It is important to identify underlying causes of falls and risk factors. The purpose is to identify the clinical status of the individual, verify and treat injuries, identify underlying causes of the fall when possible, and assist in implementing appropriate individualized risk-reduction interventions. Incomplete analysis of the reasons for a fall can result in repeated incidents. If the patient cannot tell you about the circumstances of the fall, information should be obtained from staff or witnesses. Standard "incident report" forms do not provide adequate PFA information.

Conducting a postfall huddle (after action review) as soon as possible after a fall adds to information about the circumstances of the fall. Staff at all levels should be involved, as well as the patient, to discuss the fall: what happened, how it happened, why it happened, how the outcome could be avoided the next time, what is the follow-up plan. Other components to be addressed in the PFA are presented in Box 15.7. The Department of Veterans Affairs National Center for Patient Safety provides comprehensive information about fall risk reduction, policies and procedures, and includes a postfall huddle guide. For

---

BOX 15.7 Evaluation Post Fall

Initiate emergency measures as indicated.

History
- Description of the fall from the individual or witness
- Individual's opinion of the cause of the fall
- Circumstances of the fall (trip or slip)
- Person's activity at the time of the fall
- Presence of comorbid conditions, such as a previous stroke, Parkinson's disease, osteoporosis, seizure disorder, sensory deficit, joint abnormalities, depression, cardiac disease
- Medication review
- Associated symptoms, such as chest pain, palpitations, light-headedness, vertigo, loss of balance, fainting, weakness, confusion, incontinence, or dyspnea
- Time of day and location of the fall
- Presence of acute illness

Physical Examination
- Vital signs: postural blood pressure changes, fever, or hypothermia
- Head and neck: visual impairment, hearing impairment, nystagmus, bruit
- Heart: arrhythmias or valvular dysfunction
- Neurological signs: altered mental status, focal deficits, peripheral neuropathy, muscle weakness, rigidity or tremor, impaired balance
- Musculoskeletal signs: arthritic changes, range of motion (ROM) changes, podiatric deformities or problems, swelling, redness or bruises, abrasions, pain on movement, shortening and external rotation of lower extremities

Functional Assessment
- Functional gait and balance: observe resident rising from chair, walking, turning, and sitting
- Balance test, mobility, use of assistive devices or personal assistance, extent of ambulation, restraint use, prosthetic equipment
- Activities of daily living: bathing, dressing, transferring, toileting

Environmental Assessment
- Staffing patterns, unsafe practice in transferring, delay in response to call light
- Faulty equipment
- Use of bed, chair alarm
- Call light within reach
- Wheelchair, bed locked
- Adequate supervision
- Clutter, walking paths not clear
- Dim lighting
- Glare
- Uneven flooring
- Wet, slippery floors
- Poorly fitted seating devices
- Inappropriate footwear
- Inappropriate eyewear

falls that happen outside the hospital or skilled nursing facility, individuals can complete the "Story of Your Falls" to provide PFA information (Box 15.6).

Nursing Actions: Fall Prevention

Nurses play a major role in fall prevention but fall prevention is a shared responsibility of all health care providers caring for older adults. Across settings of care, fall prevention programs incorporating multifactorial and interprofessional approaches, aimed at multiple risk factors contributing to falls, are the most effective (Gray-Miceli et al., 2017; Isaranuwatchai et al., 2017; Jackson, 2016). The focus of the program may differ according to the setting (community, hospital, home, long-term care) (Kruschke & Butcher, 2017). Engaging older adults in teaching about fall prevention is especially important during the transition from hospital to home.

Transitional care programs need to be tailored for fall risk and prevention. Homebound or semi-homebound older adults are another population at risk of falls and are 50% more likely to experience a fall than non-homebound individuals. Impaired balance was the strongest predictor for falls in this population, followed by problems moving around in the home. Recognizing and analyzing these cues is important to implement nursing actions to tailor fall prevention programs in the home setting and during transitions of care (Zhao et al., 2018).

Choosing the most appropriate actions to reduce the risk of falls depends on appropriate evaluation at various intervals depending on the individual's changing condition and tailoring interventions to individual cognitive function, language, and health literacy. A one-size-fits-all approach is not effective. Further research is needed to determine the type, frequency, and timing of interventions best suited for specific populations. The majority of research on fall-risk reduction interventions has been conducted with community-dwelling older adults and there is a need for more research on effective interventions in acute and long-term care settings. CDC's STEADI program provides excellent free materials on fall prevention for health care providers and older adults (Box 15.6).

Fall Risk Reduction Programs

Fall risk reduction programs in hospitals and long-term care settings should be designed to meet organizational needs and to match patient population needs and clinical realities of the staff. A system-level quality improvement approach, including educational programs for staff, has been reported to reduce fall rates in hospitals and nursing homes (Dykes et al., 2017; Gray-Miceli et al., 2016, 2017; Quigley et al., 2016). Suggested components of fall prevention programs are presented in Box 15.8. Some

---

BOX 15.8 Suggested Components of Fall Risk Reduction Interventions

- Adaptation or modification of the home environment
- Withdrawal or minimization of psychoactive medications
- Withdrawal or minimization of other medications
- Detection and prevention of delirium
- Management of orthostatic hypotension
- Continence programs such as prompted voiding
- Management of foot problems and footwear
- Exercise, particularly balance, strength, and gait training
- Staff and patient education

From American Geriatrics Society/British Geriatrics Society (2010). *2010 AGS/BGS clinical practice guideline: Prevention of falls in older persons, Summary of recommendations.* https://geriatricscareonline.org/application/content/products/CL014/html/CL014_BOOK001.html.

---

examples of effective programs in acute care settings include Acute Care of the Elderly units (ACE), Nurses Improving Care for Healthsystem Elders (NICHE), and the Geriatric Resource Nurse (GRN) model. The Hospital Elder Life Program (HELP) is another valuable resource in fall prevention in the hospital (Chapter 1). The optimal bundle of interventions is not established but suggested system-level interventions are presented in Box 15.9.

Group and home-based exercise programs, along with home safety interventions, reduced the rate of falls and risk of falling in community-dwelling older adults. Vision screening, medication reduction, evaluation of cardiovascular syncope and postural hypotension, providing hip protectors and other assistive devices, and education on falls and fall prevention have also been associated with decreased fall risk (Taylor-Piliae et al., 2017). Home-based Tai Chi Chuan (TCC) has been shown to reduce falls and improve physical performance among older adults in

---

BOX 15.9 System-Level Interventions for Fall Risk Reduction in Acute Care

- Nurse champions
- Teach backs (all patients and families receive education about their fall and injury risks)
- Comfort care and safety rounds
- Safety huddle post fall
- Protective bundles: Patients with risk factors for serious injury, such as osteoporosis, anticoagulant use, and history of head injury or falls, are automatically placed on high fall risk precautions and interventions to reduce risk of serious injury.
- Bundles may include interventions such as bedside mat on floor at side of bed, height-adjustable bed, helmet use, hip protectors, comfort and safety rounds.

community settings more than conventional lower extremity exercise training (Hwang et al., 2016; Li et al., 2016).

Environmental Modifications

Among community-living older adults, falls are more likely to occur during activities of daily living but occur most frequently when the individual is transferring or changing physical positions (sitting to standing, using a bathtub/shower, or walking downstairs). Environmental modifications alone have not been shown to reduce falls, but when included as part of a multifactorial program, they may be of benefit in risk reduction. A home safety assessment and home modification interventions have been shown to reduce the rates of falls, especially for individuals at high risk and those with visual impairments. However, referrals for home safety assessment are not consistently done in primary care (Phelan et al., 2016). A recent survey of community-living older adults found that approximately one-half reported never seeing a home safety checklist, an accessible and easy tool for older adults to complete (Lach & Noimontree, 2018). As part of the STEADI program, the CDC provides a comprehensive home fall prevention checklist that can be used by older adults and clinicians (Box 15.6).

In institutional settings, the patient care environment should be evaluated routinely for extrinsic factors that may contribute to falls and corrective action taken. About 50% to 70% of falls in hospitals occur while transferring between bed and chair; and 10% to 20% occur in bathrooms (Quigley et al., 2016). Patients should be able to access the bathroom or be provided with a bedside commode, routine assistance to toilet, and programs such as prompted voiding (Chapter 12). Dual-stiffness flooring, which incorporates a layer of compressible material meant to cushion falls, can reduce fractures in nursing homes (Morley, 2017).

Assistive Devices

Research on multifactorial interventions including the use of assistive devices has demonstrated benefits in fall risk reduction. Many devices are available that are designed for specific conditions and limitations. Physical therapists provide training on use of assistive devices and nurses can supervise correct use. Improper use of these devices can lead to increased fall risk. For the community-dwelling individual, Medicare may cover up to 80% of the cost of assistive devices with a written prescription. New technologies such as "smart canes" that assess gait and fall risk or that "talk" and provide feedback to the user, sensors that detect when falls have occurred or when risk of falling is increasing, and other developing assistive technologies hold the potential to improve functional ability, safety, and independence significantly for older adults (Muchna et al., 2017) (Chapter 16).

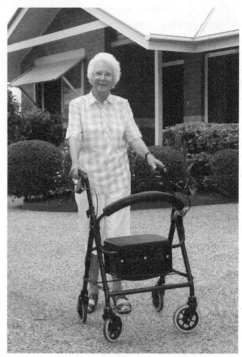

Maintaining ambulation and safety with appropriate assistive devices. (© iStock.com/pamspix.)

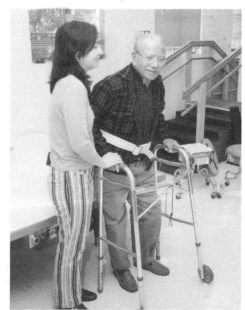

A physical therapist helping a client to ambulate. (From Igna- tavicius, D. D., Workman, M. L. (2010). *Medical-surgical nursing: Patient-centered collaborative care* (6th ed.). St Louis: Saunders.)

Safe Patient Handling

Lifting, transferring, and repositioning patients are the most common tasks that lead to injury for health care staff and patients in hospital and nursing home environments. Handling and moving patients offers multiple challenges because of variations in size, physical abilities, cognitive function, level of cooperation, and changes in condition. Evidence-based practices for safe patient handling include: (1) use of patient handling equipment/devices; (2) patient-care ergonomic assessment protocols; (3) no lift policies; (4) training on proper use of patient handling equipment/devices; and (5) patient lift teams. Examples of helpful equipment are ceiling- and floor-based dependent lifts, sit-to-stand assists, ambulation aids, motorized hospital beds, powered shower chairs, and friction-reducing devices (American Nurses Association, 2013; Campo et al., 2013). Key aspects of patient assessment to improve safety for patients and staff are presented in Box 15.10.

BOX 15.10   Tips for Best Practice

Evidence-Based Practices for Safe Patient Handling and Movement

- Ability of the patient to provide assistance
- Ability of the patient to bear weight
- Upper extremity strength of the patient
- Ability of the patient to cooperate and follow instructions
- Patient height and weight
- Special circumstances likely to affect transfer or repositioning tasks, such as abdominal wounds, contractures, pressure injuries, presence of tubes
- Specific physician orders or physical therapy recommendations that relate to transferring or repositioning patients (e.g., knee or hip replacement precautions)

From Nelson, A., Baptiste, A. (2004). Evidence-based practices for safe patient handling and movement, *Online J Issues Nurs 9*(3). http://www.seiu1991.org/files/2013/07/Audrey_Nelson_Safe_Patient_Handling.pdf.

Wheelchairs

Wheelchairs are a necessary adjunct at some level of immobility and for some individuals, but they are overused in long-term care facilities, with up to 80% of residents spending time sitting in a wheelchair every day. Often, the individual is not evaluated for therapeutic treatment and restorative ambulation programs to improve mobility and function. Improperly maintained or ill-fitting wheelchairs can cause pressure injuries, skin tears, bruises and abrasions, and nerve impingement, and contribute to falls in nursing homes. It is important that a professional evaluate the wheelchair for proper fit and provide training on proper use, and evaluate the resident for more appropriate mobility and seating devices and ambulation programs. There are many new assistive devices that could replace wheelchairs, such as small walkers with wheels and seats.

All long-term care facilities need to implement programs that promote ambulation and improve function. Brief walks and repeated chair stands four times a day improved walking and endurance in frail, deconditioned, cognitively impaired nursing home residents. If the individual is unable to ambulate without assistance, they should be seated in a comfortable chair with frequent repositioning and wheelchairs should be used for transport only. Electric scooters and wheelchairs may also be appropriate for some residents, but instruction on safe use is necessary. The GROW initiative (Getting Residents Out of Wheelchairs) (Box 15.6) was conceived by a group of health professionals to lobby against the overuse of wheelchairs in nursing homes. The program advocates for increased ambulation whenever possible and decreasing the use of wheelchairs when regular chairs could be used for stationary seating.

Osteoporosis Treatment/Vitamin D Supplementation

Practice guidelines recommend calcium and vitamin D supplements for older adults with osteoporosis to prevent fractures. Evidence of the association between calcium, vitamin D, or combined calcium and vitamin D supplements and fracture risk has not reached consistent conclusions. A recent meta-analysis reported that calcium, calcium plus vitamin D, and vitamin D supplementation were not significantly associated with a lower incidence of hip, nonvertebral, vertebral, or total fractures in community-dwelling older adults. There is evidence that these supplements may lower fracture risk for individuals living in residential institutions because of their poorer mobility, infrequent sun exposure, and poorer diet. However, findings do not support the routine use of these supplements in community-dwelling older adults (Zhao et al., 2017) (Chapter 21).

Hip Protectors

The use of hip protectors for prevention of hip fractures in high-risk individuals may be considered. There is some evidence that they may be protective when used in individuals who are at risk of hip fracture, but further research is needed to determine their effectiveness (Quigley et al., 2016). Compliance has been a concern related to the ease of application and removing them quickly enough for toileting, but newer designs that are more attractive and practical may assist with compliance issues.

Alarms/Motion Sensors/Staff Observation

Alarms, either personal or chair/bed, are often used in fall risk reduction programs. Alarms were designed to be early warning systems and there has been no research to support their effectiveness in prevention of a fall. Use of alarms may increase patient agitation, especially in individuals with cognitive impairment. Silent alarms, visual or auditory monitoring systems, motion detectors, and physical staff presence may be more effective. Continuous video monitoring has been demonstrated as an effective intervention to reduce significantly the incidence of patient falls and the likelihood of injury if the patient does experience a fall. Motion sensors inside patient rooms may be another viable, cost-efficient, unobtrusive solution to prevent and detect falls (Potter et al., 2017; Rantz et al., 2015; Sand-Jecklin et al., 2016). One of the most effective methods used in fall prevention is assessing patients' needs every 1 to 2 hours (Jackson, 2016).

The use of direct in-person observation in care of hospitalized older adults (sitters) is a common intervention utilized to prevent falls and injury. This practice is costly and has not been evaluated for effectiveness in preventing falls. "There is a need for additional, more rigorous research to quantify the extent of this practice, clarify indications for its use and discontinuation, and document outcomes of care delivered through direct observation and associated care costs. The perspectives of patients and family caregivers is needed to fully understand the true impact of direct observation practices" (Gilmore Bykovskyi et al., 2020, p. 23).

RESTRAINTS AND SIDE RAILS

Definition and History

A physical restraint is defined as any manual method, physical or mechanical device, material, or equipment that immobilizes or reduces the ability of a patient to move their arms, legs, body, or head freely. A chemical restraint is when a drug or medication is used as a restriction to manage the patient's behavior or restrict the patient's freedom of movement and is not a standard treatment or dosage for the patient's condition. Historically, restraints and side rails have been used for the "protection" of the patient and for the security of the patient and staff. Originally, restraints were used to control the behavior of individuals with mental illness considered to be dangerous to themselves or others (Evans & Strumpf, 1989).

Research over the past 35 years by nurses such as Lois Evans, Neville Strumpf, and Elizabeth Capezuti has shown that the practice of physical restraint is ineffective and hazardous. The use of physical restraints in long-term care settings was effectively addressed 25 years ago in these facilities. The Joint Commission and the CMS have focused on restraint reduction strategies in acute care over the past 10 to 15 years, but studies continue to document that it is routine practice (Lach & Leach, 2016).

Consequences of Restraints

Physical restraints, intended to prevent injury, do not protect patients from falling, wandering, or removing tubes and other medical devices. Physical restraints may actually exacerbate many of the problems for which they are used and can cause serious injury and death, and emotional and physical problems. Physical restraints are associated with higher death rates, injurious falls, nosocomial infections, incontinence, contractures, pressure injuries, agitation, and depression. Injuries occur as a result of the patient attempting to remove the restraint or attempting to get out of bed while restrained. The use of restraints is a great source of physical and psychological distress to older adults and may intensify agitation and contribute to depression.

> "I felt like a dog and cried all night. It hurt me to have to be tied up. I felt like I was nobody; that I was dirt. The hospital is worse than a jail."

Side Rails

Side rails are no longer viewed as simply attachments to a patient's bed but are considered restraints with all the accompanying concerns just discussed. Side rails are now defined as restraints or restrictive devices when used to impede a person's ability to get out of bed voluntarily if the person cannot lower them by themselves. Side rails may be seen as a barrier rather than a reminder of the need to request assistance with transfers. Restrictive side rail use is defined as two full-length or four half-length raised side rails. If the patient uses a half- or quarter-length upper side rail to assist in getting in and out of bed, it is not considered a restraint.

The proper use of side rails can be considered a means of assisting in-bed movement and getting in and out of bed (Morse et al., 2015). Side rails manufactured for use on hospital beds have been redesigned and are no longer a threat to patient entrapment but use of outmoded designs and incorrect assembly continue to be a concern. The CMS requires nursing homes to conduct individualized evaluations of residents, provide alternatives, or clearly document the need for restrictive side rails.

Restraint-Free Care

Restraint-free care is now the standard of practice and an indicator of quality care in all health care settings, although transition to that standard is still in progress, particularly in acute care settings. Physical restraint use in acute care is now predominantly in ICUs, particularly for patients with medical devices and those with delirium. Physical restraint is more likely to be used in ICUs because nurses fear tube dislodgment related to greater frequency of invasive lines and mechanical ventilation. However, physical restraints are not effective in preventing unplanned endotracheal extubation and increase its risk threefold (Hall et al., 2018). Daily evaluation of the necessity of medical devices (intravenous lines, nasogastric tubes, catheters, endotracheal tubes), and securing or camouflaging (hiding) the device, is important. Both the American Geriatrics Society and the American Board of Internal Medicine recommend that physical restraints should not be used to manage behavioral symptoms of hospitalized older adults with delirium (American Geriatrics Society, 2014). Further research is needed in ICU settings to determine the best strategies to manage delirium (Chapter 25).

Implementing best-practice nursing in fall risk reduction and restraint-free care is a complex clinical decision-making process and calls for recognition and analysis of cues to physical and psychosocial concerns contributing to patient safety, knowledge of restraint alternatives, interdisciplinary teamwork, and institutional commitment. Nursing staff can benefit from educational programs focused on correcting misperceptions related to physical restraint application and the use of alternatives (Hall et al., 2017). The use of advanced practice nurse consultation in implementing alternatives to restraints has been most

---

BOX 15.11 **Suggestions From Advanced Practice Nursing Consultation on Restraint-Free Fall Prevention Interventions**

- Compensating for memory loss (e.g., improving behavior, anticipating needs, providing visual and physical cues)
- Improving impaired mobility; reducing injury potential
- Evaluating nocturia/incontinence; reducing sleep disturbances
- Implementing restraint-free fall prevention interventions based on conducting careful individualized assessments; what works for one individual may not necessarily be effective for another.

---

effective. Important areas of focus derived from research on advanced practice nurse consultations are presented in Box 15.11. Many of the suggestions on safety and fall risk reduction in this chapter can be used to promote a safe and restraint-free environment. Some examples of fall risk reduction and alternative strategies to restraints are presented in Box 15.12.

BOX 15.12 **Tips for Best Practice**
Fall Risk Reduction and Restraint Alternatives

Individual
- Work with the interdisciplinary team; nurses cannot manage these complicated challenges alone
- Perform fall risk screening and evaluate gait, balance, and mobility and recognize the multifactorial nature of falls
- Refer to physical therapy for walking and/or strengthening programs as appropriate
- Check for postural hypotension
- Use a behavior log to track when the person in trying to get up and/or when they seem agitated
- Recognize signs and symptoms of delirium
- Evaluate ability to see and hear adequately. If individual wears glasses or hearing aid, or dentures, ensure devices are worn
- Ensure pain is well managed
- Involve family and all staff in fall-risk reduction education and activities
- Identify individuals at risk for falls (ID bracelet, door sign, red socks)

Patient room
- Evaluate ability to transfer in and out of bed and adjust height of bed for safety
- Use a concave mattress if trying to get out of bed
- Use bed boundary markers to mark the edges of the bed, such as mattress, rolled blanket, or "swimming noodles" under sheets
- Place a soft floor or a mattress by the bed to cushion any falls
- Use a water mattress to reduce movement to the edge of the bed
- Remove wheels from bed
- Clear the floor of debris or excess furniture; ensure floors are nonskid

- Place call bell within reach and make sure individual can use it (attach to patient's garment or obtain adapted call device)
- Ensure all personal items are within reach
- Ambulation devices within reach and used properly
- Trapeze or patient assist handles to enhance mobility in bed
- Make every effort to keep individual ambulatory
- Stay alert for falls especially at change of shift
- Provide diversional activities (catalogs, puzzles, therapeutic activity kit

Bathroom
- Evaluate continence and establish toileting plan, if appropriate
- Bedside commode available if needed
- Grab bars in bathroom and shower; shower chair
- Elevated toilet seat
- Clothing easy to pull down for toileting
- Make sure individual knows location of bathroom and can find (keep door open, picture of toilet on the door, clear path, night lights, light inside toilet bowl; glow-in-the-dark footprints going from bed to toilet

On the unit
- Remove environmental hazards
- Keep individual in supervised area or room with view of nursing station
- Sit in reclining chair; chair with deep seat, bean bag chair, rocker
- Provide meaningful activities
- Provide hip protectors, helmets, arm pads for at risk ambulatory individuals
- Provide a restraint management cart with alternative restraint products arranged in order of least restrictive

KEY CONCEPTS

- Falls are one of the most important geriatric syndromes and the leading cause of morbidity and mortality for people older than 65 years of age.
- The risk of falling increases with the number of risk factors. Most falls occur from a combination of intrinsic and extrinsic factors that unite at a certain point in time.
- Clinical judgment is required to recognize and analyze cues to fall risk and implement nursing actions to prevent falls. Evaluations must be ongoing and include analysis of any fall that occurs.
- Physical restraints, intended to prevent injury, do not protect patients from falling, wandering, or removing tubes and other medical devices. Physical restraints may actually exacerbate many of the problems for which they are used and can cause serious injury and death, as well as physical and emotional problems.
- Restraint-appropriate care is the standard of practice in all settings and knowledge of restraint alternatives and safety measures is essential for nurses

ACTIVITIES AND DISCUSSION QUESTIONS

1. Put your shoes on the wrong feet and then ask another student to analyze your gait.
2. Borrow a pair of bifocals from someone and then attempt to go up and down stairs.
3. Discuss falls you have had and their consequences. Consider how it might have been different if you were 80 years old.
4. Obtain a wheelchair and sit in it for 20 minutes with a restraining belt around your waist. Discuss your feelings with a partner. Reverse the process with your partner.
5. What are the major reasons individuals are restrained in ICUs and which interventions are most effective in decreasing restraint use in this setting? Are these alternatives available in the acute care setting where you study?

NEXT-GENERATION NCLEX® EXAMINATION-STYLE QUESTIONS

Ms. Parra, 68 years old, arrives in the emergency department via ambulance. The report from emergency services personnel indicate she fell in her home with loss of consciousness. The nurse obtains her history. The client states she slipped in the bathroom while getting up to urinate during the night; the need to urinate was urgent and she feels she rushed more than usual. When she fell, she hit her head on the sink and passed out. She was wearing her medical alert watch; it notified emergency services she had fallen. Ms. Parra's medical history includes hypertension and osteoarthritis in her knees.

Her medications include atenolol 50 mg daily, meloxicam 7.5 mg daily, and acetaminophen as needed. Although she has never fallen before, her daughter bought her the medical alert watch when she noticed how stiff Ms. Parra became after short periods of inactivity. Vital signs include a blood pressure of 100/68 mmHg, heart rate of 58 beats per minute, respirations of 16 breaths per minute, temperature of 99.5°F, and oxygen saturation of 98% on room air. Results of laboratory work include:

- White blood cell count: 12.5×10^3 cells/mm^3
- Hemoglobin and hematocrit: 16 g/dL and 45%
- Platelet count: 100,000 cells/mm^3
- Blood urea nitrogen/creatinine: 23 mg/dL and 1.2 mg/dL
- Sodium: 142 mEq/L
- Glucose: 100 mg/dL
- Urinalysis: Urine is amber and clear, pH 7.0, nitrite negative and leukocyte esterase +, blood 5/hpf, WBC 10/hpf, and bacteria 100,000 CFUs/mL.

Highlight the assessment data above that require follow-up by the nurse.

REFERENCES

American Geriatrics Society. (2014). Choosing wisely. https://www.choosingwisely.org/clinician-lists/american-geriatrics-society-physical-restraints-to-manage-behavioral-symptoms-of-hospitalized-older-adults/. Accessed January 2021.

American Geriatrics Society/British Geriatrics Society. (2010). *2010 AGS/BGS clinical practice guideline: prevention of falls in older persons, summary of recommendations*. https://geriatricscareonline.org/ProductAbstract/updated-american-geriatrics-societybritish-geriatrics-society-clinical-practice-guideline-for-prevention-of-falls-in-older-persons-and-recommendations/CL014.

American Nurses Association. (2013). *Safe patient handling and mobility: interprofessional national standards across the care continuum*. https://www.nursingworld.org/~498de8/globalassets/practiceandpolicy/work environment/health—safety/ana-sphmcover__finalapproved.pdf.

Booth, V., Hood, V., & Kearney, F. (2016). Interventions incorporating physical and cognitive elements to reduce falls risk in cognitively impaired older adults: a systematic review. *JBI Database System Rev Implement Rep, 14*(5), 110–135.

Booth, V., Logan, R., Harwood, R., & Hood, V. (2015). Falls prevention interventions in older adults with cognitive impairment: a systematic review of reviews. *Int J Ther Rehabil, 22*(6), 289–296.

Campo, M., Shiyko, M. P., Margulis, H., & Darragh, A. R. (2013). Effect of a safe patient handling program on rehabilitation outcomes. *Arch Phys Med Rehabil, 94*(1), 17–22.

Centers for Disease Control and Prevention (CDC). *Important facts about falls*, 2017. https://www.cdc.gov/homeandrecreationalsafety/falls/adultfalls.html.

de Vries, M., Seppala, L. J., Daams, J. G., et al. (2018). Fall-risk-increasing drugs: a systematic review and meta-analysis: I. Cardiovascular drugs. *J Am Med Dir Assoc, 19*(4), 371e1–371e9.

Dykes, P. C., Duckworth, M., Cunningham, S., et al. (2017). Pilot testing fall TIPS (Tailoring Interventions for Patient Safety): a patient-centered fall prevention toolkit. *Jt Comm J Qual Patient Saf, 43*(8), 403–413.

Evans, L., & Strumpf, N. (1989). Tying down the elderly: A review of literature on physical restraint. *J Am Geriatr Soc, 37*, 65–74.

Finucane, C., O'Connell, M. D., Donoghue, O., Richardson, K., Savva, G. M., & Kenny, R. A. (2017). Impaired orthostatic blood pressure recovery is associated with unexplained and injurious falls. *J Am Geriatr Soc, 65*, 474–482.

Gardner, R. C., Byers, A. L., Barnes, D. E., Li, Y., Boscardin, J., & Yaffe, K. (2018). Mild TBI and risk of Parkinson disease: a chronic effects of neurotrauma consortium study. *Neurology, 90*(20), e1771–e1779.

Gilmore-Bykovskyi, A., Fuhr, H., Jin, Y., et al. (2020). Use of direct in-person observation in the care of hospitalized older adults with cognitive impairment: a systematic review. *Jour Gerontol Nurs, 46*(5), 23–28.

Gopinath, B., McMahon, C. M., Burlutsky, G., & Mitchell, P. (2016). Hearing and vision impairment and the 5-year incidence of falls in older adults. *Age Ageing, 45*(3), 409–414.

Gray-Miceli, D. (2017). Impaired mobility and functional decline in older adults: evidence to facilitate a practice change. *Nurs Clin North Am, 52*, 469–487.

Gray-Miceli, D., de Cordova, P. B., Crane, G. L., Quigley, P., & Ratcliffe, S. J. (2016). Nursing home registered nurses' and licensed practical nurses' knowledge of causes of falls. *J Nurs Care Qual, 31*(2), 153–160.

Gray-Miceli, D., Mazzia, L., & Crane, G. (2017). Advanced practice nurse-led statewide collaborative to reduce falls in hospitals. *J Nurs Care Qual, 32*(2), 120–125.

Gray-Miceli, D., Ratcliffe, S. J., & Johnson, J. (2010). Use of a postfall assessment tool to prevent falls. *West J Nurs Res, 32*(7), 932–948.

Gupta, P., Aravindhan, A., Gand, A. T. L., et al. (2017). Association between the severity of diabetic retinopathy and falls in an Asian population with diabetes: the Singapore epidemiology of eye diseases study. *JAMA Ophthalmol, 135*(12), 1410–1416.

Hall, D. K., Zimbro, K. S., Maduro, R. S., Petrovitch, D., Ver Schneider, P., & Morgan, M. (2018). Impact of a restraint management bundle on restraint use in an intensive care unit. *J Nurs Care Qual, 33*(2), 143–148.

Hwang, H. F., Chen, S. J., Lee-Hsieh, J., Chien, D. K., Chen, C. Y., & Lin, M. R. (2016). Effects of home-based tai chi and lower extremity training and self-practice on falls and functional outcomes in older fallers from the emergency department-a randomized controlled trial. *J Am Geriatr Soc, 64*(3), 518–525.

Isaranuwatchai, W., Perdrizet, J., Markle-Reid, M., & Hoch, J. S. (2017). Cost-effectiveness analysis of a multifactorial fall prevention intervention in older home care clients at risk for falling. *BMC Geriatr, 17*, 199.

Jackson, K. M. (2016). Improving nursing home falls management program by enhancing standard of care with collaborative care multi-interventional protocol focused on fall prevention. *J Nurs Educ Pract, 6*(6), 84–95.

Krbot Skoric, M., Crnošija, L., Habek, M., & Pavelic, A. (2017). Postprandial hypotension in neurological disorders: systematic review and meta-analysis. *Clin Auton Res, 27*(4), 263–271.

Kruschke, C., & Butcher, H. K. (2017). Evidence-based practice guideline: fall prevention for older adults. *J Gerontol Nurs, 43*(11), 15–21.

Lach, H. W., Harrison, B. E., & Phongphanngam, S. (2017). Falls and fall prevention in older adults with early-stage dementia: an integrative review. *Res Gerontol Nurs, 10*(3), 139–148.

Lach, H., & Leach, K. (2016). Changing the practice of physical restraint use in acute care. *J Gerontol Nurs, 42*(2), 17–26.

Lach, H. W., & Noimontree, W. (2018). Fall prevention among community-dwelling older adults: current guidelines and older adult responses. *J Gerontol Nurs, 44*(9), 21–29.

Li, F., Harmer, P., & Fitzgerald, K. (2016). Implementing an evidence-based fall prevention intervention in community senior centers. *Am J Public Health, 106*(11), 2026–2031.

Lipsitz, L. A. (2017). Orthostatic hypotension and falls. *J Am Geriatr Soc, 65*, 470–471.

Martinez-Velilla, N., Herrero, A., Zambom-Ferraresi, F., et al. (2019). Effect of exercise intervention on functional decline in very elderly patients during acute hospitalization: a randomized clinical trial. *JAMA Int Med, 179*(1), 28–36.

Menz, H. B. (2016). Chronic foot pain in older people. *Maturitas, 91*, 110–114.

Morley, J. E. (2017). The future of long-term care. *J Am Med Dir Assoc, 18*, 1–7.

Morse, J. M., Gervais, P., Pooler, C., Merryweather, A., Doig, A. K., & Bloswick, D. (2015). The safety of hospital beds: ingress, egress, and in-bed mobility. *Glob Qual Nurs Res, 2*, 2333393615575321.

Muchna, A., Najafi, B., Wendel, C. S., Schwenk, M., Armstrong, D. G., & Mohler, J. (2017). Foot problems in older adults: associations with incident falls, frailty syndrome, and sensor-derived gait, balance, and physical activity measures. *J Am Podiatr Med Assoc, 108*(2), 126–139.

Musich, S., Wang, S. S., Ruiz, J., Hawkins, K., & Wicker, E. (2017). Falls-related drug use and risk of falls among older adults: a study in a US Medicare population. *Drugs Aging, 34*, 555–565.

Nishijima, D. K., Gaona, S. D., Waechter, T., et al. (2017). Out-of-hospital triage of older adults with head injury: a retrospective study of the effect of adding "anticoagulation or antiplatelet medication use" as a criterion. *Ann Emerg Med, 70*(2), 127–138e6.

Peach, T., Pollock, K., van der Wardt, V., das Nair, R., Logan, P., & Harwood, R. H. (2017). Attitudes of older people with mild dementia and mild cognitive impairment and their relatives about falls risk and prevention: a qualitative study. *PLoS One, 12*(5), Article e0177530.

Phelan, E. A., Aerts, S., Dowler, D., Eckstrom, E., & Casey, C. M. (2016). Adoption of evidence-based fall prevention practices in primary care for older adults with a history of falls. *Front Public Health, 4*, 190.

Pirker, W., & Katzenschlager, R. (2017). Gait disorders in adults and the elderly: a clinical guide. *Wien Klin Wochenschr, 129*(3-4), 81–95.

Potter, P., Allen, K., Costantinou, E., et al. (2017). Evaluation of sensor technology to detect fall risk and prevent falls in acute care. *Jt Comm J Qual Patient Saf, 43*(8), 414–421.

Quigley, P. A., Barnett, S. D., Bulat, T., & Friedman, Y. (2016). Reducing falls and fall-related injuries in medical-surgical units: one-year multihospital falls collaborative. *J Nurs Care Qual, 31*(2), 139–145.

Rantz, M., Skubic, M., Abbott, C., et al. (2015). Automated in-home fall risk assessment and detection sensor system for elders. *Gerontologist, 55*(Suppl 1), S78–S87.

Sand-Jecklin, K., Johnson, J. R., & Tylka, S. (2016). Protecting patient safety: can video monitoring prevent falls in high-risk patient populations? *J Nurs Care Qual, 31*(2), 131–138.

Schaffert, J., LoBue, C., White, C. L., et al. (2018). Traumatic brain injury history is associated with an earlier age of dementia onset in autopsy-confirmed Alzheimer's disease. *Neuropsychology, 32*(4), 410–416.

Tatum, P., Talebreza, S., & Ross, J. (2018). Geriatric assessment: an office based approach. *Am Fam Physician, 97*(12), 776–784.

Taylor-Piliae, R. E., Peterson, R., & Mohler, M. J. (2017). Clinical and community strategies to prevent falls and fall-related injuries among community-dwelling older adults. *Nurs Clin North Am, 52*, 489–497.

Torvinen-Kiiskinen, S., Tolppanen, A. M., Koponen, M., et al. (2017). Antidepressant use and risk of hip fractures among community-dwelling persons with and without Alzheimer's disease. *Int J Geriatr Psychiatry, 32*, e107–e115.

Wald, H., Ramaswamy, R., Perskin, M., et al. (2019). The case for mobility assessment in hospitalized older adults: American Geriatrics Society White Paper Executive Summary. *JAGS, 67*, 11–16.

Zhao, J. G., Zeng, X. T., Wang, J., & Liu, L. (2017). Association between calcium or vitamin D supplementation and fracture incidence in community-dwelling older adults: a systematic review and meta-analysis. *JAMA, 318*(24), 2466–2482.

Zhao, Y. L., Alderden, J., Lind, B. K., & Kim, H. (2018). A comprehensive assessment of risk factors for falls in community-dwelling older adults. *J Gerontol Nurs, 44*(10), 40–48.

16

Clinical Judgment to Promote Safe Environments

Theris A. Touhy

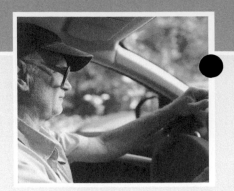

http://evolve.elsevier.com/Touhy/gerontological/

Upon completion of this chapter, the reader will be able to:
- Recognize and analyze cues to the effects of declining health, reduced mobility, isolation, and unpredictable life situations on older adults' perception of security.
- Explain the underlying vulnerability of older adults to natural disasters and the effects of extreme temperatures.
- Identify resources for disaster preparedness.
- Utilize clinical judgment to identify and evaluate nursing actions to maintain a safe environment for older adults.
- Consider the impact of available transportation and driving in relation to independence and safety.
- Discuss the use of assistive technologies to promote self-care, safety, and independence.
- Identify the components of an elder-friendly community to enhance the ability to age in place.

THE LIVED EXPERIENCE

I have been in my home for 50 years and widowed for 25 of those 50. The upkeep on my home is expensive and my resources are limited. I'm hoping I can manage to remain here, but I need some modifications to make it safe and I really don't know how to go about getting assistance to make the necessary changes.

Esther, aged 79 years

A safe environment is one in which a person is capable, with reasonable caution, of carrying out activities of daily living (ADLs) and instrumental activities of daily living (IADLs), and the activities that enrich life, without fear of attack, accident, or imposed interference. Vulnerability to environmental risks increases as individuals become less physically or cognitively able to recognize or cope with real or potential hazards.

This chapter discusses the influence of changing health and disability on safety and security. Included are vulnerability to temperature extremes, natural disasters, transportation safety, driving safety, and the role of assistive technology in enhancing independence and the ability to live safely at home. Elder-friendly communities that foster aging in place and promote safety and security are also discussed.

HOME SAFETY

The safety of older adults at home is a worldwide concern. Identification of safety issues can assist in developing measures to help individuals stay at home for longer as they age. Safety has been primarily studied in acute care and long-term care; few studies focus on safety at home and the emphasis has been on physical safety. A more holistic view is recommended and includes the following dimensions: physical, social, emotional and mental, and cognitive safety (Kivimaki et al., 2019). Actions to promote home safety must be multifaceted and individualized to the areas of identified risks. They are particularly important for older adults who are at risk of falls. Home safety assessments by occupational therapists are recommended in evidence-based protocols for fall risk reduction (Chapter 15). There are several home safety evaluation instruments that can be used to increase knowledge of safety and assist older adults and their caregivers to develop home safety plans (Box 16.1). Education about home safety is an important component of care of older adults and an integral part of discharge planning.

BOX 16.1 Resources for Best Practice

Aging 2.0: Overview of global technology innovations in aging and senior care

Aging and Technology Research Center. Online home safety self-assessment (HSSAT).

Alzheimer's Association: Checklist for home safety. https://www.alz.org/media/Documents/alzheimers-dementia-home-safety-checklist-ts.pdf

American Automobile Association: Driver improvement courses, online defensive driving course

American Association of Retired Persons: CarFit: Helping Mature Drivers Find Their Safety Fit

Centers for Disease Control and Prevention (CDC) Grand Rounds: Technology and Health: Aging Safely and More Independently: Presentations and videos on technology for older adults. https://www.youtube.com/watch?v=XRYyGtAWXnQ

Centers for Disease Control and Prevention: Personal disaster preparedness for older adults and their caregivers, COVID-19 Guidance for Older Adults.

Dementia Friendly America: National network of communities, individuals, organizations seeking to ensure communities across the U.S. are equipped to support people living with dementia and their caregivers. https://www.dfamerica.org/what-is-dfa

National Aging in Place Council: Information and resources for aging in place

National Crime Prevention Council: Safety in the Golden Years

National Institute on Aging: Age Page: Hyperthermia: Too Hot for Your Health; Hypothermia: A Cold Weather Hazard; Aging in Place: Growing Old at Home

US Fire Administration: Fire-Safe Seniors Program

US Department of Health and Human Services, Administration on Aging: Preparing for an Emergency or Disaster, Resources for Individuals, Families, and Caregivers

---

VULNERABILITY TO ENVIRONMENTAL TEMPERATURES

Extreme weather events such as heat waves, cold spells, floods, storms, and droughts are increasing across the globe. These extreme events are an emerging environmental health concern and potentially affect the health status of millions of people around the globe. More than one-half of older adults live in areas that disproportionally experience the effects of heat waves, forest fires, hurricanes, and coastal flooding (McDermott-Levy et al., 2019, p. 23). Heat-related and cold-related deaths increase with age, particularly for those aged 75 years and over.

Many older adults do not have the physical, cognitive, social, and economic resources to avoid and/or mitigate the effects of exposure to these extreme weather events. Poor housing and substandard communal living sites that lack basic necessities such as air conditioning further increase exposure to extreme weather events. Preventive measures require attentiveness to impending climate changes and protective alternatives. Early intervention in extreme temperature exposure is crucial because excessively high or low body temperatures further impair thermoregulatory function and can be lethal.

Neurosensory changes in thermoregulation delay or diminish the individual's awareness of temperature changes and may impair behavioral and thermoregulatory response to dangerously high or low environmental temperatures. These changes vary widely among individuals and are related more to general health than to age. Additionally, many drugs affect thermoregulation by affecting the ability to vasoconstrict or vasodilate, both of which are thermoregulatory mechanisms.

Other drugs inhibit neuromuscular activity (a significant source of kinetic heat production), suppress metabolic heat generation, or dull awareness (tranquilizers, pain medications). Alcohol inhibits thermoregulatory function by affecting vasomotor responses in either hot or cold weather. The ability to sense heat, to sweat, and to increase skin blood flow is reduced in healthy older adults. Risk of heat-related illnesses or injuries is increased in older adults with obesity, cardiovascular disease, respiratory disease, and diabetes, which affect normal thermoregulatory responses.

Economic, behavioral, and environmental factors may combine to create a dangerous thermal environment in which older adults are subjected to temperature extremes from which they cannot escape or that they cannot change. Caregivers and family members should be aware that individuals are vulnerable to temperature extremes if they are unable to shiver, sweat, control blood supply to the skin, take in sufficient liquids, move about, add or remove clothing, adjust bedcovers, or adjust the room temperature. A temperature that may be comfortable for a young and active person may be too cold or too warm for a frail older adult. Local governments and communities must coordinate response strategies to protect older adults. Strategies may include providing fans and opportunities to spend part of the day in air-conditioned buildings and identification of high-risk individuals.

Temperature Monitoring in Older Adults

Diminished thermoregulatory responses and abnormalities in both the production and the response to endogenous pyrogens may contribute to differences in fever responses between older and younger individuals in response to an infection. Up to one-third of older adults with acute infections may present without a robust febrile response, leading to delays in diagnosis and appropriate treatment, and increased morbidity and mortality. Careful attention to temperature monitoring in older adults is very important, and often this technical task is not given adequate consideration by professional nurses.

⚡ SAFETY ALERT

Because of thermoregulatory changes, up to one-third of older adults with acute infections may present without a febrile response. Additionally, baseline temperatures in frail older adults may be lower than the expected 98.6°F. If the baseline temperature is 97°F, a temperature of 98°F is a 1°F elevation and may be significant.

Temperatures reaching or exceeding 100.9°F are very serious in older adults and are more likely to be associated with serious bacterial or viral infections. Early recognition and analysis of cues to impaired thermoregulatory response are important and can prevent morbidity and mortality. Accurate measurement and reporting of body temperature require professional nursing supervision.

Hyperthermia

When body temperature increases above normal ranges because of environmental or metabolic heat loads, a clinical condition called heat illness, or *hyperthermia,* develops. Administration of diuretics and low intake of fluids exacerbate fluid loss and can precipitate the onset of hyperthermia in hot weather. Although most of these problems occur in the home among individuals who do not have air conditioning during temperature extremes, older adults with multiple physical problems residing in institutions may be especially vulnerable to temperature changes. LTC facilities must have emergency plans in place if power is lost and air conditioning not available.

BOX 16.2   Tips for Best Practice
Preventing Hyperthermia

- Drink 2 to 3 L of cool fluid daily and eat smaller, more frequent meals.
- Minimize exertion, especially during the warmest times of the day.
- Use A/C or go to where A/C is available (malls, library), use fans.
- Wear light loose-fitting cotton clothing and hat when outside; remove most clothing when indoors.
- Take tepid baths or showers.
- Apply cold wet compresses, or immerse the hands and feet in cool water.
- Evaluate medications for risk of hyperthermia.
- Avoid alcohol.

Individuals with cardiovascular disease, diabetes, or peripheral vascular disease and those taking certain medications (anticholinergics, antihistamines, diuretics, beta-blockers, antidepressants, antiparkinsonian drugs) are at risk. Interventions to prevent hyperthermia when the ambient temperature exceeds 90°F (32°C) are presented in Box 16.2.

Hypothermia

More than half of all hypothermia-related deaths happen in individuals over the age of 65 years. Hypothermia in older adults presents with more subtle cues and occurs more easily than in younger adults. Early recognition and implementation of nursing actions to prevent and treat are essential. Hypothermia is produced by exposure to cold environmental temperatures and is defined as a core temperature of less than 95°F (35°C). Hypothermia is a medical emergency requiring comprehensive evaluation of neurological activity, oxygenation, renal function, and fluid and electrolyte balance. When exposed to cold temperatures, healthy individuals conserve heat by vasoconstriction of superficial vessels, shunting circulation away from the skin where most heat is lost. Heat is generated by shivering and increased muscle activity, and a rise in oxygen consumption occurs to meet aerobic muscle requirements. Under normal circumstances, heat is produced in sufficient quantities by cellular metabolism of food, friction produced by contracting muscles, and the flow of blood.

Recognizing and Analyzing Cues: Hypothermia

Paralyzed or immobile individuals lack the ability to generate significant heat by muscle activity and become cold even in normal room temperatures. Individuals

BOX 16.3   Factors That Increase the Risk of Hypothermia in Older Adults

Thermoregulatory Impairment

Failure to vasoconstrict promptly or sufficiently on exposure to cold

Failure to sense cold

Failure to respond behaviorally to protect oneself against cold

Diminished or absent shivering to generate heat

Failure of metabolic rate to rise in response to cold

Conditions That Decrease Heat Production

Hypothyroidism, hypopituitarism, hypoglycemia, anemia, malnutrition, starvation

Immobility or decreased activity (e.g., stroke, paralysis, parkinsonism, dementia, arthritis, fractured hip, coma)

Thinning hair, baldness

Diabetic ketoacidosis

Conditions That Increase Heat Loss

Open wounds, generalized inflammatory skin conditions, burns

Conditions That Impair Central or Peripheral Control of Thermoregulation

Stroke, brain tumor, Wernicke's encephalopathy, subarachnoid hemorrhage

Uremia, neuropathy (e.g., diabetes, alcoholism)

Acute illnesses (e.g., pneumonia, sepsis, myocardial infarction, congestive heart failure, pulmonary embolism, pancreatitis)

Anesthesia/surgery

Drugs That Interfere With Thermoregulation

Tranquilizers (e.g., phenothiazines); sedative-hypnotics (e.g., barbiturates, benzodiazepines); antidepressants (e.g., tricyclics); vasoactive drugs (e.g., vasodilators); alcohol (causes superficial vasodilation; may interfere with carbohydrate metabolism and judgment); others (e.g., methyldopa, lithium, morphine)

who are emaciated and have poor nutrition lack insulation and fuel for metabolic heat-generating processes and therefore they may be mildly hypothermic. Circulatory, cardiac, respiratory, or musculoskeletal impairments affect either the response to or the function of thermoregulatory mechanisms. Box 16.3 presents risk factors.

Older adults with some degree of thermoregulatory impairment, when exposed to cold temperatures, are at high risk of hypothermia if they undergo surgery, are injured in a fall or accident, or are lost or left unattended in a cool place. The more severe the impairment or prolonged the exposure, the less able the thermoregulatory responses are to defend against heat loss. Unfortunately, a dulling of awareness accompanies hypothermia, and

individuals experiencing the condition rarely recognize the problem or seek assistance. For the very old and frail, environmental temperatures less than 65°F (18°C) may cause a serious drop in core body temperature to 95°F (35°C).

All body systems are affected by hypothermia, although the deadliest consequences involve cardiac arrhythmias and suppression of respiratory function. Correctly conducted rewarming is the key to good management and the guiding principle is to warm the core before the periphery and raise the core temperature by between 0.5°C and 2°C per hour. Heating blankets and specially designed heating vests are used in addition to warm humidified air by mask, warm intravenous boluses, and other measures depending on the severity of the hypothermia.

Detecting hypothermia among community-dwelling older adults is sometimes difficult because, unlike in the clinical setting, no one is measuring body temperature. For individuals exposed to low temperatures in the home or the environment, confusion and disorientation may be the first overt signs. As judgment becomes clouded, an individual may remove clothing or fail to seek shelter, and hypothermia can progress to profound levels. For this reason, regular contact with home-dwelling older adults during cold weather is crucial. For those with preexisting alterations in thermoregulatory ability, this surveillance should include even mildly cool weather. Provide education to caregivers, older adults, and families about measures to prevent hypothermia. Because heating costs are high in the United States, the Department of Health and Human Services provides funds to help low-income families pay their heating bills. Specific interventions to prevent hypothermia are shown in Box 16.4.

VULNERABILITY TO NATURAL DISASTERS

Natural disasters such as hurricanes, tornadoes, floods, wildfires, and earthquakes claim the lives of many individuals worldwide each year. In addition, human-made or human-generated disasters include chemical, biological, radiological, and nuclear terrorism and food and water contamination. Older adults are at great risk during and after disasters and have the highest casualty rate during disaster events when compared with all other age groups (Malik et al., 2018). Images of residents of assisted living and long-term care facilities sitting in waist-high water or dying because of heat extremes caused by air conditioning failures during hurricanes are a call to action to protect older adults better. The COVID-19 pandemic claimed the lives of more older adults around the world than other age groups, and the

BOX 16.4   Tips for Best Practice

Preventing Cold Discomfort and Development of Accidental Hypothermia in Frail Elders

- Maintain a comfortably warm ambient temperature no lower than 65°F. Many older adults who are frail will require much higher temperatures.
- Provide generous quantities of clothing and bedcovers. Layer clothing and bedcovers for best insulation. Be careful not to judge your patient's needs by how you feel working in a warm environment.
- Provide a head covering whenever possible—in bed, out of bed, and particularly outdoors.
- Cover patients well when in bed or bathing. The standard—a light bath blanket over a naked body—is not enough protection for older adults who are frail.
- Cover patients with heavy blankets for transfer to and from showers; dry quickly and thoroughly before leaving shower room; cover head with a dry towel or hood while wet. Shower rooms and bathrooms should have warming lights.
- Dry wet hair quickly with warm air from an electric dryer. Never allow the hair to air-dry.
- Provide as much exercise as possible to generate heat from muscle activity.
- Provide hot, high-protein meals and bedtime snacks to add heat and sustain heat production throughout the day and as far into the night as possible.

most frail in long-term care facilities were extremely vulnerable.

Older adults who are most vulnerable to natural disasters include, but are not limited to, those who depend on others for daily functioning; the medically frail; those with limited mobility; those who use medical devices requiring externally supplied electricity; those who are socially isolated or live alone; and those who are cognitively impaired or institutionalized. The older and poorer the individual, the more likely they are to be isolated and vulnerable. Older adults may be less likely to seek formal or informal help during disasters or may be unable to do this independently. Many lack access to the technology that supplies communication during emergencies. Nursing facility residents comprise a particularly vulnerable group because of their frailty, and facilities are required to have disaster plans in place.

Adopting tailored disaster preparedness plans that address the general and emergency health needs for older adults is a worldwide concern. Families caring for older adults need to have individualized emergency plans. Public health prevention planning and programs are needed to identify older adults at increased risk in the event of disasters and address their needs. Communities need to enhance preparedness and information networks among organization and agencies that serve older adults (American Red Cross and the American Academy of Nursing, 2020; Shih et al., 2018). Gerontological nurses can assist in the development of these plans and educate fellow professionals and community agencies about the special needs of older adults. Nurses can also provide educational programs and outreach on disaster preparedness to older adults and their caregivers. Box 16.1 presents resources for emergency and disaster preparedness for special populations, including older adults.

GUN SAFETY

Gun safety among older adults is relevant to medical and public health professionals, given that older adults experience changes in memory, function, and mood that may increase risks of gun-related injuries and deaths, including suicide. Older adults have the highest rates of gun ownership in the United States. Older adults also have high rates of suicide and gun access is a risk factor for suicide. Older White males have the highest suicide rate and 71% of the time they use guns (Chapter 24). Evaluating gun safety and risk of injury is important in care of older adults and questions about gun ownership should be asked as routinely as questions about driving. The 5 Ls approach is recommended for assessment of firearm safety practices (Lum et al., 2016) (Box 16.5).

TRANSPORTATION SAFETY

Adequate, affordable, and convenient transportation services are essential to health and quality of life and the ability to age in place. The lack of accessible transportation may contribute to other problems, such as social withdrawal, poor nutrition, depressive symptoms, and health decline. A "crisis in mobility" exists for many older adults because of the lack of an automobile, an inability to drive, limited access to public transportation, health factors, geographical location, and economic considerations.

BOX 16.5   5 Ls Approach to Assessing Gun Safety Practices

- **Locked:** Is there a gun present? Is it locked?
- **Loaded:** Is it loaded?
- **Little children:** Are there children present in the home?
- **Feeling Low:** Does the gun owner feel low, having suicidal thoughts?
- **Learned owner:** Has the owner had formal gun safety training?

Urban buses and subways can be physically hazardous and often dangerous for older adults. Rural and suburban areas may not have accessible transportation systems, making transportation by car essential. Even walking can be dangerous, and older adults are more likely to be injured or killed as pedestrians than as car drivers. Suggested pedestrian improvements include raised pavement markings, median islands, larger street signs with bigger lettering, increased time for pedestrian crossings, and lowered speed limits.

County, state, or federally subsidized transportation is provided in certain areas to assist individuals in reaching social services, nutrition sites, health services, emergency care, recreational centers, day care programs, physical and vocational rehabilitation centers, grocery stores, and library services. Some senior centers and assisted living facilities also offer transportation services. Although transportation can often be found for special needs, it is virtually impossible to locate transportation for pleasure or recreation and many of these services are restricted to individuals with serious physical or mental impairments.

Ride-sharing services such as Uber and Lyft can assist in providing more transportation options, but some older adults may not be able to afford these services or may not feel safe using them. Some of these transportation services are offering special services for individuals who need more assistance, such as wheelchair-accessible vehicles or a driver trained to provide additional assistance. Nurses need to inquire about the individual's access to transportation and make referrals to local social service and aging organizations (e.g., Area Agencies on Aging) to assist in finding resources and financial assistance for services.

Driving

Older adults' driving is a critical public health issue. Driving is one of the IADLs for most older adults because it is essential for obtaining necessary resources. Currently, almost half of drivers on the road are over the age of 65 years, with substantial increases predicted in the next 30 years (Wiese & Wolff, 2016). For many older adults, alternative transportation is not available and, consequently, they may continue driving beyond the time when it is safe. Driving is a highly complex activity that requires a variety of visual, motor, and cognitive skills. Age alone is not a good indicator of driving safety, but health conditions, sensory functioning, road design and traffic, and weather conditions contribute to increasing concern with driving safety as individuals age (Edwards et al., 2017; Liddle et al., 2017).

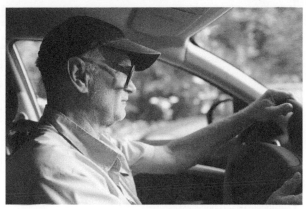

Driving is the preferred means of travel for older adults. (© iStock.com/danr13.)

Driving Safety

Older drivers typically drive fewer miles than younger drivers and tend to drive less at night, during adverse weather conditions, or in congested areas. Generally, they choose familiar routes, and fewer older drivers speed or drive after drinking alcohol than drivers of other ages. However, when compared with younger age groups, older adults have more accidents per mile driven. Driving fatalities increase with age, and the risk of death for drivers 85 years or older is ninefold greater in a crash than it is for drivers 69 years or younger (Roe et al., 2017). Improving the safety of cars through new design and adaptations should be considered for older drivers to enhance safety (Box 16.6).

BOX 16.6   Adaptations for Safer Driving

- Wider rear-view mirrors
- Pedal extensions
- Less complicated, larger, and legible instrument panels
- Electronic detectors in front and back that signal when the car is getting too close to other cars, drifting into another lane, or likely to hit center dividers or other highway infrastructure
- Technology that facilitates left turns by alerting drivers when it is safe to make the turn
- Better protection on doors
- Booster cushions for shorter-stature drivers
- "Smart" driving assistants (under development) that automatically plan a safe driving route based on the person's driving habits
- GPS devices

Modified from Dugan, E., Lee, C. (2013). Biopsychosocial risk factors for driving cessation: Findings from the Health and Retirement Study, *J Aging Health 25*, 1313–1328.

BOX 16.7   Tips for Best Practice

Safe Driving

- Include the person in all discussions about driving safety.
- Encourage the individual to conduct a self-assessment of driving abilities.
- Assess vision and hearing and ensure appropriate use of corrective lenses and hearing devices.
- Evaluate medical conditions that may interfere with driving ability (arthritis, Parkinson's disease, dementia, stroke) and ensure appropriate treatment, and adaptations that may be necessary to enhance driving safety.
- Discuss the impact of medical conditions and sensory impairments on driving safety.
- Suggest vehicle adaptations and older adult driving assessment programs if indicated.
- Encourage the individual to modify driving habits, such as not driving on unfamiliar roads, during rush hour, at dusk or at night, in inclement weather, or in heavy traffic.
- Avoid risky spots like ramps and left turns.
- Advise individual to limit night driving.
- Discuss strategies to decrease the need to drive including arranging for home-delivered groceries, prescriptions, and meals; having personal services provided in the home; asking a caregiver to obtain needed supplies or act as a copilot; and exploring community resources for transportation.
- Ask the family to have the family lawyer discuss with the individual the financial and legal implications of a crash or injury.

From National Institute on Aging: Older Drivers. https://www.nia.nih.gov /health/older-drivers#besafe. Accessed January 2021.

The legal regulations regarding driver's license renewal in older drivers and the responsibility of medical practitioners to identify unsafe drivers vary among states and countries. Driver's license renewal procedures may include accelerated renewal cycles, renewal in person rather than electronically or by mail, and vision and road tests. The issues of driving in the older adult population are the subject of a great deal of public discussion. Many older drivers and their families struggle with issues related to continued safety in driving and when and how to tell older adults that their driving safety is a concern (Box 16.7).

Driving and Dementia

Driving is one of the largest ethical issues associated with dementia. Dementia, even in the early stages, can impair the cognitive and functional skills required for safe driving. There is at least a twofold greater risk of crashes for drivers with dementia when compared with age-matched individuals without dementia (Wiese & Wolff,

2016). Many individuals early in the course of dementia are still able to pass a driving performance test, and therefore a diagnosis of dementia should not be the sole justification for revoking a driver's license. However, a recent study found that declines in driving performance probably precede problems with thinking, memory, or cognition in individuals in the later stages of preclinical Alzheimer's disease (Roe et al., 2017). Discussions about driving safety should begin when dementia is diagnosed, and driving evaluations should be conducted every 6 months or as needed as the disease progresses.

To enhance driving safety, many states have implemented the Silver Alert system. Similar to Amber Alerts for missing children, the Silver Alert is designed to create a widespread lookout for older adults who have wandered from their surroundings while driving a car. Silver Alert features a public notification system to broadcast information about missing persons, especially older adults with Alzheimer's disease or other mental disabilities, in order to help their return. Silver Alert uses a wide array of media outlets, such as commercial radio stations, television stations, and cable television, to broadcast information about missing persons. Silver Alert also uses message signs on roadways to alert motorists to be on the lookout for missing older adults and provides the car's make, model, and license plate number.

Driving Cessation

Relinquishing the mobility and independence afforded by driving one's own car has many psychological ramifications and inconveniences. Giving up driving is a major loss for an older adult both in terms of independence and pleasure as well as in feelings of competence and self-worth. The health consequences of driving cessation include social isolation, health problems, institutionalization, higher mortality, and an approximately doubled risk of depression (Davis & Ohman, 2017). Women are more likely than men to stop driving for less pressing reasons than health, and at a younger age. Older men seem to place more value on the ability to drive and on owning a car than do older women. Therefore, one can expect more stress involved with the decision not to drive for older men.

Planning for driving cessation should occur for all older adults before their mobility situations become urgent. Health care providers should encourage open discussion of issues related to driving with the older adult and their family and should identify impairments that affect safe driving, correct them when possible, and offer alternatives for transportation. Forty percent of individuals aged 50 years or older believed that their primary care provider could best determine their driving

BOX 16.8 Is it Time to Give up Driving?

We all age differently. For this reason, there is no way to set one age when everyone should stop driving. So, how do you know if you should stop? To help decide, ask yourself:

- Do other drivers often honk at me?
- Have I had some accidents, even if they were only "fender benders"?
- Do I get lost, even on roads I know?
- Do cars or people walking seem to appear out of nowhere?
- Do I get distracted while driving?
- Have family, friends, or my doctor said they're worried about my driving?
- Am I driving less these days because I'm not as sure about my driving as I used to be?
- Do I have trouble staying in my lane?
- Do I have trouble moving my foot between the gas and the brake pedals, or do I sometimes confuse the two?
- Have I been pulled over by a police officer about my driving?

If you answered "yes" to any of these questions, it may be time to talk with your doctor about driving or have a driving assessment.

From National Institute on Aging: Is it time to give up driving? https://www.nia.nih.gov/health/older-drivers#give-up. Accessed January 2021.

BOX 16.9 Safe Driving

- **S** Safety record
- **A** Attention skills
- **F** Family report
- **E** Ethanol use
- **D** Drugs
- **R** Reaction time
- **I** Intellectual impairment
- **V** Vision and visuospatial function
- **E** Executive functions

ability. But health care providers often feel unprepared to identify unfit drivers and may benefit from education about driving with dementia so that they have the skills needed to counsel patients and families (Davis & Ohman, 2017).

Voluntarily giving up a driver's license, rather than having it revoked, is associated with more positive outcomes. Specialized driving cessation support groups aimed at the transition from driver to nondriver may also be beneficial in decreasing the negative outcomes associated with this decision. "Family members require support and education about how to give feedback on driving safety in a way that ensures the message is carefully timed, received as well as possible, and supports relationships" (Liddle et al., 2017). Box 16.8 presents a self-evaluation of driving skills and safety.

❖ USING CLINICAL JUDGMENT TO PROMOTE HEALTHY AGING: DRIVING SAFETY

◆ Recognizing and Analyzing Cues: Driving Safety

Driving ability should be included in an analysis of functional abilities. Areas include an evaluation of whether an individual can drive, feels safe driving, and has a driver's license. Additional areas include evaluation of skills needed for safe driving, such as vision and hearing screening, cognitive assessment, medication review,

and an active range-of-motion tests and evaluation of strength and general mobility. These tests help to identify weaknesses that would impair an individual's ability to drive, make driving decisions, or exit the car quickly. A mnemonic, SAFE DRIVE, addresses key components in screening older drivers (Box 16.9). The American Association of Retired Persons and the American Automobile Association provide many resources for driving safety for older adults (Box 16.1). These kinds of tools can be effective in raising awareness of threats to driving.

There is no gold standard for determining driving competency, but driving evaluations are offered by driver rehabilitation specialists through local hospitals and rehabilitation centers and private or university-based driving assessment programs. Components of a thorough driving examination also include a road test. Some programs that evaluate driving ability may use a standardized computer driving simulation. The local Alzheimer's Association and Area Agency on Aging can assist in locating driving evaluation sites. State Departments of Motor Vehicles (DMVs) also conduct performance-based road tests. There is a lack of resources for driving evaluations and the evaluation is also very expensive and not covered by Medicare or insurance. More research is needed to address driving safety in older adults.

EMERGING TECHNOLOGIES TO ENHANCE SAFETY OF OLDER ADULTS

Advancements in all types of technology hold promise for improving quality of life, decreasing the need for personal care, enhancing independence, social engagement, and the ability to live safely at home and age in place (Pepito & Locsin, 2019). The costs of nursing home and assisted living are driving sales and innovation in the technology market. A growing concern related to the increasing number of older adults is the lack of both family and paid caregivers (Chapters 26 and 27). Emerging technologies will play a larger role in ensuring care for older adults in the future. Existing and emerging solutions also have the potential to make life better for caregivers and open the door for a new era of "tech-enabled caregiving" (Andruszkiewicz and Fike, 2015–2016, p. 64).

Assistive technology is any device or system that allows a person to perform a task independently or that makes the task easier and safer to perform. Assistive technology is decreasing the number of older adults who depend on others for personal care in ADLs and presents cost-effective alternatives to human services and institutionalization. Gerotechnology is the term used to describe assistive technologies for older adults and these technologies are expected to significantly influence how we live in the future. Health care technologies, robotics, telemedicine, mobility and ADL aids, and smart home technology are some examples of assistive technology (Choi et al., 2019).

Telehealth

Telehealth (telemedicine) is the use of technologies to enable clinicians to diagnose, monitor, and treat patients remotely. Telehealth offers exciting possibilities for managing medical problems in the home or other setting, reducing health care costs, and promoting self-management of illness, particularly in rural and underserved areas. A number of studies have reported that telehealth technology improves patient outcomes and decreases hospital readmissions and health care costs (Marchibroda, 2015). Telehealth can also be effective for delivering interventions designed for family caregivers (Chi & Demiris, 2017). During the COVID-19 pandemic, Medicare and other insurers began covering the cost of telehealth visits, and we can expect a great increase in the use of this technology. Nurses, particularly advanced practice nurses, are expected to play a major role in the technology.

Smart Homes

There are many exciting technologies being developed to support monitoring and management of older adults' health and homes and to support aging in place and remote caregiving (Turjamaa et al., 2019). Remote monitoring via in-home sensors allows caregivers to track daily behavior passively and be notified about deviations from daily routines. Newly evolving smart-home systems include a combination of home-control applications (e.g., appliances, lighting, security systems) and safety, health, wellness, and social connectivity technologies. These technologies can simultaneously and continuously monitor environmental conditions, daily activity patterns, vital signs, movement patterns, sleep patterns, medication adherence, and fall detection. Examples of smart-home technology adaptations include smart pill dispensers with automated reminders, smart stoves that automatically shut off when left unsupervised, smart mattresses to monitor sleep duration, body movement, and sleep cycles, sensors to measure sitting time and provide notification to promote physical activity, and virtual reality social gatherings with distant family members and friends (Choi et al., 2019).

The MEDCottage (granny-pod) is an interesting example of a smart home. The MEDCottage provides a family communication center that allows telemetry, environmental control, and dynamic interaction to off-site caregivers through smart and robotic technology. Technology inside the home includes monitoring of the person's vital signs and safety, medication reminders, and adaptive devices. The MEDCottage can be purchased or leased and temporarily placed on the caregiver's family property (http://www.medcottage.com/).

Motion and pressure sensors may be useful in the homes of older adults with cognitive impairment. These sensors can detect movement and the absence of movement. If there has been no movement for a period of time, a monitoring system is activated and a plan of action initiated depending on the person's response or lack thereof. Pressure sensors can be used under the mattress and can turn on bedside lights when the individual gets out of bed and activate an alarm if they do not return to bed in a specified period of time. Sensors placed in entry doors or GPS watches or pendants can detect if a person leaves the home, and their location, and can send messages to caregivers. SmartSoles, shoe insoles with an embedded GPS device, are being developed and may be an aid to locate individuals with dementia who wander from their home.

Robots

Robotic technology for health care is more advanced in Europe and Japan than in the United States at this time, but we can expect to see increased development and use of robotics in nursing. Already developed are robots that can help lift both individuals and objects, remind patients to take their medicine or administer the medication, check a person's vital signs, provide help in the event of a fall, and assist with baths and meals. A child-sized therapist robot on wheels with a humanlike torso is being developed for use in homes and long-term care facilities to assist with the high level of attention individuals with dementia require for safety and function. Research is ongoing to develop a humanoid nursing robot with caring function, specifically designed for the functional and practical use of older adults with dementia (Locsin et al., 2018; Miyagawa et al., 2019). Programming robots with basic skills in humanlike caring is essential because these machines are increasingly in use as health care partners-in-caring.

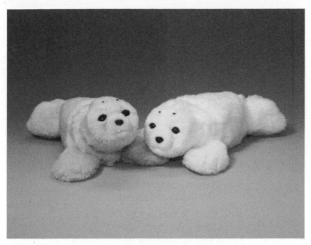

FIG. 16.1 PARO, the therapeutic robotic seal. (Used with permission from AIST JP/PARO ROBOTS US INC.)

PARO, a therapeutic robot, allows the documented benefits of animal-assisted therapy to individuals in hospitals and long-term care facilities (Fig. 16.1) (www .parorobots.com). PARO is considered a robopet (small animal-like robots that have the appearance and behavioral characteristics of pets). By interaction with people, PARO responds as if it is alive, moving its legs and head, making sounds, and responding to touch and sound. Benefits of interaction with PARO and other robopets in long-term care include increased interaction and engagement, reduction of agitation, pleasure, and comfort. Not everyone engages with robopets, and some older adults, families, and staff may not like them; therefore it is important to consult about preferences and history with pets before engaging the individual with a robopet. Robopets are not intended to replace human interaction, but there appears to be some benefit for using them as therapy for agitated or isolated individuals in long-term care (Abbott et al., 2019).

As the baby boomers and future generations age, comfort with technology will be increased, and people will seek options for better, safer, and more independence in ways not yet imagined. At this time, many of the assistive technologies can be cost prohibitive, but with advances in development they may be more accessible and affordable for more people. Issues of privacy and data sharing need consideration, and training and support for proper use of devices and application are important. Many technologies were initially designed to serve the rich and young, and later adopted for older adults without a great deal of input. Older adults and their caregivers should be involved in the design and implementation of technologies.

Many systems are complex and difficult to use, especially for individuals with limited technology and health literacy skills. "Nurses can play essential roles in designing future research to improve the design and use of mobile and connected health technologies and researching their effects on older adults' health outcomes and ability to age in place. Nurses are also in a prime position to lead interprofessional teams of engineers, computer scientists, physicians, informaticians and other health professionals and partner with patients and their families to design, develop and implement technology in a holistic manner" (Wang, 2018, p. 4).

AGING IN PLACE

Developing elder-friendly communities and providing increasing opportunities to age in place can lead to enhanced health and well-being. Aging in place is the ability to live in one's own home and community safely, independently, and comfortably, regardless of age, income, or ability level. Many state and local governments are assessing the community and designing interventions to enhance the ability of older adults to remain in their homes and familiar environments. These interventions range from adequate transportation systems to home modifications and universal design standards for barrier-free housing.

Components of an elder-friendly community include the following: (1) addresses basic needs; (2) optimizes physical health and well-being; (3) maximizes independence for the frail and disabled; and (4) provides social and civic engagement. Fig. 16.2 presents elements of an elder-friendly community. Efforts to create physical and social urban environments that promote healthy and active aging and a good quality of life are occurring worldwide.

The World Health Organization (WHO) Global Network of Age-Friendly Cities and Communities helps cities and communities become more supportive of older adults by addressing their needs across eight dimensions: the built environment, transportation, housing, social participation, respect and social inclusion, civic participation and employment, communication, and community support and health services (WHO, 2018). The Dementia Friendly America movement is a growing initiative in the United States to foster the ability of people living with dementia to remain in the community and engage and thrive in day-to-day living (Box 16.1).

A majority of older midlife and older adults want to age in place and want to stay in their own homes or, if that is not possible, stay in their communities as they grow older. However, for many older adults, the ability to find affordable, physically accessible, and well-located homes in their community is a significant

Addresses Basic Needs

- Provides appropriate and affordable housing
- Promotes safety at home and in the neighborhood
- Ensures no one goes hungry
- Provides useful information about available services

Promotes Social and Civic Engagement

- Fosters meaningful connections with family, neighbors, and friends
- Promotes active engagement in community life
- Provides opportunities for meaningful paid and voluntary work
- Makes aging issues a community-wide priority

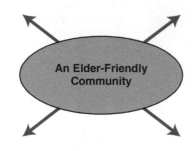

An Elder-Friendly Community

Optimizes Physical and Mental Health and Well-Being

- Promotes healthy behaviors
- Supports community activities that enhance well-being
- Provides ready access to preventive health services
- Provides access to medical, social, and palliative services

Maximizes Independence for Frail and Disabled

- Mobilizes resources to facilitate "living at home"
- Provides accessible transportation
- Supports family and other caregivers

FIG. 16.2 Essential elements of an elder-friendly community. (From AdvantAge Initiative, Center for Home Care Policy and Research, Visiting Nurse Service of New York.)

challenge. Only 1% of US housing units have all five components of what are known as "universal design" features: no-step entry; single floor living; extra-wide doorways and halls; accessible electric controls and switches; and level-style doors and faucet handles. Remodeling an existing home to install these accessibility features is expensive and many cannot afford to remodel. There is also a lack of affordable and accessible rental units and federally subsidized housing for older renters. The racial and ethnic diversity of the growing number of older adults in the United States also has significant implications. New models of housing for older adults are growing across the country and hold promise to help address the crisis in housing and support aging in place. As the baby boomers age, we can expect to see more innovative housing movements that create successful opportunities for healthy aging in the community and provide a range of options for older adults beyond what is available now.

- Transportation for older adults is critical to their physical, psychological, and social health.
- Driving safety for older adults is an important issue, and health care professionals must be knowledgeable about assessment, safety interventions, and transportation resources.
- Technology advances hold promise for improving quality of life, decreasing need for personal care assistance, and enhancing independence and ability to live safely. Nurses can play essential roles in designing future research to improve the design and use of mobile and connected health technologies and researching their effects on older adults' health outcomes and ability to age in place.
- Efforts to make communities more elder-friendly are underway across the globe. New and innovative ideas for aging in the community will continue to change living options for older adults.

KEY CONCEPTS

- Recognizing and analyzing cues to older adult's vulnerability during natural disasters and taking action to develop preventive and supportive responses to enhance safety are important nursing responsibilities.
- Thermoregulatory changes, chronic illness, and medications may predispose the older adult to hypothermia and hyperthermia. Careful attention must be paid to temperature monitoring and provision of adequate heat and cooling in weather extremes.

ACTIVITIES AND DISCUSSION QUESTIONS

1. Which actions are important to prevent hypothermia in older adults who are frail?
2. Evaluate the safety of your living quarters or the living quarters of your parents/grandparents.
3. What plans does your community have to provide for the safety of older adults during disasters and weather-related events?
4. Which types of support does your community provide to assist older adults age safely age in place?

NEXT-GENERATION NCLEX® EXAMINATION-STYLE QUESTIONS

Mrs. Walters, an 82-year-old female, resides in a secure dementia unit. She has a history of peripheral vascular disease, hypertension, asthma, hypothyroidism, osteoarthritis, and vascular dementia. She is no longer ambulatory and spends most days sitting in her wheelchair in the atrium looking at the birds and flowers. She is 5′ 8″ and weighs 110 pounds (BMI 16.72). Her hemoglobin 10.8 g/dL and hematocrit 32%, albumin 3.2 g/dL, BUN 26 mg/dL, creatinine 1.5 mg/dL, and TSH 4.12 mU/L. Mrs. Walters blood pressure is 145/86 mmHg, pulse of 88 beats per minute, respirations 16 breaths/min, oral temperature of 97.3°F, and oxygen saturation 95%. Her medications include aspirin 81 mg daily, valsartan 160 mg daily, levothyroxine 150 µg daily, acetaminophen 750 mg every 8 hours, and citalopram 20 daily.

Use an X for the nursing actions listed below that are **Indicated**, **Contraindicated**, or **Non-Essential** for the client's care at this time.

Intervention	Indicated	Contraindicated	Non-Essential
Monitor body temperature			
Keep environmental temperatures at 65°F			
Cover with thick blanket when transporting to shower			
Allow hair to air dry			
Provide high protein meals and snacks			
Minimize exertion			
Drink 2 L fluid a day			

REFERENCES

Abbott, R., Orr, N., McGill, P., et al. (2019). How do "robopets: impact the health and well-being on residents in care homes? A systematic review of qualitative and quantitative evidence. *Int J Older People Nursing*, e12239.

American Red Cross and the American Academy of Nursing: closing the gaps: advancing disaster preparedness, response and recovery for older adults, January 2020. https://www.redcross.org/content/dam/redcross/training -services/scientific-advisory-council/253901-03%20BRCR -Older%20Adults%20Whitepaper%20FINAL%201.23.2020.pdf.

Andruszkiewicz, G., & Fike, K. (2015–6). Emerging technology trends and products: how tech innovations are easing the burden of family caregiving. *Generations, 39*(4), 64–68.

Chi, N. C., & Demiris, G. (2017). The roles of telehealth tools in supporting family caregivers. *J Gerontol Nurs, 43*(2), 3–5.

Choi, Y., Lazar, A., Demiris, G., et al. (2019). Emerging smart home technologies to facilitate engaging with aging. *Jour Geron Nurs, 45*(12), 41–48.

Davis, R. L., & Ohman, J. M. (2017). Driving in early-stage Alzheimer's disease: an integrative review of the literature. *Res Gerontol Nurs, 10*(2), 86–100.

Edwards, J. D., Lister, J. J., Lin, F. R., Andel, R., Brown, L., & Wood, J. M. (2017). Association of hearing impairment and subsequent driving mobility in older adults. *Gerontologist, 57*(4), 767–775.

Kivimaki, T., Stolt, M., Charalambous, A., & Suhonen, R. (2019). Safety of older people: an integrative review. *Int J Older People Nurs, 15*(1). https://doi.org/10.1111/opn.12285.

Liddle, J., Gustafsson, L., Mitchell, G., & Pachana, N. A. (2017). A difficult journey: reflections on driving and driving cessation from a team of clinical researchers. *Gerontologist, 57*(1), 82–88.

Locsin, R., Tanioka, T., Yashura, Y., et al. (2018). Humanoid nurse robots as caring entities: a revolutionary probability? *Int J Nurs Studies, 3*(2), 146.

Lum, H., Flaten, H., & Betz, M. (2016). Gun access and safety practices among older adults. *Curr Gerontol Geriatr Res.* doi: 10.1155/2016/2980416. Epub 2016 Feb 2.

Malik, S., Lee, D. C., Doran, K. M., et al. (2018). Vulnerability of older adults in disasters: emergency department utilization by geriatric patients after Hurricane Sandy. *Disaster Med Public Health Prep, 12*(2), 184–193.

Marchibroda, J. M. (2015). New technologies hold great promise for allowing older adults to age in place. *Generations, 39*(1), 52–54.

McDermott-Levy, R., Kolanowski, A., Fick, D., & Mann, M. (2019). Addressing the health risks of climate change in older adults. *Our Gerontol Nurs, 45*(11), 21–29.

Miyagawa, M., Yasuhara, Y., Tanoika, T., et al. (2019). The optimization of humanoid robot's dialog in improving communication between humanoid robot and older adults. *Intelligent Control and Automation, 10*(3), 118–127.

Pepito, J., & Locsin, R. (2019). Constantino: Caring for older persons in a technologically advanced nursing future. *Health, 11*(5). https://m.scirp.org/papers/92368.

Roe, C. M., Babulal, G. M., Head, D. M., et al. (2017). Preclinical Alzheimer's disease and longitudinal driving decline. *Alzheimers Dement (NY), 3*(1), 74–82.

Shih R. A., Acosta J. D., Chen E. K., et al. (2018). Improving disaster resilience among older adults, Rand Corporation Research Report. https://www.rand.org/pubs/research_reports/RR2313.html.

Turjamaa, R., Pehkonen, A., & Kangasniemi, M. (2019). How smart homes are used to support older people: an integrative review. *Int J Older People Nurs, 14*, e12260. https://doi.org/10.1111/opn.12260.

Wang, J. (2018). Mobile and connected health technologies for older adults aging in place. *J Gerontol Nurs, 44*(6), 3–5.

World Health Organization (2018). *Global network for age-friendly cities and communities.* https://extranet.who.int/agefriendlyworld /who-network/. Accessed January 2021.

Wiese, L. K., & Wolff, L. (2016). Supporting safety in the older adult driver: a public health nursing opportunity. *Public Health Nurs, 33*(5), 460–471.

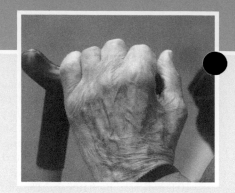

17

Living With Chronic Illness

Kathleen Jett

http://evolve.elsevier.com/Touhy/gerontological/

LEARNING OBJECTIVES

Upon completion of this chapter, the reader will be able to:
- Differentiate between the cues associated with chronic and acute illness.
- Discuss the factors that influence the experience of chronic illness.
- Identify strategies and action to improve care for those with chronic conditions.
- Discuss models to maximize the outcomes of self-care management of chronic illness.
- Discuss strategies and actions to maximize wellness in the presence of chronic illness.

THE LIVED EXPERIENCE

Just because you think you understand my disease doesn't mean you understand me. You do not know how I experience my illness. I am unique. I think and feel and behave in a combination that is a reflection of who I am underneath all that.

Judith, 87 years old

During the past century, a major shift has occurred in the leading causes of death for all age groups—from infectious diseases and acute illnesses to acute exacerbations of chronic diseases. The number of individuals who live with chronic illnesses is increasing rapidly and is influenced by many factors—from advances in medical sciences in treating illness and prolonging life to the "globalization" of lower-income countries as diets become unhealthy, exercise decreases, and people are exposed to tobacco smoke (World Health Organization [WHO], 2018).

This escalation in the numbers of persons with chronic illnesses is a global health concern. Each year 26 million persons over the age of 69 years die of a noncommunicable disease, especially one of the cardiovascular diseases. Many of these deaths are preventable, especially for persons living in low- and middle-income countries (WHO, 2018).

Six in 10 adults in the United States have at least one chronic disease and 4 in 10 have two or more. Heart disease, cancer, chronic lung disease, stroke, Alzheimer's disease, diabetes, and chronic kidney disease are not only common but are seen primarily in older adults (CDC, 2019). In 2016, 38% of all persons over the age of 65 years had none or one chronic condition, 47% had two or three, and 15% had at least four chronic conditions (Administration for Community Living [ACL], 2018). Vulnerable and socially disadvantaged people of any age get sicker and die sooner once they acquire a chronic illness. A host of social determinants, especially education, age, income, gender, and ethnicity, influence the level of illness.

Diminished quality of life is a major personal cost of living with chronic conditions for both the individual and their family and significant others. Disability is common, especially for those with advanced heart disease or arthritis. In turn, this disability results in social costs in terms of reduced financial productivity.

This chapter addresses chronic illness as a life experience and discusses how gerontological nurses can work with the person through secondary and tertiary prevention strategies, that is, promptly observing any cues suggestive of any new problems or exacerbations of chronic problems and maximizing function and quality of life while promoting healthy aging.

ACUTE ILLNESS

Before chronic disorders can be discussed, their relationship to acute illness must be addressed. They cannot be separated in the health of older adults because so many conditions are intricately intertwined. A previously stable chronic condition can and often does worsen when an acute illness occurs. For example, an episode of pneumonia may trigger acute congestive heart failure even if the failure had been present but controlled before the pneumonia. During the COVID-19 pandemic, those at highest risk of dying were those with underlying conditions such as diabetes and heart disease, both more common in later life.

Sudden changes in the functional, physiological, cognitive, psychological, or spiritual status of an older adult call for immediate and prompt nursing and medical attention to determine the possibility of an acute and hopefully reversible condition. A person with cognitive impairments attributable to dementia may suddenly become more confused or less alert than usual and found to have a urinary tract infection or constipation. Once the acute condition is treated, the person may return to their prior state, i.e., living with the chronic condition. Unfortunately, because physiological reserves are diminished in healthy aging (see Chapter 4), it takes longer to "bounce back," or the person may never fully return to their prior state of health and/or dies unexpectedly (Box 17.1).

BOX 17.1 Walking on Air

I have been walking about 4 miles a day for most of my life, but over the last year it has been becoming more difficult. The bottoms of my feet tingle and sometimes it just doesn't feel like I can feel the ground as well and I am afraid I will miss a bump in the sidewalk and fall. My doctor says it is because my diabetes is getting worse. I don't quite understand that; I have had it for 20 years.

Helena at 86 years of age

CHRONIC ILLNESS

"Chronic health problems are not fixable with shiny new technology, and do not promise the suspense, exhilarating hope, and dramatic ending that acute medical crises often do. They simply continue day after day, [they are] often invisible or misunderstood" (Hodges et al., 2001,

BOX 17.2 Tips for Best Practice
Assessing Frailty

Frailty is characterized by marked vulnerability to adversity. It is loosely defined as evidence of three of the following: unexplained weight loss, self-reported exhaustion, weak grip strength, slow walking speed, and low activity. It is better to ask specifically about each one of these symptoms. Many people consider the signs as "just a normal part of aging." To provide a method of quantifying frailty as far as possible, a number of scales have been developed and some of them tested. Most are available free of charge for educational and professional practice use.

p. 390). Chronic illnesses are those that occur slowly and progress slowly. They are the result of a combination of genetic, physiological, and behavioral factors (WHO, 2018). They have an irreversible presence and may be hidden to outsiders. The presence of a chronic illness may be as little as an inconvenience or as great as an impairment of one's ability to perform even the most basic self-care activities (see Chapter 8). According to a 2017 survey of the US Census Bureau, some type of disability was reported by 35% of those at least 65 years of age and 46% of those over 75 had at least some difficulty in physical functioning (Fig. 17.1) (ACL, 2018).

For those with multiple chronic illnesses who are also frail (Box 17.2), the nurse is called upon to minimize the effect of any of the complications of the geriatric syndromes (Box 17.3). The syndromes are often hard to explain, and recognition of related cues may be delayed. Many overlap and appear as clusters. They are also often interwoven with both acute and chronic conditions each complicating the other. For example, a person with dementia and osteoporosis develops a urinary tract infection, and although they may have been ambulatory, they fall and break a bone before cues indicating the first acute condition are noticed or treatment

BOX 17.3 Most Common Conditions Referred to as "Geriatric Syndromes"[a]

- Falls and gait abnormalities
- Frailty
- Delirium
- Urinary incontinence
- Sleep disorders
- Pressure injuries
- Malnutrition
- Sarcopenia

[a]From multiple sources.

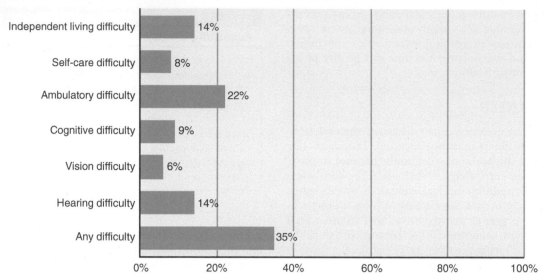

FIG. 17.1 Percentage of persons over the age of 65 years with a disability, 2017. Administration for Community Living [ACL]: *Profile of older Americans: 2017.* https://acl.gov/sites/default/files/Aging%20and%20Disability%20in%20America/2018OlderAmericansProfile.pdf.

is effective. The subsequent hospitalization for the fall may lead to acute delirium as a result of the combination of the infection, the fall, and the necessity of being in an unfamiliar environment. The delirium may lead to death (see Chapter 25). The gerontological nurse must be particularly attentive to any cues indicating change in the older adult and to analyze these promptly with knowledge of normal changes with aging and the potential syndromes that can occur or were already present. Prompt prioritization of hypotheses is necessary with action taken to minimize poor outcomes.

If not triggered by an acute event such as a seizure or a stroke, the onset of a chronic disease or a disability may be insidious and cues identified only during a wellness health screening. The person may have long periods of remission, times when symptoms appear under control and the person is functioning at the highest level possible. Many continue to work and perform their usual activities and roles. The cues suggestive of illness may only be identified when symptoms reach a level noticeable to the person (e.g., diminishing sensation to the feet, indicating years of hyperglycemia) (see Chapter 20) or to others (e.g., memory loss); or when the damage caused by the condition results in an acute event, such as an acute myocardial infarction (heart attack) indicative of many years of untreated, undertreated, or unknown hypertension (see Chapter 22).

As of 2018, more than two out of every three older Americans have multiple chronic conditions. At all ages, the health status of Hispanics, Asian Americans, Blacks, and other minority population groups, such as American Indians/Alaska Natives and Native Hawaiians/Other Pacific Islanders, lags behind that of non-Hispanic Whites. For a variety of reasons, older adults in these groups experience the effects of health disparities more than younger people. Language barriers, reduced access to health care, historically low economic status, and different cultural norms can be major challenges to promoting health in an increasingly diverse older population (Chapter 2) (KFF, 2020).

Symptoms of chronic illness interfere with many normal activities and routines, make medical regimens necessary, disrupt patterns of living, and frequently make it necessary for the individual to incorporate significant lifestyle changes. Physical suffering, loss, worry, grief, depression, functional impairment, and increased dependence on family or friends are among the potential negative consequences of chronic illnesses.

The current generation of persons 65 years and older is living longer with more chronic diseases. A dramatic example of this phenomenon is the changing trajectory for persons with human immunodeficiency virus (HIV). Only a short time ago, those infected with HIV died quickly of acquired immunodeficiency syndrome (AIDS) because of delayed diagnoses and absence of treatment. Since the advent of HIV-specific antiviral medications, more persons are living into later life with HIV. It is one more chronic disease that will be superimposed on hypertension, diabetes, dementia, and other disorders that commonly develop with aging.

Prevention

It is perhaps most accurate to say that many of the chronic diseases in late life are the result of our lifestyle choices at an earlier age. Most people in their sixties and seventies today can remember eating (or "smoking") candy in the shape of tiny cigarettes in imitation packaging when they were children. In doing so, they were emulating their parents and celebrities. Smoking tobacco early in life was often condoned rather than criticized. This is one of the explanations for the high levels of heart and lung disease in older adults following years of tobacco exposure as children and younger adults.

Preventive practices were not emphasized until the very youngest of the Baby Boomers (born between approximately 1947 and 1964) became older (see Chapter 2). The document *Healthy People 2000* (CDC, 2015a) was published in 1990, and a national agenda for the achievement of improving the health of the nation was proposed. This was updated with *Healthy People 2010* (CDC, 2015b) and with *Healthy People 2020* (Office of Disease Prevention and Health Promotion [ODPHP], 2019). At the time of writing, *Healthy People 2030* was not yet available. The 2020 edition is the first one that adds a section specific to improving the health of older adults. In 2018, a document was published focusing on strategies for healthy aging (CDC, 2018).

In a document that builds on the *Healthy People* work, the *State of Aging and Health in America* provides intermittent status updates of 15 different indicators. The report of 2013 (most recent edition) indicates that some areas have exceeded goals: (1) leisure time in the past month, (2) reduced obesity, (3) reduced smoking, (4) taking medications for diagnosed high blood pressure, (5) had mammogram within past 2 years, and (6) had timely colorectal cancer screenings. However, many other goals remain unmet, including no state having met the 2020 goal for flu or pneumonia vaccinations (CDC, 2013).

Many chronic illnesses and their associated acute events are not inevitable consequences of aging. They may be prevented through healthy lifestyle choices at any age, with the reduction of modifiable risk factors for disease later in life (Box 17.4). The use of preventive strategies has the potential to reduce morbidity (associated disability) and premature mortality (death sooner than would have occurred without the condition). As the emphasis continues to shift toward healthy lifestyle choices, it is anticipated that future cohorts of older adults, especially the youngest Baby Boomers, will be healthier and more functional longer than their predecessors.

THEORETICAL FRAMEWORKS FOR CHRONIC ILLNESS

Several theoretical frameworks have been used to understand the effect of chronic illness and help nurses recognize and analyze cues to the presence and progression of chronic illness, including the Chronic Illness Trajectory (Corbin and Strauss, 1992; Strauss and Glaser, 1975) and the Shifting Perspectives Model (Paterson, 2001). The outcomes of chronic disease may be improved through prompter and evidence-based analyses.

Chronic Illness Trajectory

The trajectory model, originally conceptualized from research conducted by Strauss and Glaser (1975) and later expanded by Corbin and Strauss (1992), has long aided health care providers to better understand the realities of chronic illness and its effect on individuals. According to this theoretical approach, chronic illness is viewed from a life course perspective or along a trajectory. In this way, the course of a person's illness can be viewed as an integral part of the person's life rather than as an isolated event. The nurse's response is then holistic rather than isolated. The time between the diagnosis of an illness and death is divided into eight phases for the purpose of identifying hypotheses and developing strategies and action (Table 17.1). The shape and stability of the trajectory are influenced by the combined efforts, attitudes, and beliefs held by the older person, family members, and significant others, and the involved health care providers (Box 17.5). Although it appears linear, it is instead fluid as crises reappear and are addressed and as instability becomes stable again until this is no longer possible.

The Shifting Perspectives Model of Chronic Illness

The Shifting Perspectives Model (Paterson, 2001) is derived from a synthesis of qualitative research findings of living with chronic illness as an ongoing, continually shifting process in which the person moves between the perspectives of wellness in the foreground and illness in the foreground. This model is more reflective of an "insider" perspective on chronic illness as opposed to the more traditional "outsider" view. At any point in

---

BOX 17.4 Modifiable Risk Factors for the Development of Chronic Diseases

- Smoking or exposure to second-hand smoke
- Excessive alcohol use
- Lack of physical exercise
- Poor nutrition
- Obesity

TABLE 17.1 The Chronic Illness Trajectory and Nursing Reponses

Phase	Definition
1. Pretrajectory	Before the illness course begins, the preventive phase, no signs or symptoms present
2. Trajectory onset	Signs and symptoms are present, includes diagnostic period
3. Crisis	Life-threatening situation
4. Acute	Active illness or complications that require hospitalization for optimal management
5. Stable	Controlled illness course/symptoms
6. Unstable	Illness course/symptoms not completely controlled by regimen but not requiring or desiring hospitalization
7. Downward	Progressive decline in physical/mental status characterized by increasing disability/symptoms
8. Dying	Active decline in physical/mental status characterized by increasing disability/symptoms Immediate weeks, days, hours preceding death

Examples of goals that nurses might establish include the following:

1. To assist a client in overcoming a plateau by increasing adherence to a regimen so that they might reach the highest level of functional ability possible within limits of the disability
2. To assist a client in making the attitudinal and lifestyle changes that are needed to promote health and prevent disease
3. To assist a client who is in a downward trajectory to be able to maintain sense of self and receive expert palliative care
4. To assist with advance care planning to ensure wishes are met
5. To assist the client who is in an unstable phase to gain greater control over symptoms that are interfering with their ability to carry out everyday activities

BOX 17.5 Key Points in the Chronic Illness Trajectory Framework

- The majority of health problems in late life are chronic.
- Chronic illness and its management often profoundly affect the lives and identities of both the individual and significant others.
- The acute phase of illness management is designed to stabilize physiological processes and return to a state of stability.
- Maintaining stability is central in the work of managing chronic illness.
- A primary care nurse often has the role of coordinator of the multiple resources that may be needed to promote quality of life at any point along the trajectory.

Chronic illness contains elements of both illness and wellness, and people live in the "dual kingdoms of the well and the sick" (Donnelly, 2003, p. 6). The illness in the foreground is triggered when threats to control occur or are perceived. As signs and symptoms of disease progress and become noticeable to the person, they may lack the skills or knowledge to manage them, or have intense fear of suffering and loss or fear of the potential burden the illness may cause to others. However, the illness in the foreground has a protective function and may foster conservation of energy and help a person learn more about the illness and try to adjust and come to terms with it (Paterson, 2001).

Those who are able to bring wellness to the foreground in the face of chronic illness exhibit courage and resilience and are able to develop strategies and draw on resources to adjust to the changes that are occurring and those that are anticipated. When wellness is in the foreground, the focus is centered more on the self and others and less on the disease and its consequences. The illness becomes part of who a person is rather than how they define themselves (Box 17.6). The illness is seen as an opportunity for growth and meaningful changes in relationships with the environment and others. This perspective is fostered by learning as much as possible about the illness, creating supportive environments, paying attention to the person's own patterns of response to the illness, and sharing knowledge of the disease with others. With this perspective, focus can be on the

BOX 17.6 Wellness in the Foreground

In nursing we often automatically put the illness in the foreground when we discuss a patient as "The stroke in Room 212." The nurse can promote a wellness perspective in the presence of chronic disease by just slightly changing the way we view patients to "Mr. Jones in room 212 who had a stroke yesterday."

time, illness or wellness may take precedence over the other, but the goal is to move toward the highest level of well-being even in the presence of illness through appropriate actions on the part of nurses and all involved in the persons' lives.

A person's perspective of the chronic illness is neither right nor wrong but reflects their needs and situation. How people perceive the chronic illness at any given time influences how they interpret and respond to the disease and situations affected by the illness (Lindqvist et al., 2006; Paterson, 2001).

emotional, psychological, spiritual, and social aspects of life while still attending to disease management and the effects of the illness on the person's life. Paterson (2001) suggests that the shifting perspectives model calls for understanding the person's perspective and the reasons the person varies in their attention to symptoms; the nurse supports persons at either perspective.

❖ USING CLINICAL JUDGMENT TO PROMOTE HEALTHY AGING: CHRONIC ILLNESS

The goals of caring for persons with chronic disease are to minimize worsening, provide comfort when this is not possible, and always be alert for cues suggesting an added, reversible condition requiring prompt treatment. A multimodal strategy is always necessary, including expert medical and nursing care and social, psychological, and spiritual support. Regardless of the setting, from acute care to home care, the nurse is usually the person who ensures that the best care of all types is provided, including functional rehabilitation (see Chapter 6).

◆ Recognizing and Analyzing Cues

Nursing care of older adults with a chronic illness is a holistic and interactive process. In no other situation is it more important to be alert to cues related to all aspects of a person: physiological, psychological, social, spiritual, and functional. Tools can be found throughout the text that can be used to facilitate this, both comprehensive (see Chapter 8) and specific related to the chronic condition and development of an acute event (e.g., fall; Chapter 15). Each aspect of the person is affected by the presence of the disease in the context of the person's culture (see Chapter 3).

Because a chronic disease is an evolving situation, so is the analysis of cues and the development of hypotheses. Nursing skills are needed to conduct ongoing evaluation of outcomes, continued careful observation, periodic reevaluation, alert watchfulness, and, most importantly, discussion and collaboration with older adults about their perceptions, the meaning of their illness, and their plans (see the LEARN Model in Chapter 3 for help with this). At all times the awareness of the normal changes of aging inform the observations regarding clinical judgment gaps between the existing patient self-care abilities and needed self-care resources.

◆ Nursing Actions

Caring for patients with chronic illness consists of addressing acute events that are superimposed on underlying conditions. It is curing what can be cured, providing comfort, at the same time as assuring that the person receives optimal, evidence-based care for that which is chronic. Individuals with chronic conditions require care that is coordinated across time and settings centered on their needs, values, and preferences. The nurse is often the person to teach self-management skills if appropriate. This includes teaching strategies to minimize long-term complications and how to get help when needed. Health care providers, including nurses, must understand the specific illness adequately enough to know the fundamental differences between episodic acute illness to be cured and exacerbations of the chronic conditions, always within the context of normal aging. Solutions leading to actions must take into consideration all of the information learned in cue analysis to work with the individual and significant others to help the person develop personal goals and achieve whenever outcomes possible.

The western medical care model and models of public health have come a long way in addressing infectious and episodic illness, e.g., Polio, measles, influenza. However, they have not been effective in dealing with the complexity of chronic illness. In particular, the training, education, and skill of today's health care personnel have been inadequate in providing evidence-based care to older adults with chronic illnesses. The last updated version of *Healthy People* (2020) notes the need for improved training with a new objective aimed toward improving the health of older adults by increasing the proportion of the health care work force with geriatric certification.

Nursing roles may include direct caregiver, resource person, advisor, teacher, facilitator, and student (of the person who usually has years of experience dealing with the ups and downs of the illness) (Box 17.7). Gerontological nurses are care coordinators regardless of setting; they help older adults and their families navigate the maze of disparate financing and delivery

---

BOX 17.7 Nursing Roles in Caring for Persons With Chronic Illness

- **Counselor:** Listen to the story and come to know the person and what gives him or her meaning in life. Help person set realistic goals and expectations. Focus on potential rather than limitations.
- **Educator:** Regarding the illness, its management, and skills required for effective self-care.
- **Nursing practice:** Ongoing with a focus on prevention of complications. Ensure delivery of the highest-quality evidence-based medical and nursing care at all times.
- **Coordinator:** Assist with obtaining access to resources. Refer appropriately and when needed. Refer and coordinate palliative care as needed.

- Long-term and uncertain nature of the illness
- Costs associated with care including preventive and long-term personal care
- Little coordination of care across the continuum
- Lack of health care professionals with expertise in geriatrics and chronic care
- Focus of health care system on acute and episodic care
- Continued disparities in health care outcomes for vulnerable groups

systems that are complex and confusing and where care is often fragmented, ineffective, and costly (Box 17.8).

Gerontological nurses develop and work with self-management programs to help persons with chronic illnesses function as independently as possible and prevent unnecessary hospitalizations. A number of innovative models are either being tested or planned that have the potential to improve the lives of persons with chronic diseases (http://www.innovations.cms.gov/initiatives/index .html). Other ongoing models include the Geriatric Resources for Assessment and Care of Elders model (GRACE) for low-income older adults (AHRQ, 2017), the Guided Care Results (Hostettler et al, 2016), and the well-established Program of All-Inclusive Care for the Elderly (PACE) (Medicaid, n.d.) (Box 17.9).

BOX 17.9 **Characteristics of Successful Chronic Illness Management Models**

- Interdisciplinary team of health care professionals, often led by a nurse
- Ability to conduct initial and intermittent comprehensive assessments
- Skill in the development of a comprehensive care plan that is individualized, incorporates evidence-based protocols, and is culturally appropriate
- Adequate funding to implement the plan over time
- Actively engages the patient and family caregivers in care
- Proactive monitoring of the patient's clinical status and ability and willingness to modify the care plan as needed
- Success in facilitating transitions across settings
- Facilitation of the patient's access to community resources

◆ Evaluating Outcomes

Nurses work toward the achievement of the outcomes established by the *Healthy People* documents to prepare individuals for a healthier later life and to enhance health and wellness for those already in later life. Progress is not measured in attempts to achieve cure, but rather in prompt responses to new acute events and maintenance of a steady state or regression of the chronic condition while remembering that the condition does not define the person.

Nursing's response of caring instead of curing brings the highest level of expertise to assist people in adapting, continuing to grow, and attaining a level of wellness and wholeness despite their illness and, ultimately, their functional limitations. Gerontological nurses know that understanding and caring for those with chronic illnesses and long-term disabilities require close caring relationships in order to accompany the person on their journey with hope, courage, and joy, day after day and year after year.

Healthy aging does not mean the absence of disease; rather, it means moving toward wellness in the presence of disease. Someone once said that a chronic illness is like a grain of sand in an oyster; either it irritates and creates a pearl or the oyster just dies. Some nursing actions are aimed at helping create that pearl.

KEY CONCEPTS

- Declines in mortality, increasing medical expertise, and sophisticated technological developments have resulted in a great increase in the survival of the very old with multiple chronic disorders.
- The effects of chronic illness range from mild to life-limiting, with each person responding to unique circumstances in unique ways.
- The Chronic Illness Trajectory and the Shifting Perspectives Model of Chronic Illness offer useful frameworks in observing cues to exacerbations of chronic illness, analyzing these cues and ultimately designing nursing actions to improve or stabilize health outcomes.
- People with chronic illnesses can achieve some level of wellness, and the role of the nurse is varied and critical.
- The goals of promoting healthy aging include rapidly responding to cues suggestive of the emergence of an acute and curable illnesses, minimizing risk of exacerbations of the chronic disease, encouraging health promotion, and, in the presence of disease, alleviating symptoms, delaying or avoiding the development of complications, and focusing on the outcome of maximizing function and quality of life.
- New models of cost-effective care are needed that increase access and improve outcomes and quality of life for persons with chronic illness. Nurses are particularly well prepared to assume major roles in care of those with chronic illness.

ACTIVITIES AND DISCUSSION QUESTIONS

1. What type of education and counseling might the nurse provide to a 30-year-old person in anticipation of a healthier late life?
2. What would be the most devastating loss to you, should you develop a chronic condition that affects your day-to-day life?
3. Which nursing actions assist a person with chronic illness to deal with loss? Practice or role-play various ways that these issues can be addressed.
4. How would you encourage an individual toward a goal of maximal participation in self-care to improve health outcomes?
5. What would be the measures of wellness during chronic illness?

REFERENCES

Administration for Community Living [ACL]. (2018). *Profile of older Americans*. https://acl.gov/aging-and-disability-in-america/data-and-research/profile-older-americans.

AHRQ [Agency for Healthcare Research and Quality]. (2017). *GRACE team care*. https://www.ahrq.gov/workingforquality/priorities-in-action/grace-team-care.html.

Centers for Disease Control and Prevention (CDC). (2013). *The state of aging and health in America*. https://www.cdc.gov/aging/pdf/state-aging-health-in-america-2013.pdf.

Centers for Disease Control and Prevention (CDC). (2015a). *Healthy People 2000*. http://www.cdc.gov/nchs/healthy_people/hp2000.htm.

Centers for Disease Control and Prevention (CDC). (2015b). *Healthy People 2010*. http://www.cdc.gov/nchs/healthy_people/hp2010.htm.

Centers for Disease Control (CDC). (2018). *Healthy aging in action*. https://www.cdc.gov/aging/pdf/healthy-aging-in-action508.pdf.

Centers for Disease Control and Prevention (CDC). (2019). *About chronic disease*. https://www.cdc.gov/chronicdisease/about/index.htm.

Corbin, J. M., & Strauss, A. (1992). A nursing model for chronic illness management based upon the trajectory framework. In P. Woog (Ed.), *The chronic illness framework: The Corbin and Strauss nursing model*. New York: Springer.

Donnelly, G. (2003). Chronicity: Concepts and reality. *Holist Nurs Pract, 8*(1), 1–7.

Hodges, H. F., Keeley, A. C., & Grier, E. C. (2001). Masterworks of art and chronic illness experiences in the elderly. *J Adv Nurs, 36*(3), 389–398.

Hostetter, M., Klein, S., McCarthy, D., Hayes, S. (2016). *Guided Care: A structured approach to proving comprehensive primary care for complex patients*. https://www.commonwealthfund.org/publications/case-study/2016/oct/guided-care-structured-approach-providing-comprehensive-primary.

KFF [Kaiser Family Foundation]. (2020). *Disparities in health and health care: Five key questions and answers*. https://www.kff.org/disparities-policy/issue-brief/disparities-in-health-and-health-care-five-key-questions-and-answers/.

Lindqvist, O., Widmark, A., & Rasmussen, B. (2006). Reclaiming wellness-Living with bodily problems, as narrated by men with advanced prostate cancer. *Cancer Nursing, 29*(4), 327–337.

Medicaid: *Program of all-inclusive care for the elderly*, n.d. https://www.medicaid.gov/medicaid/ltss/pace/index.html.

Office of Disease Prevention and Health Promotion (ODPHP): *Healthy People 2020*. http://www.healthypeople.gov/.

Paterson, B. L. (2001). The shifting perspectives model of chronic illness. *J Nurs Scholarsh, 33*(1), 21–26.

Strauss, A., & Glaser, B. (1975). *Chronic illness and the quality of life*. St Louis: Mosby.

World Health Organization (WHO). (2018). *Noncommunicable diseases*. https://www.who.int/en/news-room/fact-sheets/detail/noncommunicable-diseases.

18

Clinical Judgment to Promote Relief From Pain

Kathleen Jett

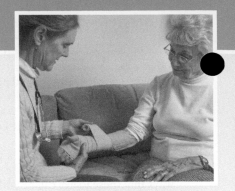

http://evolve.elsevier.com/Touhy/gerontological/

THE LIVED EXPERIENCE

Ms S. had cancer and was in severe pain most of the time. When she was referred to the local hospice, the nurse assessed the level of pain, the type of pain, and the level of relief that was acceptable. After a careful titration of her medications, it was found that only a long-acting morphine provided her comfort and an improved quality of life. However, at the dose needed she also hallucinated, seeing several puppies in the room with her. When asked if she wanted to reduce the dosage to eliminate this side effect, she responded, "No—I'll keep the puppies, I know they are not real and they don't hurt anything. I'd rather have them with me than the pain."

Helen, age 93

In a study reported by the National Institutes of Health more than half (53%) of older adults reported pain in the previous month and 75% of them reported pain in more than one place (Hulla et al., 2019). The percentage of those with pain living in long-term care facilities is expected to be higher.

Pain is a subjective sensation of physical, psychological, or spiritual distress. It is a multidimensional phenomenon, and the types of pain are usually intertwined with one another. Physical pain is intensified when accompanied by any of the other types of pain. It has many consequences, including questioning the meaning of one's life (Box 18.1).

How pain is expressed is influenced by the unique history of the individual and the meaning they ascribe to it. Some are only able to express pain in terms of "not feeling well"; others are highly articulate but controlled; still others are highly vocal and expressive. It is important for nurses to realize that an individual will respond to pain in a way that reflects their own cultural expectations and understanding of acceptable behavior (Box 18.2). How we respond to pain is part of who we are—part of our very core. Even the words we use to describe it are personal. Pain may be referred to as an ache, a hurt, a "pester," a nuisance, a bother, and so forth, with the language and the willingness to express it a manifestation of the person's relationship to whom they are speaking. The communication of pain is not always straightforward, complicating a nurse's ability to attend to related cues. Some do not, cannot, or will not

BOX 18.1 Tips for Best Practice

Potential Impact of Persistent Pain in the Older Adult

Depression and anxiety

Sleep disturbances

Loss or worsening of physical function and fitness

Loneliness attributable to loss of social support/withdrawal from social activities

Loss of ability to perform usual role activities

Loss of ability to perform prior leisure activities

Potential for drug/alcohol abuse or misuse

Delayed healing

Increased falls

Impaired cognition

Impaired nutrition

Behavioral changes

Reduced quality of life

Adapted from several sources.

BOX 18.2 Examples of Possible Effect of Culture on Expressions of Pain

Stoic and unemotive

"Grin and bear it" approach—withdrawn, prefers to be alone

When asked about pain, it is minimized

Generalized to northern European and Asian heritage

Emotive

Wants others around to validate feelings

Readily cries out in pain

Generalized to Hispanic, Middle Eastern, Mediterranean

Data from Carteret, M. (2010). *Cultural aspects of pain management.* http://www.dimensionsofculture.com/2010/11/cultural-aspects-of-pain-management; Peacock, S., Patel, S. (2008). Cultural influences on pain, *Reviews in Pain 1*(2), 6–9.

verbalize their pain in ways that the nurse understands (see Chapter 2). Instead, the nurse must be alert to the cues that suggest that pain or discomfort is present (see Special Circumstances described below).

For many years there was a commonly held belief that older adults experienced pain less often than younger persons and that those with dementia had the least amount of pain. There is now a significant amount of research that refutes this. There appears to be an increase in sensitivity to pain that is caused by pressure but not to that evoked by heat. The pain caused by hard surfaces against sensitive areas, e.g., pressure injuries, may be more intense in an older person than one who is younger. An older adult may also have

a delayed self-recognition of some types of pain. For example, when there is a delay responding to hot surfaces such as heating pads used for pain relief, a serious burn can occur even before the heat is perceived (Tumi et al., 2017).

Achieving the outcome of pain relief is now part of evidence-based practice (Horgas, 2017a; The Joint Commission, 2020). Health care providers, especially nurses, are expected to promptly and correctly recognize and analyze cues suggestive of pain and take action to address these in a culturally appropriate manner. In this chapter, the types of pain are briefly reviewed and considered in the context of aging. The barriers to comfort are discussed, especially for those with cognitive impairments. Finally, solutions and actions that are used by prescribing providers and nurses to promote comfort are proposed.

ACUTE AND PERSISTENT PAIN

The most common type of pain in later life is persistent, also referred to as "chronic." Pain may be differentiated as nociceptive, neuropathic, idiopathic, or mixed types (Box 18.3). The most common causes of persistent pain in later life is musculoskeletal in nature and the result of degenerative joint disease (Bruckenthal, 2017; Horgas, 2017b) (see Chapter 21). However, persons with all levels of cognition experience acute pain at times.

BOX 18.3 Types of Physical Pain Sensations

- **Nociceptive pain** is associated with injury to the skin, mucosa, muscle, or bone and is usually the result of stimulation of pain receptors. This type of pain arises from tissue inflammation, trauma, burns, infection, ischemia, arthropathies (rheumatoid arthritis, osteoarthritis, gout), nonarticular inflammatory disorders, skin and mucosal ulcerations, and internal organ and visceral pain from distention, obstruction, inflammation, compression, or ischemia of organs. Nociceptive mechanisms usually respond well to common analgesic medications and nonpharmacological interventions.
- **Neuropathic pain** involves a pathophysiological process of the peripheral or central nervous system and presents as altered sensation and discomfort. This type of pain may be described as stabbing, tingling, burning, or shooting.
- **Mixed or unspecified pain** usually has mixed or unknown causes. A compression fracture causing nerve root irritation, common in older people with osteoporosis, is an example of a mix of nociceptive and neuropathic pain.

Acute Pain

Acute pain in late life is essentially the same as it is in earlier life: temporary, postoperative, procedural, or posttraumatic (e.g., fractures). It is a universal experience for older adults, attributable to increased risk of traumatic injury (e.g., falls). Most importantly, as a person ages, it is much more likely that acute pain will be superimposed on preexisting persistent pain.

Persistent Pain

Persistent pain is that which lasts beyond an expected duration, at least 3–6 months. Most pain in later life is of this type and described as moderate to severe. Osteoarthritic back and neck pain are the most common causes of nociceptive pain in later life (Horgas, 2017b). Persistent pain may develop insidiously as a disease progresses such as with cardiovascular disease or diabetes or may be a sequela to an episode of acute pain. For example, after the acute neuropathic pain of an outbreak of shingles, a postherpetic neuralgia with pain of varying intensities may last a lifetime. More than 50%–75% of older adults living in the community are thought to be living with persistent pain, 50% of which is untreated or undertreated. The number of those living in long-term care facilities with pain is estimated at 75%–80% and 80% of these untreated or undertreated (Hulla et al., 2019).

Persistent pain may vary in intensity throughout the day or with changes in activity. For example, persons with depression usually feel the worst emotional pain in the morning with a lessening as the day progresses (see Chapter 24). For those with the nociceptive pain of rheumatoid arthritis, pain is the most intense in the morning with slow but limited improvement with movement (see Chapter 21). Neuralgias occur frequently from long-standing diabetes, peripheral vascular disease, and other syndromes such as stroke, and iatrogenic side effects of treatment such as chemotherapy. For most of those at late life the only outcome possible may be to lessen pain rather than resolve it. In doing so, the person's quality of life and independence may be maximized (Galicia-Castillo & Weiner, 2019).

BARRIERS TO PROVIDING COMFORT TO OLDER ADULTS IN PAIN

Providing expert care to those in pain is a considerable challenge for gerontological nurses. The barriers are many. The oldest adults may underreport pain and undertreat themselves because of the cost of the medications, the belief in an associated stigma, the association of pain to normal burdens of "old age," or the fear of addiction. The nurse and patient may have incongruent personal beliefs and expectations of how pain is expressed. Both are influenced by their beliefs about pain

---

BOX 18.4   Barriers to Pain Management in Older Adults

Health Care Professional Barriers
Lack of education regarding pain assessment and management
Concern regarding regulatory scrutiny
Belief that pain is a normal part of aging
Belief that cognitively impaired older adults have less pain
Personal beliefs and experiences with pain
Inability to accept the person's report of pain without "objective" signs

Older Adults and Family Barriers
Concern that the person will not be believed
Fear of being a "bad patient" if complaining
Fear of the meaning of the pain, e.g., that the person has cancer
Fear of addiction
Fear of side effects of treatments
Financial limitations
Concern that the pain is not important to the health care provider /nurse
Fear of medication side effects
Belief that pain is a normal part of the aging
Belief that nothing can be done to adequately relieve pain
Coexistence of sensory or cognitive deficits

Health Care System Barriers
Cost
Time
Policy regarding opioid use
Systemic bias

Modified from multiple sources.

---

and its expression. The influences come from the nurse's personal experiences, professional experiences, and culture-associated beliefs.

As a result of these and other barriers (Box 18.4), the recognition of cues is often inadequate and ultimately result in undertreatment of pain, especially for those residing in nursing homes or living with dementia. The Centers for Medicare and Medicaid Services (CMS) have tried to address this issue by requiring periodic pain assessment of residents using standardized instruments. The results must be used to revise the plan of care/action and outcomes (CMS, 2019; Galicia-Castillo & Weiner, 2019).

Special Circumstances: Pain in Older Adults With Cognitive and Communication Limitations

Study after study has shown that older adults who are cognitively impaired receive less pain medication for the same conditions and situations that would be painful to those without impairments (Horgas, 2017a). Yet there is no convincing evidence that peripheral transmission of the sensation of pain to the brain is altered by dementia (Ahn & Horgas, 2013; Epplin et al., 2014). However, those with cognitive impairments may not understand what they are feeling, why they are feeling it, or where it is coming from. Their expressions of pain are most likely different than others. Research has suggested that older people with mild to moderate cognitive impairment can provide valid reports of pain using self-report scales if the cues are recognized by the nurse and other caregivers (Box 18.5).

People with more severe impairment or loss of language skills for whatever reason may not be able to communicate the presence of pain in a manner that is easily understood. Cues to the possibility of pain include changes in behavior, alterations in ambulation, agitation, aggression, increased confusion, or passivity (Ahn & Horgas, 2013). When the person who is usually active and talkative becomes passive or withdrawn, pain should be suspected. Achieving an outcome of comfort for those who cannot express themselves requires careful observation of behavior for subtle changes (Box 18.6).

BOX 18.6   **Pain Cues in the Person With Communication or Cognitive Limitations**

Changes in Behavior
Restlessness and/or agitation or reduction in movement
Repetitive movements
Unusually cautious movements, guarding

Activities of Daily Living
Sudden resistance to help from others
Decreased appetite
Decreased sleep

Vocalizations
Person groans, moans, or cries for unknown reasons
Person increases or decreases usual vocalizations

Physical Changes
Pleading expression
Grimacing
Pallor or flushing
Physical tension such as clenching teeth or hands
Diaphoresis (sweating)
Increased pulse, respirations, or blood pressure

❖ USING CLINICAL JUDGMENT TO PROMOTE HEALTHY AGING: PAIN

Gerontological nurses and nursing assistants are usually the most attuned to the needs of patients and can become skilled at the recognition of cues suggestive of pain in older adults. The nurse is responsible for assuring that the patient is comfortable and has the highest possible health-related quality of life regardless of cognitive or functional status or disease state. Care of the person in pain begins with assessment and continues through to the evaluation of the effectiveness of the interventions.

◆ Recognizing and Analyzing Cues

Care of the person thought to be in pain or expressing pain (or other word that is consistent with the person's preference) always begins with a complete analysis of all available cues such as the environment, history, and physical findings to determine whether there are any treatable causes, such as a urinary tract infection. If there are no cues correlating to pain or the pain persists after actions have been completed, the analysis is repeated realizing that the previous hypotheses was insufficient to achieve the desired outcomes. There are a number of excellent assessment guidelines that can be used with older adults in pain. Particularly useful guidance can be found at https://geriatricpain.org/pain-assessment and https://consultgeri.org/try-this/general-assessment/issue-7. It is also possible to use a mnemonic OLD CART (onset, location, duration, characteristics, aggravating and relieving factors, and treatment already used) to ensure that all cues have been reviewed (Box 18.7).

Onset: "When did it start?" If the pain has been persistent the answer to this question is likely to be vague, such as "A few months ago." With older adults, relative time may be more useful: "Was it troubling you before…. (your birthday, a particular holiday, etc.)"

Location: Do not forget to ask about where the pain is, where it starts, and if it goes (radiate) anywhere else.

BOX 18.7   **Basic Pain Assessment**

1. **Self-report of pain intensity (rating):** _____
2. **OLD CART**
   Onset: _____
   Location: _____
   Duration: _____
   Characteristics: _____
   Aggravating factors: _____
   Relieving factors: _____
   Treatment previously tried: _____
3. **Comfort level goal:** _____

Having a drawing of a body is very helpful; this often becomes part of the person's medical record.

Duration: With the recognition of onset (previous) it may appear that duration can be estimated, but more detail relative to the pain at the time of the assessment is needed. "Do you have pain now?" "Do you have pain every day?" "All day or a certain time of the day?" "Have you ever had this before?"

Characteristics: Verbal descriptors should be obtained, that is, a description of how the pain feels, such as burning, tingling, or stabbing or aching or dull. This information contributes to the diagnosis of the type of pain (e.g., neuropathic pain is almost always described as "burning," "tingling," or "shooting"). Is it affecting function, sleep, appetite, activity, mood, relationships with others? Does the pain awaken the person from sleep? A significant number of persons with pain are chronically sleep deprived and depressed (Lee & Oh, 2019).

For those who are able to express themselves, numerical rating scales (NRS) are used most often: the person is asked to rate their pain on a scale of 1 (or "0") to 10, with 1 being no pain and 10 the worst imaginable. For example, they are asked what is the worst it has ever been, and what is it today, now, and this week (Fig. 18.1). Most persons have this level of numerical ability. It should be noted that the use of numbers differs by culture and individuals. There may be specific numbers with specific meanings (e.g., "lucky number") that may skew this assessment (Booker, 2015).

Written or visual analog scales have been developed; most can be used cross-culturally or with persons with limited English proficiency. For those without numerical ability, a drawing of a ladder can be used and the person asked to put their pain where it would be on the ladder (top = worst). Scales using a series of facial expressions such as the revised Faces Pain Scale (FPS-R) have also been used (Fig. 18.2). Although some have been tested more broadly than others, the uniqueness of emotional expression associated with culture cannot be assumed (Booker, 2015). However, the use of scales may help those who would otherwise not report pain directly. Although many scales have been clinically tested, not everyone agrees which is best to use with the older population (Taylor et al., 2005).

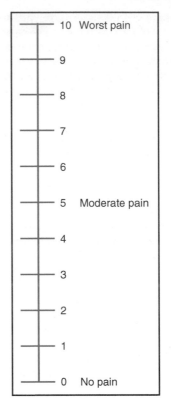

FIG. 18.1 Example of a numeric rating/visual analog scale (can also be verbally administered).(From Pasero, C., & McCaffery, M. (2011). *Pain assessment and pharmacologic management*, St Louis: Elsevier.)

Aggravating factors: "What makes it worse?" Try to be as specific as possible. Remember that pain affects a person's physical, psychological, and spiritual well-being, often all at the same time (Chapter 3).

Relieving factors: "What have you tried to make it better (include prescribed medication, herbs and supplements, over-the-counter drugs, alcohol, and street drugs)?" "What do you think is needed to stop the pain?" This could be correcting a failure as previously mentioned or re-establishing balance of some kind (Chapter 3). If this type of pain has occurred in the past, be sure to ask what helped before.

FIG. 18.2 Example of a face pain-rating scale. (From Swartz, M. H. (2014). *Textbook of physical diagnosis* (7th ed.) St Louis: Elsevier.)

For persistent pain, it is recommended to go a step further to ask, "If your pain could not be relieved completely, what would be an acceptable level?" The nurse may be very surprised at the high levels of pain that people have become accustomed to living with. For example, a person who is not outwardly expressive and does not "appear" to be in pain may describe it as 8 out of 10 when an analog scale is offered.

Regular, repeated assessments, use of standardized tools with consistent documentation, and communication are the most important components of pain management. This leads to the ability to adjust the hypotheses, strategies, action, and outcomes as soon as needed. This should be done consistently and expertly in the promotion of comfort. For more information on pain assessment, see the *Try This* materials available on the website for the Hartford Institute for Geriatric Nursing (https:// consultgeri.org/tools/try-this-series).

RECOGNIZING AND ANALYZING CUES: PAIN IN THOSE WITH COGNITIVE OR COMMUNICATION LIMITATIONS

When a person has cognitive impairments or difficulty with communication, recognizing and analyzing often subtle cues is particularly challenging and an alternative approach is needed. In nursing homes, the certified nursing assistants (CNAs) play an important role in observing discomfort in the older adults they may know better than anyone else.

Herr and a number of colleagues maintain information and reviews of tools to assess pain in both cognitively intact and cognitively impaired older adults (Herr & Decker, 2004). Several of the tools and a plethora of information can be found on the website www.geriatricpain .org. The *Pain Assessment in Advanced Dementia Scale* (PAINAD) and the *Pain Assessment Checklist for Seniors with Limited Ability to Communicate* (PACSLAC) are recommended for use with persons with cognitive or communication limitations. They are complementary to the Minimum Data Set 3.0 (MDS 3.0), which is already required for use in skilled nursing facilities (see Chapter 8). If a person cannot describe their pain (including by pointing to location), it is recommended that both tools be used to determine the presence or absence of cues related to possible pain based on behavior initially, in the determination of outcomes, and at intervals thereafter.

The PAINAD is a simple, short, focused tool that has been found to demonstrate sensitivity to change over time or in response to an action/intervention (Goebel et al., 2019; Warden et al., 2003) (Table 18.1). Four behaviors are rated by an observer on a scale of 0 to 2: breathing when not speaking, negative vocalizations, facial expression and body language, and whether the person can be comforted. The tool is described in detail online including

TABLE 18.1 Pain Assessment in Advanced Dementia (PAINAD)

Items	0	1	2	Score
Breathing independent of vocalization	Normal	Occasional labored breathing Short period of hyperventilation	Noisy labored breathing Long period of hyperventilation Cheyne-Stokes respirations	
Negative vocalization	None	Occasional moan or groan Low level of speech with a negative or disapproving quality	Repeated calling out Loud moaning or groaning Crying	
Facial expression	Smiling or inexpressive	Sad Frightened Frowning	Facial grimacing	
Body language	Relaxed	Tense Distressed pacing Fidgeting	Rigid Fists clenched Knees pulled up Pulling or pushing away Striking out	
Consolability	No need to console	Distracted or reassured by voice or touch	Unable to console, distract, or reassure	
			TOTAL[a]	

[a]Total scores range from 0 to 10 (based on a scale of 0 to 2 for five items), with a higher score indicating more severe pain (0 = no pain, 10 = severe pain). From Warden, V., Hurley, A.C., Volicer, V. (2003). Development and psychometric evaluation of the Pain Assessment in Advanced Dementia (PAINAD) Scale, *J Am Med Dir Assoc 4*, 9–15.

sources of videos to demonstrate its use. It is in use in its original form internationally. (https://geriatricpain.org/sites/geriatricpain.org/files/wysiwyg_uploads/painad_tool_with_logo_updated3.pdf).

The Pain Assessment Checklist for Seniors with Limited Ability to Communicate (PACSLAC) includes four domains of observation: facial expression, activity/body movement, social/personality/mood, and physiological/sleeping/eating/vocal. The CNA in any care setting can use the PACSLAC to observe cues suggestive of pain (Fuchs-Lachelle & Hadjistavropoulos, 2004). Detailed instructions and downloads of the PACSLAC are available online in various formats. Understanding what the person is trying to communicate through their behavior is an essential skill for all staff caring for older adults with communication limitations.

Nursing Actions: Promoting Comfort

The desired outcomes of pain management in older adults are comfort, maintenance of the highest level of functioning and self-care possible, and balance of the risks and benefits of the various treatment options. Careful use of pharmacological and nonpharmacological approaches helps to achieve these goals. A holistic approach is necessary because of the complex and pervasive nature of pain in later life. Nursing actions associated with pain management in older adults are highly complex for a number of reasons, including age-related physiological changes that result in altered drug absorption and excretion, the number of comorbid conditions that may be present, and the common polypharmacy that is found (Chapter 9).

Reducing suffering calls for first addressing any potentially reversible causes, such as a urinary tract infection or a fracture. If pain persists, the nurse and nursing assistant intervene with expert and prompt nonpharmacological strategies. To minimize suffering, only a short trial of nonpharmacological strategies is used before pharmacological interventions are added. Because of the nature of pain in older adults it is most likely that a combination will be needed.

Promoting comfort requires multiple actions, including careful listening, unconditional positive regard, ongoing support, and mobilization of resources. Use of pillows for support or body positioning, appropriate and comfortable seating and mattresses, frequent rest periods, and pacing of activities to balance activity and rest may all be necessary.

At the same time nurses should encourage older adults to stay as active as possible within their comfort range. Nurses learn the cues indicating the person's ability to cope with pain and work within those parameters. When a person has pain with a specific activity (e.g., as in rehabilitation or psychotherapy), anticipation anxiety may decrease both the motivation and the ability to participate fully. In this case, the plan of care may include both pharmacological and nonpharmacological interventions such as relaxation before the scheduled activity. Administering an effective short-acting medication 30 to 60 minutes before the activity may be the action needed to lessen or eliminate the fear of discomfort and enhance the individual's capacity for maximal participation and achievement of the best outcomes possible. It is equally important to treat the person for pain prior to sleep because optimal physical and cognitive functioning the next day is partially mediated by quality sleep (Lee & Oh, 2019) (Chapter 13).

Nurses should encourage older adults and their significant others to take an active role in pain management. After the cues suggestive of pain are identified, a diary of self-assessed levels of pain including the times and strategies and actions used to attempt to find comfort, their effect and the duration of benefit is very helpful. This information helps establish patterns that may be useful in improving comfort by adjusting activity, providing medications at the right times, and promoting control of some aspect of their life. A pain graph provides a visual picture of the highs and lows of the pain. The diary should be reviewed with the nurse and other care providers to adjust dosages or timing of activities for optimal pain management.

Nonpharmacological Strategies

Nurses have a long history of comforting patients through nonpharmacological measures. This may be either in the form of a caring and supportive relationship or through the use of specific techniques performed by the nurse or at the recommendation of the nurse. Several methods that are commonly used with older adults are briefly reviewed here, but it must be acknowledged that this represents only a small sample of what is available (Box 18.8).

BOX 18.8   Research Note

In a study of 141 person residing in a skilled long-term care facility, the used of warmed blankets placed over residents was found to decrease both pain and as-needed analgesic use.

Kovach, C. R. , Putz, M., Guslek, B., McInnes, R. (2019). Do warmed blankets change pain, agitation, mood or analgesic use among nursing home residents? *Pain Management Nurs 20*(6), 526-531.

Cutaneous stimulation. Massage and application of heat and cold are actions nurses have long provided to promote comfort. Heat and cold temporarily interrupt the transmission of pain impulses to the cerebral pain center; however, caution must be used in consideration of the cause and type of pain. Heat provides comfort but will also increase the circulation to the area and therefore is contraindicated in occlusive vascular disease and in non-expansive tissue such as bursae (some joints), where it may increase pain (Cherian et al., 2016). Intermittent application of cold packs is especially recommended for pain related to muscle strain, a common complaint in older patients. Extra care must be taken when applying heat and cold to older skin to prevent skin damage because of normal age-related thinning (see Chapter 4). There should always be a cloth barrier of some kind between the heat/cold source and the skin.

Massage is usually provided by licensed massage therapists. It has many benefits, including relaxing tight, painful muscles. Neither Medicare nor most other health insurance plans pay for this and it can be very expensive. If massage is used, older adults should be encouraged to see a therapist with special skills working with older bodies! Massage, cold, and deep heat are often part of the strategies and actions performed by registered physical therapists. When medically indicated, Medicare may cover some or all the costs.

Several forms of cutaneous nerve stimulation involve the application of small amounts of electricity to the skin to achieve the same purpose. The best known of these is TENS (transcutaneous electrical nerve stimulation) and is thought to work by reducing inflammatory cytokines in the blood (do Carmo Almeida et al., 2018). Although it has been found to reduce pain only by a small amount (Tao et al., 2018), patients often reported anecdotally that at least they were doing "something" for their pain.

Acupuncture and acupressure. Pain is perceived when impulses pass through the theoretical pain gate in the spine and the sensation is registered in the brain, which in turn signals the central mechanism of the brain to return counter-impulses to close the gate. Acupuncture uses tiny needles inserted along specific meridians or pathways in the body (National Center for Complementary and Integrative Health [NCCIH], 2016). Acupressure is pressure applied with the thumbs or tip of the index finger at the same locations. It is thought that acupuncture and acupressure stimulate nerve clusters that cause the "pain gate" to close more quickly or that trigger the release of the body's own opiate substances, enkephalins (endorphins). Acupuncture and acupressure have been used for thousands of years and scientific evidence of their effectiveness in the treatment of persistent pain is growing. There is evidence that acupuncture is especially effective for specific conditions (i.e., pain associated with back, neck, and shoulder; osteoarthritis; and chronic headaches) and can reduce the need for opioids (Johns Hopkins, 2019). Medicare covers the cost of a limited number of acupuncture sessions when prescribed specifically for chronic low back pain.

Touch. Some say the use of touch therapies is a legacy in nursing in promoting pain-relieving outcomes. Over the years, different kinds of touch have been formalized to include those referred to as Healing Touch, Therapeutic Touch, Reiki, and others. When combined with purposeful relaxation, touch may decrease anxiety, reduce muscle tension, and help relieve pain. The acceptability of touch varies considerably by individual and culture. Some touch may never be acceptable, such as cross-gender touch in strict Muslim or Orthodox Jewish traditions (Attum et al., 2019). A culturally sensitive nurse always requests permission before touching a patient in any way (Chapter 3).

Biofeedback. Biofeedback is a cognitive-behavioral strategy that has been used to control pain. It is based on the theory that an individual can learn voluntary control over some body processes and alter them by changing the physiological correlates appropriate to them. Training and equipment of some type are needed to learn how to alter one's body response to the painful sensation through biofeedback. It requires full cognitive functioning and manual dexterity for self-treatment and therefore cannot be used by all older adults.

Distraction. Distraction is a behavioral strategy that temporarily lessens the perception of pain by drawing the person's attention away from it. In some instances, the individual is able to become completely unaware of the pain; in other instances, the intensity of pain is significantly diminished. Pain messages are more slowly transmitted to the pain center in the brain and therefore less pain is felt. The most common forms of distraction include slow rhythmical breathing, slow rhythmical massage, rhythmical singing or tapping, active listening, guided imagery, and humor.

Relaxation, meditation, and imagery. As a behavioral strategy, relaxation enables the quieting of the mind and the muscles, providing the release of tension and anxiety. Relaxation should be adjunctive to all pharmacological interventions and for all types of pain. Meditation and imagery are two methods of promoting relaxation. Several studies have shown that guided imagery can decrease pain perception.

Pharmacological Interventions

A pharmacological approach to pain relief is aimed at altering sensory transmission to the brain, specifically to the cerebral cortex. This is most effective when the treatment plan involves teamwork between the person and the health care providers (especially nurses), caregivers, and significant others, and used to supplement nonpharmacological measures when they are not sufficiently effective on their own. In some cultures, the patient is not the decision-maker regarding treatment. With permission of the older adult, a tribal elder, oldest son, or others may need to be consulted first (see Chapter 3).

The American Geriatrics Society is the source for multiple resources related to care of the older adult in pain and continues to service as a resource to all health professionals caring for older adults (www.geriatrics-careonline.org) (Box 18.9). When generating solutions inclusive of pharmacological agents, those that are the least likely to cause dangerous side effects should be used first. However, more complex and potentially dangerous agents are added or used until the outcome of pain relief to the extent possible is reached. Topical, injectable (e.g. steroids), oral analgesics (nonopioid and opioid agents) and adjuvant medications (antidepressants, anticonvulsants, and herbal preparations, including cannabinoids) have all been found to have a role in addressing both acute and persistent pain in older adults. Several age-related changes and common conditions always need to be considered, especially reduced kidney function, increased fat to muscle ratio, and decreased gastric motility (see Chapter 4) (Marcum et al., 2016).

In gerontological nursing it is essential that medications are started at the lowest dose possible. However, it is equally as important for the doses to be titrated up as needed to the level that pain is relieved to a point that is acceptable to the patient and the relief is *continuous*. Too often, while a low dose is started, increases are delayed, and suffering is unnecessarily prolonged. The adage "Start low, go slow, *but go!*" is important to remember.

Nonopioid analgesics. The choice of medication given for the relief of pain begins with understanding the type of pain that is being experienced, especially the distinction between neuropathic and nociceptive. For pain related to acute inflammation, localized medication such as lidocaine or prednisone can be highly effective when injected into a joint or a trigger point by a skilled clinician. Topical preparations such as nonsteroidal anti-inflammatory drugs, lidocaine, and

capsaicin (a derivative of red pepper) are often used for neuropathic pain, such as that which occurs during and following a shingles outbreak or for diabetic neuropathy. They are also used for nociceptive pain such as that caused by osteoarthritis. Skin must be intact and the area watched for signs of irritation. Because of the normal age-related thinning of the skin and frequency of dehydration quick observation of new cues indicating irritation is especially important.

Acetaminophen (Tylenol) is considered safe and effective when used properly for nociceptive pain such as osteoarthritis and back pain. It is not an anti-inflammatory. It can be used "round the clock" as long as the maximum dose is not exceeded. Acetaminophen is often considered a first-line oral/systemic approach unless contraindicated as in persons who are taking the anticoagulant warfarin (Horgas, 2017a; Marcum et al., 2016). It must be used with caution if the person is also taking a medication that induces cytochrome P450, common in later life (Box 18.10).

Nonsteroidal anti-inflammatory drugs (NSAIDs) are widely used across all ages. When persistent pain is from inflammation, one of the NSAIDs or cyclooxygenase-2 (COX-2) inhibitor (Celebrex) is sometimes used. However, older adults are at significantly higher risk of adverse drug effects from oral NSAIDs than younger adults, especially those with heart or renal disease, with preexisting gastric irritation, or with low albumin levels (Box 18.11). Side effects for non-aspirin formulations include myocardial infarction or stroke and can occur as soon as the first week of use (FDA, 2015). NSAIDs in topical formulations (e.g., diclofenac gel or solution) can be used as an alternative with fewer side effects but slower onset of action.

BOX 18.11   Possible Side Effects or Adverse Drug Reactions to NSAIDs

Indigestion/dyspepsia
Abdominal pain
Nausea
Gastrointestinal bleeding
Increased blood pressure
Myocardial infarction
Stroke

Adapted from Stanos, S. (2013). Osteoarthritis guidelines: A progressive role for topical NSAID *J American Osteopathic Association 113*(2),123–127.

BOX 18.12   Possible Adverse Events When Older Adults Are Prescribed Opioids

Sedation
Gait disturbance
Imbalance
Dizziness
Falls
Nausea
Pruritis
Constipation

BOX 18.13   Tips for Best Practice

At any time that an opioid is prescribed the nurses should expect the older adult to become constipated. Scheduled preventive strategies should be immediately initiated.

Co-administration of any of the protective gastric agents available (histamine-2 [H$_2$] antagonists or proton pump inhibitors) may be helpful and reasonable, especially for persons at a higher risk of gastrointestinal bleeding. NSAIDs cannot be used by persons taking anticoagulants such as warfarin and should not be taken by persons with hypertension.

Opioid analgesics. The use of opioids is part of the "step-wise" approach that should always be considered in attempts to achieve the outcome of pain relief in older adults, but always with caution. The frailer the person, the more caution is needed. Acute traumatic physical pain is usually easily controlled by common analgesic medications, especially a short course of opioids. In the hospital setting an analgesic pump controlled by the patient is used for a restricted period. At the same time, the older a person is, the more likely it is that they will have an adverse reaction (see Chapter 9). For example, most analgesics cause sedation, which increases the risk of falls, delirium, and any of the geriatric syndromes (see Chapter 17).

Opioid analgesics effectively treat both acute and persistent physical pain and have a very important role in the management of the latter. Prior to their use it must be determined that there is no alternative that has an equivalent or greater likelihood of proving relief adequate to restore function and improve quality of life. It should also be known whether the individual has an increased risk of opioid-related adverse effects (Galicia-Castillo & Weiner, 2019). In older adults, opioids may produce a greater analgesic effect, a higher peak effect, and a longer duration of effect when compared with younger adults, attributable in part to prolonged half-lives (see Chapter 9). However, responses to opioids are highly individualized, especially in older adults. Depending on the metabolism of the particular medication, a standard dose in one person may prove toxic yet have no effect in another (see Chapter 9). The recommendation is to start with the lowest anticipated effective dose, monitor the response frequently, and titrate slowly to the point when the desired outcome is achieved (Bruckenthal, 2017).

Side effects should be expected and can be transient or treatable (Box 18.12) (Dowell et al., 2016). They may be lessened or prevented when the prescribing provider works closely with the patient and nurse to attend to cues carefully and try to address potential side effects in advance (e.g., constipation, etc.) (Box 18.13). With the possible exception of oxycodone, sedation and impaired cognition often occur when opioid analgesics are started or when doses are increased and lessen over time. This often causes great concern from patients, families, and nurses but is usually temporary. Appropriate safety precautions should be instituted to minimize the risk of falling.

Although many of the opioid pain relievers can be used cautiously in later life, *the use of meperidine (Demerol) is absolutely contraindicated* (AGS, 2019). The metabolites of meperidine can quickly produce confusion, psychotic behavior, and seizures. The same can be said for pentazocine (Talwin) and the nonopioid methadone.

Adjuvant drugs. There are several drugs developed for other purposes that have been found to be useful in the management of pain, sometimes alone, but more often in combination with an analgesic; these are referred to as adjuvant medications.

Adjuvant medications are thought to be most effective for neuropathic pain syndromes such as postherpetic neuralgia and diabetic nephropathy. The pain is described as sharp, shooting, piercing, or burning. Currently there are several medications that are approved by the FDA for the treatment of neurogenic pain syndromes.

Antidepressants: The tricyclic antidepressants such as nortriptyline had been used as adjuvant for many years.

However, they all have a high potential for increased sedation, cognitive dysfunction, orthostatic hypotension and anticholinergic effects. SSRIs (selective serotonin reuptake inhibitors) and SNRIs (selective noradrenalin reuptake inhibitors) are sometimes used to effect pain relief. However, older adults are much more sensitive to the individual drug's side effects. Venlafaxine (Effexor) has been found to be effective for some. However, higher doses are required and hypertension can occur. Duloxetine (Cymbalta) may be the safest and especially effective for diabetic peripheral neuropathic pain (Marcum et al., 2016).

Anticonvulsants: Although the mechanism is unknown, several anticonvulsants, e.g., lamotrigine (Lamictal) gabapentin (Neurontin) and pregabalin (Lyrica), have been found to be helpful in the treatment of persistent neuropathic pain such as peripheral neuropathy, common in later life (Vinik et al., 2018). Although they are not without possible side effects, they have been found to be safer for older adults than several other medications.

Cannabis and cannabinoids are being used with increased frequency as they become legal for use across the United States. In a study reported in Medscape from a presentation at the 2019 American Academy of Neurology, about half of the participants aged 75 and older reported pain relief. However, its use is still quite controversial and much more research is needed (Cassels, 2019). Several normal changes with aging need to be considered, i.e., reduced hepatic clearance and increased body fat may significantly alter the products' metabolism when compared with use with younger adults. Potential side effects especially important to older adults are altered cognition and gait instability (Cassels, 2019; Minerbi et al., 2019; Romero-Sandoval et al., 2018).

Pain Clinics

The use of opioids has greatly increased over the last few years and, along with this, death as a result of overdoses, especially in younger adults. There are multiple reasons for the increased use, including a failure to address pain adequately in a comprehensive manner and inadequate skills of the provider. Pain clinics, when available, offer much to those in pain.

Pain clinics provide a specialized, often comprehensive, multidisciplinary approach to the management of pain that has not responded to that which can be provided in general practice. The research related to the use of pain clinics by older adults has been limited. However, their use should be encouraged when appropriate. Pain clinics may be inpatient, outpatient, or both. They are generally one of three types: syndrome-oriented, modality-oriented, or comprehensive. Syndrome-oriented centers focus on a specific persistent pain problem, such as headache or

arthritis (Weiner et al., 2019). Modality-oriented clinics focus on a specific treatment technique, such as relaxation or acupuncture/acupressure. Comprehensive clinics tend to be larger and associated with medical centers in urban areas. These centers often utilize an integrated health approach including any or all of the strategies described previously.

The goals of the pain clinic are: to decrease pain intensity to a tolerable limit or eliminate it, if possible; to improve functionality and activities of daily living (ADLs); to increase involvement in family and social activities; to decrease depression. This is accomplished by improving quality and frequency of contact with patients and analysis of any presenting cues, modifying hypotheses as necessary, assisting in minimizing analgesic adverse reactions, selecting nonpharmacological strategies, and evaluating and improving optimal outcomes associated with treatment. Nurses should be familiar with the types of pain management clinics available in their communities to provide the patient and family with the information needed to make decisions regarding their access.

Nurses must also recognize that only one out of ten pain clinics are in rural areas in the United States. Almost 4% of opioid-related deaths occur in these areas, with pain experts many miles away. The reasons are many and the solutions few (Benson & Aldrich, 2019).

Evaluating Outcomes

Gerontological nurses, older adults, and significant others should work together to promote comfort for the person in pain through nonpharmacological and pharmacological strategies and actions working in harmony (Box 18.14). Evaluation of the outcome of the pain relief

---

BOX 18.14 General Principles of Pharmacological Management of Pain in Older Adults

1. When pain is assessed, negotiate a pain relief or comfort goal with the patient.
2. Be aware of other conditions that may affect assessment and management of pain.
3. Anticipate age-associated, but unpredictable, differences in sensitivities and toxicities related to medication use.
4. Always start at a low dose and slowly titrate to around-the-clock pain relief.
5. Use the least-invasive possible route of administration first.
6. Plan timing of medication administration to meet the needs of the patient.
7. Never use placebos.
8. Consider complementary, nonpharmacological, and pharmacological approaches.

strategies requires repeated search for cues/reassessment of a person's functional and cognitive status and comfort level. Cues indicative of comfort include relaxation of skeletal muscles that were tense and rigid during pain, an increase in activity level, an increase in sense of self-worth, improved concentration, focus, attention span, regardless of baseline cognitive status. The individual is better able to rest, relax, and sleep.

The evaluation of the outcomes of pain relief is also measured with the same instruments used in the initially for a means of comparison. Re-evaluations of the frequency and intensity of pain and response to pharmacological and nonpharmacological interventions are done. Adjustments to nursing actions are based on repeated analyses of cues and continue until the desired outcome is reached and maintained. In doing so, health is promoted at any stage of life and wellness.

It has now been shown that a combination of pharmacological and nonpharmacological interventions/actions appears to be most effective in the relief of both acute and persistent pain in later life. Helping persons find relief from pain is to encourage whatever strategies have been effective in the past without causing harm. This is particularly applicable for older adults with a lifetime of experience managing their own pain and that of others. In some cases, what is now referred to as complementary and alternative or integrative medicine (CAM) is the formalization of strategies that people have used for years. More and more of what is considered CAM (e.g., acupuncture) is gaining acceptance by insurers such as Medicare.

Regardless of the care setting or role played, nurses have a responsibility to let go of their own expectations and promote comfort to those who are suffering, regardless of the cause and manner of expression of this suffering. The best gerontological nursing care is that provided in a nonjudgmental manner always with the goal of comfort—not just to lessen pain but to make every attempt to relieve it safely and prevent its reoccurrence.

KEY CONCEPTS

- The absence of expressed pain does not necessarily imply comfort. Comfort is a state of ease and satisfaction of bodily needs and self-worth, unique to each person.
- The experience of pain is not limited to that which is of physical origin. Pain related to psychological or spiritual factors can have the same effect and is often combined with that arising from physical causes.
- The recognition of pain is influenced by many misconceptions, myths, and stereotypes about pain and how it is expressed.

- Culture, ethnicity, family, and individual characteristics all influence a person's tolerance and expression of pain as well as the acceptance of actions that may provide relief.
- The cues to discomfort in older adults with cognitive or communication problems include increased levels of confusion, restlessness, aggression, or withdrawal.
- Some pain medications are more appropriate than others for use with older adults.
- Chronic, i.e., persistent pain predominates in the lives of many older adults.
- Various combinations of pharmacological and nonpharmacological pain control can be effective but must be individually designed with the older adults and others involved in the decision-making process.

ACTIVITIES AND DISCUSSION QUESTIONS

1. Select a culture other than your own and research how pain is expressed by persons who hold traditional beliefs in that culture.
2. How does the recognition of cues and the development of hypotheses related to providing comfort to those in pain differ in cognitively impaired older people?
3. What nonpharmacological therapy is available and how can each type work with the other to achieve the outcome of pain relief?
4. What areas of the country has the greatest "problem with opioids" and why?
5. In what circumstances has the dramatic increase in opioid use in recent years affected older adults?

NEXT-GENERATION NCLEX® EXAMINATION-STYLE QUESTIONS

Yesterday, Mrs. Aurbach, a 94-year-old survivor of the Ravensbrück concentration camp, was found on the blue mat next to her low bed. Today, her left wrist is swollen and purple. She is restless, grimaces, and withdraws her left wrist when it is touched. A portable X-ray image was negative for fracture. Mrs. Aurbach is bedridden with end-stage dementia. She also has a history of hypertension and osteoporosis. Her medications include atenolol 25 mg daily and acetaminophen 500 mg every 4 hours as needed for pain. She is 5′ 8″ and weighs 125 pounds (BMI 19 kg/m^2). Vital signs include a blood pressure of 110/68 mmHg, heart rate of 66 beats per minute, respirations of 16 breaths per minute, temperature of 97.5°F, and oxygen saturation of 98% on room air. Results of laboratory work include:

- White blood cell count: 13.5×10^3 cells/mm^3
- Hemoglobin and hematocrit: 12 g/dL and 36%
- Platelet count: 200,000 cells/mm^3
- Blood urea nitrogen/creatinine: 22 mg/dL and 1.0 mg/dL
- Sodium: 144 mEq/L
- Glucose: 90 mg/dL
- Urinalysis: Urine is amber and clear, pH 7.0, nitrite + and leukocyte esterase +, blood 5/hpf, WBC 5/hpf, and bacteria 75,000 CFUs/mL.

Use an X to indicate which actions listed in the left column would be included in this client's plan of care.

Actions	Plan of Care
Elevate left hand/wrist on pillow while in bed	
Request the client keep a pain diary	
Encourage the client to participate in restorative activities	
Use touch, such as gentle back massage, prior to bed	
Have client's preferred music genre playing in room	
Monitor client for increased restlessness and agitation	
Use numeric pain scale	

REFERENCES

Ahn, H., & Horgas, A. (2013). The relationship between pain and disruptive behaviors in nursing home residents with dementia. *BMC Geriatr, 13*, 14.

American Geriatrics Society (AGS). (2019). Beers Criteria Update Expert Panel: American Geriatrics Society 2019 updated Beers criteria for potentially inappropriate medication use in older adults. *J Am Geriatr Soc, 67*(4), 674–694.

Attum, B., Waheed, A., & Shamoon, Z. (2019). Cultural competence in the care of Muslim patients and their families. *StatPearls,* June 15.

Benson, W. F., & Aldrich, N. (2019). Rural older adults hit hard by opioid epidemic, *Aging Today.* https://www.asaging.org/blog/rural-older-adults-hit-hard-opioid-epidemic.

Booker, S. (2015). The state of "cultural validity" of self-report pain assessment tools in diverse older adults. *Pain Med, 16*, 232–239.

Bruckenthal, P. (2017). Pain in the older adult. In H. M. Fillit, K. Rockwood, & J. Young (Eds.), *Brocklehurst's textbook of geriatric medicine and gerontology* (8th ed., pp. 789–810). Philadelphia: Elsevier.

Cassels, C. (2019). Medical cannabis safe, effective for neurologic symptoms in the elderly. *Medscape.* May 6. https://www.medscape.com/viewarticle/912624#vp_1.

Centers for Medicare and Medicaid Services (CMS). (2019). *Quality measures.* https://www.cms.gov/Medicare/Quality-Initiatives-Patient-Assessment-instruments/NursingHomeQualityInits/NHQIQualityMeasures.html.

Cherian, J. J., Jauregui, J.J., Leichliter, A. K., et al. (2016). The effects of various physical non-operative modalities on the pain in osteoarthritis of the knee. *Bone Joint J, 98-B*(1 Suppl A), 89–94.

do Carmo Almeida, T. C., Dos Santos Figueiredo, F. W., Barbosa Filho, V. C., de Abreu, L. C., Fonseca, F. L. A., & Adami, F. (2018). Effects of Transcutaneous Electrical Nerve Stimulation on proinflammatory cytokine: systemic review and meta-analysis. *Mediators Inflamm* eCollection, 1094352, 2018.

Dowell, D., Haegerich, T. M., & Chou, R. (2016). CDC guideline for prescribing opioids for chronic pain – United States. *MMWR Reccomm Report, 65*(No. RR-1), 1–49.

Epplin, J. J., Higuchi, M., Gajendra, N., et al. (2014). Persistent pain. In R. J. Ham, P. D. Sloan, & G. A. Warshaw, et al. (Eds.), *Primary care: A case-based approach* (6th ed., pp. 306–314). Philadelphia: Elsevier.

Food and Drug Administration [FDA]. (2015). *FDA drug safety communication: FDA strengthens warning that non-aspirin nonsteroidal anti-inflammatory drugs (NSAIDs) can cause heart attacks or strokes.* https://www.fda.gov/drugs/drug-safety-and-availability/fda-drug-safety-communication-fda-strengthens-warning-non-aspirin-nonsteroidal-anti-inflammatory.

Fuchs-Lachelle, S., & Hadjistavropoulos, T. (2004). Development and preliminary validation of the Pain Assessment Checklist for Seniors with Limited Ability to Communicate (PACSLAC). *Pain Manag Nurs, 5*(1), 37–49.

Galicia-Castillo, M. C., & Weiner, D. K. (2019). Treatment of persistent pain in older adults, *UpToDate.* https://www.uptodate.com/contents/treatment-of-persistent-pain-in-older-adults.

Goebel, J. R., Ferolito, M., & Gorman, N. (2019). Pain screening in the older adult with delirium. *Pain Manag Nurs, 20*(6), 519–525.

Herr, K. (2010). Pain in the older adult: An imperative across all health care settings. *Pain Manag Nurs, 11*(2 Suppl), S1.

Herr, K., & Decker, S. (2004). Assessment of pain in older adults with severe cognitive impairment. *Ann Longterm Care, 12*(46).

Horgas, A. L. (2017a). Pain management in older adults. *Nurs Clinics of N America, 52*(4), e1–e7. https://www.ncbi.nlm.nih.gov/pubmed/29080585.

Horgas, A. L. (2017b). Pain assessment in older adults. *Nurs Clinics of N America, 52*(3), 375–385.

Hulla, R., Vanzzini, N., Salas, E., Beyers, K., Garner, T., et al. (2019). Pain management in the elderly. *Practical Pain Management, 17*(1). https://www.practicalpainmanagement.com/treatments/pain-management-elderly.

Johns Hopkins: Acupuncture, 2019. https://www.hopkinsmedicine.org/health/wellness-and-prevention/acupuncture.

Lee, M. K., & Oh, J. H. (2019). The relationship between pain and physical function Mediating role of sleep quality, depression, and fatigue. *J Geron Nurs, 45*(7), 46–54.

Marcum, Z. A., Duncan, N. A., & Makris, U. E. (2016). Pharmacotherapies in geriatric chronic pain management. *Clin Geriatr Med, 32*(4), 705–724.

Minerbi, A., Hauser, W., & Fitzcharles, M. A. (2019). Medical cannabis for older adults. *Drugs Aging, 36*(1), 39–51.

National Center for Complementary and Integrative Health (NCCIH): Acupuncture in depth, 2016. https://nccih.nih.gov/health/acupuncture/introduction.

Romero-Sandoval, E. A., Fincham, J. E., Kolano, A. L., Sharpe, B. N., & Alvarado-Vazquez, P. A. (2018). Cannabis for chronic pain: challenges and considerations. *Pharmacotherapy, 38*(6), 651–662.

Tao, H., Wang, T., Dong, X., Guo, Q., Xu, H., & Wan, Q. (2018). Effectiveness of transcutaneous electrical nerve stimulation for the treatment of a migraine: a meta-analysis of randomized control trial. *J Headache Pain, 19*(1), 42.

Taylor, L., Harris, J., Epps, C., et al. (2005). Psychometric evaluation of selected pain-intensity scales for use with cognitively impaired and cognitively intact older adults. *Rehabil Nurs, 30*, 55–61.

The Joint Commission. (2020). *Pain management standards for accredited organizations*. https://www.jointcommission.org/topics/pain_management_standards_hospital.aspx.

Tumi, H. E., Johnson, M. I., Dantas, P. B. F., Maynard, M.J., & Tashani, O.A. (2017). Age-related changes in pain sensitivity in healthy humans: A systematic review of the literature. *European J of Pain, 21*(6), 955–964.

Vinik, A., Casellini, C., Nevoret, M. L.: Diabetic neuropathies. *Endotext* online, Table 7, updated Feb 2018. https://www.ncbi.nlm.nih.gov/books/NBK279175/table/diab-neuropathies.medication/.

Warden, V., Hurley, A. C., & Volicer, L. (2003). Development and psychometric evaluation of the Pain Assessment in Advanced Dementia (PAINAD) scale. *J Am Med Dir Assoc, 4*(9).

Weiner, D. K., Gentili, A., Rossi, M., Coffey-Vega, K., Rodriguez, K. L., et al. (2020). Aging back clinics- a geriatrics syndrome approach to treating chronic low back pain in older adults: results of a preliminary randomized controlled study. *Pain Med, 21*(2), 274–290.

19

Clinical Judgment to Enhance Hearing and Vision

Theris A. Touhy

http://evolve.elsevier.com/Touhy/gerontological/

LEARNING OBJECTIVES

Upon completion of this chapter, the reader will be able to:
- Describe the impact of hearing and vision changes on quality of life and function.
- Describe the importance of health education and screening for hearing and vision problems.
- Identify effective communication strategies for older adults with vision and hearing impairment.
- Utilize clinical judgment to recognize and analyze cues and identify and evaluate nursing actions to enhance hearing and vision.
- Gain awareness of assistive devices to enhance vision and hearing.

THE LIVED EXPERIENCE

One of the great frustrations is the matter of eyesight. One can get used to large print and hope for black letters on white paper, but why do modern publishers seem to prefer the shiny, slick off-white paper and pale ink in minuscule print? Thank goodness for restaurants with lighted menus and my new iPhone with a bright light. And my new prescription glasses have not restored my ability to cut my own toenails without danger of wounding myself.

Lyn, age 85

This chapter discusses changes in hearing and vision with age, diseases that affect vision, and adaptations to enhance communication for those with vision and hearing impairments. While vision and hearing loss is discussed separately in the chapter, it is important to note the prevalence of older adults reporting both hearing and vision loss. An estimated 30% of those aged 80 years and older have dual sensory loss (DSL). Older adults with a single sensory deficit (either vision or hearing) can rely on the intact sensory function to compensate. Those with DSL lack this compensatory capability and this increases challenges and poor outcomes. Research and public policies mainly address either hearing or vision loss. More attention must be paid to the design of nursing actions to assist individuals experiencing DSL (Ge et al., 2021). *Healthy People 2020* (US Department of Health and Human Services [USDHHS], 2012) has set goals for vision and hearing (Box 19.1).

VISUAL IMPAIRMENT

Incidence and Prevalence

Vision loss is not an inevitable part of the aging process, but age-related changes contribute to decreased vision (Chapter 4). Even older adults with good visual acuity (20/40 or better) and no significant eye disease show deficits in visual function and need accommodations to enhance vision and safety. As we age there is a higher risk of developing age-related eye diseases and other conditions (hypertension, diabetes) that can result in vision losses if left untreated.

♥ BOX 19.1   Healthy People 2020

Objectives Vision and Hearing—Older Adult

- Increase the proportion of adults who have had a comprehensive eye examination, including dilation, within the past 2 years.
- Reduce visual impairment caused by diabetic retinopathy, glaucoma, cataract, and macular degeneration.
- Increase the use of vision rehabilitation services by persons with visual impairment.
- Increase the use of assistive and adaptive devices by persons with visual impairment.
- Increase the proportion of persons with hearing impairment who have ever used a hearing aid or assistive listening device or who have cochlear implants.
- Increase the proportion of adults 70 years of age who have had a hearing examination in the past 5 years.
- Increase the number of persons who are referred by their primary care physician or other health care provider for hearing evaluation and treatment.
- Increase the proportion of adults bothered by tinnitus who have seen a health care professional.

From US Department of Health and Human Services, Office of Disease Prevention and Health Promotion (2012). *Healthy People 2020*. http://www.healthypeople.gov/2020.

Vision loss is a leading cause of age-related disability. More than two-thirds of those with visual impairment are older than 65 years of age and adults older than 80 years account for 70% of the cases of severe visual impairment. The World Health Organization (WHO, 2020) defines visual impairment as visual acuity worse than 20/70 but better than 20/400 (legal blindness) in the better eye, even with corrective lenses.

Visual impairment worldwide has decreased since the 1990s as a result of increased availability of eye care services (particularly cataract surgery), promotion of eye care education, and improved treatment of infectious diseases. However, vision impairment is a major public health problem across the globe that is expected to increase substantially with the aging of the population. Rates of blindness and visual impairment in disadvantaged, minority populations, particularly Blacks and Latino subpopulations who have an increased prevalence of diabetes and hypertension, are expected to increase even further. In the United States, the leading causes of visual impairment are cataracts, glaucoma, diabetic neuropathy, and age-related macular degeneration (AMD). Globally, uncorrected refractive errors (myopia, hyperopia, or astigmatism), glaucoma, and unoperated cataract are the leading causes of visual impairment.

Consequences of Visual Impairment

Visual problems have a negative impact on quality of life, equivalent to that of life-threatening conditions such as heart disease and cancer. Loss of vision impacts an individual's quality of life and ability to function in most daily activities such as driving, reading, maneuvering safely, dressing, cooking, taking medications, and participating in social activities. Decreased vision has also been found to be a significant risk factor for falls and other accidents and is associated with cognitive decline and depression, increased risk of institutionalization, and death. "Vision loss not only severely impairs one's ability to be independent and self-sufficient, but it also has a 'snowball effect' on the health and well-being of older adults, families, caregivers, and society at large. This cumulative effect is severely underestimated." (International Federation on Ageing, 2012, p. 4).

Prevention of Visual Impairment

Many age-related eye diseases have no symptoms in the early stages but can be detected early through a comprehensive dilated eye examination. However, knowledge about eye disease and treatments remains inadequate among both laypersons and medical professionals. Socioeconomic position and educational position are important social determinants that may influence access to and use of effective and appropriate eye care, thus influencing disease identification and treatment (MacLennan et al., 2014; Zhang et al., 2013).

At all ages, attention to eye health and protection of vision are important (Box 19.2). Prevention and treatment of eye disease are important priorities for nurses and other health professionals. The National Eye Health Education Program (NEHEP) of the National Eye Institute (NEI) provides a program for health

BOX 19.2   Promoting Healthy Eyes

- Do not smoke.
- Eat a diet rich in green, leafy vegetables and fish.
- Exercise.
- Maintain normal blood pressure and blood glucose measurements.
- Wear sunglasses and a brimmed hat anytime you are outside in bright sunshine.
- Wear safety eyewear when working around your house or playing sports.
- See an eye care professional routinely.

From the National Eye Institute, National Eye Health Education Program: *Make vision health a priority*. http://www.nei.nih.gov/healthyeyestoolkit/pdf/VisionAndHealth_Tagged.pdf.

BOX 19.3   Resources for Best Practice

Vision Impairment

- **CDC:** Keep an Eye on your Visual Health. https://www.cdc.gov /features/healthyvision/index.html: Educational materials, videos illustrating vision with AMD, glaucoma, diabetic retinopathy
- **Eye Care America:** https://www.aao.org/eyecare-america: On -line referral center for eye care resources
- **National Eye Health Education Program (NEHEP) and National Eye Institute (NEI):** https://www.nei.nih.gov/learn -about-eye-health/resources-for-health-educators: Educational and professional resources, vision and aging program: *See Well for a Lifetime Toolkit,* vodcasts on common visual problems, videos on eye disease (https://nei.nih.gov/videos).
- **National Federation for the Blind:** https://www.nfb.org/: Educational information, resources
- **Vision Aware (American Foundation for the Blind):** https:// www.visionaware.org/default.aspx: Resources for independent living with vision loss, Getting started kit for people new to vision loss, How to walk with a guide.

professionals with evidence-based tools and resources that can be used in community settings to educate older adults about eye health and maintaining healthy vision. Educational materials and outreach activities targeted to populations at high risk for eye diseases, including Blacks, American Indians, Alaska natives, Hispanics/ Latinos, and individuals with diabetes and a family history of glaucoma are available (NEI, NEHEP, 2019a) (https://www.nei.nih.gov/learn-about-eye-health /resources-for-health-educators/vision-and-aging -resources/see-well-lifetime-toolkit) (Box 19.3).

DISEASES AND DISORDERS OF THE EYE

Cataracts

A cataract is an opacification (cloudiness) in the eye's normally clear crystalline lens, causing the lens to lose transparency or scatter light. Cataracts can occur at any age (babies can be born with them), but they are most common later in life. In the United States, about 70% of people over the age of 75 years have cataracts. Older adults with diabetes are 60% more likely to develop cataracts than individuals without diabetes (https://www.nei.nih.gov /learn-about-eye-health/resources-for-health-educators). Cataracts are categorized according to their location within the lens: nuclear, cortical, and posterior subcapsular (in the rear of the lens capsule). Nuclear cataracts are the most common type and their incidence increases with age and cigarette smoking. Cortical cataracts also are more common with age and their development is related to a lifetime of exposure to ultraviolet light.

Recognizing and Analyzing Cues: Cataracts

Cataracts form painlessly over time. The most common symptom is cloudy or blurred vision. Everything becomes dimmer, as if seen through glasses that need cleaning. Other symptoms include glare, halos around lights, poor night vision, a perception that colors are faded or that objects are yellowish, and the need for brighter light when reading. The red reflex may be absent or may appear as a black area. Fig. 19.1A illustrates normal vision; Fig. 19.1B illustrates the effects of a cataract on vision. The National Eye Institute provides videos on eye disorders and eye health (Box 19.3).

Treatment of Cataracts

The treatment of cataracts is surgical and cataract surgery is the most common surgical procedure performed in the United States. The surgery involves removal of the lens and placement of a plastic intraocular lens (IOL). Most often, cataract surgery involves only local anesthesia and is done on an outpatient basis. If the eye is normal except for the cataract, surgery will improve vision in 95% of cases. Significant postsurgical complications such as inflammation, infection, bleeding, retinal detachment, swelling, and glaucoma are rare. Individuals with medical problems such as diabetes and other eye diseases are most at risk of complications.

Nursing Actions: Presurgical and Postsurgical Cataract Removal

Nursing actions when caring for a person experiencing cataract surgery include preparing the individual for significant changes in vision and adaptation to light and ensuring that the individual has received adequate counseling regarding realistic postsurgical expectations. Most people experience a small amount of discomfort after surgery. Some redness, scratchiness, or discharge from the eye may occur during the first day after surgery. There may also be a few black spots or shapes (floaters) drifting through the field of vision. Vision remains blurred for several days or weeks and then gradually improves as the eye heals.

If the person has bilateral cataracts, surgery is performed first on one eye with the second surgery on the other eye a month or so later to ensure healing. Following surgery, the individual needs to avoid heavy lifting, straining, and bending at the waist. Eye drops may be prescribed to aid healing and prevent infection. Teaching fall prevention techniques and ensuring home safety modifications are also important because some research suggests that the risk of falls increases after

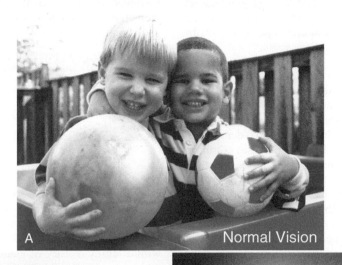

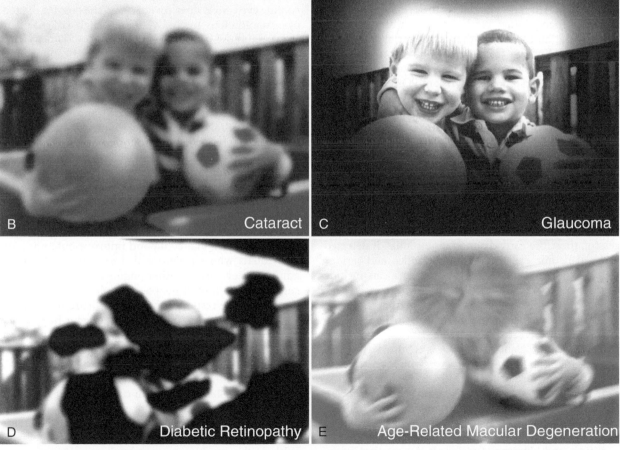

FIG. 19.1 (A) Normal vision. (B) Simulated vision with cataracts. (C) Simulated vision with glaucoma. (D) Simulated vision with diabetic retinopathy. (E) Simulated vision with age-related macular degeneration (AMD). (From National Eye Institute, National Institutes of Health, 2015.)

surgery, particularly between first and second cataract surgeries. The vision imbalance that can occur if the person has one "good" eye and one "bad" eye contributes to the risk of falls.

Glaucoma

Glaucoma is a group of diseases that can damage the optic nerve. Glaucoma is the second leading cause of blindness in the United States. Glaucoma affects as many as 2.3 million Americans aged 40 years and older and 6% of those older than 65 years. Because the most common form of the condition, primary open-angle glaucoma (POAG), affects side vision first, it may remain unnoticed for years. At least half of all persons with glaucoma are unaware they have the disease.

Individuals at higher risk of glaucoma include Blacks over the age of 40 years; people with a family history of glaucoma; and everyone over 60 years, especially Mexican Americans. The condition is four times more common in Hispanics and five times more common in Blacks than Whites. Blacks are at risk of developing glaucoma at an earlier age than other racial and ethnic groups and blindness from glaucoma is four to five times more common than among Whites. Type 2 diabetes is associated with an 82% higher risk of POAG. Other risk factors include trauma to the eye, severe myopia, or previous eye surgeries. Other high-risk groups are individuals with a history of corticosteroid use, trauma to the eye, myopia, or previous eye surgeries. Some genetic variants may be associated with elevated IOP; thus family history is an important risk factor. Research is currently being done into genes that could explain how glaucoma damages the eye (NEI, 2019a).

The damage to the optic nerve in glaucoma is irreversible and regenerative attempts have been unsuccessful, therefore early diagnosis is essential. If detected early, glaucoma can usually be controlled and serious vision loss prevented. Signs of glaucoma can include headaches, poor vision in dim lighting, increased sensitivity to glare, "tired eyes," impaired peripheral vision, a fixed and dilated pupil, and frequent changes in prescriptions for corrective lenses (Fig. 19.1C).

Angle-closure glaucoma is not as common as POAG and occurs when the angle of the iris causes obstruction of the aqueous humor through the trabecular network. Individuals with smaller eyes, Asians, and women are most susceptible. It may occur as a result of infection or trauma. IOP rises rapidly accompanied by redness and pain in and around the eye, severe headaches, nausea and vomiting, and blurring of vision. It is a medical emergency and blindness can occur in 2 days. Treatment is an iridectomy to ease pressure. Many drugs with anticholinergic properties, including antihistamines, stimulants, vasodilators, and sympathomimetics, are particularly dangerous for individuals predisposed to acute-closure glaucoma.

> ### ⚡ SAFETY ALERT
>
> Redness and pain in and around the eye, severe headaches, nausea and vomiting, and blurring of vision occur with angle-closure glaucoma. It is a medical emergency and blindness can occur in 2 days.

A dilated eye examination and tonometry are necessary to diagnose glaucoma. Adults over the age of 65 years should have annual eye examinations with dilation and those with medication-controlled glaucoma should be examined at least every 6 months. Annual screening is also recommended for Blacks and other individuals with a family history of glaucoma who are older than 40 years. Although standard Medicare does not cover routine eye care, it does cover 80% of the cost for dilated eye examinations for individuals at high risk of glaucoma and those with diabetes.

Management of glaucoma involves medications (oral or topical eye drops) to decrease IOP and/or laser trabeculoplasty and filtration surgery. Medications reduce eye pressure either by decreasing the amount of aqueous fluid produced within the eye or by improving the flow through the drainage angle. Beta-blockers are the first-line therapy for glaucoma followed by prostaglandin analogues. Second-line agents include topical carbonic anhydrase inhibitors and α_2-agonists. The patient may need combinations of several types of eye drops.

There is ongoing research on the development of a contact lens to deliver glaucoma medication in a continuous-release dose that may become an option for the treatment of glaucoma and improve outcomes for individuals who struggle with imprecise, difficult to administer eye drops. Other ongoing research findings suggest vision loss in people with glaucoma is caused by an immune response to early exposure to bacteria, which can elevate eye pressure and trigger heat shock proteins. While further research is needed, targeted manipulation of the immune response in the eye may help eliminate the disease (Glaucoma Research Foundation, 2020).

In the hospital or long-term care setting, it is important to obtain a medical history to determine whether the person has glaucoma and to ensure that eye drops are given according to the person's treatment regimen. Without the eye drops, eye pressure can rise and cause an acute exacerbation of glaucoma. Usually medications can control glaucoma, but laser surgery (trabeculoplasty) and filtration surgery may be recommended for some types of glaucoma. Surgery is usually recommended only if necessary to prevent further damage to the optic nerve.

Diabetic Eye Disease

Diabetic eye disease includes diabetic retinopathy (DR) and diabetic macular edema (DME). Cataracts and glaucoma are also more prevalent in individuals with diabetes. All forms of diabetic eye disease have the potential to cause severe vision loss and blindness (NEI, 2019c).

Diabetic Retinopathy

Diabetes has become an epidemic in the United States and DR occurs in both type 1 and type 2 diabetes mellitus (Chapter 20). Risk increases the longer an individual has diabetes. Almost all people with type 1 diabetes will eventually develop retinopathy. People with type 2 diabetes are less likely to develop more advanced retinopathy than those with type 1. Chronically high blood sugar from diabetes is associated with damage to the tiny blood vessels in the retina, leading to DR. Blood and lipid leakage leads to macular edema and hard exudates (composed of lipids). In advanced disease, new fragile blood vessels form and hemorrhage easily. Because of the vascular and cellular changes accompanying diabetes, there is often also rapid worsening of other pathologic vision conditions (Fig. 19.1D).

Recognizing and Analyzing Cues: Diabetic Retinopathy

Early detection and treatment of diabetic DR is essential. There are no symptoms in the early stages of DR. The disease often progresses unnoticed until it affects vision. Bleeding from abnormal retinal blood vessels can cause the appearance of "floating" spots that sometimes clear on their own. Without prompt treatment, bleeding often recurs, increasing the risk of permanent vision loss. Early signs are seen in the fundoscopic examination and include microaneurysms, flame-shaped hemorrhages, cotton wool spots, hard exudates, and dilated capillaries. Constant, strict control of blood glucose levels, cholesterol levels, and blood pressure measurements and laser photocoagulation (LPC) treatments can halt progression of the disease.

Annual dilated fundoscopic examination of the eye is recommended beginning 5 years after diagnosis of diabetes type 1 and at the time of diagnosis of diabetes type 2. Nurses need to provide education to individuals with diabetes about the risk of DR, the importance of early identification, and good control of diabetes. An increased likelihood of falls has been reported in individuals with mild to moderate nonproliferative DR. Fall prevention education should be provided to individuals with early-stage disease (Gupta et al., 2017). Some

experts are encouraging mass screening efforts. There is good treatment that can reverse vision loss and improve vision, but individuals must have access to screenings and eye examinations.

Diabetic Macular Edema (DME)

DME is the buildup of fluid (edema) in a region of the retina called the macula. DME is the most common cause of visual loss attributable to diabetes and the leading cause of legal blindness. The disease affects 1 in 25 adults aged 40 years and older with diabetes and the incidence is higher in Blacks and Hispanics. About half of people with DR will develop DME. People with a history of high blood pressure and atherosclerosis are also at a high risk of developing DME. Although it is more likely to occur as DR becomes worse, it can happen at any stage of the disease. Symptoms include blurred vision, loss of contrast, and patches of vision loss, which may appear a black dots or lines "floating" across the front of the eye (Genentech, 2017).

Treatment includes medications (often cortisone-type drugs), anti-VEGF (vascular endothelial growth factor) injection therapy, and laser therapy to cauterize leaky blood vessels and to reduce accumulated fluid within the macula. Anti-VEGF therapy (Lucentis) is used alone or in conjunction with laser treatment to treat DR in individuals with DME. The treatment appears to be well tolerated but requires about 12 to 15 injections into the eye over 36 months (NEI, 2019c).

Strict control of blood glucose, cholesterol, and blood pressure values, completion of annual dilated retinal examinations, and education about eye disease and diabetes are essential. However, in a recent study, only 44.7% of adults 40 years and older with DME reported that they were told by a physician that diabetes had affected their eyes and 59.7% had received a dilated eye examination in the past year. Approximately 55% of individuals with DME are unaware they have the condition (Genentech, 2017). Advances in stem cell technology and tissue engineering in the past several years have opened the possibility of replacing lost retinal neurons that occur as a result of DR, as well as glaucoma and AMD (Levin et al., 2017).

Detached Retina

A retinal detachment can occur at any age but is more common after the age of 40 years. Emergency medical treatment is required or permanent visual loss can result. There may be small areas of the retina that are torn (retinal tears or breaks) and will lead to retinal detachment. This condition can develop in persons with cataracts or recent cataract surgery or trauma, or it can occur spontaneously. Symptoms include a gradual increase in the number of floaters and/or light flashes in the eye. It also manifests as a curtain coming down over the person's field of vision. Small holes or tears are treated with laser surgery or a freeze treatment called *cryopexy*. Retinal detachments are treated with surgery. More than 90% of individuals with a retinal detachment can be successfully treated, although sometimes a second treatment is needed. However, the visual outcome is not always predictable and may not be known for several months following surgery. Visual results are best if the detachment is repaired before the macula detaches and immediate treatment of symptoms is therefore essential (NEI, 2019b).

Age-Related Macular Degeneration

AMD is the most common cause of new visual impairment among people aged 50 years and older, although it is most likely to occur after the age of 60 years (NEI, 2019c). The prevalence of AMD increases drastically with age, with more than 15% of White women older than age 80 years having the disease. Whites and Asian Americans are more likely to lose vision from AMD than Blacks or Hispanics/Latinos. With the number of affected older adults projected to increase over the next 20 years, AMD has been called a growing global epidemic.

AMD is a degenerative eye disease that affects the macula, the central part of the eye responsible for clear central vision. The disease causes the progressive loss of central vision, leaving only peripheral vision intact. The early and intermediate stages usually start without symptoms and only a comprehensive dilated eye examination can detect AMD. Objects may not appear to be as bright as they used to be and individuals may attribute their vision problems to normal aging or cataracts.

As AMD progresses, a blurred area near the center of vision is a common symptom. Over time, the blurred areas may grow larger and blank spots can develop in the central vision. AMD does not lead to complete blindness, but the loss of central vision interferes with everyday activities such as the ability to see faces, read, drive, or do close work, and can lead to impaired mobility, increased risk of falls, depression, and decreased quality of life (NEI, 2019c) (Fig. 19.1E).

AMD results from systemic changes in circulation, accumulation of cellular waste products, atrophy of tissue, and growth of abnormal blood vessels in the choroid layer beneath the retina. Fibrous scarring disrupts nourishment of photoreceptor cells, causing their death and loss of central vision. Risk factors for AMD are similar to those for coronary artery disease (hypertension, atherosclerosis), inflammation, and diet. High glycemic diets are associated with AMD onset and progression (Rowan et al., 2017). Smoking doubles the risk of AMD.

Individuals with a family history of AMD are at higher risk. At least 20 genes have been identified that affect the risk of developing AMD and many more genetic risk factors are suspected.

There are three stages of AMD, defined in part by the size and number of drusen under the retina. An individual can have AMD in one eye only or have one eye with a later stage than the other. Not everyone with early AMD will develop the later stage of the disease. In individuals with early AMD in one eye and no signs of AMD in the other eye, about 5% will develop advanced AMD after 10 years. For people who have early AMD in both eyes, about 14% will develop late AMD in at least one eye after 10 years. Having late AMD in one eye puts an individual at increased risk of late AMD in the other eye.

In late AMD, there is vision loss attributable to damage to the macula. There are two types of late AMD: geographic atrophy (dry AMD) and neovascular AMD (wet AMD). Neovascular AMD occurs when abnormal blood vessels behind the retina start to grow under the macula. These new blood vessels are fragile and often leak blood and fluid, which raise the macula from its normal place at the back of the eye. With wet AMD, the severe loss of central vision can be rapid and many people will be legally blind within 2 years of diagnosis.

Screening and Treatment of AMD

Early diagnosis is the key. An Amsler grid (Fig. 19.2) is used to determine clarity of vision. A perception of wavy lines is diagnostic of beginning macular degeneration. In the advanced forms, the person may see dark or empty spaces that block the center of vision. People with AMD are usually taught to test their eyes daily using an Amsler grid so that they will be aware of any changes. AMD occurs less in individuals who exercise, avoid smoking, and consume a diet high in green, leafy vegetables and fruits. In early AMD, adopting some of these habits may help keep vision longer (NEI, 2019c).

The NEI Age-Related Eye Disease Studies (AREDS/AREDS2) found that daily intake of certain high-dose vitamins and minerals can slow progression of the disease in individuals with intermediate AMD and those with late AMD in one eye. Supplementation with these formulations will not help people with early AMD and will not restore vision already lost. Individuals should discuss the supplementation with AREDS formulations with their eye care professional.

Treatment of wet AMD includes photodynamic therapy (PDT), LPC, and anti-VEGF therapy. In 2010, the FDA approved an implantable telescope (IMT) to help individuals 65 years of age and older with vision loss attributable to AMD. The IMT helps individuals with advanced AMD by enlarging objects in the center

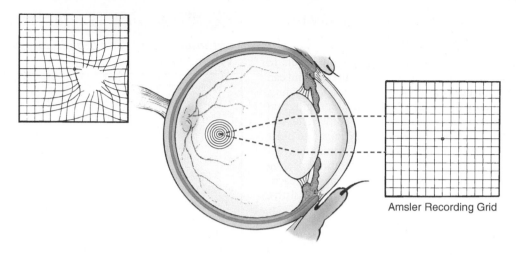

FIG. 19.2 Macular degeneration: distortion of center vision, normal peripheral vision. (Illustration by Harriet R. Greenfield, Newton, MA.)

of the visual field (Duffy, 2020). Lucentis and Avastin (anti-VEGF therapy) are biological drugs that are the most common form of treatment in neovascular AMD. Abnormally high levels of a specific growth factor occur in eyes with wet AMD and promote the growth of abnormal blood vessels. Anti-VEGF therapy blocks the effect of the growth factor. These drugs are injected into the eye as often as once a month and can help slow vision loss from AMD and, in some cases, improve sight. PDT with laser treatment is also used to manage AMD (NEI, 2019c).

Charles Bonnet Syndrome

Charles Bonnet syndrome (visual hallucinations) is a common side effect of vision loss in individuals with AMD. Individuals may see simple patterns of colors or shapes or detailed pictures of people, animals, buildings, or landscapes. Sometimes these images fit logically into a visual scene but often they do not. Nurses are cautioned to understand the syndrome and not attribute symptoms to cognitive impairment or mental illness.

The condition is similar to phantom limb syndrome, a condition in which individuals with a missing limb still feel their fingers or toes or experience itching. Similarly, when the brain loses input from the eye, it may fill the void by generating visual images on its own. The syndrome often goes away a year to 18 months after it begins. Interventions to lessen the symptoms include adequate lighting and encouraging the individual to blink, close the eyes, or focus on a real object for a few moments.

Dry Eye

Dry eye is not a disease of the eye but is a frequent complaint among older adults. Tear production normally diminishes as we age. The condition is termed *keratoconjunctivitis sicca*. It occurs most commonly in women after menopause. There may be age-related changes in the mucin-secreting cells necessary for surface wetting, in the lacrimal glands, or in the meibomian glands that secrete surface oil, and all of these may occur at the same time. The individual will describe a dry, scratchy feeling in mild cases (xerophthalmia). There may be marked discomfort and decreased mucus production in severe situations.

Medications can cause dry eye, especially anticholinergics, antihistamines, diuretics, beta-blockers, and some hypnotics. Sjögren syndrome is a cell-mediated autoimmune disease whose manifestations include decreased lacrimal gland activity. The problem is diagnosed by an ophthalmologist using a Schirmer tear test, in which filter paper strips are placed under the lower eyelid to measure the rate of tear production.

A common treatment is artificial tears or a saline gel, but dry eyes may be sensitive to them because of preservatives, which can be irritating. The ophthalmologist may close the tear duct channel either temporarily or permanently. Other management methods include keeping the house air moist with humidifiers, avoiding wind and hair dryers, and using artificial tear ointments at bedtime. Vitamin A deficiency can be a cause of dry eye and vitamin A ointments are available for treatment.

❖ USING CLINICAL JUDGMENT TO PROMOTE HEALTHY AGING: VISION

Vision impairment is common among older adults in connection with aging changes and eye diseases and can significantly affect communication, functional ability, safety, and quality of life. To promote healthy aging and quality of life, nurses who care for older adults in all settings can improve outcomes for visually impaired older adults by identifying vision changes, adapting the environment to enhance vision and safety, communicating appropriately, and providing appropriate health teaching and referrals for prevention, treatment, and assistive devices.

◆ Nursing Actions: Enhancing Vision

General principles in caring for persons with visual impairment include the following: use warm incandescent lighting; increase intensity of lighting; control glare by using shades and blinds; suggest yellow or amber lenses to decrease glare; suggest sunglasses that block all ultraviolet light; recommend reading materials that have large, dark, evenly spaced printing; and select colors with good contrast and intensity. Color contrasts are used to facilitate location of items. Sharply contrasting colors assist the partially sighted. For instance, a bright towel is much easier to locate than a white towel hanging on a beige wall. If you think of the colors of the rainbow, it is more likely that people will see reds and oranges better than blues and greens. Fig. 19.3 beautifully illustrates the use of color in a nursing home in Copenhagen, Denmark. Box 19.4 presents Tips for Best Practice in care for older adults with visual impairment.

BOX 19.4   Tips for Best Practice

Communicating With Individuals Who Have Visual Impairment

- Identify adequacy of vision.
- Make sure you have the person's attention before speaking.
- Clearly identify yourself and others with you.
- Position yourself at the person's level when speaking.
- Ensure adequate lighting and eliminate glare.
- When others are present, address the visually impaired person by prefacing remarks with their name or a light touch on the arm.
- Select colors for paint, furniture, pictures with rich intensity (e.g., red, orange).
- Use large, dark, evenly spaced printing and contrast in printed materials (e.g., black marker on white paper).
- Use a night light in bathroom and hallways and use illuminated switches.
- Do not change room arrangement or the arrangement of personal items without explanations.
- If in a hospital or nursing home, use some means to identify patients who are visually impaired and include visual impairment in the plan of care.
- Use the analogy of a clock face to help locate objects (e.g., describe positions of food on a plate in relation to clock positions, such as meat at 3 o'clock, dessert at 6 o'clock).
- Label eyeglasses and have a spare pair if possible; make sure glasses are worn and are clean.
- Be aware of low-vision assistive devices such as talking watches, talking books, and magnifiers, and facilitate access to these resources.
- If the person is blind, ask the person how you can help. If walking, do not try to push or pull. Let the person take your arm just above the elbow, and give directions with details (e.g., the bench is on your immediate right); when seating the person, place their hand on the back of the chair.

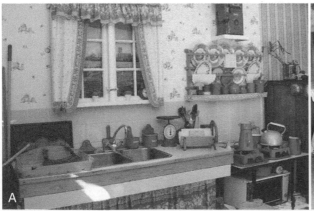 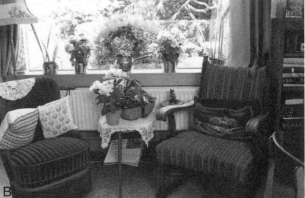

FIG. 19.3 (A) Reminiscence kitchen. (B) Sitting room. (Højdevang Sogns Plejejem, Copenhagen, Denmark. Photos courtesy Christine Williams, PhD, RN.)

◆ Special Considerations in Long-Term Care Settings

Visual impairment among nursing facility residents ranges from 3% to 15% higher than for adults of the same age living in the community (Johnson & Record, 2014). Cataracts and AMD are the most frequent causes of impaired vision. Information on eye diagnoses was often lacking in medical records and staff were often unaware of vision impairment. Cognitive and hearing impairments often accompany visual impairment and can severely affect communication, safety, functional status, and quality of life.

Recommendations to improve care of the visually impaired in nursing facilities are that individuals should have an eye examination prior to entering the nursing home and information on visual aids that the individual uses (glasses, need for lighting, optical aids) needs to be in the plan of care. Ongoing evaluation of vision is important and if function declines, a referral made to an ophthalmologist is indicated. Treatments to improve visual acuity such as cataract removal, if needed, should be accessible. Even in individuals with dementia who have clinically significant cataracts, surgery was found to improve visual acuity, to slow the rate of cognitive decline, to decrease neuropsychiatric symptoms, and to reduce caregiver stress (Cassels, 2014).

Although it may sound like common sense, it is especially important that individuals who wear glasses are wearing them and that the glasses are cleaned regularly. It is also important to ask the person or the person's family/significant other whether the person routinely wears glasses and whether the person is able to see well enough to function. There is limited research on visual impairment in nursing homes and assisted living facilities in spite of the scope of the concern and the need for improved interventions.

◆ Low-Vision Optical Devices

Technology advances in the past decade have produced some low-vision devices that may be used successfully in the care of the visually impaired individual. These devices are grouped into devices for "near" activities (such as reading, sewing, and writing) and devices for "distance" activities (such as attending movies, reading street signs, and identifying numbers on buses and trains). Nurses can refer individuals with low vision or blindness to vision rehabilitation services, which may include assistance with communication skills; counseling; independent living and personal management skills; independent movement and travel skills; training with low-vision devices; and vocational rehabilitation. It is important to be familiar with agencies in your community that offer these services. Persons with severe visual impairment may qualify for disability and financial and

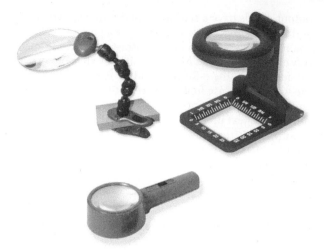

Magnifiers. (Reprinted with permission from Carson Optical.)

social services assistance through government and private programs including vision rehabilitation programs.

An array of low-vision assistive devices is now available, including insulin delivery systems, talking clocks and watches, large-print books, magnifiers, telescopes (handheld or mounted on eyeglasses), electronic magnification through closed circuit television or computer software, and software that converts text into artificial voice

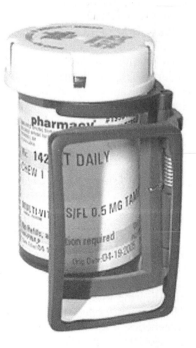

Prescription bottle magnifier. (Reprinted with permission from Carson Optical.)

output. iPods have a setting for audio menus; Microsoft and Apple computer programs allow a person to change color schemes, select a high-contrast display, and magnify and enlarge print. Many websites also have an option for audio text. The e-Reader product from Kindle allows the user to increase font sizes up to 40 points in e-books and offers a Text-to-Speech feature. The iPad from Apple can enlarge text up to 56 points and includes VoiceOver, a feature that reads everything displayed on the screen for you, making it fully usable for people with low to no vision. More and more mobile phones have speech-enabled features and the Jitterbug phone comes with a live operator whose actions can be directed. As individual needs are unique, it is recommended that before investing in vision aids, the individual consult with a low-vision center or low-vision specialist. Other vision resources are presented in Box 19.3.

HEARING IMPAIRMENT

Although both vision and hearing impairment significantly affect all aspects of life, Oliver Sacks (1989), in his book *Seeing Voices*, presents a view that blindness may in fact be less serious than loss of hearing. Hearing loss interferes with communication with others and the interactional input that is necessary to stimulate and validate. Helen Keller was most profound in her expression: "Never to see the face of a loved one nor to witness a summer sunset is indeed a handicap. But I can touch a face and feel the warmth of the sun. But to be deprived of hearing the song of the first spring robin and the laughter of children provides me with a long and dreadful sadness" (Keller, 1902). Both hearing and vision impairments have a significant effect on the social and daily lives of older adults. Hearing impairment in particular is a burden on social life and vision impairment strongly impacts everyday tasks (Haanes et al., 2019).

Hearing loss is the third most prevalent chronic condition and the foremost communicative disorder of older adults in the United States. Hearing loss is an underrecognized public health issue. Nearly two-thirds of adults aged 70 years and older have a hearing loss significant enough to impair daily communication. In all age groups, men are more likely than women to be hearing impaired and Black Americans have a lower prevalence of hearing impairment than either White or Hispanic Americans (Lin & Whitson, 2017).

Age-related hearing loss (ARHL) is a complex disease caused by interactions between age-related changes (Chapter 4), genetics, lifestyle, and environmental factors. Factors associated with hearing loss include noise exposure, ear infections, smoking, and chronic disease (e.g., diabetes, chronic kidney disease, heart disease)

BOX 19.5   Promoting Healthy Hearing

- Avoid exposure to excessively loud noises.
- Avoid cigarette smoking.
- Maintain blood pressure/cholesterol levels within normal limits.
- Eat a healthy diet.
- Have hearing evaluated if any changes are noticed.
- Avoid injury with cotton-tipped applicators and other cleaning materials.

(Bainbridge & Wallhagen, 2014). Hearing loss may not be an inevitable part of aging and increased attention is being given to the links between lifestyle factors (e.g., smoking, poor nutrition, hypertension) and hearing impairment (Box 19.5).

Consequences of Hearing Impairment

The broad consequences of hearing loss have functional and clinical significance and should not be viewed as something a person accepts as part of aging. Hearing loss diminishes quality of life and is associated with multiple negative outcomes, including decreased function, miscommunication, depression, falls, loss of self-esteem, safety risks, poor cognitive function, and possible increased health service utilization secondary to unmet health care needs (Wallhagen & Strawbridge, 2017). Failures in clinical communication are considered to be the leading cause of medical errors and ARHL has a negative effect on clinical communication across both hospital and primary care clinical settings (Cohen et al., 2017). ARHL has also been linked with late-life cognitive disorders and correcting hearing loss may have a long-term protective effect against cognitive decline (Logroscino & Panza, 2016).

Hearing loss increases feelings of isolation and may cause older adults to become suspicious or distrustful or to display feelings of paranoia. Because older adults with hearing loss may not understand or respond appropriately to conversation, they may be inappropriately diagnosed with dementia. Older adults who are hospitalized are at risk of adverse outcomes such as being labeled confused, experiencing a loss of control, heightened fear and anxiety, and misunderstanding the plan of care (Funk et al., 2018). All of these consequences of hearing impairment further increase social isolation and decrease opportunities for meaningful interaction and stimulation.

Types of Hearing Loss

The two major forms of hearing loss are *conductive* and *sensorineural*. Sensorineural hearing loss results from damage to any part of the inner ear or the neural pathways to the brain. Presbycusis (also called age-related hearing loss or ARHL) is a form of sensorineural hearing loss that is related to aging and is the most common form of hearing loss. Presbycusis progressively worsens with age and is usually permanent. The cochlea appears to be the site of pathogenesis, but the precise cause of presbycusis is uncertain. Other causes of sensorineural hearing loss include hereditary or genetic factors, viral or bacterial infections, noise exposure, head trauma, and ototoxic medications (Meyer & Hickson, 2020).

Noise-induced hearing loss (NIHL) is the second most common cause of sensorineural hearing loss among older adults. Direct mechanical injury to the sensory hair cells of the cochlea causes NIHL, and continuous noise exposure contributes to damage more than intermittent exposure. NIHL is permanent but considered largely preventable. The rate of hearing impairment is expected to rise because of the growing number of older adults and also because of the increased number of military personnel who have been exposed to blast exposure in combat situations. NIHL may be reduced through the development of better ear-protection devices, education about exposure to loud noise, and emerging research into interventions that may protect or repair hair cells in the ear, which are key to the body's ability to hear (National Institute on Deafness and Other Communication Disorders [NIDCD], 2017).

Recognizing and Analyzing Cues: Presbycusis

Presbycusis is a slow, progressive hearing loss that affects both ears equally. Because of its slow progression, many individuals ignore their hearing loss for years, considering it "just part of aging." Identification of signs, symptoms, and behaviors indicative of hearing loss is important so that negative consequences can be prevented. Only about 10% to 25% of Americans with hearing loss wear hearing aids, depending on the extent of the loss (Strawbridge & Wallhagen, 2017). It is common to hear older adults deny hearing impairment and accuse others of mumbling. Their spouse or significant other, however, often voices frustration over the hearing loss long before the individual acknowledges it.

One of the first signs of presbycusis is difficulty hearing and understanding speech in noisy environments. A hallmark of presbycusis is difficulty separating the incoming speech signal from background noise (Cohen et al., 2017). Presbycusis begins in the high frequencies and later affects the lower frequencies. High-frequency consonants are important to speech understanding. Changes related to presbycusis make it difficult to distinguish among some of the sibilant consonants such as z, s, sh, f, p, k, t, and g.

People often raise their voices when speaking to a hearing-impaired person. When this happens, more consonants drop out of speech, making hearing even more difficult. Without consonants, the high-frequency–pitched language becomes disjointed and misunderstood. Older adults with presbycusis have difficulty filtering out background noise and often complain of difficulty understanding women's and children's speech (higher pitched) and conversations in large groups. Sensorineural hearing loss is treated with hearing aids and, in some cases, cochlear implants.

Conductive Hearing Loss

Conductive hearing loss usually involves abnormalities of the external and middle ear that reduce the ability of sound to be transmitted to the middle ear. Otosclerosis, infection, perforated eardrum, fluid in the middle ear, tumors, or cerumen accumulations cause conductive hearing loss. Cerumen impaction is the most common and easily corrected of all interferences in the hearing of older adults (Fig. 19.4).

Cerumen interferes with the conduction of sound through air in the eardrum. The reduction in the number and activity of cerumen-producing glands results in a tendency toward cerumen impaction. Long-standing impactions become hard, dry, and dark brown. Individuals at particular risk of impaction are Blacks, individuals who wear hearing aids, and older men with large amounts of ear canal tragi (hairs in the ear) that tend to become entangled with the cerumen. One-third to two-thirds of nursing home residents and patients older than 65 years have cerumen impaction (Sun, 2017).

It is very important to assess the ears for cerumen impaction in primary care evaluation and among long-term care residents (Schwartz et al., 2017). When hearing loss is suspected or a person with existing hearing loss experiences increasing difficulty, it is important first to check for cerumen impaction as a possible cause.

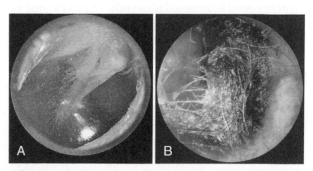

FIG. 19.4 (A) Normal eardrum. (B) Eardrum impacted with cerumen. ((A) From Ball, J. W., Dains, J. E., Flynn, F. A., et al. (2015). *Seidel's guide to physical examination* (8th ed.). St Louis: Mosby. (B) From Swartz, M. H. (2014). *Textbook of physical diagnosis* (7th ed.). Philadelphia: Saunders.)

After accurate evaluation, if cerumen removal is indicated, it may be removed through irrigation, cerumenolytic products, or manual extraction (Schwartz et al., 2017).

> ## ⚡ SAFETY ALERT
>
> Do not attempt ear lavage or cerumen removal if the person has a history of ear surgery, ruptured tympanic membrane, otitis externa (swimmer's ear), or ear trauma. Use sterilized equipment to avoid infection and spreading bacteria and use caution in patients with diabetes because of an increased risk of infection.

Hearing Aids

A hearing aid is a personal amplifying system that includes a microphone, an amplifier, and a loudspeaker. There are numerous types of hearing aids with either analog or digital circuitry. The size, appearance, and effectiveness of hearing aids have greatly improved (decreasing stigma), and many can be programmed to meet specific needs. Digital hearing aids are smaller and have better sound quality and noise reduction, and less acoustic feedback; however, they are expensive. Completely-in-the-canal (CIC) hearing aids fit entirely in the ear canal. These types of devices are among the most expensive and require good dexterity. Some models are invisible and placed deep in the ear canal and replaced every 4 months. New hearing aids can be adjusted precisely for noisy environments and telephone usage through software built into smartphones.

Most individuals can obtain some hearing enhancement with a hearing aid but among adults aged 70 years and older, fewer than one in three have ever used a hearing aid (Kimball et al., 2017). The kind of device chosen depends on the type of hearing impairment and the cost, but most users will experience hearing improvement with a basic to midlevel hearing aid. The investment in a good hearing aid is considerable and a good fit is critical. Accessibility and affordability of hearing care are massive barriers for those with hearing impairment. The average cost of bilateral hearing aids in the United States is $4700 and requires several visits to a hearing professional's office. The cost of hearing aids is usually not covered by health insurance or Medicare, another barrier to purchase.

The way hearing aids are regulated and sold is also a deterrent to use. The National Academies of Sciences, Engineering, and Medicine (2016) made the following recommendations for hearing health care: (1) include options for more coverage for hearing care under Medicare; (2) eliminate the regulation for medical evaluation prior to hearing aid purchase; (3) create a new regulatory classification for hearing aids that could be sold over the counter for adults with mild to moderate hearing loss (Lin & Whitson, 2017; Warren & Grassley, 2017).

Adjustment to Hearing Aids

Nearly 50% of people who purchased hearing aids either never began wearing them or stopped wearing them after a short period. Factors contributing to low hearing aid use after purchase include difficulty manipulating the device, annoying loud noises, being exposed to sensory overload, developing headaches, and perceiving stigma. Hearing aids amplify all sounds, making things sound different. ARHL is like any other physical impairment and requires counseling, rehabilitative training, patient education, environmental accommodations, and patience. The Internet may be a valuable tool for aural rehabilitation and for improving adjustment to hearing aids and communication (Lewis, 2014). More research about factors that influence the decision to seek help for hearing loss is needed (Wallhagen & Strawbridge, 2017).

It is important for nurses who work with individuals wearing hearing aids to be knowledgeable about their care and maintenance and teach the individual, family, or formal caregiver proper use and care. Recent research findings report that only a minority of staff in long-term care facilities receive training on the use and care of hearing aids and few believe they have sufficient knowledge about the hearing aids used by residents, including how to change hearing aid batteries (Haanes et al., 2019). Many older adults experience unnecessary communication problems when in the hospital or nursing home because their hearing aids are not inserted and working properly, need batteries, or because they are lost. Additionally, individuals who wear hearing aids often come to the hospital in emergent situations without their hearing aids or do not bring them because they fear they will be lost or broken (Kimball et al., 2018).

Cochlear Implants

Cochlear implants are increasingly being used for older adults with sensorineural loss who are not able to gain effective speech recognition with hearing aids. Thorough assessment of hearing loss is necessary to determine whether a cochlear implant may be indicated. Cochlear implants are safe and well tolerated and improve communication. A cochlear implant is a small, complex electronic device that consists of an external portion that sits behind the ear and a second portion that is surgically placed under the skin (Fig. 19.5). Unlike hearing aids that magnify sounds, the cochlear implant bypasses damaged portions of the ear and directly stimulates the

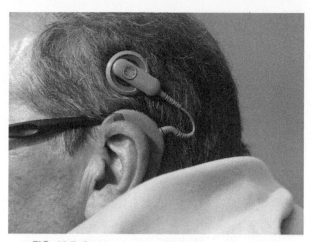

FIG. 19.5 Cochlear implant. (© iStock.com/Gannet77.)

auditory nerve. Hearing through a cochlear implant is different from normal hearing and takes time to learn or relearn. Most insurance plans cover the cochlear implant procedure. The transplant carries some risk because the surgery destroys any residual hearing. Therefore, cochlear implant users can never revert to using a hearing aid. Individuals with cochlear implants need to be advised to never have an MRI (magnetic resonance imaging) because it may dislodge the implant or demagnetize its internal magnet.

Assistive Listening and Adaptive Devices

Assistive listening devices (also called personal listening systems) should be considered as an adjunct to hearing aids or used in place of hearing aids for people with hearing impairment. These devices are available commercially and can be used to enhance face-to-face communication and to better understand speech in large rooms such as theaters, to use the telephone, and to listen to television. Many movie theaters have both sound amplifiers and personal subtitle devices available. Hearing loop conduction systems are newer technology and consist of a copper wire that is installed around the periphery of a room or other venue to transmit the microphone or TV sound signal to hearing aids and cochlear implants that have "telecoil" receivers (built into most hearing aids and cochlear implants). Sound from the microphone or TV is received but not background noises. This transforms the hearing aid into loudspeakers delivering sound for a person's own hearing loss. These devices are widely used in Europe and becoming more available in the United States in places such as theaters, churches, subway information booths, taxi back seats, and home TV rooms.

Other examples of assistive listening and adaptive devices include text messaging devices for telephones and closed-caption television, now required on all televisions with screens 13 inches and larger. Alerting devices, such as vibrating alarm clocks that shake the bed or activate a flashing light, and sound lamps that respond with lights to sounds, such as doorbells and telephones, are also available. Special service dogs ("hearing dogs") are trained to alert people with a hearing impairment about sounds and intruders. Dogs are trained to respond to different sounds, such as the telephone, smoke alarms, alarm clock, doorbell/door knock, and name call, and lead the individual to the sound.

The use of computers and email also assists individuals with hearing impairment to communicate more easily. Programs such as Skype and FaceTime are also beneficial because they may allow the person to lip read and to adjust volume. Pocket-sized amplifiers (available at retail stores) are especially helpful in improving communication in health care settings and nurses in a clinical setting should be able to obtain appropriate devices for use with hearing-impaired individuals. A recent study reported that these devices are safe and easy to use in inpatient settings and both patients and nurses were very satisfied with their use (Kimball et al., 2018).

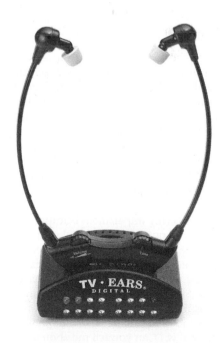

Voice-clarifying headset system for TV listening. (With permission from TV Ears, Inc.)

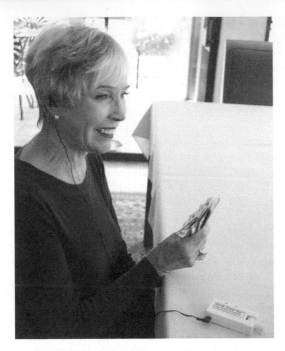

Pocket-sized amplifier. (With permission from Sonic Technology Products, Inc.)

❖ USING CLINICAL JUDGMENT TO PROMOTE HEALTHY AGING: HEARING

◆ Recognizing and Analyzing Cues: Hearing Impairment

Hearing impairment is underdiagnosed and under-treated in older adults. There is a low rate of hearing screening in primary care in spite of the high prevalence of hearing loss among older adults. Older adults may be initially unaware of hearing loss because of the gradual manner in which it develops and, therefore, may not report any problems. Screening for hearing impairment and appropriate treatment are essential parts of primary care for older adults (Wallhagen & Strawbridge, 2017). In hospitals and long-term care facilities, bedside screening for hearing impairment is important.

Nurses should note any nonverbal signs of a hearing deficit (e.g., cupping the ear, turning the head to one side when asked questions, or misunderstanding questions). Ask the individual directly whether they have a hearing impairment. Since many individuals are unaware of or deny hearing impairment, the screening should include a short discussion rather than yes-or-no questions. A suggested question is: "Can you tell me about any problems you have with hearing or misunderstanding questions?" The individual should also be asked their preferred

BOX 19.6 Do I Have a Hearing Problem?

- Do I have a problem hearing on the telephone?
- Do I have trouble hearing when there is noise in the background?
- Is it hard for me to follow a conversation when two or more people talk at once?
- Do I have to strain to understand a conversation?
- Do many people I talk to seem to mumble (or not speak clearly)?
- Do I misunderstand what others are saying and respond inappropriately?
- Do I have trouble understanding the speech of women and children?
- Do people complain that I turn the TV volume up too high?
- Do I hear a ringing, roaring, or hissing sound a lot?
- Do some sounds seem too loud?

From National Institute on Deafness and Other Communication Disorders (2014). *Hearing loss and older adults.* http://www.nidcd.nih.gov/health/hearing/pages/older.aspx#2.

method for enhancing hearing such as writing or using personal sound amplifiers (Funk et al., 2018). Obtaining information from the significant other about hearing problems can also be useful. Self-assessment instruments (Box 19.6) and the Hearing Handicap Inventory for the Elderly Screening Version (HHIT-S) can also be included (Box 19.7).

BOX 19.7 Resources for Best Practice

Hearing Impairment

- **American Tinnitus Association:** Listen to the sounds of tinnitus; patient and professional information
- **Experience hearing loss:** Unfair hearing test: https://www.youtube.com/watch?v=9vqY7cJpwRs
- **Hartford Institute for Geriatric Nursing:** Hearing Handicap Inventory for the Elderly: Screening Version (HHIE-S). https://consultgeri.org/try-this/general-assessment/issue-12.
- **National Institute on Deafness and Other Communication Disorders (NIDCD):** https://www.nidcd.nih.gov/health/hearing-ear-infections-deafness: Hearing loss and older adults patient information; Interactive hearing test; "It's a noisy planet: protect their hearing"; resources for health professionals.
- **National Institute Health (NIH):** Senior Health: Hearing Loss (patient information)
- **U Iowa Cosmay Gero Resources:** Nursing Management of Hearing Impairment in Nursing Facility Residents. https://www.uiowacsomaygeroresources.com/Nursing-Management-of-Hearing-Impairment-in-Nursin-p/956.htm.

Physical examination includes examining the external ear to determine any evidence of infection and using an otoscope to visualize the inner ear, looking for any possible causes of conductive hearing loss, such as cerumen impaction or foreign objects. Inspect the tympanic membrane for integrity. Question the individual about prolonged noise exposure, past ear injuries, and the use of potentially ototoxic medications. Depending on findings, the patient may need to be referred for follow-up by a specialist. Results of a recent study reported that the finger rub test showed high sensitivity and requires little time and no special equipment, making it an effective screening tool in primary care (Strawbridge & Wallhagen, 2017).

◆ Nursing Actions: Enhancing Hearing

Nursing actions are based on history and examination findings and may include referral to an audiologist, education on hearing loss (including prevention and consequences), hearing aids, assistive listening devices, and communication techniques. If cerumen impaction is found, cerumen removal may be indicated according to protocol. Providing education to individuals and family members about hearing loss, how it affects a person's communication, why it is important to address hearing loss early in the process, what hearing aids can and cannot do, and alternatives to the use of hearing aids is important and may enhance the effective use of hearing health care services (Wallhagen & Strawbridge, 2017).

There are many evidence-based resources available that can be used to educate the patient and family and assist the nurse in designing educational materials (Box 19.7). Using the information presented in this chapter, nurses can play an important role in providing older adults the information they need to improve their hearing and avoid the negative consequences of untreated hearing loss. Effective communication strategies when working with individuals who are hearing-impaired are presented in Box 19.8.

TINNITUS

Tinnitus is defined as the perception of sound in one or both ears or in the head when no external sound is present. It is often referred to as "ringing in the ears" but may also manifest as buzzing, hissing, whistling, cricket chirping, bells, roaring, clicking, pulsating, humming, or swishing sounds. The sounds may be constant or intermittent and are more acute at night or in quiet surroundings. The most common type is high-pitched tinnitus with sensorineural loss; less common

---

BOX 19.8   Tips for Best Practice

Communicating With Individuals Who Have Hearing Impairment

- Never assume hearing loss is caused by old age until other causes are ruled out (infection, cerumen buildup).
- Inappropriate responses, inattentiveness, and apathy may be symptoms of a hearing loss.
- Gain the individual's attention before beginning to speak. Look directly at the person at eye level before starting to speak.
- Determine whether hearing is better in one ear than another and position yourself appropriately.
- If a hearing aid is used, make sure it is in place and batteries are functioning.
- Keep hands away from your mouth and project voice by controlled diaphragmatic breathing.
- Avoid conversations in which the speaker's face is in glare or darkness; orient the light on the speaker's face.
- Careful articulation, moderate speed of speech, and lower tone are helpful.
- Label the chart, note on the intercom button, and inform all caregivers that the patient has a hearing impairment.
- Use nonverbal approaches: gestures, demonstrations, visual aids, and written materials.
- Pause between sentences or phrases to confirm understanding.
- Reduce background noise (e.g., turn off television, close door).
- Utilize assistive listening devices such as pocket talker.
- Verify that the information being given has been clearly understood. Be aware that the person may agree to everything and appear to understand what you have said even when they did not hear you (listener bluffing).
- Share resources for the hearing-impaired and refer as appropriate.

From Adams-Wendling, L., Pimple, C. (2008). Evidence-based guideline: Nursing management of hearing impairment in nursing facility residents. *J Gerontol Nurs 34*(11), 9–16.

---

is low-pitched tinnitus with conduction loss such as is seen in Ménière's disease. Tinnitus affects about one in five people. Tinnitus is the number one service-related disability for US veterans military personnel and is the leading cause of service-connected disability of veterans returning from Iraq or Afghanistan (American Tinnitus Association, 2017).

The exact physiological cause or causes of tinnitus are not known, but there are several likely factors that are known to trigger or worsen tinnitus. Exposure to loud noises is the leading cause of tinnitus and the exposure can damage and destroy cilia in the inner ear. Once damaged, the cilia cannot be renewed or replaced. Other possible causes of tinnitus include head and neck trauma, certain types of tumors, cerumen accumulation, jaw misalignment, cardiovascular disease, and ototoxicity from medications. More than 200 prescription and nonprescription medications list tinnitus as a potential side effect, aspirin being the most common. There is some evidence that caffeine, alcohol, cigarettes, stress, and fatigue may exacerbate the problem.

Nursing Actions: Tinnitus

Some persons with tinnitus will never find the cause; for others the problem may arbitrarily disappear. Hearing aids can be prescribed to amplify environmental sounds to obscure tinnitus and there is a device that combines the features of a masker and a hearing aid, which emits a competitive but pleasant sound that distracts from head noise. Therapeutic modes of treating tinnitus include transtympanal electrostimulation, iontophoresis, biofeedback, tinnitus masking with alternative sound production (white noise), cochlear implants, and hearing aids. Some have found hypnosis, cognitive behavioral therapy, acupuncture, and chiropractic, naturopathic, allergy, or drug treatment to be effective.

Other nursing actions include discussions with the client regarding times when the noises are most irritating and having the person keep a diary to identify patterns. Assess medications for possibly contributing to the problem. Discuss lifestyle changes and alternative methods that some have found effective. Also, refer clients to the American Tinnitus Association for research updates, education, and support groups (Box 19.8).

KEY CONCEPTS

- Vision loss is a leading cause of age-related disability.
- The leading causes of visual impairment in the United States are diseases that are common in older adults: age-related macular degeneration (AMD), cataracts, glaucoma, and diabetic retinopathy.
- Many causes of visual impairment are preventable, therefore attention to keeping eyes healthy throughout life and early recognition and analysis of cues to vision impairment is essential in the detection of eye disease.
- Nurses who care for visually impaired older adults in all settings can improve outcomes by evaluating vision changes, adapting the environment to enhance vision and safety, communicating appropriately, and providing appropriate health teaching and referrals for prevention, treatment, and assistive devices.
- Age-related hearing impairment is a complex disease caused by interactions among age-related changes, genetics, lifestyle, and environment.
- *Presbycusis* (also called age-related hearing impairment or ARHI) is a form of sensorineural hearing loss that is related to aging and is the most common form of hearing loss.
- Hearing loss diminishes quality of life and is associated with multiple negative outcomes including decreased function, increased likelihood of hospitalizations, miscommunication, depression, falls, reduced self-esteem, safety risks, and cognitive decline.
- Screening for hearing loss is an essential component when examining older adults.
- Nurses need to know how to operate hearing aids and assist individuals with hearing impairment to access assistive listening devices to enhance communication.

ACTIVITIES AND DISCUSSION QUESTIONS

1. How can nurses enhance awareness and education about vision and hearing disorders?
2. What is the role of a nurse in the acute care setting in screening and assessment for vision and hearing deficits and eye diseases?
3. What type of resources could a nurse in any setting offer to an older adult who has vision and hearing loss?
4. Which of the various sensory/perceptual changes of aging would you find most difficult to handle?

NEXT-GENERATION NCLEX® EXAMINATION-STYLE QUESTIONS

Mrs. Hoang, 82 years old, was diagnosed with age-related macular degeneration (ARMD) 15 years ago during a routine eye examination. She has developed progressively blurred central vision, making it difficult to read, watch TV, knit, and participate in other craft projects. She has an 80-pack/year history of smoking; she quit 15 years ago. She states her mother had ARMD. She is 5′6″and weighs 225 pounds (BMI 36.31 kg/m^2). She has a history of hypertension and hypercholesterolemia. Mrs. Hoang's medications include a daily multivitamin containing lutein and omega-3 fatty acids, atenolol 50 mg twice a day, ezetimibe 10 mg daily, and acetaminophen occasionally for headaches. She tells the nurse she is frustrated at the continued loss of her vision and has stopped attending the senior center bingo night and arts and craft night because of her low vision. She scores 8 on her short-form Geriatric Depression Scale (GDS), indicating depression. Her blood pressure is 125/80 mmHg, her heart rate is 78 beats per minute, her respirations are 16 breaths per minute and her temperature is 97.2°F. The nurse discusses resources that are available from low vision and rehabilitation services and answers Mrs.

Hoang's questions. A 3-month follow-up appointment is scheduled.

For each client finding, use an X to indicate whether the teaching concerning low vision and rehabilitation services was Effective (helped to meet expected outcomes), Ineffective (did not help to meet expected outcomes), or Unrelated (not related to the expected outcomes). Only one selection can be made for each client finding.

Client Finding	Effective	Ineffective	Unrelated
Score on GDS is 8			
Wears a talking watch			
Has magnifier but still does not attend bingo night			
Has electronic magnification for TV and computer			
BMI 33.89 kg/m²			
Has access to audio books			

REFERENCES

American Tinnitus Association. (2017). *Understanding the facts.* Tinnitus. https://www.ata.org/understanding-facts.

Bainbridge, K., & Wallhagen, M. (2014). Hearing loss in an aging American population: Extent, impact, management. *Annu Rev Public Health, 35,* 139–152.

Cassels, C. (2014). Cataract surgery may cut cognitive decline in dementia. *Medscape Medical News.* http://www.medscape.com/viewarticle/828188.

Cohen, J. M., Blustein, J., Weinstein, B. E., et al. (2017). Studies of physician-patient communication with older patients: how often is hearing loss considered? A systematic literature review. *J Am Geriatr Soc, 65,* 1642–1648.

Duffy, M. (2020). The implantable miniature telescope (IMT) for end-stage macular degeneration. https://visionaware.org/your-eye-condition/age-related-macular-degeneration-amd/new-fda-approved-implantable-telescope-for-end-stage-amd/. Accessed February 2021.

Funk, A., Garcia, C., & Mullen, T. (2018). Original research: understanding the hospital experience of older adults with hearing impairment. *Am J Nurs, 118*(6), 28–34.

Ge, S., Belza, B., & Wallhagen, M. (2021). Imagine a world with limited sound and light. *Jour Gerontol Nurs, 47*(1), 3–4.

Genentech. (2017). *Retinal diseases fact sheet.* https://www.gene.com/stories/retinal-diseases-fact-sheet.

Glaucoma Research Foundation. (2020). *New medication systems for glaucoma.* https://www.glaucoma.org/treatment/new-medication-delivery-systems-for-glaucoma.php.

Gupta, P., Aravindhan, A., Gand, A. T. L., et al. (2017). Association between the severity of DR and falls in an Asian population with diabetes: the Singapore epidemiology of eye diseases study. *JAMA Ophthalmology, 135*(12), 1410–1416.

Haanes, G., Hall, E., & Eilertsen, G. (2019). Acceptance and adjustment: a qualitative study of experiences of hearing and vision impairments and daily life among oldest old recipients of home care. *International Journal of Older People Nursing, 14*(3). doi.org/10.1111/opn.12236. https://www.ncbi.nlm.nih.gov/pubmed/31099486.

International Federation on Ageing. (2012). *The high cost of low vision: the evidence on ageing and the loss of sight.* https://www.ifa-fiv.org/publication/vision/the-high-cost-of-low-vision-the-evidence-on-ageing-and-the-loss-of-sight/.

Keller, H. (1902). *The story of my life.* Garden City, NY: Doubleday.

Kimball, A. R., Roscigno, C. I., Jenerette, C. M., Hughart, K. M., Jenkins, W. W., & Hsu, W. (2018). Amplified hearing device use in acute care settings for patients with hearing loss: a feasibility study. *Geriatr Nurs, 39,* 279–284.

Lewis, T. (2014). Hearing impairment. In R. Ham, P. Sloane, & G. Warshaw et al. (Eds.), *Primary Care Geriatrics* (ed 6, pp. 291–300). Philadelphia: Elsevier Saunders.

Lin, F. R., & Whitson, H. E. (2017). The common sense of considering the senses in patient communication. *J Am Geriatr Soc, 65,* 1659–1660.

Logroscino, G., & Panza, F. (2016). The role of hearing impairment in cognitive decline: need for the special sense assessment in evaluating cognition in older age. *Neuroepidemiology, 6*(46), 290–291.

MacLennan, P. A., McGivin, G., Jr., Heckemeyer, C., et al. (2014). Eye care use among a high-risk diabetic population seen in a public hospital's clinics. *JAMA Ophthalmology, 132*(2), 162–167.

Meyer, C., & Hickson, L. (2020). Nursing management of hearing impairment in nursing facility residents. *Jour Gerontol Nurs, 46*(7), 15–21.

National Academies of Sciences, Engineering, and Medicine. (2016). *Hearing health care for adults: priorities for improving access and affordability.* Washington, DC: The National Academies Press.

National Eye Institute, National Eye Health Education Program. (2019a). *At a glance: Glaucoma.* https://nei.nih.gov/health/glaucoma/glaucoma_facts.

National Eye Institute, National Eye Health Education Program. (2019b). *Retinal detachment.* https://www.nei.nih.gov/learn-about-eye-health/eye-conditions-and-diseases/retinal-detachment.

National Eye Institute. (2019c). *Facts about age-related macular degeneration.* https://nei.nih.gov/health/maculardegen/armd_facts.

National Eye Institute, National Eye Health Education Program: *Vision and aging: See Well for a Lifetime Toolkit.* https://nei.nih.gov/nehep/programs/visionandaging/toolkit.

Other Communication Disorders (NIDCD): *Hearing, ear infections, and deafness.* https://www.nidcd.nih.gov/health/hearing-ear-infections-deafness. Accessed December 2017.

Rowan, S., Jiang, S., Korem, T., et al. (2017). Involvement of a gut-retina axis in protection against dietary glycemia-induced age-related macular degeneration. *Proceedings of the National Academy of Science USA, 114*(22), E4472–E4481.

Schwartz, S., Magit, A., Rosenfeld, R., et al. (2017). Clinical practice guideline (update): earwax (cerumen impaction). *Otolaryngol Head Neck Surg, 156*(1S), S1–S29.

Strawbridge, W. J., & Wallhagen, M. I. (2017). Simple tests compare well with a hand-held audiometer for hearing loss screening in primary care. *J Am Geriatr Soc, 65,* 2282–2284.

Sun G: Dealing with cerumen impaction, *Medscape Nurses,* 2017. https://www.medscape.com/viewarticle/875560_print. Accessed December 2017.

US Department of Health and Human Services. (2012). Office of Disease Prevention and Health Promotion: *Healthy People 2020*. http://www.healthypeople.gov/2020.

Wallhagen, M., & Strawbridge, W. (2017). Hearing loss education for older adults in primary care clinics: benefits of a concise educational brochure. *Geriatr Nurs, 38*(6), 527–530.

Warren, E., & Grassley, C. (2017). Over-the-counter hearing aids: the path forward. *JAMA Intern Med, 177*(5), 609–610.

World Health Organization (2020). Blindness and vision impairment. https://www.who.int/news-room/fact-sheets/detail/blindness-and-visual-impairment. Accessed February 2021.

Zhang, X., Beckles, G. L., Chou, C. F., et al. (2013). Socioeconomic disparity in use of eye care services among US adults with age-related eye diseases: National Health Interview Survey, 2002 and 2008. *JAMA Ophthalmology, 131*(9), 1198–1206.

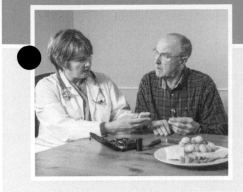

20

Metabolic Disorders

Kathleen Jett

LEARNING OBJECTIVES

Upon completion of this chapter, the reader will be able to:

- Explain the risks and complications of endocrine disorders in older adults.
- Describe the recognition and analyses of cues necessary when screening and monitoring persons with diabetes.
- Identify the unique aspects of diabetes management in older adults.
- Develop strategies and actions to maximize outcomes in older adults with endocrine disorders.
- Discuss the nurse's role in caring for persons with endocrine disorders.
- Propose a reason for the significantly higher rate of diabetes among those more than 75 years of age when compared with those between 50 and 74 years old.

THE LIVED EXPERIENCE

I can see that Anna is going to need a lot of help learning to manage her diabetes. I know now that I have already overwhelmed her with brochures and information. She just looked frightened to death, and she just has a mild elevation in blood sugar; it could probably be controlled with diet and exercise. I will call her tomorrow and see how she is doing.

Anna's gerontological clinical nurse specialist

The endocrine system works with multiple body organs to regulate and integrate body activities through the release of hormones. Among other things, the hormones provide cell metabolism and energy balance. Although the exact relationship between normal changes with aging and changes in endocrine function is unknown, they are most likely attributable to normal age-related reduced immune function (see Chapter 4). Because of the large number of older adults who are affected, the gerontological nurse should have a working knowledge of these conditions to provide the care needed to optimize health outcomes and thereby promote healthy aging. In this chapter the most common endocrine disorders, thyroid disease and diabetes mellitus, are reviewed.

THYROID DISEASE

The thyroid is a small gland in the neck that stores and secretes thyroid hormones, which regulate metabolism and affect nearly every organ in the body. Although only a small percentage of persons in the United States have thyroid disease, the prevalence increases significantly with age. A few people older than 65 years of age have hyperthyroidism, but up to a quarter, predominantly women, have hypothyroidism (Papaleontiou & Esfandiari, 2017). Thyroid disorders are fairly easy to diagnose in younger adults, but as a person ages, especially if frail, many of the cues mirror those of other common health problems (Box 20.1). These may be nonspecific, atypical, or absent. They may be incorrectly attributed to normal aging, to

---

BOX 20.1   Symptoms of Hypothyroidism: Differences in Older Adults Compared With Younger Adults

Probably Less Common in Older Adults
Fatigue
Weakness
Depression
Dry skin
Constipation

Significantly Less Common in Older Adults
Weight gain
Cold intolerance
Muscle cramps

From Campbell, J. W. (2013). Thyroid disorders. In R. J. Ham, P. D. Sloane, G. A. Warshaw, et al. (Eds.), *Ham's primary care geriatrics: A case-based approach* (6th ed., p. 442). St Louis: Elsevier.

---

another disorder, or to side effects of medications when the problem is a life-threatening thyroid disturbance. The cues may be only recognized when the person is screened for depression, anxiety, functional or cognitive changes, or cardiac disease.

Blood tests are used to make a diagnosis of a thyroid disturbance with the measurement of thyroid-stimulating hormone (TSH), free T3 (triiodothyronine), and free T4 (thyroxine) levels.

Hypothyroidism

The most common thyroid disturbance in older adults is hypothyroidism, that is, the failure of the thyroid gland to produce an adequate amount of the hormone thyroxine. The onset is often subtle, is slow in development, and is thought to be caused most frequently by chronic autoimmune thyroiditis. It may be iatrogenic, resulting from radioiodine treatment, a subtotal thyroidectomy, or medications. It can also be caused by a pituitary or hypothalamic abnormality. There is a strong family association (ATA, 2020).

⚡ SAFETY ALERT

Amiodarone is an antidysrhythmic agent that is still in use. It is associated with multiple toxicities including thyroid disease. All persons taking amiodarone must be monitored regularly for hypothyroidism (AGS, 2019).

An older adult may report heart palpitations, slowed thinking, gait disturbances, fatigue, weakness, or cold intolerance. These and other cues are often evaluated for

other causes before the possibility of hypothyroidism is considered. An elevated TSH level combined with a low free T4 (FT4) measurement indicates that the pituitary is working extra hard to make the thyroid secrete thyroxine when it may not be able to do so (Papaleontiou & Esfandiari, 2017). The treatment is to replace the missing thyroxine, in the form of the medication levothyroxine; *armor thyroid is contraindicated in older adults* (AGS, 2019). The usual dose in an older adult is 0.025 mg (25 µg) and it is rarely necessary to advance to a higher dose. It takes 4–6 weeks to effect changes in thyroid function and changes in the laboratory findings, therefore it is incorrect to increase the dose at more frequent intervals. If a dose is increased rapidly, it could be life threatening. Generics (e.g., levothyroxine) are not always equivalent to trade formulations (e.g., Synthroid). Unfortunately, many Medicare drug plans only cover generic formulations. The person should be advised to work with their pharmacist to try to ensure that a consistent generic is dispensed.

Hyperthyroidism

Hyperthyroidism is an excessive amount of thyroxine in the body. Although it does not occur often, women are more likely to develop it than men (Papaleontiou & Esfandiari, 2017). Graves' disease is the most common cause in later life, but the incidence of multi-nodular goiter increases with age. It can also result from ingestion of iodine or iodine-containing substances, such as those found in some seafood, radiocontrast agents, the medication amiodarone, or when too high a dose of levothyroxine is prescribed or taken. The same blood tests are done: this time the TSH level would be very low and the FT4 level would be normal and the T3 low in a younger person, but an isolated low TSH is common in older adults. FT4 levels are also closely associated with protein levels in the blood. If the protein level is too low, the FT4 level will be artificially low, making diagnosis difficult, especially in the large number of medically frail persons with hypoproteinemia (ATA, 2020).

Compared with hypothyroidism, the onset of hyperthyroidism may be quite sudden. The cues in older adults include unexplained atrial fibrillation, heart failure, constipation, anorexia, muscle weakness, and other vague complaints. Cues indicative of heart failure or angina may cloud the clinical presentation and prevent the correct medical diagnosis. The person may be misdiagnosed as being depressed or having dementia. Physical cues include tachycardia, tremors, and weight loss. In later life a condition known as apathetic thyrotoxicosis, rarely seen in younger persons, may occur in which the usual hyperactivity is replaced with slowed movement and depressed affect. If left untreated, it will increase the speed of bone loss and is as life threatening as hypothyroidism.

❖ USING CLINICAL JUDGMENT TO PROMOTE HEALTHY AGING: THYROID DISEASE

The achievement of optimal outcomes related to thyroid disturbances is largely one of careful pharmacological intervention and, in the case of hyperthyroidism, one of surgical or chemical ablation. As advocates, nurses can ensure that a thyroid screening test be done anytime potential cues are present, including when addressing any symptoms that are "vague."

◆ Recognizing and Analyzing Cues

Nurses caring for frail elders must be attentive to the possibility that with the cues of atrial fibrillation, anxiety, dementia, or depression may be indicative of a thyroid disturbance. Although little can be done to prevent thyroid disturbances, organizations such as the Monterey Bay Aquarium have launched campaigns to inform consumers of the iodine and mercury found in seafood, both of which are toxic to the thyroid (http://www.seafoodwatch.org).

◆ Nursing Actions

The nurse may be instrumental in working with the person and family to understand both the seriousness of the problem and the need for very careful adherence to the prescribed regimen. If an older adult is hospitalized for acute management of a thyroid disorder, the life-threatening nature of both the disorder and the treatment can be made clear so that advanced planning can be done that will account for all possible outcomes. At the same time, those with a prolonged acute illness may have transient thyroid disturbances that resolve at the same time as the illness does.

A nurse should work with the person and significant others in the correct self-administration of medications (Box 20.2). The nurse who is responsible for the administration of levothyroxine must take care to follow these same instructions especially for those who are fed artificially.

◆ Evaluating Outcomes

Negative outcomes/complications of thyroid disease occur both as the result of treatment and as the result of failure to diagnose or treat in a timely manner. Thyroxine increases myocardial oxygen consumption; therefore, the elevations found in hyperthyroidism produce a significant risk for atrial fibrillation and exacerbation of angina in persons with preexisting heart failure or may precipitate acute congestive heart failure (see Chapter 22). Although surgery is often the treatment in younger persons with hyperthyroidism, it is rarely appropriate for older adults because of the increase in operative risks in later life. Instead,

---

BOX 20.2   Appropriate Administration of Levothyroxine

Levothyroxine should always be taken early in the morning, on an empty stomach, and at least 30 minutes before a meal. It should be taken with a full glass of water to ensure it does not begin to dissolve in the esophagus. It cannot be taken within 4 hours of anything containing a mineral, such as calcium (including fortified orange juice), antacids, or iron supplements. It is always dosed in micrograms, and care must be taken that it is not confused with milligrams. Twenty-five μg/day (0.25 mg) is the most common dose used in adults older than 50 years of age. The same brand of levothyroxine should be used with each refill.

---

antithyroid medications are used, but the risk of poor outcomes is increased because of the likelihood of coexisting cardiac and neurological disorders (ATA, 2020).

For those with hypothyroidism, myxedema coma is a life-threatening potential outcome/complication of untreated hypothyroidism in older patients. If the disease is not detected early, even with the best treatment, death may ensue. Rapid replacement of the missing thyroxine is not possible because of the risk of drug toxicity. To maximize outcomes, synthetic levothyroxine is usually begun at the lowest dose possible (usually 25 μg), and search for cues of complications is ongoing. Changes in dose are guided by the results of the TSH laboratory test. Unfortunately it takes 6–8 weeks for any changes in TSH (and therefore thyroid function) to be evident.

DIABETES

Diabetes mellitus (DM) is a syndrome of disorders of glucose metabolism resulting in hyperglycemia. The three main types of diabetes are type 1 and type 2 and gestational diabetes, which may occur during pregnancy. Either the body resists the effects of insulin or doesn't produce the insulin needed to move glucose into the cells (type 1) or it doesn't produce enough insulin to meet the needs of the body (type 2), as in the case of obesity. In other words, insulin is available, but the cells, especially in the muscles, liver, and fat, are not able to use it. This is referred to as insulin-resistant diabetes and affects 90% to 95% of the more than 34 million with the disease. (Centers for Disease Control and Prevention [CDC], 2019a). DM is now viewed on a continuum from asymptomatic prediabetic insulin resistance, to mild postprandial hyperglycemia and/or mild fasting hyperglycemia, to diagnosable diabetes. Because glucose is necessary for life, DM is a potentially life-threatening condition.

More than 50% of all Americans have DM. This includes approximately 25% of all older adults (women

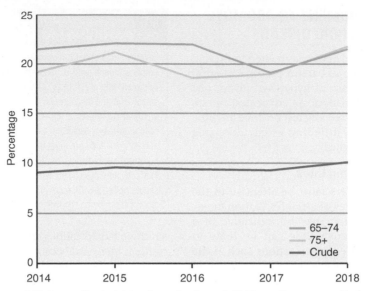

FIG. 20.1 Diagnosed Diabetes, Total, Adults Over the Age of 65 Years, Percentage, National. From CDC. https://gis.cdc.gov/grasp/diabetes/DiabetesAtlas.html.

more often than men) compared with 9.4% of those in the general population (ACL, 2019; CDC, 2020; Sinclair et al., 2017) (Fig. 20.1). Many others have the disease but have not yet been diagnosed. Twenty-four million persons at least 65 years of age have prediabetes (CDC, 2020). This high risk and rate of DM are associated with

normal changes with aging leading to insulin resistance and glucose intolerance. It is estimated that slightly over 46% of those over 75 years of age have prediabetes and still have a chance to prevent the disease from fully developing (Sinclair et al., 2017).

There is a wide variation of the prevalence of diabetes among ethnic/racial groups and subgroups (Table 20.1). American Indian/Alaskan Native, Hispanic, non-Hispanic Black, Asian American, and non-Hispanic White rank in order of prevalence from highest to lowest. However, an important caveat is the diversity within any one group. For example, persons of Chinese descent have a rate of about 5.6% compared with 12.6% among Asian Indians. Those from Central and South America have a prevalence of 8.3%, but this value increases to 14.4% among persons from Mexican Americans (American Diabetes Association [ADA], 2020).

❖ USING CLINICAL JUDGMENT TO PROMOTE HEALTHY AGING: DIABETES

Clinical judgment when caring for older adults in any setting includes the early recognition of potential cues—of prediabetes, disease, and the early signs of poor outcomes. Unfortunately, older adults may often have diabetes for a long time before it is diagnosed. In later life it is a chronic disease that even when the person appears healthy and has glycemic control, the older body will ultimately suffer damage, especially the cardiovascular system. Because of the high prevalence and incidence of DM in later life,

TABLE 20.1	Diabetes by Race/Ethnicity
Race/Ethnicity	Percentage of Adults Diagnosed With Diabetes
Non-Hispanic whites	8.0
Asian Americans	8.0
Chinese	4.3
Filipinos	8.9
Asian Indians	11.2
Other Asian Americans	8.5
Hispanics	12.5
Central and South Americans	8.5
Cubans	9.0
Mexican Americans	13.8
Puerto Ricans	12.0
Non-Hispanic blacks	10.9
American Indians/Alaskan Natives	15.1

Data from American Diabetes Association (April 2018). *Statistics about diabetes*. https://www.diabetes.org/resources/statistics/statistics-about-diabetes?referrer=https%3A//www.google.com/.

BOX 20.3   **Signs of End-Organ Damage in DM**

Decreased visual acuity
Paresthesia
Neuropathy
Heart disease
Stroke
Periodontal disease

From Razzaque, I., Morley, J. E., Nau, K. C., et al. (2013). Diabetes mellitus. In R. J. Ham, P. D. Sloane, G. A. Warshaw, et al. (Eds.), *Ham's primary care geriatrics: A case-based approach* (6th ed., pp. 431–439). St Louis: Elsevier.

BOX 20.5   **Factors Contributing to Increase Incidence of Hypoglycemia in Older Adults**

Multiple comorbidities
Presence of geriatric syndromes
Frequency of frailty
Polypharmacy
Long duration of illness
Prevalence of renal and hepatic disease

whenever risk factors or potential cues are present, diagnostic testing should be done. There is an online quiz for those who wish to know their risk of developing diabetes at http://www.doihaveprediabetes.org.

◆ Recognizing and Analyzing Cues

The onset of type 2 diabetes mellitus (T2DM) in later life is usually insidious with few if any recognizable cues until there is already end-organ damage (e.g., blindness) or an acute event occurs (e.g., stroke) (Box 20.3). Older adults with T2DM often have other health issues, including problems with the metabolism of lipids and proteins. Cues more specific in the older population are changes in functional abilities (Box 20.4). Both the diagnosis and the care provided to those with diabetes in later life are considerably complex.

The classic cues suggestive of diabetes include thirst and excessive urination as the body tries to reduce the relative concentration of glucose in the blood. Yet both hypoglycemia and hyperglycemia appear to be well tolerated in later life and there may be no early warning signs until the person is found to be in a life-threatening (hyperosmolar nonketotic) coma. For unknown reasons diabetic coma is more common among older Blacks. It

BOX 20.4   **Diabetes-Related Functional Disabilities in Later Life**

Mobility impairment
Falls
Incontinence
Cognitive impairments
Muscle weakness
Fatigue
Weight loss

From Razzaque, I., Morley, J. E., Nau, K. C., et al. (2013). Diabetes mellitus. In R. J. Ham, P. D. Sloane, G. A. Warshaw, et al. (Eds.), *Ham's primary care geriatrics: A case-based approach* (6th ed., pp. 431–439). St Louis: Elsevier.

is not unusual to find asymptomatic older persons with fasting glucose levels of ≥300 mg/dL or as low as 50 mg/dL. In older adults, the early cues may be dehydration, confusion, or delirium instead; death may result when these are mistaken as worsening dementia (Razzaque et al., 2013). Instead of urinary frequency, the high amount of glucose in the urine may cause incontinence.

Hypoglycemia (blood glucose level <60 mg/dL) is more common in older adults with diabetes and can occur from many causes, especially overly "tight" glycemic control with insulin. There are multiple factors contributing to an increased incidence of hypoglycemia in older adults (Box 20.5). Cues in older adults include tachycardia, palpitations, diaphoresis, tremors, pallor, and anxiety. Later cues may include headache, dizziness, fatigue, irritability, confusion, hunger, visual changes, seizures, and coma. Many of these can be and are confused with those of dementia (Sinclair et al., 2017). Immediate care involves giving the patient glucose either orally or intravenously.

Medical diagnosis requires the results of two of three possible tests on two different days. Prediabetes is indicated when the fasting plasma glucose (FPG) (not finger stick) level is 100–125 mg/dL or the hemoglobin A1c (HgbA1c) value is 5.7% to 6.4%. Diabetes is diagnosed with a FPG of ≥126 mg/dL or an HgbA1c ≥6.5%. If a person has a random blood glucose measurement of ≥200 mg/dL and symptomatic, no further testing is necessary (CDC, 2019b). The glucose tolerance test (GTT) used sometimes in younger adults and children is rarely used in this population.

Once a diagnosis has been made, the nurse continues to observe and analyze cues indicating changing health status. A full analysis of functional cues is necessary for documentation of a baseline. Smoking status, nutritional status, weight history, and exercise history are lifestyle choices that can provide clues leading to the development of realistic hypotheses and strategies leading to actions. Recognizing cues indicative of economic resources helps establish the person's ability to purchase the equipment, materials, and foods that are needed to maintain glycemic control. This is especially important for older adults who have very limited incomes. Cues related to access to transportation provides information about the ability to obtain the foods necessary for a diabetic diet and health care. History of alcohol and tobacco use provides cues to risk of complications, especially cardiovascular.

Nurses need to recognize and analyze the earliest cues to complications. This requires careful and repeated measurement of blood pressure, visual acuity, gross neurological function, and depression. Distant vision can be checked with a Snellen chart and near vision with a newspaper. The skin and feet should be thoroughly inspected for any cues, such as corns, calluses, blisters, cracks, or fungal infections, each time the person is seen by a health care professional or changes care settings.

◆ Nursing Actions

Nurses have a vital role in multiple aspects of preventing and minimizing diabetes complications and thereby maximize outcomes. A nurse can participate in early detection/recognition through screening of persons both in the community and residential settings such as nursing homes and assisted living centers. Because of a close association of DM and heart disease, all persons with an elevated blood pressure (treated or untreated) should be screened for DM at least every 3 years. More frequent screening is individually determined based on both risk factors and life expectancy. A nurse can promote healthy aging by helping people understand and reduce modifiable risk factors as appropriate (see Box 20.6).

BOX 20.6   Risk Factors for Diabetes Mellitus

- **Nonmodifiable Risk Factors**
  - High-risk population
  - More than 45 years of age
  - First-degree relative (parent, sibling, child) with DM
  - Previous gestational DM or having had a child with a birth weight >9 pounds
  - History of cardiovascular disease of any kind
  - Taking atypical antipsychotics or glucocorticoids
- **Modifiable Risk Factors**
  - Blood pressure ≥140/90 mmHg
  - Prediabetes
  - Overweight or obese: body mass index (BMI) >25 kg/m2
  - Undesirable lipid levels: high-density lipoproteins (HDLs) ≤35 mg/dL or triglycerides ≥250 mg/dL
  - Inactivity

Other nursing actions to promote healthy aging may differ from those used with younger adults because of the multiple factors that confound decision-making in later life, including comorbid conditions, life expectancy, and ability to comply with needed strategies and actions. If the person is frail, management is difficult, and if there is not a consistent caregiver (if needed) or they have not obtained the necessary diabetes education on behalf of, or with, the older adult, diabetes control may be impossible.

Promoting healthy aging in older adults with diabetes requires an array of actions and an effective interdisciplinary team. Optimizing outcomes requires expertise in medication use, diet, exercise, counseling, and the ability to find ways to support while empowering. The care team includes the person, their care partner, the bedside and office nurses, nutritionists, pharmacists, podiatrists, ophthalmologists, physicians or nurse practitioners, and counselors. If the person's disease is hard to control, endocrinologists are involved, and as complications develop, more specialists, such as nephrologists, cardiologists, and wound care specialists, are required. Nurses with a special interest in diabetes can become certified diabetic educators.

The actions implemented are based on life expectancy and the recognition of the importance of cardiovascular health-promoting strategies. The benefits of better control of blood pressure and lipids can be seen in 2 to 3 years. In comparison, research has indicated that it may take 8 years of glycemic control before benefits are seen. A discussion of expectations, potential longevity, and life choices takes on special meaning as the person approaches the end of life.

◆ Nursing Action: Diabetes Self-Management (DSM)

The skills and actions needed for self-management are many, and the nurse and dietitian are often the cornerstones of related education (Box 20.7). The nurse encourages and supports an older adult and significant others while they struggle with a complicated and very serious disease (Beck et al., 2017).

Experiential learning and mastery are important to successful self-management of DM. However, there are multiple factors related to aging that can affect the outcome (Box 20.8). Standards have now been established for diabetes self-management education (DSME) with the cost covered by many insurance companies including Medicare. Medicare pays 100% of the initial 10 hours of education and 2 hours each year after that. Limited diabetic supplies are now covered by Medicare as well (see Chapter 7).

DSM includes self-monitoring blood glucose (SMBG). Older adults with arthritis, low vision, or peripheral

BOX 20.7   Evidence-Based Practice

Minimal Self-Care Skills Needed for the Person With Diabetes

Glucose Self-Monitoring
- Obtaining a blood sample correctly
- Using the glucose monitoring equipment correctly
- Troubleshooting when results indicate an error
- Recording the values from the machine
- Understanding the timing and frequency of the self-monitoring
- Understanding what to do with the results
- Knowing signs and symptoms of high and low blood glucose level and what to do about either one

Medication Self-Administration
Where Appropriate, Insulin Use
- Selecting appropriate injection site
- Using correct technique for injections
- Disposing of used needles and syringes correctly
- Storing and transporting insulin correctly

Oral Medication Use
- Knowing drug, dose, timing, and side effects
- Knowing drug-drug and drug-food interactions
- Recognizing side effects and knowing when to report

Foot Care and Examination
- Selecting and using appropriate and safe footwear

Handling Sick Days
- Understanding the effects illness and new medications may have on glycemic control

Note: See also http://www.niddk.nih.gov/health-information/health-communication-programs/ndep/health-care-professionals/guiding-principles/principle-03-provide-self-management-education-support/Pages/default.aspx.

BOX 20.8   Interaction Between Diabetes and the Aging Process

1. A decline in visual acuity can affect an individual's ability to read printed educational material, medication labels, markings on a syringe, and blood glucose monitoring devices.
2. Auditory impairments can lead to difficulty in hearing instructions.
3. Altered taste can affect food choices and nutritional status.
4. Poor dentition or changes in the gastrointestinal system can lead to difficulties with food ingestion and digestion needed to maintain a stable diet.
5. Altered ability to recognize hunger and thirst may lead to weight loss, dehydration, and increased risk for hyperosmolar nonketotic syndrome.
6. Unrecognized changes in hepatic or renal function occur more frequently in later life and affect anti-hyperglycemic drug dosing.
7. Arthritis or tremors can affect the ability to self-administer medications and to use monitoring devices.
8. Polypharmacy complicates medication choices.
9. Diabetes and chronic disease-related depression reduce the motivation for self-management.
10. Cognitive impairment and dementia decrease self-care ability and necessitate a care-partner who has complete diabetes education and can act on behalf of the person as needed.
11. Low levels of education and low health literacy call for modifications in the method of teaching about diabetes care.
12. Reduced access to care because of financial limitations or geographic isolation can occur

neuropathy (regardless of cause) will have difficulties with the mechanics of SMBG and will require creative teaching, perhaps enlisting friends or neighbors in the tasks that are necessary; however, new technologies and drug delivery systems are being designed to make these tasks easier. Daily foot care and foot examination should be discussed and demonstrated. Persons who are not particularly flexible will have difficulty reaching and inspecting their feet, and a family member or friend can be asked to do this. If vision is adequate, checking can also be done by placing an unbreakable mirror on the floor to examine sole and toes. A nurse teaches foot care to reduce the risk of amputation. A person with diabetes needs to understand that wearing good shoes that fit well is essential. Those with Medicare and severe diabetic foot disease may be eligible (at least annually) for one pair of specially made shoes or inserts (Medicare, n.d.).

Nursing actions related to teaching include helping the person learn about the disease and its effects and knowing what affects blood glucose levels, such as eating high-carbohydrate foods and skipping meals. All of those involved in the day-to-day life of older adults with DM should have a list of warning cues of both high and low blood glucose levels, especially one that reflects those they typically experience, and know that extra SMBG (analyses of the cues) should be done any time the person feels clammy or cold, sweaty, shaky, or confused, which are all signs of low blood glucose level. An identification bracelet is highly recommended, especially because of the quick misdiagnosis that can occur if the person is found to be confused and mistakenly believed to have dementia.

◆ Nursing Action: Nutrition

Adequate and appropriate nutrition is a key aspect in maximizing health outcomes for a person with diabetes. An initial nutrition assessment with a 24-hour recall will provide some clues to the person's dietary habits and style of eating. This may not be possible for persons who are independent but have some memory limitations. It is always necessary to know who shops for and prepares the food and, at the very least, this person is included in all aspects of nutrition-related education. If the person is from an ethnic group different from that of the nurse, they will need to learn about the usual ingredients and methods of food preparation to be able to incorporate these into the development of dietary strategies. Ideally, all persons with diabetes should have what is referred to as "medical nutrition therapy" by a registered dietitian who is a certified diabetic educator, on an annual basis. This service is covered by Medicare (see earlier section on Diabetes Self-Management [DSM]).

All evidence-based guidelines focus on a healthy diet with attention to an adequate variety of foods with portion control. Recommended daily caloric intake ranges from 1600 to 2000 calories for women and from 2000 to 2600 calories for men over 60 years of age, depending on activity level. The goal is to keep the glucose level under control through multiple strategies, including balancing exercise with eating, losing weight (if overweight), and by limiting saturated fats, sodium, baked goods, and beverages with added sugar in the diet (National Institute of Diabetes and Digestive and Kidney Diseases [NIDDK], 2016). Carbohydrates are included, but these are restricted to those that are full grain. There is detailed and consumer-friendly dietary information on many websites, including that of the NIDDK at https://www.niddk.nih.gov/health-information/diabetes. Working with older adults to change dietary habits formed over a lifetime can be difficult but not impossible.

◆ Nursing Action: Exercise

Daily exercise is an important aspect of therapy for T2DM because it decreases blood glucose level by increasing insulin production and decreasing insulin resistance. Walking is an inexpensive and beneficial way to exercise. Unfortunately, in some communities, environmental conditions prevent walking in one's neighborhood, especially for older adults who live in areas of extremes of climates or in communities with high crime rates. Walking in a location that is climate controlled and environmentally safe such as an indoor shopping mall has proven to be a good alternative. Those who have limited mobility can still do chair exercises or, if possible, use exercise machines that permit sitting and holding on for support.

Exercise in conjunction with an appropriate diet may be sufficient actions to maintain blood glucose levels within acceptable limits. An intensive exercise program should not be started until the person has had a physical examination, including a stress test and electrocardiogram (ECG). A physician or nurse practitioner and a diabetic educator will then have the cues necessary to develop a safe and individualized exercise action plan. If the person is using insulin, exercise must be done on a regular rather than an erratic basis and blood glucose level should be tested before and after exercise to avoid hypoglycemia.

◆ Nursing Action: Medications

Care of older adults with DM requires that the bedside or community nurse develop a knowledge base of the most commonly used medications. These include antiglycemic and preventive (cardiac) adjuvant therapy, such as angiotensin-converting enzyme (ACE) inhibitors and aspirin. All have demonstrated to improve outcomes. Oral medications are the mainstay of pharmacological treatment of T2DM in later life. The sulfonylureas have been used the longest but also present the greatest risk for hypoglycemia and in most cases are considered inappropriate for use in older adults (American Geriatrics Society [AGS], 2019). The biguanide metformin (Glucophage) is frequently prescribed for both diabetes and prediabetes. It has been found to be very safe and effective but can only be used by people with good renal function. It is not recommended for use in persons over 80 years of age (Veterans Administration/Department of Defense [VA/DoD], 2017). Renal function must be monitored periodically and whenever there is a dose change. Several other classes of antiglycemic drugs are used, all with their own risks and levels of effectiveness.

If oral medications do not produce an adequate outcome (usually lowering the post-prandial blood glucose level to <200 mg/dL), then insulin may be added. It is important to note that the use of insulin by someone with T2DM does not "convert" them to a type 1 diabetic, because the diagnosis is made on the type of disorder rather than on the treatment. The current practice is to use long-acting formulations: the ongoing use of sliding-scale dosing is considered inappropriate in older adults (AGS, 2019). The same DSM skills/actions used by all persons with diabetes are required with additional skills specific to the use of insulin. For those who can afford them, insulin pens require less manual dexterity and visual acuity.

If any other medications are prescribed, it must be done carefully. The effect of drugs on blood glucose level must be given serious consideration because a number of medications commonly used in later life adversely affect blood glucose levels, especially psychotropics, antibiotics, and steroids. Therefore, older adults should ask whether a newly prescribed medication affects their diabetes therapy and should always check with their primary care provider or pharmacist before taking any over-the-counter medications.

◆ Evaluating Outcomes

The healthy aging outcomes in older adults with diabetes are to maintain the best health that is realistically possible and to ensure that evidence-based care is received (Boxes 20.9 and 20.10). The ideal outcomes for older adults with diabetes is glycemic (blood glucose) control to the level appropriate to their overall health status and early recognition and treatment of pending poor outcomes/complications, especially those associated with cardiovascular disease (Box 20.11).When untreated or undertreated, complications develop more quickly and more severely in older adults, especially as a result of the common comorbid diseases and disorders (Box 20.12).

Although the same types of complications occur in both older and younger adults, the risk of death from heart disease or stroke is higher in later life (NIDDK, 2017). Functional declines are more likely unless proactive measures are taken to promote wellness. Diabetes is associated with a high rate of depression and those who are depressed have a higher mortality than others. Older adults and those

---

BOX 20.10 Healthy People 2020

Goals for Persons With Diabetes or Pre-Diabetes

- Reduce annual number of new cases
- Reduce death rate
- Reduce number of lower extremity amputations
- Improve glycemic control
- Improve lipid control
- Increase the proportion of persons with controlled hypertension
- Increase the number of persons with at least annual dental, foot, and dilated eye examinations
- Increase the proportion of persons with at least biannual glycosylated hemoglobin measurement
- Increase the proportion of persons who obtain an annual microalbumin measurement
- Increase the number of persons who perform self-monitoring of blood glucose levels at least twice a day
- Increase the number of persons who receive formal diabetes education
- Increase the number of persons who have been diagnosed with diabetes mellitus
- Increase preventive measures in persons at high risk or with prediabetes

Data from US Department of Health and Human Services, Office of Disease Prevention and Health Promotion. (2019). *Healthy People 2020: Diabetes: Objectives,*. http://www.healthypeople.gov/2020/topics-objectives/topic/diabetes/objectives.

---

with diabetes have also been found to have increased mortality associated with the COVID-19 pandemic, which was first found in the United States in January 2020.

With aging there is a higher tolerance for elevated levels of circulating glucose, making hyperglycemia harder to detect. It is not unusual to find persons with fasting glucose levels of 200 to 600 mg/dL. If higher than 600 mg/dL the condition is referred to as hyperosmolar

---

BOX 20.9 Evidence-Based Practice

Minimal Standards of Medical/Nursing Care for the Person With Diabetes

At Each Visit
- Monitor weight and BP
- Inspect feet
- Review self-monitoring glucose record
- Review/adjust medications as needed
- Review self-management skills/goals
- Assess mood

Quarterly Visits
- Obtain hemoglobin A1c measurement (biannually if stable)

Annual Visits
- Obtain fasting lipid profile and serum creatinine values
- Obtain albumin-to-creatinine ratio
- Refer for dilated eye examination
- Perform foot exam for evidence of neuropathy
- Refer to dentist for comprehensive exam and cleaning

Immunizations
- Check for receipt of both pneumococcal vaccinations (PCV13 and PPSV-23). PPSV-23 repeated as appropriate
- Assess for COVID-19 vaccination
- Obtain high-dose influenza vaccine annually

BOX 20.11 Minimizing Cardiovascular Risk in Persons With Diabetes

Eat a healthy diet (lower carbohydrate, lower sodium)
Get regular exercise (at least 150 minutes moderate intensity / week)
Keep BP <140/90 mmHg for most people
Stop smoking
Maintain a HgbA1c <7% for most people
Attain and maintain acceptable lipid levels:
- Cholesterol <200 mg/dL
- LDL <100 mg/dL
- HDL >35 mg/dL
- Triglycerides <250 mg/dL

BOX 20.12   Complications of DM More Common in Older Adults

Dry eyes

Dry mouth

Confusion

Incontinence

Weight loss

Anorexia

Dehydration

Delirium

Nausea

Delayed wound healing

From Razzaque, I., Morley, J. E., Nau, K. C., et al. (2013). Diabetes mellitus. In R. J. Ham, P. D. Sloane, G. A. Warshaw, et al. (Eds.), *Ham's primary care geriatrics: A case-based approach* (6th ed., pp. 431–439). St Louis: Elsevier.

hyperglycemic syndrome (HHS) leading to coma. Most often caused by an infection, coma can also be triggered by medications that are frequently prescribed to older adults: thiazide diuretics, beta blockers, glucocorticoids, and some atypical antipsychotics. Other possible outcomes include renal injury, blindness, focal neurological deficits, and delirium. The latter is easily misdiagnosed in older adults, especially those with baseline cognitive impairments. Those who suffer coma are disproportionately Blacks, Native Americans, and Latino(a) individuals (Adeyinka and Kondamudi, 2020). Older adults in a coma or with hypotension have higher mortality than younger adults and therefore it is always a medical emergency.

The HgbA1c test is used to monitor the outcome of treatment since it is an indicator of the average plasma glucose level over the previous 90 days (Table 20.2).

TABLE 20.2   Hemoglobin A1c Readings Compared With the Calculated Estimated Average Glucose (eAG)

A1c (%)	eAG (mg/dL)
6	126
7	154
8	183
9	212
10	240
11	269
12	298

Adapted from American Diabetes Association: Understanding A1C, 1995–2020. https://www.diabetes.org/a1c.

However, there is newer information suggesting that because of genetic differences, the HgbA1c value may not be a true measurement of glucose level in some subpopulations. Persons of African, Mediterranean, or Southeast Asian descent may have a hemoglobin variant that makes the A1C unreliable. It is also unreliable in persons with kidney failure or liver disease (NIDDK, 2018).

The American Diabetes Association now recommends that the degree of glycemic control be based on the condition of the person rather than a universal number. For healthy older adults with a reasonably long life expectancy (10–15 years), an A1C of 7.5% is reasonable, compared with 7.0% in younger adults. However, for those who are very medically fragile, whose life expectancy is limited, or those among the oldest, a higher A1C (8.0%–8.5%) and flexibility may be more appropriate, with an emphasis on quality of life rather than length of life. Tight control of glucose levels in the very frail may lead to life-threatening hypoglycemia (Spero, 2019; VA/DOD, 2017).

❖ CLINICAL JUDGMENT WHEN CARING FOR OLDER ADULTS WITH DIABETES IN LONG-TERM CARE SETTINGS

Many of the persons cared for by gerontological nurses in long-term care facilities have diabetes. In this setting the nurse may be responsible for most or all the actions that would otherwise be the responsibility of the patient or a home caregiver. Cues related to altered nutritional status, intake and output, exercise, and skin integrity must be recognized and analyzed early. A nurse should regularly observe for cues of hypoglycemia and hyperglycemia as well as evidence of complications. Nursing actions often involve decision-making related to medication selection, especially insulin dosage change. Nurses ensure that evidence-based practice is followed. Nurses monitor the outcome of diet, exercise, and medication use and encourage self-care whenever possible.

▍KEY CONCEPTS

- Cues suggestive of endocrine disorders in the older adult may be vague or attributed to other medical conditions or even considered as part of "old age."
- Although thyroid disorders only affect a small number of persons, the incidence increases with age and is life threatening when not treated appropriately.
- Any time a person evidences cues for depression, atrial fibrillation, dementia, or confusion a thyroid disturbance should be considered.

- Very low doses of thyroid replacement are usually adequate in older adults. When dose changes are necessary, they must be made very slowly.
- The person's life expectancy and the risks and benefits of treatment are considered when determining the desired outcomes related to the appropriate level of glycemic control in the older adult with DM.
- Achieving optimal outcomes for older adults with diabetes is a comprehensive team effort and should include the individual as much as they can realistically participate. If this is not possible, the caregiver, if not the nurse, will need to ensure that the medical regimen is followed and is effective.
- Caring for persons with DM includes working with them to reduce their risk of complications, especially cardiovascular diseases.

ACTIVITIES AND DISCUSSION QUESTIONS

1. What are the risks and complications of DM for older adults?
2. What are the risks of treatment of older adults with DM?
3. State the components of diabetes management and explain what each component entails.
4. Describe the nurse's role in the management of endocrine disorders in older adults.

REFERENCES

Adeyinka, A., & Kondamudi, N. P. (2020). Hyperosmolar hyperglycemic nonketotic coma (HHNC, hyperosmolar hyperglycemic nonketotic syndrome). *StatPearls*. https://www.ncbi.nlm.nih.gov/books/NBK482142/.

Administration for Community Living (ACL). (2019). *Diabetes awareness month*. https://acl.gov/news-and-events/acl-blog/recognizing-national-diabetes-awareness-month.

American Diabetes Association (ADA). (2020). *Statistics about diabetes*. http://www.diabetes.org/diabetes-basics/statistics/.

American Geriatrics Society (AGS). (2019). American Geriatrics 2019 updated Beers Criteria® for potentially inappropriate medication use in older adults. *J Am Geriatr Soc, 67*(4), 674–694.

American Thyroid Association (ATA). (2020). *Older patients and thyroid disease*. https://www.thyroid.org/thyroid-disease-older-patient/.

Beck, J., Greenwood, D. A., Blanton, L., Bollinger, S. T., Butcher, M. K., et al. (2017). National standards for diabetes self-management education and support. *Diabetes Care, 40*(10), 1409–1419.

Centers for Disease Control and Prevention (CDC). (2020). *National diabetes statistics report*. https://www.cdc.gov/diabetes/data/statistics/statistics-report.html.

Centers for Disease Control and Prevention (CDC). (2019a). *Type 2 diabetes*. https://www.cdc.gov/diabetes/basics/type2.html.

Centers for Disease Control and Prevention (CDC). (2019b). *Getting tested*. https://www.cdc.gov/diabetes/basics/getting-tested.html.

Medicare: *Therapeutic shoes and inserts*, n.d. https://www.medicare.gov/coverage/therapeutic-shoes-inserts.

National Institute of Diabetes and Digestive and Kidney Diseases (NIDDK). (2016). *Diabetes diet, eating, & physical activity*. https://www.niddk.nih.gov/health-information/diabetes/overview/diet-eating-physical-activity.

NIDDK. (2018). *The A1C test and diabetes*. https://www.niddk.nih.gov/health-information/diabetes/overview/tests-diagnosis/a1c-test#affected.

NIDDK. (2017). *Diabetes, heart disease, and stroke*. https://www.niddk.nih.gov/health-information/diabetes/overview/preventing-problems/heart-disease-stroke#lower.

Papaleontiou, M., & Esfandiari, N. E. (2017). Disorders of the thyroid. In H. M. Fillit, K. Rockwood, & J. Young (Eds.), *Brocklehurst's textbook of geriatric medicine and gerontology* (pp. 731–741). Philadelphia: Elsevier.

Razzaque, I., Morley, J. E., Nau, K. C., et al. (2013). Diabetes mellitus. In RJ Ham, PD Sloane, & GA Warshaw (Eds.), *Primary care geriatrics, A case-based approach* (ed 6). Philadelphia: Elsevier.

Sinclair, A. J., Abdelhafiz, A. H., & Morley, J. E. (2017). Diabetes mellitus. In H. M. Fillit, K. Rockwood, & J. Young (Eds.), *Brocklehurst's textbook of geriatric medicine and gerontology* (pp. 747–756). Philadelphia: Elsevier.

Spero, D. (2019). *Elderly A1C targets*. https://www.diabetesselfmanagement.com/blog/elderly-a1c-targets-older-people-relaxed-glucose-goals/.

Veterans Administration/Department of Defense: *VA/DOD Clinical practice guideline for the management of type 2 diabetes mellitus*, 2017. https://www.healthquality.va.gov/guidelines/CD/diabetes/VADoDDMCPGFinal508.pdf.

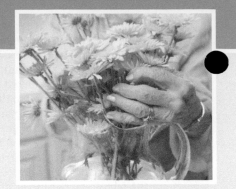

21

Bone and Joint Problems

Sandra Saint-Eloi, Kathleen Jett

http://evolve.elsevier.com/Touhy/gerontological/

LEARNING OBJECTIVES

Upon completion of this chapter, the reader will be able to:

- Describe the most common bone and joint problems affecting older adults.
- Discuss the potential dangers of osteoporosis.
- Recognize postural cues that suggest the presence of osteoporosis.
- Explain some effective strategies to prevent or slow the progression of osteoporosis.
- Compare the differing cues associated with common arthritic conditions.
- Describe a nurse's responsibility when developing strategies to maximize outcomes for a person with arthritic conditions.
- Name several actions leading to the outcome of healthy aging in a person with pain and disability from joint and bone disorders.

THE LIVED EXPERIENCE

I was always so athletic; I can't understand how I have become so crippled up. Now I understand what my grandmother used to say about the weather affecting her rheumatism. I can feel it when a storm is coming.

Mabel, age 80

I don't know how folks with arthritis can stand being uncomfortable so much of the time. I know Mabel takes medications, but she still seems to be in a lot of pain and has so much trouble moving about. I try to be as gentle as possible when I help her.

Elva, student nurse

MUSCULOSKELETAL SYSTEM

A healthy musculoskeletal system not only allows the body to be upright but also is necessary for carrying out the most basic activities of daily living (ADLs) (Chapter 8). For some, later life is an opportunity to explore the limits of their ability and become master athletes. For others, it is a time of significant restriction in movement. However, both athletes and nonathletes must deal with the challenges of one or more of the musculoskeletal problems commonly encountered in later life.

Gerontological nurses recognize the needs of older adults with musculoskeletal problems and work to promote outcomes leading to the healthiest bones and joints possible. In this chapter we discuss osteoporosis, several forms of arthritis, and the cues to recognize their presence. The analyses of these cues lead to prioritized hypotheses for that individual and strategies and actions to promote health while aging.

OSTEOPOROSIS

In the normal process of growth, bones increase in structural density and strength through the accumulation of calcium and other minerals (bone mineral density) at the same time they are weakened as calcium and minerals return (are resorbed) into the bloodstream. Peak bone mass is reached at about 30 years of age. After that, resorption and the subsequent loss of bone mineral density (BMD) is minimal at first but accelerates with aging. For women, the period of fastest loss of BMD is in the 5 to 7 years immediately following menopause.

Osteoporosis means *porous bone*. Primary osteoporosis is so common in women that it is sometimes thought to be part of the normal aging process. Secondary osteoporosis is caused by another disease, such as Paget's disease, or by medications, such as long-term steroid use. In *osteopenia*, BMD has been lost but not to the extent it is in osteoporosis. Both are characterized by deterioration of the bone structure and changes in posture (Fig. 21.1).

More than 53 million Americans either have osteoporosis or are at risk of it because of low BMD, the majority of whom are women (NIH, 2018). Over 70% of those over the age of 80 years have some level of reduced BMD or osteoporosis worldwide. In developed countries it affects only 2%–8% of men and 9%–38% of women. Black women have a higher BMD than Whites but have similar risk of fractures (Porter & Varacallo, 2020). Osteoporosis is a silent disorder; the person may never know they have it until suffering a fracture. Many fractures are the result of trauma. Other fractures are classified as "fragility fractures"; these are non- or low-traumatic fractures resulting from an activity that would not normally cause one, such as falling from a standing height or from coughing, sneezing, or laughing (National Osteoporosis Guideline Group, 2018).

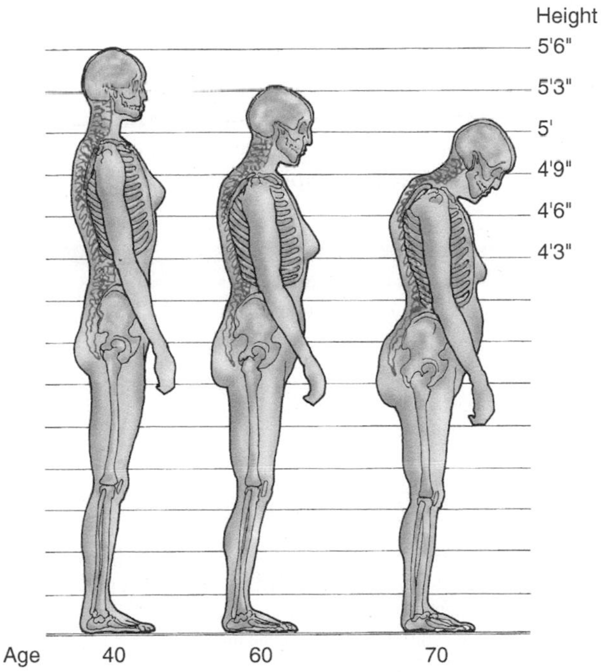

BMD is measured with a dual-energy x-ray absorptiometry (DEXA) scan. Osteoporosis is presumed in older adults with nontraumatic (fragility) fractures. The US Preventive Services Task Force (USPSTF) recommends that all women 65 years of age or older and younger women with significant risk factors (e.g., family history) be screened for osteoporosis. There is insufficient evidence for or against screening in men (USPSTF, 2018). For those at risk or taking FDA-approved treatment, Medicare will pay for a DEXA scan every 2 years and more frequently if medically necessary (Centers for Medicare and Medicaid Services [CMS], 2019).

FIG. 21.1 Age-related changes in the spine as a result of bone loss. (From Ignatavicius, D. D., & Workman, M. L. (2016). *Medical-surgical nursing: Patient-centered collaborative care* (8th ed.). St Louis: Elsevier.)

❖ USING CLINICAL JUDGMENT TO PROMOTE HEALTHY AGING: SKELETAL DISORDERS

◆ Recognizing and Analyzing Cues

Prior to a fracture, cues suggestive of progressive loss of BMD are a loss of 3 inches or more in height and/or kyphosis (see Fig. 21.1). The nurse may be the first person to identify these cues. At the same time, the nurse may recognize cues in the person's lifestyle or characteristics that put them at risk for osteopenia or osteoporosis (Box 21.1). With the treatments and interventions now available, some osteoporosis can be reduced in severity or at least stabilized.

◆ Nursing Actions

Nursing actions to prevent or minimize a person's risk of osteoporosis in later life include teaching younger adults about the need for a diet rich in calcium and exposure to ultraviolet light for the production of vitamin D by the skin. The latter must be tempered by awareness of the risk of skin cancer from excessive exposure (Chapter 14). Nurses should always recommend persons of any age prioritize strategies to reduce all modifiable risk factors possible (Box 21.1). Nursing actions will include facilitating smoking cessation if appropriate, diet counseling regarding the need to achieve and maintain an ideal body weight (based on age), and education about the maintenance

BOX 21.1   Risk Factors for Osteoporosis

Nonmodifiable Factors
Gender (female)
Race (White)
Age
Family history of osteoporosis

Modifiable Factors
Weight (underweight)
Diet (low calcium, excessive caffeine, ethyl alcohol)
Hormonal deficiencies
Activity level (low)
Medications (steroids, anticonvulsants, thyroid preparations)
Cigarette smoking

of bone strength and flexibility through weight-bearing exercise.

As the person ages, especially for women approaching menopause, nurses should participate in the responsibility of ensuring that screening (DEXA scans) is done as appropriate and that preventive behaviors continue. If screening indicates osteopenia, the nursing actions are prioritized to helping the person realize the need to continue preventive strategies and receive pharmacological therapy as appropriate. The World Health Organization provides an osteoporosis risk assessment tool (FRAX) that can be completed and used to predict an individual's 10-year probability of a fracture (https://www.sheffield.ac.uk/FRAX/tool.aspx?country=23).

If screening or a fracture leads to the diagnosis of osteoporosis, the same strategies are used to prevent worsening with added pharmacological intervention. Nurses act to advocate for the older adult to receive appropriate and timely treatment to potentially reduce the likelihood of a poor outcome, i.e., new or repeat fractures and risk of fall related death (Chapter 15). All the nursing actions associated with prevention and in the presence of osteopenia also apply to osteoporosis. Nurses conduct home safety inspections and education regarding injury prevention strategies (detailed in Chapters 15 and 16). Weight-bearing physical activity, such as brisk walking or carrying light weights, helps to maintain bone mass by applying mechanical force to the spine and long bones. Muscle-building exercises help to maintain skeletal architecture by improving general muscle strength, flexibility, thigh strength, and overall coordination. Yoga and tai chi can help improve balance. While this will not reduce the development of osteoporosis, it can reduce the risk of a fall (Porter & Varacallo, 2020).

Nurses should provide information about the sites most vulnerable to injury. Explanation should be given about changes in the upper spine that occur when vertebrae are weakened and about the pain that can result from strain on the lower spine when effort is needed to compensate for balance and height changes attributable to alteration of the upper spine. An assortment of print and interactive educational materials for both the lay and professional audience can be found at http://www.niams.nih.gov/Health_Info/Bone/Osteoporosis/default.asp.

For optimal bone mass in later life, a healthy diet is necessary, especially one with adequate calcium and vitamin D intake earlier in life (see Chapter 10). The diet during adolescence and young adulthood is a key to healthy bones later. A balanced diet that includes food sources providing the recommended amount of calcium is best (Box 21.2). However, because of age-related changes in the gastrointestinal tract, calcium supplementation is usually necessary.

Women more than 50 years of age should ingest 1200 mg of calcium per day (men 1000 mg/day); for both men and women older than age 70, 1200 mg of calcium a day is recommended from combined dietary and supplementary sources (NIH/NORBDRC, 2018). The two most common forms are calcium carbonate and calcium citrate. Calcium carbonate has the highest amount of available calcium but it must be taken with food. Calcium citrate can be taken at any time. Both products interact with a number of medications, and nurses need to be aware of this when scheduling or recommending a dosing schedule. The dose is best spread over the course of the day (for example, 400 mg of calcium three times a day).

Constipation, already a problem for many as they age, is worsened by calcium supplementation and may reduce

BOX 21.2   Sources of Calcium

Dairy products (e.g., yogurt, milk, cheese)
Chinese cabbage or bok choy
Tofu (calcium fortified)
Soymilk (calcium fortified)
Orange juice (calcium fortified)
Dried figs
Cheese pizza
Green, leafy vegetables (e.g., broccoli, brussels sprouts, mustard greens)
Beans/legumes
Tortillas
Cooked soybeans
Sardines or salmon, shrimp with edible bones
Nuts (especially almonds)
Bread, cereals (fortified)

From National Institutes of Health. (2019). *A guide to calcium rich food.* https://ods.od.nih.gov/factsheets/Calcium-Consumer/.

the person's willingness to take it. Nursing actions include working with the person to develop an effective bowel regimen to prevent this untoward outcome. Strategies usually include stool softeners and plenty of water (e.g., a full glass of water with at least each dose of calcium).

Six hundred international units (600 IU) of vitamin D supplementation until the age of 70 years is recommended, with an increase to 800 IU a day thereafter. However, many older adults require at least 1000 IU a day to achieve a therapeutic blood level of 50 nmol/L to 125 nmol/L (NIH Office of Dietary Supplements, 2020). Combined calcium–vitamin D supplements can be found in solid, liquid, and chewable forms. Older adults are at particularly high risk of vitamin D deficiencies because of changes in the skin that reduce the ability to synthesize vitamin D efficiently. For those who are homebound or live in institutional settings or cold climates where the skin is covered, the reduced opportunities for sunlight exposure only increase the risk of deficiencies and the need for supplementation.

Patient teaching includes discussion of the factors that inhibit calcium absorption (e.g., excess alcohol, protein, or salt) or enhance excretion (e.g., caffeine; excess fiber; phosphorus in meats, sodas, and preserved foods) and the influence of the body's response to stress (decreased calcium absorption, increased excretion of calcium in the urine).

> ## ⚡ SAFETY ALERT
>
> Neither calcium nor any other product containing a metal may be taken at the same time as thyroid preparations. They will chemically bind together and the levothyroxine with be inactivated.

There are several medications currently available for both preventing the development of osteoporosis and slowing its progression. They increase bone mass, reduce bone turnover, or both and are available in oral and injectable forms and are taken daily, weekly, or quarterly (Mayo, 2020). Calcitonin is available in a spray formulation. Only the subcutaneous Prolia (every 6 months) and Forteo (daily) have been found to reverse BMD loss but can only be used in unique circumstances and are very expensive. Nurses either administer these medications or teach patients/significant others how to do so.

The effectiveness of the class of drugs called bisphosphonates longer than 5 years is unknown. The nurse is often the person to notice that this time period has been reached. Nursing education also includes the appropriate way to take prescribed medications and their side effects. Adequate intake of calcium and vitamin D and must be taken with all the prescribed treatments currently available.

> ## ⚡ SAFETY ALERT
>
> Because of the seriousness of the risk of esophageal erosion, bisphosphonates must be taken on an empty stomach, with a full glass of water, and with the person completely upright for 0.5 to 1 hour after ingestion. They are not appropriate for the person with memory loss or for anyone who cannot be depended upon to comply with these directions.

The medication Evista is used as a substitute for estrogen as a bone protector and decreases the risk of breast cancer. It is approved for both the prevention and the treatment of bone loss, but it can cause hot flashes and coagulation disorders and is contraindicated for use by anyone with a history of a deep venous thrombosis (DVT) or who is taking blood thinners.

THE ARTHRITIS

Arthritis is the term used to apply to more than 100 musculoskeletal conditions. It is significantly more common in women in all age groups and increases dramatically after about 45 years of age. From 2013 to 2015, an estimated 54.4 million American adults were told by a doctor that they had gout, lupus, or fibromyalgia. This number is expected to rise to 78.4 million by 2040, and 43.2% of these have an arthritis-associated disability. The prevalence increases with age (Centers for Disease Control and Prevention [CDC], 2018). Many over the age of 65 years will have radiographic evidence of osteoarthritis (OA) even if they are asymptomatic. The osteoarthritic joint is one in which the normal soft and resilient cartilaginous lining becomes thin and damaged.

There is considerable racial and ethnic variability in prevalence (Table 21.1). The most common forms of arthritis that the gerontological nurse will encounter are

TABLE 21.1 Prevalence of Arthritis by Race/Ethnicity

Race/Ethnicity	Prevalence
Non-Hispanic White	22.6%
Non-Hispanic Black	22.2%
Hispanic/Latino(a)	15.4%
Asian	11.8%
American Indian/Alaskan Native	24.4%

From Barbour, K. E., Helmick, C. G., Theis, K. A., et al. (2017). Prevalence of doctor-diagnosed arthritis and arthritis-attributable activity limitation—United States, 2013–2015, *MMRW 66*, 246–253.

TABLE 21.2   Comparison of Osteoarthritis, Rheumatoid Arthritis, and Gout

	Osteoarthritis	Rheumatoid Arthritis	Gout
Onset	Insidious	More acute in older adults than in younger adults	Sudden/acute
Classic symptoms	Stiffness of joint resolved in less than 20 minutes after rest	Stiffening lasting more than 20–30 minutes after rest	Acute pain
Classic signs	Affects distal interphalangeal joints, knees, hips, and vertebrae	Affects proximal joints; may be systemic	Inflammation, especially at the base of the great toe
Key management	Initial treatment may be nonpharmacological such as heat and exercise; later acetaminophen and NSAIDs	Use of DMARDs as soon as diagnosis is made	NSAIDs

DMARDs, Disease-modifying antirheumatic drugs; *NSAIDs,* non-steroidal anti-inflammatory drugs.

OA, polymyalgia rheumatica (PMR), giant cell arteritis (GCA), rheumatoid arthritis (RA), and gout (Table 21.2).

Recognizing and Analyzing Cues: Osteoarthritis

OA, the most common type of arthritis, is a degenerative joint disorder. Risk factors include genetic predisposition (family history), local inflammation, and mechanical forces such as prior injury or overuse.

In classic OA the primary cue is stiffness with inactivity that is relieved by activity. At the same time activity may lead to pain relieved by rest. Persons will report the stiffness is greatest after the disuse during sleep but should resolve within 30 minutes of use. A later cue, pain at rest, develops as the disease advances and more joints become involved. The nurse will often be able to palpate crepitus (that is, the sensation of crunching or popping) as the joint is moved, indicating joint instability and deterioration. The joint will eventually enlarge as osteophytes develop, range of motion is reduced, and deformities occur (Fig. 21.2). Cues for OA are most often found in the knees, fingers (especially base of the thumb), and hips (CDC, 2020). The neck (cervical spine) and the lower back (lumbar spine) may also be

What Areas Does Osteoarthritis Affect?

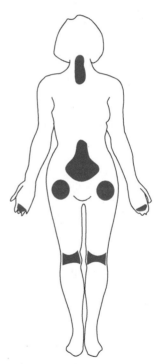

FIG. 21.3 Common locations for osteoarthritis. (From National Institutes of Health. (2019). *Handout on health: Osteoarthritis.* http://www.niams.nih.gov/hi/topics/arthritis/oahandout.htm.)

affected (Fig. 21.3). OA is found in the shoulders less often. Depression, anxiety, and decreased functional status are all associated with OA.

Nursing Actions

Nursing actions in the care of persons with OA or at risk of OA are directed to assuring early detection,

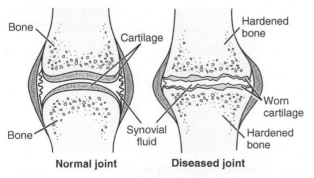

FIG. 21.2 Normal joint and diseased joint.

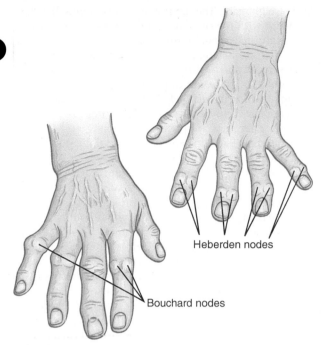

FIG. 21.4 Hand deformities in arthritis. (From McCance, K. L., & Huether, S. E., (Eds.). (2014). *Pathophysiology: The biologic basis for disease in adults and children* (7th ed.). St Louis: Elsevier.)

maintaining comfort, and preserving function and thereby independence. When assessing the musculo-skeletal system, a nurse should examine the joints and muscles for tenderness, swelling, warmth, and redness. The hands are examined for the presence or absence of osteophytes. If they appear in the proximal interpha-langeal joints, they are called Bouchard's nodes and Heberden's nodes in the distal joints; the latter much less common than the former (Fig. 21.4). The nurse questions their effect on function and the presence of pain.

Both passive and active range of motion is evaluated. How far can the person reach and bend all joints without assistance? The degrees of flexion, extension, rotation, abduction, and adduction are measured and documented. The testing of passive range of motion must go only to the point of discomfort and never to that of inducing pain. Ask whether there are any activities of daily living (ADLs) or instrumental activities of daily living (IADLs) that are limited or not possible because of musculoskeletal issues. For example, can the person comb their hair or tie a shoe; can a woman fasten her bra; can food and other needed materials be taken from cabinets; is the person able to get up and down from the toilet, open medicine bottles, and hold and use eating utensils safely?

Pain is a cue that the disease is progressing. Heat may be applied superficially or deeply to provide significant relief. Ultrasound provides deep heat and is usually administered by physical therapists. Hot packs, hydrotherapy, and radiant heat provide superficial heat. Liquid paraffin baths can be purchased in most drug stores for submerging the hands to provide deep heat and temporary relief.

Although acetaminophen (Tylenol) is the drug of choice for intermittent OA pain, many patients self-report that they prefer one of the nonsteroidal anti-inflammatory products such as naproxen sodium. In most cases opioids will eventually be necessary (see Chapter 18). Several complementary and alternative medicine (CAM) interventions are used by persons around the globe to attempt to treat the pain associated with musculoskeletal problems, especially osteoarthritis. Among the most popular is the use of the dietary supplement glucosamine and chondroitin sulfate. There is now a growing body of evidence that finds there is improvement in pain or function of joints when these products are used. There is some evidence that Devil's Claw (*Harpagophytum*) may also be helpful for some pain in osteoarthritis (NCCIH, 2016).

When pain can no longer be controlled or function is impaired to the point that quality of life is unacceptable, a joint replacement procedure (arthroplasty) may be performed for osteoarthritis in knees or hips. These are often highly successful and restore the person to their previous or higher level of functioning. In select cases, joint replacement surgery is recommended for even the very old when pain cannot be controlled through other means (see Chapter 18). The nurse is involved in the preoperative, perioperative periods, and rehabilitation to assist in helping the person working toward the outcome of learning to use the new joint and return to (hopefully) full function.

Rheumatoid Arthritis

Rheumatoid arthritis (RA) is a chronic, systemic, inflammatory joint disorder. It is considered an autoimmune disease in which products from the inflamed lining of the joint invade and destroy the cartilage and bone within the joint. It affects about 1.5 million people, or 0.6% of the US adult population and most often starts in midlife between 40 and 60 years of age (NIAMS, 2019a).

The natural course of RA is highly variable, with good and bad days. The disease may last a few months or years or may become a chronic condition with progressive damage to the joints. Although the cause of RA is unknown, a combination of sex hormones (e.g., estrogen), genes, and environmental factors may be involved (NIAMS, 2019b).

Recognizing and Analyzing Cues: RA

RA is characterized by pain and swelling in symmetrical joints (for example, both hands, both sides of the hip). The joints are warm and tender. It generally affects the small joints of the wrist, the ankle, or the hand, although it can affect large joints as well. The most significant cue to detection is stiffness in the affected joint that lasts longer than 30 minutes, compared with less than 30 minutes in OA. RA is a systemic disease; therefore, other possible cues are generalized fatigue and malaise and occasional unexplained fevers. Weight loss is common.

Nursing Actions: RA

In the past, nonsteroidal anti-inflammatory drugs (NSAIDs) were used for treatment early in the disease and RA-specific drugs were "saved" for later. However, it has been found that prompt treatment may halt or slow the damage (Mian et al., 2019). Persons diagnosed with RA are usually under a rheumatologist's care, which involves aggressive therapy primarily using a class of drugs called disease-modifying antirheumatic drugs (DMARDs) and the newer biological response modifiers and janus kinase inhibitors. All the DMARDs are potentially toxic and are administered with care by a registered nurse, such as the charge nurse in a nursing home, or by a physician. Nurses provide expert education regarding the use of the medications. Nursing actions include providing comfort and support while monitoring the progression of the disease and the effectiveness, side effects, and potential toxicity of pharmacological treatment (Box 21.3). Because RA is an inflammatory condition, heat can never be used. However, the application of cold packs can decrease muscle spasm, decrease swelling, and relieve inflammatory pain.

Attention should also be given to diet (see Chapter 10). With the decreases in activity associated with pain in all forms of arthritis, it is easy for the person to gain weight. Excess weight significantly increases the pressure and wear and tear on the joints, leading to less activity and more weight gain. The nurse and the registered dietitian can work with the person to identify realistic strategies for weight management and the development of meal plans that are personally and culturally acceptable but still balanced and healthy.

Regular exercise can improve flexibility and muscle strength, which in turn help support the affected joints, reduce pain, and reduce falls. Walking, swimming, and water aerobics are preferred by many, and the latter is often available in senior centers, public pools, and YMCAs in many communities.

Nurses work with persons with either RA or OA to develop strategies to minimize disability by protecting their joints from stress and, in doing so, possibly decrease pain and improve balance and function. Canes, crutches, walkers, collars, shoe orthotics, and corsets can relieve joint pressure and help support the person with muscle and joint weakness or resultant orthopedic abnormalities. A shoe lift can improve lumbar pain. A knee brace is useful if there is lateral instability (the knee "gives out"). The person can avoid carrying packages by their fingers or can use utensils and household equipment with larger rather than smaller grips if their hands are affected. Preventing the exposure of affected joints to cold environmental temperatures may provide further protection. The person is encouraged to wear leggings, gloves, or scarves as necessary while outside.

Polymyalgia Rheumatica and Giant Cell Arteritis

PMR is one of the more common inflammatory diseases seen in older adults, especially those over 50 years of age, with the highest incidence between 70 and 80 years of age. For unknown reasons, PMR may occur at the same time as giant cell arteritis (GCA). Their causes are unknown, but they are associated with aging, environmental triggers, immune disorders, and genetic factors (National Institute of Arthritis and Musculoskeletal and Skin Diseases [NIAMS], 2016a).

Giant cell arteritis (also known as *temporal arteritis*) is primarily an acute inflammation of the arteries of the scalp in the temporal area but medium to large vessels may be involved as well. The inflammation causes restricted blood flow and may cause very serious and permanent damage such as stroke or blindness.

Recognizing and Analyzing Cues: PMR and GCA

Although PMR may appear as suddenly as overnight, it often develops slowly. Classic cues are stiffening and pain beginning in the neck and upper arms and possibly evolving to the pelvic and pectoral girdles, flu-like symptoms such as fatigue and a low-grade fever. Pain is usually greatest at night and in the early morning, but usually without joint inflammation. It usually resolves on its own in 1 to 2 years.

BOX 21.3 Partial List of Potential Side Effects of Medications Used to Treat Rheumatoid Arthritis

- Nonbiological DMARDs: upset stomach, nausea, diarrhea, stomatitis, rash (may be very serious); liver, kidney, or lung problems
- Biological DMARDS: Redness, swelling, itching, bruising where injection given; sinusitis, headache, nausea, diarrhea
- Rare but serious side effects of either: Infection such as tuberculosis, fungal infections such as yeast, pneumonia, listeria, cancer (especially lymphoma)

From National Institute of Arthritis and Musculoskeletal and Skin Diseases. https://www.ncbi.nlm.nih.gov/books/NBK115126/pdf/Bookshelf_NBK115126.pdf.

Like PMR, early cues suggestive of GCA are flu-like symptoms such as fatigue, loss of appetite, and fever. Other cues specifically related to enlarged, inflamed arteries in the head include headaches, pain and tenderness over the temples, double vision or vision loss, dizziness, or problems with coordination. Pain may also affect the jaw and tongue, especially when eating and opening the mouth to chew. GCA can cause serious problems such as visual loss or stroke if not treated promptly (NIAMS, 2016b). *Sudden changes in vision are always a medical emergency.*

Nursing Actions: PMR and GCA

The most important strategy in addressing these conditions is prompt recognition and hypotheses prioritization. Initial treatment is high-dose steroids and later low-dose steroids continuing for years or indefinitely. Heat is absolutely contraindicated in those with GCA.

Gout

Gout is a common form of inflammatory arthritis seen primarily in men at mid-life and beyond. It rarely affects young adults or women prior to menopause. It appears to result from the accumulation of needle-shaped uric acid crystals in a joint. Uric acid is produced when purines found in food break down. The development of gout and the body's response to uric acid accumulation are highly individualized. It is important to note that some people have elevated levels of uric acid and do not get gout, a clinical picture described as asymptomatic hyperuricemia, and others have gout and low levels of uric acid. The uric acid level itself does not result in a diagnosis of gout.

Gout typically starts with an acute attack that may be triggered by alcohol, foods, medications, or trauma to the joint. After an acute attack, gout may become chronic with periodic acute "attacks" if preventive actions are not taken. Some persons are at higher risk and those with gout are more likely to develop other health problems, especially cardiac and renal. Risk factors include alcohol abuse, high blood pressure, a diet high in purines, drinking beverages with high-fructose corn syrups such as sodas (Box 21.4), and certain medications, especially thiazide diuretics, salicylates (e.g., aspirin), niacin (large amounts), and ciclosporins (NIAMS, 2020).

Recognizing and analyzing cues: Gout

The person typically complains of sudden and *exquisite* or *severe* pain in the affected joint, often starting in the middle of the night during sleep. The most common cue is a joint that is bright purple-red, hot, and too painful to touch. The proximal joint of the great toe is the most typical site, although sometimes the ankle, the knee, the wrist, or the elbow is involved. A nurse practitioner may

BOX 21.4 Examples of Foods High in Purines

Asparagus
Game meat
Beef kidneys
Gravy
Brain
Herring, mackerel, and sardines
Sweetbread
Mushrooms
Dried beans and seeds
Scallops

order an ultrasound or take a sample of fluids from the joints.

If left untreated or undertreated, tophi may develop (a build-up of urate crystals) in the joints and in organs. The cue that indicates long-standing gout is the appearance of these tophi as palpable white lumps under the skin.

Nursing Actions: Gout

The most common treatment for an acute attack is an over-the-counter anti-inflammatory drug such as ibuprofen; however, nonsteroidal anti-inflammatories are associated with a high risk of adverse drug events in older adults and cannot be taken by those with hypertension (see Chapter 9). For some, corticosteroids are necessary. If there is still no relief, colchicine is used as a last resort and with much caution in older adults (NIAMS, 2020). As with RA, an important nursing action is to help the person develop strategies to protect the joint during the acute attack, as well as to prevent another acute attack and the development of chronic gout. Strategies to optimize these outcomes include the avoidance of risk-elevating drugs or of foods that are high in purine and alcohol, both of which increase uric acid levels; also, medications can be used either to decrease uric acid production (e.g., allopurinol) or to increase its excretion (e.g., probenecid) (American Society of Health-System Pharmacists [ASHP], 2020). Finally, nurses should strategize with the person to find a way to drink enough nonalcoholic liquids to help flush the uric acid through the kidneys (2 L/day if not contraindicated).

❖ USING CLINICAL JUDGMENT TO PROMOTE HEALTHY AGING: BONE AND JOINT PROBLEMS

Gerontological nurses have a direct impact on promoting musculoskeletal health in a number of ways. They are active at all levels of health promotion and disease prevention (Box 21.5).

Box 21-5 Healthy People 2030

Goals for Musculoskeletal Wellness

- Reduce the proportion of adults with provider-diagnosed arthritis who experience a limitation in activity due to arthritis or joint symptoms.
- Reduce the proportion of adults with provider-diagnosed arthritis who experience severe or moderate joint pain.
- Reduce the proportion of adults with provider-diagnosed arthritis who are limited in their ability to work for pay due to arthritis.
- Increase the proportion of adults with provider-diagnosed arthritis who receive health care provider counseling for physical activity or exercise.

Data from US Department of Health and Human Services, Office of Disease Prevention and Health Promotion. (n.d.). Healthy People 2030. https://health.gov/healthypeople/search?query=arthritis.

◆ **Evaluating Outcomes**

The outcomes for all the different forms of musculoskeletal problems are accurate diagnosis and treatment as soon as possible, pain control, return to prior functional ability, and minimizing the development of disabilities, injury, or even a fall-related death (Table 21.3).

The nurse acts as an advocate for achieving these outcomes and for minimizing iatrogenic complications of medication management. In administering medications, the nurse minimizes adverse outcomes by paying close attention to blood pressure, renal, and liver function and notifies the physician or nurse practitioner of any change so that the dosages can be adjusted. The nurse revises hypotheses through ongoing reevaluation of therapeutic approaches and patient teaching. Pain management and the minimization of disability are interconnected. In joint replacement, outcomes depend on the timing of surgery, the number of procedures that the surgeon has performed, the nursing care received, and the patient's

TABLE 21.3 Prevalence of Arthritis-Related Activity Limitation Among Adults by Race/Ethnicity

Race/Ethnicity	Prevalence
Non-Hispanic White	40.1%
Non-Hispanic Black	48.6%
Hispanic/Latino(a)	44.3%
Asian	37.6%
American Indian/Alaskan Native	51.6%

From Barbour, K. E., Helmick, C. G., Theis, K. A., et al. (2017). Prevalence of doctor-diagnosed arthritis and arthritis-attributable activity limitation—United States, 2013–2015, *MMRW 66*, 246–253.

medical status before and after the surgery, and the ability to participate in rehabilitation.

Nurses work with the older adult and an occupational therapist to achieve outcomes to maintain or improve the ability to perform activities of daily living as independently as possible. It cannot be overstated that ongoing treatment from accredited physical therapists is necessary for persons with musculoskeletal problems to achieve the outcome of retained joint use and maximum independence for as long as possible.

KEY CONCEPTS

- Most people over the age of 40 years have osteoarthritis to some extent.
- Osteoporosis can become a crippling problem for many older adults, especially women. Although it cannot be completely prevented, it can be minimized by early self-care actions: weight-bearing exercise and therapeutic calcium and vitamin D intake.
- The most serious outcomes of osteoporosis are fractures and are associated with high mortality.
- The cues suggestive of rheumatoid arthritis are swelling, inflammation, intense pain, and distortion of the joints.
- Gout is both an acute and a chronic condition. One of the goals of treatment with gout is to minimize the likelihood of a future attack.
- Individuals have found certain types of complementary and alternative interventions very helpful for joint disorders and chronic discomfort.

ACTIVITIES AND DISCUSSION QUESTIONS

1. What are the most effective ways of preventing osteoporosis?
2. What lifestyle issues would you discuss with an individual with advanced osteoporosis?
3. What are the differences in cues between osteoarthritis and rheumatoid arthritis?
4. What advice would you give someone who is experiencing joint pain and mobility limitations?
5. Which of your favorite activities would be difficult if you were afflicted with osteoarthritis?

NEXT-GENERATION NCLEX® EXAMINATION-STYLE QUESTIONS

Mrs. Anderson, 65 years old, arrives at the senior health center for her "Welcome to Medicare" preventive visit. She has a 25-pack/year history of smoking, but she quit smoking 15 years ago. She is married and lives in a two-story home in an established neighborhood. Her two adult children live nearby and visit often. She enjoys spending time with her grandchildren. Mrs. Anderson has a history of hypothyroidism and takes levothyroxine 112 µg daily but is otherwise healthy; she also takes a multivitamin and calcium + D each day. She states she went through menopause about 10 years ago and no longer experiences hot flashes or other symptoms. Her vital signs include a blood pressure of 115/82 mmHg, heart rate of 84 beats per minute, respiration rate of 14 breaths per minute, and temperature of 97.6°F. Her dual-energy X-ray absorptiometry scan yielded a T score of -3.0 (a T score of -1.0 or above = normal bone density).

Based on the client's condition, the client's priority need will be to prevent _____1_____. Essential strategies to prevent injury include ____2_____ and _____3_____.

Options for 1	Options for 2 and 3
Osteopenia	Smoking cessation
Hormonal deficiencies	Home safety inspection
Fractures	Weight gain
Decreased calcium absorption	Education regarding injury prevention
Esophageal erosion	Osteoporosis screening

REFERENCES

American Society of Health-System Pharmacists (ASHP): *Probenecid*, 2020. https://www.nlm.nih.gov/medlineplus/druginfo/meds/a682395.html.

Centers for Disease Control and Prevention (CDC): *Arthritis data and statistics*, 2018. http://www.cdc.gov/arthritis/data_statistics/index.htm.

Centers for Disease Control and Prevention (CDC): *Osteoarthritis*, 2020. https://www.cdc.gov/arthritis/basics/osteoarthritis.htm.

Centers for Medicare and Medicaid Services (CMS): *Preventive services chart*, 2019. https://www.cms.gov/Medicare/Prevention/PrevntionGenInfo/medicare-preventive-services/MPS-QuickReferenceChart-1.html#BONE_MASS.

Mayo Clinic Staff: *Osteoporosis treatment: Medications can help*, 2020. http://www.mayoclinic.org/diseases-conditions/osteoporosis/in-depth/osteoporosis-treatment/art-20046869?pg=1.

Mian, A., Ibrahim, F., & Scott, D. L. (2019). A systematic review of guidelines for managing rheumatoid arthritis. *BMC Rheumatology, 3*(42), EJournal.

National Center for Complementary and Integrative Health: *Osteoarthritis: in depth*, 2016. https://www.nccih.nih.gov/health/osteoarthritis-in-depth.

NIAMS (National Institute of Arthritis and Musculoskeletal and Skin Diseases): *Polymyalgia rheumatica*, 2016a. https://www.niams.nih.gov/health-topics/polymyalgia-rheumatica/advanced#tab-overview.

NIAMS: *Giant cell arteritis*, 2016b. https://www.niams.nih.gov/health-topics/giant-cell-arteritis/advanced#tab-treatment.

NIAMS: *Handout on health: rheumatoid arthritis*, 2019a. http://www.niams.nih.gov/Health_Info/Rheumatic_Disease/default.asp. Accessed June 2020.

NIAMS: *Overview of gout*, 2020. https://www.niams.nih.gov/health-topics/gout/advanced#tab-overview.

NIH/NORBDRC (National Institutes of Health/National Osteoporosis and Related Bone Disorders Resource Center): *Bone health for life: Osteoporosis overview*, 2018. https://www.bones.nih.gov/sites/bones/files/pdfs/osteopoverview-508.pdf.

NIH/Office of Dietary Supplements: *Vitamin D*, 2020. https://ods.od.nih.gov/factsheets/VitaminD-HealthProfessional.

National Osteoporosis Foundation: *Calcium and vitamin D*. https://www.nof.org/patients/treatment/calciumvitamin-d.

Porter, J. L., & Varacallo, M (2020). Osteoporosis. *StatPerls* [Internet]. March 15. https://www.ncbi.nlm.nih.gov/books/NBK441901/.

US Preventive Services Task Force (USPSTF): *Osteoporosis to Prevent Fractures: Screening*, 2018. https://www.uspreventiveservicestaskforce.org/uspstf/document/evidence-summary1/osteoporosis-screening.

22

Cardiovascular and Respiratory Disorders

Kathleen Jett

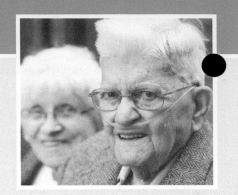

http://evolve.elsevier.com/Touhy/gerontological/

LEARNING OBJECTIVES

Upon completion of this chapter, the reader will be able to:
- Identify the most common types of cardiovascular and respiratory diseases occurring in late life.
- Discuss how cues, actions, and outcomes for cardiovascular and respiratory diseases in older adults may differ from those for younger adults.
- Suggest actions geared toward the outcomes of minimizing the risk for cardiovascular and respiratory disease.
- Discuss the cues suggestive of community-acquired pneumonia and explain how they may differ in one who is a frail older adult.
- Propose how the nurse works with older adults in the consideration of nursing actions in the presence of pneumonia.

THE LIVED EXPERIENCE

I went down to the clinic and told them that I felt kind of strange all night, just a little pressure in the middle of my chest but otherwise the same as always. It was amazing how fast the nurse practitioner sent me to the emergency room. I had been having something they called "angina" and didn't even know it! They said I could have died and I am not quite ready for that.

Milly, age 93

We keep trying to tell dad he needs to stop smoking or it is going to kill him! He coughs all the time and gets one infection after another. All he says is, "I've been smoking all of my life, why should I stop now?"

Maria, daughter of José, age 59

Caring for older adults often means caring for persons with cardiovascular disease (CVD), respiratory problems, or both. These two systems are interconnected: a problem in one is likely to result in, or complicate, a problem in the other. When a nurse is addressing a cardiac problem, the respiratory system is also addressed, and vice versa. For example, pneumonia may trigger heart failure. The outcomes of nursing actions frequently overlap as well. One carefully planned action must address several systems at the same time and achieve outcomes that meet basic physiological, psychological, and spiritual needs while promoting healthy aging in the face of very serious illnesses.

CARDIOVASCULAR DISEASE (CVD)

The American Heart Association identifies the major cardiovascular diseases as hypertension (HTN); coronary heart disease (CHD), including acute myocardial infarction (STEMI or NSTEMI) and angina; and heart failure (HF). Although the numbers of deaths from heart disease have decreased, they remain the number one cause of death for all racial and ethnic groups in the United States except Asian or Pacific Islanders, for whom it is second to cancer (Heron, 2019). The rate of deaths increases dramatically with age partly because of normal changes with aging (see Chapter 4) but more often from the rising incidence of hypertension and diabetes (Chapter 20). Older adults also undergo most CVD-related procedures, but treatment approaches, frequency of diagnosis, and disease-associated mortality are highly variable by ethnicity and sex. Black men still have a higher mortality than other racial/ethnic groups and may persist even with equal access to care (Youmans et al., 2019).

Hypertension

Hypertension (HTN) is the most common chronic cardiovascular disease encountered by gerontological nurses. Both the definition of and the overall guidelines for treatment of HTN in "older adults" has varied widely by organization. In 2017, the American College of Cardiology and the American Heart Association recommended a goal of less than 130/90 mmHg for those at least 65 years of age. In 2018, this guideline was changed to less than140/90 mmHg. **In 2017, the American College of Physician/American Association of Family Guidelines proposed a target of BP less than 150/90 mmHg and the 2017 guidelines proposed an SBP of less than120 mmHg for those over 75 years of age** (Benetos et al., 2019)

Systolic blood pressure increases slightly with age, with a leveling off or decrease in the diastolic pressure for persons about 60 years of age and older. Older adults most often have isolated systolic hypertension, that is, an elevation in only the systolic reading. This is quite different from the younger person, who is more likely to have an elevation in just the diastolic, or in both.

Although often treatable, and in some cases preventable, the rate of HTN has increased in the last 15 years, especially for women; significant disparities between racial and ethnic groups persist. Although some factors are not modifiable, others are within control of the individual to reduce this disparity and the risk for hypertension-associated heart disease (Box 22.1).

A consistent research finding is that a lifetime risk of developing hypertension in those 55–60 years old is over

BOX 22.1 Modifiable Factors to Minimize Risk of Heart Disease

- Control blood pressure.
- Maintain healthy triglyceride and cholesterol levels.
- Prevent or control diabetes.
- Cease or never use tobacco products/reduce exposure to pollutants including tobacco smoke.
- Eat a healthy diet and maintain or attain acceptable weight.
- Engage in regular exercise.
- Control alcohol intake (one drink daily for women and two for men).
- Reduce stress and treat depression.

90% (Benetos et al., 2019). Older persons with HTN have an absolute higher risk of stroke, cognitive impairment, and cardiac disease such as atrial fibrillation, and heart failure. Poorly controlled HTN can also lead to chronic renal insufficiency, end-stage renal disease, and peripheral vascular disease (Potter & Myint, 2017).

Heart Disease

The beating heart, like other muscles, needs oxygen and other nutrients to survive. Like all other muscles, the heart receives its oxygen from adjacent arteries rather than from the blood passing through it.

Heart disease (HD) is also often referred to as coronary heart disease (CHD) and coronary artery disease (CAD). It develops from a number of causes including *atherosclerosis* or "hardening of the arteries" or when cholesterol and other fats stick to the arterial walls impeding smooth flow of blood within the vessels. As a result, oxygen reaching heart tissue is limited or absent and damage to the muscle occurs (ischemia). Among other things, HD is also a direct consequence of chronic, untreated, or inadequately treated hypertension (Aronow, 2017). The extent to which one suffers from HD is significantly affected by a personal history of exposure to smoke and pollutants, blood pressure control, and the coexistence of diabetes or a family history of diabetes.

Angina is short-lived ischemia and resolves on its own or with the ingestions of nitroglycerine and subsequent relaxation and dilation of the blood vessels. A more serious and often permanent blockage is referred to as an acute myocardial infarction (AMI) that is STEMI (ST-elevation myocardial infarction) or a NSTEMI (Non-ST-elevation myocardial infarction), the latter more common in women (Mehta et al., 2016).

Death from HD, specifically from an AMI, has been more common in women since 1984. However, for the last 20 years the survival rate among older women is improving and attributed to the increased awareness of the differences in the cues suggestive of acute cardiac event in older women compared with older men and the use of evidence-based guidelines (Mehta et al., 2016).

Atrial Fibrillation

Atrial fibrillation (AF or afib) is the most common type of arrhythmia (irregularity). The contractions of the atria and ventricles are not coordinated, resulting in a heartbeat that is too slow, fast, or irregular; a rapid and irregular heartbeat affects 2.7–6.1 million Americans. It contributes to 158,000 deaths a year. The irregularity of heartbeat may have some type of pattern or be completely random; it may occur once, intermittently, or persistently. Because the pulsations of the heart in AF are irregular, when the time between the beats is prolonged there is always a risk of pooling of blood in the atria. This pooling increases the risk of the development of tiny emboli. If an embolus leaves the heart, the risk of stroke is very high.

Although it occurs in about 2% of younger adults, it affects about 9% of those at least 65 years of age, the majority of whom are of European descent. There are many causes including indications of advanced heart failure, diabetes, alcohol abuse, HD, hypertension, and thyroid disease (CDC, 2020a). It is associated with a heightened risk for dementia and stroke-related mortality (Da Silva et al., 2019).

Heart Failure

Heart failure (HF) is a disease of the heart muscle in which it is damaged or malfunctions and can no longer pump enough blood to meet the needs of the body. Causes of HF may include long-term hypertension, fever, hypoxia, anemia, metabolic disease, and infection. If the underlying problem (e.g., hypertension) is poorly controlled, further damage leads to increasingly severe HF, known as congestive heart failure (CHF). Lifestyle choices such as an unhealthy diet, smoking, and lack of exercise aggravate the development of heart disease and the extent of damage, especially for those who have a family (genetic) history of heart disease. Affecting more than 6.5 million Americans, CHF contributes to 1 in 8 deaths (CDC, 2019b).

⚡ SAFETY ALERT

One of the major ways that cardiac conditions differ from other chronic problems in older adults is that when they become acute, they can do so very rapidly, and often necessitate acute hospitalization and intensive treatment followed by rehabilitation. Many other chronic disorders are managed at home.

❖ USING CLINICAL JUDGMENT TO PROMOTE HEALTHY AGING: CVD

As with the preparation for any analyses of cues related to CV diseases, obtaining a pertinent history of the events leading up to and including the presentation of the health problem(s) is essential, whether the history is from the patient or a friend or family member. As discussed in Chapter 8, working with older adults to document a medical history can be especially taxing and prolonged simply because of the length of the preexisting illness, comorbidities, and the vagueness of cues. Nursing actions are preventive: early screening, teaching how to stay healthy, and when a diagnosis is made, working with the person to prevent complications.

Through these actions, the nurse works with the persons to improve outcomes at best and to minimize the likelihood of poor outcomes at the very least.

◆ Recognizing and Analyzing Cues: HTN

Cues leading to the diagnosis of HTN in most persons are recognized during health screening or examination for another problem when related complications have already developed, referred to as "end-organ damage," especially to the heart. Diagnosis in younger adults is most often made from readings taken in the office with a minimum of two readings at different times. More readings may be necessary because of the variability inherent with the less compliant vasculature associated with normal aging. The BP is measured in both arms and the highest is considered in diagnosis and evaluation of treatment.

In 2015, the US Preventive Services Task Force found that ambulatory blood pressure monitoring (ABPM) or home blood pressure monitoring (HBPM) have been found to be much more accurate (Box 22.2). All adults at least 40 years of age should be screened at least once a year. Consideration of more frequent screenings should be made for those at high risk (i.e., smokers, those who are obese, and those of Black descent). At the time of writing, these recommendations were in the process of being updated (USPSTF, 2020) (Box 22.3).

BOX 22.2 Tips for Best Practice
Home Measurement of Blood Pressure

- Observe the technique that the person uses in the measurement of blood pressure, in both arms, using their personal home device.
- Duplicate the measurement using the same device, but with the nurse conducting the measurement.
- Measure the BP using either a reliable and tested BP cuff or a cuff and a stethoscope.
- If there is a discrepancy even with a person using a good technique, counsel the person regarding the replacement of the home device.

BOX 22.3 Evidence-Based Practice
Screening for Hypertension

Office measurement of blood pressure is done with a manual or automated sphygmomanometer. Proper protocol is to use the mean of two measurements taken while the patient is seated. Allow for ≥5 min between entry into the office and blood pressure measurement. Use an appropriately sized arm cuff and place the patient's arm at the level of the right atrium, with the patient's legs uncrossed and the patient not speaking. The measurements must be in contralateral arms. Multiple measurements over time have better positive predictive value than a single measurement.

◆ Recognizing and Analyzing Cues: HD

The cues suggestive of HD are also often vague (e.g., fatigue, edema) and are not brought to the attention of a medical provider but may be "mentioned" to the nurse (Box 22.4). It is not uncommon for older adults to have "silent MI" and the cues are not found until the time of death or when an electrocardiogram (ECG) is performed for some other purpose, such as during an Annual Medicare Wellness Visit (Chapter 7).

An acute event, i.e., an acute myocardial infarction (AMI), may be the first cue. In younger adults, especially men, it is described as gripping chest pain and radiation to the shoulder, left arm, or jaw and a heart attack is immediately suspected. In women (Box 22.5) and in older adults, if present at all, the cues are more likely to be mild and may be localized to the back or the abdomen or manifest as a sensation of nausea or heartburn, but they are nonetheless just as serious as typical AMI cues.

BOX 22.4 Signs of Potential Exacerbation of Illness in an Older Adult With Coronary Heart Disease

- Light-headedness or dizziness
- Disturbances in gait and balance
- Loss of appetite or unexplained loss of weight
- Inability to concentrate or shortened attention span
- Changes in personality or mood
- Changes in grooming habits
- Unusual patterns in urination or defecation
- Vague discomfort, frequent bouts of anxiety
- Excessive fatigue, vague pain
- Withdrawal from usual sources of pleasure

BOX 22.5 Cues Suggestive of Chest Pain Differs by Sex

The signs of an acute myocardial infarction in women, especially older women, have been found to be noticeably different from those in men. Women are more likely to report shortness of breath, weakness, fatigue, indigestion, and a sense of dread. Risk factors that influence women more than men are major life stressors and events, sense of loss of control, and the illness or death of significant others.

Data from Mehta, L. S., Becker, T. M., DeVon, H. A., et al. (2016). Acute myocardial infarction in women: A scientific statement from the American Heart Association, *Circulation, 133*(9), 916–147.

◆ Recognizing and Analyzing Cues: AF

If a younger adult has AF, they are more likely to have it in the absence of other diseases; in an older adult it is most often a complication of another disease such as HD. In many cases, AF itself is completely asymptomatic and cues are only identified by the nurse or other practitioner as part of a thorough auscultation of the heart. If potential cues are observable to the person, they are often vague, such as fatigue. In the presence of other underlying heart disease, the cues may be difficult to attribute specifically to AF. The fatigue may be incorrectly attributed to "old age," their underlying HD, or the onset of frailty. People occasionally report the sensation of "palpitations," intermittent shortness of breath, or nonspecific chest pain, especially if the fibrillation is intermittent.

◆ Recognizing and Analyzing Cues: HF

Although the cues indicating heart failure are based on which side is damaged (right or left), both sides of the heart are often affected by the time one reaches late life.

At all times when working with an older population, gerontological nurses should observe for cues of fatigue, but also shortness of breath, the person's inability to lie flat without getting short of breath (orthopnea), waking up at night gasping for air, weight gain, and swelling in the lower extremities. Dyspnea may occur at rest or on exertion (DOE) or it may appear intermittently at night (paroxysmal nocturnal dyspnea). The dyspnea may be relieved by sitting up, sleeping on multiple pillows, or with the head of the bed elevated. If a cough is present, it is worse at night. The New York Heart Association provides a clear classification of the cues of severity of HF, from symptom-free to severely disabled (Box 22.6).

Nurses should be particularly alert for the atypical cues of either the presence of or exacerbations of cardiovascular disease in older adults. The person may appear confused or delirious; begin falling; or complain of insomnia or urinary frequency at night (nocturia). They may complain of dizziness or may have syncope (fainting). More often, the nurse will notice that the person has the "droops," or malaise and a subtle decline in activity tolerance or functional or cognitive abilities.

For older adults in the acute or long-term care setting, monitoring vital signs and kidney function has special meaning because of the high potential of long-standing comorbid conditions, especially diabetes. Instructions for assessment and care of residents of a long-term care facility with heart disease can be purchased from the University of Iowa College of Nursing Evidence-Based Practice Guidelines (https://www.uiowacsomaygerore-sources.com/).

BOX 22.6   New York Heart Association Functional Classification of Heart Failure Symptoms

Class I: Asymptomatic

Cardiac disease without associated limitations of physical activity

Ordinary activity does not cause undue fatigue, palpitations or shortness of breath.

Class II: Mild Heart Failure

Slight limitation of physical activity

Comfortable at rest

Ordinary activity causes fatigue, palpitations, or shortness of breath.

Class III: Moderate Heart Failure

Marked limitation in physical activity

Comfortable at rest

Less than ordinary activity causes fatigue, palpitations, or shortness of breath.

Class IV: Severe Heart Failure

Inability to carry out any physical activity without discomfort

Some symptoms occur at rest

Increased discomfort with any activity

Adapted from Dolgin, M., Fox, A. C., Gorlin, R., & Levin, R. I. (1994). *New York Heart Association Criteria Committee: Nomenclature and criteria for diagnosis of diseases of the heart and great vessels.* (9th ed.). Boston, MA: Lippincott, Williams, and Wilkins. https://www.heart.org/en/health-topics/heart-failure/what-is-heart-failure/classes-of-heart-failure.

◆ Nursing Actions: HTN

In most cases, preventing or controlling hypertension is the key action to prevent the development of cardiovascular disease in later life. Although the best outcomes can only be achieved through risk reduction earlier in life, modifiable factors can be addressed at any time to minimize the likelihood of poor outcomes or delay their onset. Nursing actions include promoting an overall healthy lifestyle: cease or avoid smoke and other pollutants, a balanced diet (e.g. DASH diet), a healthy weight, regular exercise, and emotional modulation.

When introducing such strategies, nurses must have a clear understanding of the difficulties involved in attempts to alter practices that have occurred over a lifetime and are not easily changed by "education." The nurse's role in these instances is to discuss lifestyle practices in a nonjudgmental manner; providing acceptance, encouragement, resources, information, and affirmation of both the difficulty of making changes, the person's right to choose, and the consequences of the choices. The LEARN Model of communication (see Chapter 3)

may be particularly useful for persons from any culture or background.

◆ Nursing Actions: HD

A key action specific to the reduction of disability and death related to HD is to teach all persons the warning signs of an impending heart attack, the effective and accurate use of automatic defibrillators (AEDs), and the importance of responding quickly in an emergency. When aggressive treatment is no longer effective and HD has advanced to HF, a change of focus to palliative care is appropriate and may include a referral to a hospice agency or palliative care service (see Chapter 28).

◆ Nursing Actions: AF

Either medications or a procedure called cardioversion are used in an attempt to restore regular heart action in the presence of fibrillation. However, some are either not effective or have unacceptable side effects or drug–food interactions. In later life, anticoagulation therapy remains the gold standard for treatment with a goal of reducing the incidence of stroke. Many older adults are prescribed warfarin (e.g., Coumadin, Jantoven). Warfarin is highly effective but must be monitored closely and regularly to ensure that the level of anticoagulation is within a range that is effective at the same time the risk of bleeding is minimized (see Chapter 9). The nurse is usually the person to do this using a point-of-care instrument to measure coagulation status and effectiveness of the warfarin. It does interact with many foods and medications and at times must be measured often. Vitamin K is the reversal agent and can quickly inactivate the effects of warfarin.

New medications are the non–vitamin K antagonist oral anticoagulant or NOACs direct thrombin inhibitor dabigatran (Pradaxa) and Xa inhibitors apixaban (Eliquis), rivaroxaban (Xarelto), and the newest edoxaban (Savaysa). Reversal agent are either available or in development for each of the NCOAs. There are several medical conditions that make one preferable to another (AHA/ACC, 2019). A person who is taking an anticoagulant should be directed to seek prompt emergency support with any obvious bleeding or the potential of bleeding (e.g., trauma to the head following a fall).

Nurses have important roles in helping patients understand the dangers and benefits of anticoagulation therapy, the impact of medication/food/herb/nutritional supplement interactions (see Chapter 9), and the need for strict adherence to the prescribed dosing regimen and prompt emergency care if even the potential for need is considered.

◆ Nursing Actions: HF

Although there is no cure for HF except a heart transplant, nursing actions to assist persons with HF to maximize their cardiovascular health outcomes have been found to be highly effective (Pl & Hu, 2016; Riley, 2015) (Box 22.7). Education includes information about healthy eating, an exercise plan consistent with the person's cardiovascular ability, and other measures as needed such as how to balance rest and activity and the correct and safe use of supplemental oxygen as needed for persons with CHF. The specific interventions depend on the severity of the disease and the desire for either palliative or the level of aggressive care that is possible.

Evidence-based guidelines for the care of older adults with cardiovascular disease can be purchased from the University of Iowa College of Nursing Evidence-Based Practice Guidelines (https://www.uiowacsomaygeroresources.com/). Unfortunately, little is known about appropriate actions when working with very fragile older adults with CHF, including those who are residing in long-term care facilities. A more careful risk–benefit analysis must be performed related to actions and outcomes in this setting. For someone with a limited life expectancy, the significant side effects of many medications and limited food choices may result in an undesirable or unacceptable decrease in quality of life.

Disability can progress rapidly after an acute event or episode of illness, especially if the person believes that any exertion overtaxes the heart and will cause a relapse or death. To prevent this, cardiac exercise rehabilitation programs are designed to address the physical, mental, and spiritual needs and overall health of the person and their family. Typical programs begin with self-management education and light activity progressing to moderate activity under the supervision of a rehabilitation nurse and physical therapist. For those who are more physically compromised, it is necessary to identify energy-conserving measures applicable to their daily tasks with the goal of maximizing independence.

The nurse and the person with CVD must be cautious about exercise. For those who have had an AMI of any kind, exercise-related orthostatic hypotension is more likely to occur as a result of the combination of prescribed medications and age-related decreases in baroreceptor responsiveness, which controls the body's ability to respond to the need for changes in blood pressure (see Chapter 4). Thermoregulation decreases with age, and exercise intensity must be reduced in hot, humid climates (see Chapter 13). A healthy alternative is to encourage "mall walking" in local covered and climate-controlled shopping centers or other settings. In some locations this has become a social event as well as a safe way to exercise.

◆ Evaluating Outcomes

It is now recognized that the functional status and level of frailty of the individual in late life must be considered before determining treatment goals for those with heart disease. This includes systolic and diastolic goals in hypertension, the aggressiveness of actions related to heart disease and heart failure, and the risks and benefits of anticoagulation therapy. For persons with CVD, the goals of therapy are to relieve symptoms, improve quality of life, reduce mortality and morbidity, and slow or stop progressive loss of function as far as possible (Box 22.8).

BOX 22.7 Skills Required for Promoting Healthy Aging in the Person With Cardiovascular Disease

- Knowing appropriate technique for obtaining a blood pressure measurement
- Monitoring response to prescribed exercise
- Administering medications and evaluating their effects correctly
- Monitoring for signs and symptoms of changes in cardiovascular condition
- Monitoring diet and also fluid intake and output
- Monitoring weight (either daily, biweekly, or weekly)
- Auscultating heart and lung sounds and oxygen saturation
- Monitoring laboratory values
- Educating patient and caregivers related to all of the above
- Providing palliative care (see Chapter 28)

 BOX 22.8 Healthy People 2030

Heart Disease Objectives

- Increase control of high blood pressure
- Increase the proportion of adults whose risk for cardiovascular disease was addressed
- Increase the proportion of adult heart attack survivors who are referred to a rehabilitation program
- Reduce coronary heart disease deaths

From US Department of Health and Human Services, Office of Disease Prevention and Health Promotion. (2020). *Healthy People 2030. Heart disease and stroke.* https://health.gov/healthypeople/objectives-and-data/browse-objectives/heart-disease-and-stroke.

RESPIRATORY DISORDERS

The normal physical changes with aging (see Chapter 4) result in a greater risk of respiratory problems, and when they occur, there is a higher risk for death in older persons than in younger persons (see Chapter 4, Fig. 4.4). Diseases of the respiratory system are identified as infectious, acute or chronic, and involving the upper or lower respiratory tract. They are further defined as either *obstructive* (preventing airflow because of obstruction) or *restrictive* (narrowing of the respiratory structures causing a decrease in total lung capacity).

Other than asthma, almost all chronic obstructive pulmonary diseases in late life arise from tobacco use or exposure to tobacco and other pollutants earlier in life. Although asthma may be triggered by environmental factors at any time, there are strong genetic and allergic factors that contribute to its occurrence. A nurse's actions focus on helping the person with any respiratory disorder maintain function and quality of life, while being vigilant for early signs of infection, which become increasingly atypical in aging.

Chronic Obstructive Pulmonary Disease

Chronic obstructive pulmonary disease (COPD) is a catch-all term used to encompass those long-term conditions that affect airflow. It includes asthma, bronchitis, and emphysema, and as a group remains in the top 10 causes of death for both older men and women, in all racial and ethnic groups in the United States (Heron, 2019).

Older adults with advanced COPD can expect to have periods of worsening of symptoms and functioning between periods of control. During periods of acute illness, medication changes are usually needed. Persons who have well-developed skills in self-management will often begin to deal with the changes before consulting a health care provider. Hospitalization is always a possibility with COPD exacerbations, especially when the person has or is suspected of having an infection. Those with preexisting respiratory problems are at especially high risk for COVID-related mortality.

Recognizing and Analyzing Cues: COPD

The observable cues vary with the type of COPD. For example, persons with emphysema have little sputum production and appear flushed because they are able to get enough oxygen into the lungs but have problems with exhalation. In asthma, constrictions of the bronchial tubes keep air from exiting the lungs unless an effort is made. On the other hand, persons with chronic bronchitis have chronic thick sputum production, a frequent cough, and are pale and somewhat cyanotic because of low oxygen levels (hypoxia) associated with having difficulty getting oxygen into the lungs. The critical gerontological nursing action is to watch the person with COPD very closely for the earliest cues of infection, worsening of any underlying heart disease, or changes in cognition or functional status.

The major cues indicating an acute episode of emphysema or chronic bronchitis are worsening dyspnea and increased volume or change in the color of sputum. The dominant cues indicating an acute episode of asthma are shortness of breath and wheezing. Multiple factors, including viral or bacterial infections, air pollution or other environmental exposures, or changes in the weather can trigger an acute change in the health of persons with a chronic respiratory disease.

Pneumonia

Pneumonia is a bacterial or viral lower respiratory tract infection that causes the lung tissue to become inflamed. Pneumonia and associated viral illness are anywhere from the fourth to the seventh leading causes of death for persons older than 65 years of age, depending on race and ethnicity (Heron, 2019). Pneumonia is classified either as a *community-acquired disease* (CAD) or as a *hospital-acquired condition* (HAC) (nosocomial), beginning while a patient is in a hospital or other institutional setting such as a nursing home. In nursing homes, the most frequent causes of pneumonia are from aspirations of colonized oral secretions or from reflux of stomach contents from a feeding tube or other oral intake.

Factors that increase risk of pneumonia include the normal changes brought on by aging (Box 22.9; Chapter 4, Fig. 4.4). Older adults with comorbid conditions such as alcoholism, asthma, COPD, or heart disease or those who live in communal settings or are homeless are particularly susceptible. Dental caries and periodontal disease are common in late life and both predispose a person to develop pneumonia as a secondary infection. However, many cases of pneumonia can be either prevented or the lethality lessened by receipt of the two pneumonia immunizations available and the annual influenza immunization and COVID immunization.

BOX 22.9   Evidence-Based Practice

Several Factors Increasing the Risk for Pneumonia

Worsening of another health condition at the same time
Respiratory rate >30 breaths/min
Systolic BP <70 mmHg
Pulse rate >125 beats/min
Temperature <95°F
Current heart disease
Altered mental status
Age >50 years
Male gender
Living in a communal setting such as a nursing home

Mortality is further reduced by effective, appropriate, and prompt nursing and medical actions.

Recognizing and Analyzing Cues: Pneumonia

The usual cues of pneumonia such as a cough (with or without sputum), fatigue, and dyspnea may be initially (and incorrectly) attributed to something else, such as the underlying COPD or medications. However, the older adult with pneumonia also "looks sick," may have body aches, and a fever. Atypical signs in later life may include falling, mental status changes or signs of confusion, general deterioration, weakness, or anorexia and be incorrectly attributed to the appearance of a *geriatric syndrome* (see Chapter 17). When a person appears to have pneumonia, an abnormal chest x-ray, fever, and elevated white blood count would be expected. However, these cues may be delayed in an older adult, and if treatment is not started until they are present, it may be too late, and the result may be death attributable to sepsis. For the best possibility of survival of a frail elderly person with pneumonia, very prompt actions are necessary as soon as an infection is determined to be a reasonable explanation for a sudden change (Hope-Gill and Pink, 2017; Jett, 2006). Detailed algorithms for pneumonia severity are now available (e.g., PORT/PSI score; SMART-COP; DRIP score; CURB-65, etc.).

❖ USING CLINICAL JUDGMENT TO PROMOTE HEALTHY AGING: RESPIRATORY

Recognizing and Analyzing Cues

Cues suggestive of respiratory problems in older adults focus on the objective observations of oxygen saturation, sputum production, respiratory rate, and the subjective reports of dyspnea or shortness of breath, reduced functional status, and compromised quality of life. When respirations exceed about 20 per minute, the person with COPD is experiencing a worsening of their baseline illness, and prompt response by the nurse is necessary. It is not unusual for older adults with a history of COPD to have oxygen saturation rates between 90% and 95%; when it drops below this, there is always cause for urgent concern. Rates below 88% are almost always respiratory emergencies, and the person may be advancing to a state of respiratory failure. In an older adult, especially one who is frail or with multiple comorbid conditions, COPD can advance quite rapidly. The standard used for the diagnosis of COPD is referred to as the Global Initiative for Chronic Obstructive Lung Disease (GOLD) diagnostic criteria (Potnek, 2019) (see https://bestpractice.bmj.com/topics/en-us/7/criteria).

Only persons experiencing a problem can really tell us what it is like for them. Visual analog scales and numeric rating scales, similar to those used to assess pain, may be helpful (see Chapter 18). Persons can be asked how they would rate their breathing, from 1 (no dyspnea) to 10 (the worst dyspnea they can imagine), and so on.

When a bacterial infection is suspected in an older adult and treatment is desired, it is never appropriate to use a "wait and see" approach. As previously noted, elevations in temperature or in white blood cell count may not occur until the person is septic, and chest x-ray examinations in debilitated persons are often falsely negative at the beginning of respiratory tract infections because of the frequency of dehydration. Patients and their families should be told the seriousness of these or other changes in condition in older adults. More timely diagnosis calls for sensitive attention to cues of exacerbations of COPD or an infection by the person, the nurse, and the other health care providers.

The analysis of cues requires detailed information related to the history of the current illness, especially pertinent to a cough and exposure to others. When did it start? How long are the episodes of coughing? Is there any associated pain? What seems to make it better and what makes it worse? Is the person using anything to treat the cough? Is the person smoking (and how much) or exposed to smoke or other respiratory irritants? If the cough is productive, what is the color, texture, and odor of the mucus? Has the color changed? Does the color change according to the time of the day? A darker color in the morning with later clearing is typical of many persons with chronic bronchitis. If the person says, "I don't know what the color is—I swallow it," asking about any change in taste of the sputum is also a cue suggestive of worsening from baseline. Pulmonary function testing is most definitive in terms of lung capacity but not always available and cannot be done in persons with cognitive impairments if the ability to follow instructions is compromised. Box 22.10 presents the key aspects of a respiratory assessment.

◆ Nursing Actions

The most important nursing action when working with someone with COPD or pneumonia is to help them stop smoking and avoid environments where they are exposed to smoke and other pollutants or potential infection. For an older adult who has smoked for 60 or more years or lives with a smoker or in an environment with poor air quality, this will be particularly difficult.

Education is the nursing action that is part of every aspect of care of older adults with COPD or pneumonia (Box 22.11). The person is taught secretion clearance techniques and breathing retraining, how to recognize

BOX 22.10 Respiratory Assessment

History
Family
Past medical
Symptoms

Physical Assessment Includes
Overall body configuration (e.g., posture, chest symmetry, shape)
Respirations, including ease of ventilation, use of accessory muscles
Detailed description of level of dyspnea per activity
Oxygenation (pulse oximetry, skin color, capillary refill, pallor)
Sputum (color, amount, consistency)
Palpation, percussion, and auscultation
Functional status
Cognitive status
Mood
Discussion of wishes for treatment and advance planning
Presence or absence of a living will and designated health care surrogate

BOX 22.11 Instructions for Persons With Chronic Obstructive Pulmonary Disease

Nutrition
Eat small, frequent meals with high protein and caloric content.[a]
Select foods that do not require a lot of chewing or cut food in bite-size pieces to conserve energy.
Unless contraindicated (e.g., hyponatremia) drink 2 to 3 L of fluid daily.[a]
Weigh self at least twice each week and report change as directed (usually 5 pounds).

Activity Pacing to Conserve Energy
Plan exertion during the best periods of the day.
Arrange regular rest periods.
Allow plenty of time to complete activities.
Schedule sexual activity around best breathing time of day.
　Use prescribed bronchodilators 20 to 30 minutes before sexual activity.
　Use a sexual position that does not require pressure on the chest or support of the arms.

General Instructions
Participate in regular exercise.[a]
Select and wear clothing and shoes that are easy to put on and remove.
Avoid indoor and outdoor pollutants.
Avoid exposure to others with illness.
Obtain an annual influenza immunization if not allergic.
Obtain pneumococcal immunizations as appropriate.
Notify health care provider of changes:
　Temperature elevation
　Sputum color or amount produced
　Increased shortness of breath

[a]As prescribed.

the cues suggesting the onset or exacerbation of illness or infection; how to maintain adequate nutrition; how to use an inhaler, nebulizer, and a peak flow meter, and how to clean their equipment. Teaching the importance of good oral care afterward will reduce the likelihood of the development of an oral fungal infection or aspiration, especially in those who are otherwise debilitated. Patients and caregivers are taught the safe use of oxygen. The dangers of smoking while oxygen is in use or present must be made very clear. Nursing actions may also include educating the person and family about the type of exercise that is beneficial, how to pace activities, and instruction on how best to continue sexual activity if desired. Each of these areas calls for sensitive teaching and indicates specific strategies that will help older adults engage in self-care. Except in severe cases, nursing actions can occur at home with home health or in a skilled nursing facility, if oxygen therapy, parenteral fluids, and antibiotics can be administered.

Dietary education addresses the reason for monitoring weight and the signs of malnutrition. Weight loss can occur rapidly because of the energy expenditure needed to breathe while eating. A sense of being full early in the meal (early satiety) is caused by congestion in the abdomen and flattening of the diaphragm. Anorexia occurs because of sputum production and gastric irritation from the use of bronchodilators and steroids. Monitoring nutrition and helping the person obtain nutritional consultation is the nurse's responsibility in all settings. The nurse ensures that a person recovering from pneumonia is adequately nourished and hydrated while monitoring fluid volume. Older adults with coexisting heart disease are at high risk of fluid overload.

Mobilizing an older person and referring him or her for physical and occupational therapy to prevent or stop functional decline should occur as soon as the person's condition allows. *Activity and exercise tolerance* are usually assessed by the occupational and respiratory therapists and activities are prescribed to increase endurance and improve respiratory status. Exercise may be done with or without oxygen as a supplement to maintain an oxygen saturation of at least 88% for enough time to benefit from the exercise. The person should be informed that in many cases sexual activity is still possible and education and counseling information can be provided, either by the rehabilitation nurse or by a professional medical counselor.

Medications are used to treat infection and control dyspnea, cough, and sputum production. As with any medication teaching, the nurse makes sure that the person knows the purpose and the correct dosage and regimen of any medication they are taking, its side effects, and what to do if complications occur (see Chapter 9). Inhalers are difficult for those with limited manual dexterity and/or strength, such as with arthritis in the hands. However, special adaptive devices are available, and handheld or masked nebulizers are used for both severe disease and for those whose cognitive limitations prevent the use of inhalers.

Economic issues are always a concern for persons with chronic diseases (see Chapter 7). A number of medications are used and can be very expensive, especially when needed for an indefinite period of time as they are for COPD. A gerontological nurse should know how older adults will obtain their medications if they no longer drive or are on a very limited income.

Medicare coverage for oxygen and equipment such as nebulizers is determined by their oxygen saturation rates (<88% which improves with oxygen); supplemental oxygen is never covered by insurance for comfort only, but is usually provided to hospice patients. The expense of therapy for persons with a limited income or no insurance (see Chapter 7) will interfere with the adequacy of therapy and result in feelings of anxiety and a focus on the lowest-level biological needs.

As it is for those with cardiovascular problems, *rehabilitation* is an important aspect of maximizing quality of life for the person with respiratory problems. An older adult with COPD would be considered a candidate for pulmonary rehabilitation as long as they have pulmonary reserve and stable heart disease. The programs for older adults with COPD consist of drug therapy, reconditioning exercises, and counseling.

Preventive nursing actions related to immunizations are important aspects of care of persons with respiratory problems. Adults older than 65 years of age and those with chronic conditions should receive both pneumococcal vaccinations unless contraindicated. CDC now recommends that the nurse first administer the 13-valent (PCV13) pneumococcal vaccine (Prevnar) when a person turns 65 years of age. It provides protection against 13 bacteria not previously covered by the older pneumococcal vaccine (Pneumovax) with the added protection against several strains of *Streptococcus pneumoniae*, the most lethal form of community-acquired pneumonia rarely effectively treated in an outpatient setting. Pneumovax (PPSV23) provides protection against 23 pneumococcal bacteria not covered by PCV13. It is

given 1 year after the PCV13 and at least 5 years after any previous PPSV23 (CDC, 2020b). There are potential side effects of each of these and nurse actions include informing persons of these prior to administration. The immunization against the coronavirus (COVID-19) should be received as soon as it is available to the person. All of these vaccines are 100% covered by Medicare.

Annual influenza immunizations (also covered at 100%) are an important part of illness prevention in older adults, but most especially important for those with COPD. Normally one is received each fall. In years when there is a particularly intense infection outbreak in the fall, an additional dose may be recommended by public health officials.

If an older adult fails to improve or deteriorates in either setting, then hospitalization is often necessary even if only palliative care is desired. If the person is hospitalized, prolonged rehabilitation may be necessary, most often in a skilled nursing facility. Pharmacological and mechanical (e.g., intubation) treatment of infection is individually tailored based on the health status of the person before the infection, concurrent health problems, expected outcomes of treatment, where treatment will be provided, and the wishes of the patient. One of the most important questions a nurse asks is whether hospitalization is desired. If so, preparation for what will happen is helpful, e.g., possible need for IV therapy and intubation. If hospitalization is declined by the patient and/or health care surrogate (Chapter 7), the consequences of this must also be discussed and documented. The ultimate decision regarding the extent of elected treatment is always emotionally charged.

◆ Evaluating Outcomes

As with CVD, many chronic respiratory diseases in late life cannot be cured. Nursing actions and strategies are both curative and palliative in nature. The optimal desired outcomes are stabilizing the disease, reducing the risk of exacerbations and hospitalizations, promoting maximal functional capacity, and preventing premature disability. A multidisciplinary team of health professionals works collectively to help older adults achieve the following goals:

- Maximize the level of independence.
- Improve function in their environment as much as possible.
- Minimize the number of hospitalizations and need for hospitalization.
- Increase exercise tolerance.
- Increase self-esteem and self-care skills.
- Maximize quality of life and comfort.

The number of goals achieved depends on many factors, including extent of illness, coexisting conditions,

BOX 22.12 **Healthy People 2030**

Goals for Those With Respiratory Disease

Reduce the rate of hospital admissions for pneumonia among persons 65 and over

Reduce the number of COPD-related deaths in adults

Reduce COPD-related emergency room visits in adults

From US Department of Health and Human Services, Office of Disease Prevention and Health Promotion. (2020). Respiratory diseases. *Healthy People 2030*. https://health.gov/healthypeople/objectives-and-data/browse -objectives/respiratory-disease.

and quality of health care available. For those recovering from pneumonia, the rehabilitative period is often prolonged in older adults. Finally, the nurse can be aware of the pertinent outcomes put forth in the document *Healthy People 2030* and play a part in helping the nation to achieve them (Box 22.12).

KEY CONCEPTS

- Heart disease is the most common cause of death for most persons in the United States.
- The underlying cause of the majority of cardiovascular and pulmonary disease is smoking.
- Pneumonia and influenza are particularly important health problems for those older than 65 years of age and significantly more so for those who are frail, immunocompromised, have human immunodeficiency virus (HIV), or are otherwise decompensated.
- Mortality associated with pneumonia can be minimized through nursing actions that promote the acceptance and administration of pneumonia and influenza vaccinations and excellent oral hygiene.
- The outcome for older adults with cardiac and respiratory disorders is not curative. It is to relieve symptoms, to improve the quality of life, to reduce mortality, to stabilize or slow the progression of the disease, to reduce the risk of exacerbation, and to maximize functional capacity.
- There is a high correlation between heart disease and diabetes.

ACTIVITIES AND DISCUSSION QUESTIONS

1. How are heart failure and congestive heart failure different in older adults compared with younger adults?
2. How is the recognition and analyses of cues in older adults with cardiovascular and respiratory problems different from that of younger adults?

3. What is the range of possible outcomes of pneumonia in older adults and how would you address these with the patient and significant others?
4. What preventive measures can be instituted to prevent or lessen the severity of pneumonia?

NEXT-GENERATION NCLEX® EXAMINATION-STYLE QUESTIONS

Mr. Fletcher, 72 years old, is admitted to the medical department. When the nurse completes his history, he reports he has had increased difficulty sleeping for the past two weeks or more. He denies any changes in diet or nighttime routine. He sleeps on two pillows and gets up to urinate two or three times a night. He does admit he is up more often than before. He states he is tired all the time and no longer feels like going for his walks. When he tried yesterday, by the time he had walked a block he could not catch his breath. Mr. Fletcher is concerned that even though he feels worn out, he still cannot sleep. His blood pressure is 155/88 mmHg, pulse is 100 beats per minute and irregular, respirations are 20 breaths per minute, and his temperature is 98.4°F; his oxygen saturation on room air is 96%. When asked to step on the scale, Mr. Fletcher tells the nurse he thinks he has put on weight because he feels puffy. He weighs 185 pounds and is 5'8" tall. He has a history of hypertension and Type 2 diabetes and takes lisinopril/hydrochlorothiazide 20 mg/25 mg daily and metformin 850 mg twice a day.

Highlight the assessment findings above that require immediate follow up by the nurse.

REFERENCES

AHA/ACC. (2019). *AHA/ACC/HRS Focused update on the 2014 guideline for management of patients with atrial fibrillation,* 2019. https://www.acc.org/~/media/Non-Clinical/Files-PDFs-Excel -MS-Word-etc/Guidelines/2019/2019-Afib-Guidelines-Made -Simple-Tool.pdf.

Aronow, W. S. (2017). Diagnosis and management of coronary artery disease. In H. M. Fillit, K. Rockwood, & J. Young (Eds.), *Brocklehurst's Textbook of geriatric medicine and gerontology* (8th ed., pp. 278–287). Philadelphia: Elsevier.

Benetos, A., Petrovic, M., & Strandberg, T. (2019). Hypertension management in older and frail older patients. *Circulation Research, 124*(7), 1045–1060.

Centers for Disease Control and Prevention (CDC). (2019). *Heart failure.* https://www.cdc.gov/dhdsp/data_statistics/fact_sheets /fs_heart_failure.htm.

Centers for Disease Control and Prevention (CDC). (2020a). *Atrial fibrillation.* https://www.cdc.gov/dhdsp/data_statistics/fact _sheets/fs_atrial_fibrillation.htm.

CDC. (2020b). Pneumococcal disease. https://www.cdc.gov/pneumococcal/about/index.html.

Da Silva, R. M. F. L., Miranda, C. M., Liu, T., Tse, G., & Roever, L. (2019). Atrial fibrillation and risk of dementia: Epidemiology, mechanisms, and effect of anticoagulation. *Frontiers in Neuroscience, 13*, 18. ePub 2019 Jan 31. https://www.ncbi.nlm.nih.gov/pmc/articles/PMC6365433/.

Heron, M. (2019). Deaths: Leading causes for 2017. *National Vital Statistics Reports, 68*(6). https://www.cdc.gov/nchs/data/nvsr/nvsr68/nvsr68_06-508.pdf.

Hope-Gill, B., & Pink, K. (2017). Nonobstructive lung disease and thoracic tumors. In Fillit, H. M., Rockwood, K., & Young, J. (Eds.), *Brocklehurst's Textbook of geriatric medicine and gerontology* (8th ed., pp. 371–380). Philadelphia: Elsevier.

Jett, K. F. (2006). Examining the evidence: Knowing if and when to transfer a resident with pneumonia from the nursing home to the hospital or subacute unit. *Geriatric Nursing, 27*(5), 280.

Mehta, L. S., Beckie, T. M., DeVon, H. A., Grines, C. L., Krumholz, H. M., et al. (2016). Acute myocardial infarction in women: a scientific statement from the American Heart Association. *Circulation, 133*(9), 916–947.

Pl, H.-Y., & Hu, X. (2016). Nursing care in old patients with heart failure: current status and future perspectives. *Journal Geriatric Cardiology, 13*(5), 387–390.

Potnek, M. F. (2019). Assessment and management of suspected chronic obstructive pulmonary disease in the primary care setting. *JNP, 15*(10), 701–708.

Potter, J., & Myint, P. (2017). Hypertension. In H. M. Fillit, K. Rockwood, & J. Young (Eds.), *Brocklehurst's Textbook of geriatric medicine and gerontology* (ed. 8, pp. 295–306). Philadelphia: Elsevier.

Riley, J. (2015). The key roles for the nurse in acute heart failure management. *Card Fail Review, 1*(2), 123–127.

US Preventive Services Task Force [USPSTF]. (2020). *Hypertension in adults: Screening.* https://www.uspreventiveservicestaskforce.org/uspstf/draft-recommendation/hypertension-in-adults-screening.

Youmans, Q. R., Hastings-Spaine, L., Princewill, O., Shobayo, T., & Okwuosa, I. S. (2019). Disparities in cardiovascular care: past, present, and solutions. *Cleveland Clinic J Med, 86*(9), 621–632.

23

Neurological Disorders

Kathleen Jett

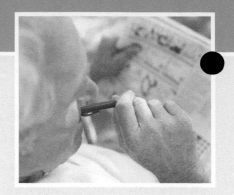

LEARNING OBJECTIVES

Upon completion of this chapter, the reader will be able to:
- Differentiate a transient ischemic attack from a stroke.
- Differentiate a hemorrhagic stroke from an embolic stroke and understand the differences in the nursing actions needed to achieve the best outcomes.
- Identify strategies and actions to decrease the likelihood of a stroke.
- Recognize early cues suggestive of the neurodegenerative disorders Parkinson's disease and Alzheimer's disease.
- Develop nursing actions to promote safety in persons with neurological disorders.
- Suggest ways to optimize communication with persons with communication difficulties attributable to a neurological impairment.

THE LIVED EXPERIENCE

People come up to me and talk to me like I should know them, and I know I should but it is just getting harder and harder to recognize them.

Henry, age 82

I just don't understand what she is trying to tell me. I know it must be very frustrating for her to feel kind of trapped inside and not being able to speak, but I am frustrated too, not knowing what she needs!

Angela, a new nurse

Neurological disorders occur in older adults more than any other age group. In this chapter we discuss two of these: Parkinson's and Alzheimer's diseases. We have also chosen to include the cerebrovascular conditions of the transient ischemic attack (TIA) and stroke. Although these are vascular in origin, their effects are universally neurological, and the implications for nursing actions for all conditions covered herein are similar. All have the potential to significantly impair a person's function and affect every aspect of life at some point. Parkinson's and Alzheimer's diseases are neurodegenerative in nature in that they are terminal conditions and characterized by a progressive decline in function ultimately resulting in death.

The nurse plays an active role in helping the person and significant others navigate the health care system with outcomes focused on rehabilitation whenever possible and comfort always. The goal is to maintain maximal function for as long as possible. Nursing actions may occur in acute care, long-term care, and rehabilitation settings, as well as in the person's home.

CEREBROVASCULAR DISEASE

Cerebrovascular diseases are interruptions in blood supply to the brain resulting in neurological damage. They are either ischemic or hemorrhagic in nature and manifest as either strokes or transient ischemic attacks

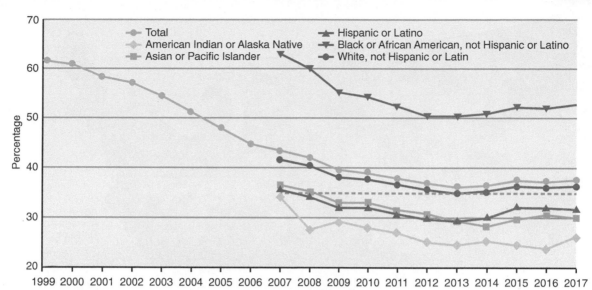

FIG. 23.1 Stroke deaths by race/ethnicity. (From https://www.healthypeople.gov/2020/topics-objectives/topic/heart-disease-and-stroke/national-snapshot.)

(TIAs). Because the initial cues are similar but the outcomes are different, the rapid identification of the specific diagnosis takes precedence and must happen before any treatment can occur.

Stroke is a leading cause of death worldwide. Most occur in persons older than 65 years of age, but there is considerable difference in race/ethnicity (Fig. 23.1). Black Americans are twice as likely as Whites to have a stroke and have the highest rate of associated death. Nonetheless the rate of stroke has been decreasing in all groups except those who self-identify as Hispanic in which there has been an increase since 2013. Each year almost 800,000 people in the United States have a stroke, and one person dies from a stroke every 40 minutes (Centers for Disease Control and Prevention [CDC], 2020a); however, there are significant regional differences. The southeast portion of the United States is known as the "stroke belt" (Fig. 23.2).

Ischemic Events

Most cerebrovascular events are ischemic in nature (87%). The four main causes are high blood pressure, high cholesterol, smoking, obesity, and diabetes (CDC, 2020b). A stroke, or "brain attack," is the result of a blockage of the blood supply to a section of the brain with resultant damage from lack of oxygen (anoxia) to the area beyond the blockage. An ischemic stroke is one with neurological cues lasting at least 24 hours without treatment. A TIA is ischemic but clinically different from a stroke in that all the neurologically associated cues begin to resolve within minutes and are completely resolved within 24 hours. However, more than one-third of persons who suffer a TIA and do not receive treatment have a major stroke within 1 year; 10% to 15% of these persons will have a major stroke within 3 months (CDC, 2020).

Hemorrhagic Events

Hemorrhagic strokes are less frequent than ischemic events but much more life threatening. They are primarily caused by uncontrolled hypertension and less often by malformations of the blood vessels (e.g., aneurysms). Although the exact mechanism is not fully understood, it appears that in some people chronic hypertension causes thickening of the vessel wall, microaneurysms, and necrosis. When damage to the vessel accumulates, a spontaneous rupture may occur. The rupture may be large and acute or may be small with a slow leaking of blood into the adjacent brain tissue. Resolution of the event can occur only when the sources of the bleeding is treated and excess blood and damaged tissue are either resorbed or removed.

❖ USING CLINICAL JUDGMENT TO PROMOTE HEALTHY AGING: CEREBROVASCULAR EVENTS

◆ Recognizing and Analyzing Cues

The first cues of both strokes and TIAs are acute neurological deficits consistent with the part of the brain affected and the type of event. Unilateral motor weakness

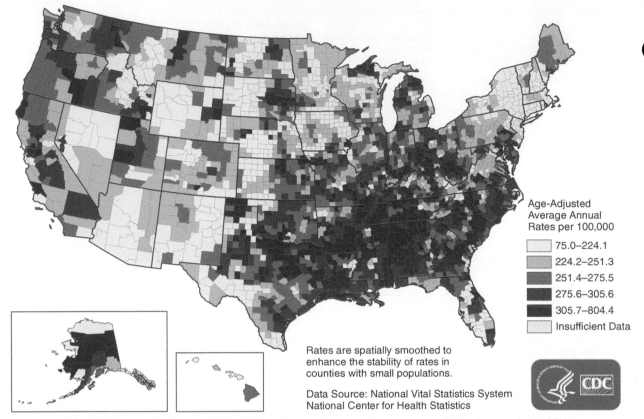

Age-Adjusted
Average Annual
Rates per 100,000

☐	75.0–224.1
☐	224.2–251.3
☐	251.4–275.5
■	275.6–305.6
■	305.7–804.4
☐	Insufficient Data

Rates are spatially smoothed to
enhance the stability of rates in
counties with small populations.

Data Source: National Vital Statistics System
National Center for Health Statistics

FIG. 23.2 Stroke death rates, 2015–2017, total population age 65+, by county. (https://www.cdc.gov/dhdsp
/maps/national_maps/stroke65_all.htm.)

is common regardless of the type of stroke. Neurological
cues may include alterations in sensory and visual function, coordination, cognition, and language. Persons
with a hemorrhage have more dramatic neurological
changes, including seizures and a more depressed level
of consciousness. If a person is unresponsive following
a stroke, they are unlikely to survive (Boss & Huether,
2019). Nausea and vomiting suggest increased cerebral
edema in response to an event of any type. Because TIAs
are highly transient in nature, they often resolve on their
own and health care is not sought. Instead, the person
reports (often to the nurse), "I think I had a small stroke
last week/month," etc. Type and damage are differentiated by computed tomography (CT) scan or magnetic
resonance imaging (MRI).

◆ Nursing Actions

Key nursing actions related to cerebrovascular health
are to teach others how to minimize their risk of strokes,
how to recognize the signs of a stroke, and when to seek
immediate emergency care (Box 23.1). Nurses recognize

**BOX 23.1   Quick Assessment of the
Person Who May Be Having a Stroke**

If you think someone may be having a stroke, act F.A.S.T. and do the
following simple test:

F—Face: Ask the person to smile. Does one side of their face droop?

A—Arms: Ask the person to raise both arms. Does one arm drift
downward?

S—Speech: Ask the person to repeat a simple phrase. Is the person's
speech slurred or strange?

T—Time: If you observe any of these signs, call 911 immediately.

---

persons who are at high risk or stroke-prone at home,
in the community, or at the health facilities where
they work. Nurses work with individuals and groups
to reduce their stroke risk (Box 23.2). Helping persons
stop smoking, control their blood pressure and diabetes,
control their weight, and remain as active as possible are
the most important things the person can do to reduce
the risk.

BOX 23.2 Leading Controllable Risk Factors for Stroke

Control blood pressure
Never smoke or quit smoking
Control diabetes
Diet with five or more servings of fruits and vegetables
Avoid obesity
Maintain optimal cholesterol

Adapted from American Heart Association. (2018). *Stroke risk factors you can control, treat and improve.* https://www.stroke.org/en/about-stroke/stroke-risk-factors/stroke-risk-factors-you-can-control-treat-and-improve.

BOX 23.3 Assessment of the Person Following a Cerebrovascular Event

General
Vital signs
Cardiovascular
Respiratory
Abdominal

Neurological
Level of arousal, orientation, attention
Speech (dysarthria, dysphasia)
Cranial nerves
Motor strength
Coordination
Sensation
Gait (if possible)

An individual's relative risk both before and after the age of 80 years can be calculated using the information available through the National Institute for Neurological Diseases and Stroke (NINDS, 2019) and other sites such as https://www.uclahealth.org/stroke/stroke-risk-calculator.

All actual or potential cerebrovascular events are considered emergencies and should be treated as such (see Safety Alert). For ischemic strokes caused by an embolism, the compromised circulation to the brain must be restored rapidly. This is done in emergency departments through *intravenous therapy* to dissolve the clot using recombinant tissue plasminogen activator (tPA) if the facility is equipped to do so. Nursing actions include obtaining consent for the treatment, administering it, and monitoring the patient during and after for any signs of bleeding.

⚡ SAFETY ALERT

Intravenous therapy using recombinant tissue plasminogen activator (tPA) is only indicated for ischemic occlusive (usually embolic) strokes documented with a CT scan or MRI within 3 hours of the onset of the event. Newer evidence indicates that it can still be useful 4.5 hours from "last known normal" (Powers et al., 2018).

If a person has had a hemorrhagic stroke and it is misdiagnosed, the bleeding is rapidly accelerated by the tPA and the person will die. The initial response to the hemorrhagic stroke is to find a means to stop the bleeding if possible and rapidly replace the blood loss. Nursing actions include participating in this process and observing carefully for any cues indicating a change in the patient's condition.

In the acute period the nurse carefully recognizes and analyzes all possible cues related to the person's health (Box 23.3). The actions are repeated often to recognize, analyze, and document areas of progress, areas of need, and signs of complications. Nursing actions can minimize the risk of aspiration by keeping the head of the bed elevated and performing frequent oral care/hygiene. Nurses attempt to reduce the development of DVTs using pneumatic compression devices, compression stockings, and the administration of low-molecular-weight heparin as prescribed. Early complications of a simple stroke include extension of the amount of damage and recurrence; brain edema could result in obstructive hydrocephalus (NHLBI, n.d).

Rehabilitation begins in the acute care setting when the nurse encourages early mobilization. The nurse works in tandem with the range of rehabilitation professionals, especially physical, occupational, and speech therapists, both inpatient and outpatient. If the person has developed dysphagia, eating may be a problem and a nasogastric (NG) tube may be considered to provide artificial nutrition. If this is anticipated to be a persistent problem, the patient and family may elect to have a semi-permanent percutaneous endoscopic gastrostomy (PEG) tube inserted directly into the stomach. If the person is going home, nursing actions include teaching about the use, care, and danger associated with artificial nutrition, especially aspiration pneumonia.

The actions of the gerontological rehabilitation nurse include the prevention and minimization of disability, that is, the promotion of healthy aging in persons with significant functional limitations following a stroke. Rehabilitation occurs in rehabilitation hospitals, in long-term care facilities, and at home depending on the location of the neurological damage, the extent of the damage, available support system, and the endurance of the person. Recovery may take as little as a few months or as long as years. The use of antithrombotic/

BOX 23.4 Resources for Stroke Rehabilitation and Support

National Stroke Association: 1-800-STROKES
American Heart Association: www.heart.org
American Stroke Association: https://www.stroke.org/en
American Academy of Neurology: www.aan.com

anticoagulants (e.g., aspirin, warfarin), blood pressure and lipid control in persons with heart disease is an attempt to reduce the risk of stroke and has proven to prevent recurrent cardioembolic strokes and TIAs (see Chapter 22). Management is usually preventive and rehabilitative. Nursing action may be palliative if this is consistent with the person's pre-stated wishes.

Nursing care following a stroke is extremely complex; it is often coordinated by a rehabilitation nurse and includes a diverse multidisciplinary team. It may include a spiritual advisor or indigenous healer as the person copes with the associated losses (see Chapter 28). It always includes the person's significant other(s) who may be involved with helping to meet daily needs as necessary. Support services of many kinds are now available in a variety of locations (Box 23.4).

◆ **Evaluating Outcomes**

In the ideal situation, the outcomes related to cerebrovascular health would be the prevention of an acute event from ever occurring. Unfortunately, gerontological nurses will work with many older adults who have already experienced cerebrovascular events, yet their health outcomes can still be maximized by ensuring that modifiable factors mentioned previously are addressed whenever possible. Nurses work to prevent multiple potential iatrogenic complications such as skin breakdown, falls, and increased confusion or delirium from medications and infections.

After a TIA resolves, there should be no residual effect other than an increased chance of recurrence and the increased risk of stroke. The potential long-term outcomes of a stroke range from neurological changes noticeable only by the person to paralysis or hemiparesis limiting or eliminating certain voluntary movements on the side of the body opposite to the brain injury. Speech may be limited by dysarthria, dysphagia, or aphasia. If paralysis or hemiparesis occurs, spasticity can develop or unusually tight muscles in the affected limb(s) lead to contractures if it is not managed well and even sometimes when it is. Pain in the affected side is not an uncommon outcome and may be treated with medications specific for neuropathic pain (see Chapter 18). Medications, added to minimize the potential limitations of the stroke,

also significantly increase the risk of falls. Poor outcomes include blood clots (deep vein thrombosis [DVT]) in the affected limb, pressure injuries, aspiration pneumonia (see Chapter 22), and urinary tract infections. Post-stroke depression is common and can negatively affect both rehabilitation and mortality.

Striving for the best outcomes means that the nurse recognizes cues suggestive of changes in mental status and respiratory functioning and ensures and maximizes the capacity for self-care, especially related to mobility, activity, eating, fluid intake, and continence. The nurse is alert for problems with sleep, constipation, and depression. The nurse acts as an advocate, providing post-stroke recommendations regarding participation in support groups for both the person and the person's significant others or caregivers. A gerontological nurse is expected to take an active role in improving outcomes and quality of life of older adults with cerebrovascular disorders, especially those with functional and/or cognitive limitations. Finally, maximizing outcomes means that the gerontological nurse helps older adults and those who love them cope with the changes inherent in these disorders, including grief support (see Chapter 28).

NEURODEGENERATIVE DISORDERS

The neurodegenerative disorders of Parkinson's and Alzheimer's diseases discussed here occur in older adults more than any other age group. Both are terminal conditions and characterized by a progressive decline in function. The declines may be barely noticeable in the beginning, with slight exacerbations and remissions, but the ultimate trajectory is always a downward slope (Chapter 17). The impairments ultimately become so severe that the person cannot meet even their most basic self-care needs. However, there are nursing actions that promote the healthiest aging possible for older persons, for their significant others, and for those who will be providing care.

The evaluation leading to a diagnosis of a presumed neurodegenerative disorder is initiated by the person, significant other, or a health care provider when changes are noted in comparison with a prior state of cognition or function. In the case of Alzheimer's disease, memory is always impaired, and with Parkinson's disease, physical stability is always impaired. In both conditions the cues are often slow to appear and difficult to analyze, delaying medical diagnosis and therefore treatment.

Clinical judgment in neurological disorders always begins with the recognition and analysis of all potentially reversible causes for the changes such as delirium, infection, vitamin deficiencies, or endocrine disturbances. If a reversible cause is not found or the cues remain after treatment, further hypotheses testing is needed to make a diagnosis, to establish a baseline, and to develop nursing actions to maximize outcomes. Recognizing relevant cues in those with neurological changes becomes increasingly complex when the person has other confounding chronic diseases, is very frail, or has sensory limitations.

Parkinson's Disease

It is estimated that nearly 1 million people in the United States have Parkinson's disease (PD) and 10 million worldwide; 60,0000 more Americans are diagnosed each year. Most are diagnosed after the age of 60 years and only 4% develop it before the age of 50 years, termed "early onset" and often inherited. Men are 1.5 times more likely than women to have PD at any age (Parkinson's Foundation, 2020). PD is the second most common neurodegenerative disease after Alzheimer's disease. In very late stages, the person may also develop Parkinson's dementia, especially those who develop the disease after the age of 70 years (Meara, 2017).

PD is typically a slowly progressing *movement disorder* that is the result of destruction of the cells in the brain that produce the neurotransmitters norepinephrine and dopamine and the accumulation of Lewy bodies especially in the substantia nigra area of the brain. Dopamine plays a major part in controlling movement.

The exact cause of most PD is unknown but thought to be a combination of factors including exposure to viruses and toxins such as pollutants (including smoking) and external factors such as repeated head trauma (Box 23.5). The later the onset, the more rapid the detcrioration (Meara, 2017). Older adults are also more likely to the develop Parkinson-like symptoms as side effects of antipsychotic medications. Any older adult receiving these medications should be routinely screened for extrapyramidal symptoms (EPSs), which resemble PD (see Chapter 9).

BOX 23.5 Genetics and Parkinson's Disease

Although the exact trigger is not yet known for the body's destruction of the neurons in the brain, scientists have identified several genes that are linked to familial Parkinson's disease (PD). If the LRRK2 or SNCA genes are considered autosomal dominant in which only one copy of the gene is necessary for the person to develop PD; a parent with PD is likely. PARK7, PINK1, and PRKN are autosomal recessive genes. Two copies are necessary, usually one from each PD free parent.

From US National Library of Medicine. (2019). *Parkinson's disease.* https://ghr.nlm.nih.gov/condition/parkinson-disease#diagnosis.

❖ CLINICAL JUDGMENT TO PROMOTE HEALTHY AGING: PD

◆ Recognizing and Analyzing Cues

PD has both motor and nonmotor cues. Some of the nonmotor cues are largely associated with reduced levels of norepinephrine and may be recognized long before the motor signs associated with reduced dopamine. Analyses of the early cues may not lead to the hypothesis of possible PD, delaying treatment and initiation of nursing actions. Micrography (small handwriting), loss of smell, sleep disturbances, constipation, and reduced facial expression may predate more classic motor cues by many years.

The major motor signs of PD are *resting tremor, muscular rigidity, bradykinesia, and akinesia.* The resting tremor (hands, arms, legs, jaw, or head) may disappear briefly during voluntary movement. The tremors that accompany PD may produce embarrassing movements such as spilling food when eating in public. They are not present during sleep but increase with stress and anxiety.

Although motor cues may be recognized as unilateral at first, they always become bilateral (NIA, 2017). Movements are stiff, slowed, and reduced (e.g., seen when trying to get out of a chair). Difficulties swallowing, chewing, and speaking require very specific preventive nursing actions and work with an interprofessional team. Drooling, a common problem with those with PD, is a socially unacceptable "behavior" in some societies. The expressionless face, slowed movement, and soft, monotone speech or aphasias of either PD or AD may give the impression of apathy, depression, and disinterest, and therefore others are discouraged to continue long-time relationships. A sensitive nurse is aware that the visible cues produce an undesired façade that may hide an alert and responsive individual who wishes to interact but is trapped in a body or brain that no longer cooperates. It is important to see beyond the disease to the person within and provide nursing actions that enhance hope and promote the highest quality of life despite disease. Whitney (2004) found that learning what gives persons purpose and meaning in life and helping them understand what is happening to their bodies can assist people to cope with their losses.

Muscular rigidity results in "cogwheel" movements; smooth movement alternating with resistance with either passive or active range of motion. Severe muscle cramps may occur in the toes or hands because of the lack of free and regular movement. Bradykinesia, or slowed movement, is common, affecting a person's ability to perform fine motor tasks such as using eating utensils. When combined with tremors, the effect on a person's loss of the ability to perform day-to-day self-care functions independently can be quite dramatic.

To prepare those with PD for anticipated changes in muscular flexibility, early training in relaxation such as modified yoga techniques and exercises may be helpful. Tai chi has been found to increase balance skills (Gao et al., 2014; Li et al., 2014). Exercise, including walking, moving all of the joints, and improving balance, needs to be included early in the course of PD treatment; physical therapy evaluation and treatment are important. Rigidity of facial muscles and bradykinesia affect eating ability, nutrition, swallowing, and communication. Occupational therapy can assist with adaptive equipment such as weighted utensils, nonslip dinnerware, and other self-care aids. Speech therapy is beneficial for dysarthria, dysphagia, and aphasia (see later in this chapter). Patients can be taught facial exercises and swallowing techniques.

As muscular rigidity and bradykinesia worsen, all the striated muscles will ultimately be affected. A person with PD will sit for long periods or lie motionless with few shifts in position and few changes in facial expression (Meara, 2017). The pain may be related to rigidity, contractures, dystonia, and central-pain syndromes seen in those with PD.

Difficulties with gross movement and positioning is of special importance to independent functioning and safety. Downward gaze becomes more difficult, and there is an involuntary flexion of the head and neck, a stooped posture, and postural instability. Rigidity combined with bradykinesia (slowed movement) and akinesia (lack of spontaneous movement) leads to the characteristic gait consisting of very short steps and minimal arm movements (festination). Initiating and restarting movement is difficult (freezing) later in the disease, but once it starts, the person moves forward with small steps and a forward lean, increasing the person's risk for falling (see Chapter 15). Turning is difficult and may require many steps. If the person becomes unbalanced, correction is very slow. These and other changes in function have the potential to decrease the quality of life (Box 23.6). Lack of spontaneous movement makes the person at high risk of pressure injuries.

Later, a nurse will recognize autonomic cues that include postural hypotension, urinary incontinence, sexual dysfunction, and abnormalities in sweating. Still later in the disease neuropsychiatric and cognitive problems may be seen, such as apathy, depression, psychosis, hallucinations, and, in some cases, dementia (Meara, 2017).

As a result of the complexity of health for many later in life, diagnosis may be one of exclusion and therefore has a higher than preferable risk of misdiagnosis. The diagnosis is then tested by a "challenge test" in which a person with symptoms is given a dose of levodopa. If there is a significant and rapid improvement, the diagnosis of PD

> **BOX 23.6   Other Symptoms Experienced by People With Parkinson's Disease**
>
> Frequent changes in body temperature
> Problems with blood pressure
> Dizziness
> Fainting
> Frequent falls
> Sensitivity to heat and cold
> Sexual dysfunction
> Urinary incontinence
> Constipation
> Poor sense of smell
> Sialorrhea (drooling)

---

is thought to be confirmed. Early falls, poor response to levodopa, symmetry of motor symptoms, lack of tremor, and early autonomic dysfunction (e.g., incontinence) suggest other illnesses (Meara, 2017).

The presence of cues and their intensity vary from person to person; some become severely disabled early in the disease and others experience only minor motor disturbances until much later. However, the number of changes and the degree to which they will affect a person's life and function will always increase over time.

◆ Nursing Actions

The most common approaches used with a person with PD are pharmacological and preventive. Medication given to treat the rigidity associated with PD is levodopa-carbidopa, the combination drug designed to increase the dopamine level in the brain and prevent the speed of its breakdown.

> **⚡ SAFETY ALERT**
>
> Levodopa-carbidopa must be taken on an empty stomach (i.e., 30–60 minutes before a meal or 45–60 minutes after a meal) for it to be effective. It is given on a set schedule to prevent fluctuations in symptom control.

Persons who are stable on levodopa-carbidopa are often followed by their primary care providers. However, when it is no longer effective or additional treatment is necessary, they are cared for by neurologists specializing in movement disorders whenever possible. Medication therapy is complicated and must be closely supervised. Hypotension, dyskinesia (involuntary movements), dystonia (lack of control of movement), hallucinations, sleep disorders, and depression are common side effects of both the disease and the medications used to treat it.

Deep brain stimulation (DBS) of the subthalamic nucleus may be used in patients who have not responded to drug therapy or have intractable motor fluctuations, dyskinesias, or tremor. However, cognitive impairment is a major contraindication and is already present in many older adults with PD (Meara, 2017). Exercise therapy and speech therapy for patients with dysarthria should be considered.

ALZHEIMER'S DISEASE

One in ten, or more than 5 million, Americans have AD; however, this number increases significantly with age. Eighty percent are 75 years of age or older. Two-thirds of these are women. This has not been found to be associated with biological or social differences, but rather with "survivor bias" (i.e., there are just more women in later life). Blacks are twice as likely as Whites and Hispanics are 1.5 times as likely as Whites to have Alzheimer's or another dementia. It is projected that almost 14 million Americans will have AD by 2050 (Alzheimer's Association [AA], 2020). It is the fifth leading cause of death in persons at least 65 years of age in the United States. Although AD rarely occurs in persons younger than 60 years of age, it is not a normal part of aging and should never be accepted as such. It is expected that the actual number of persons *diagnosed* will grow as they take advantage of the free annual wellness visit now available through the Affordable Care Act, where cognitive screening is part of the overall assessment (see Chapter 8).

Persons with AD have an increased number of beta-amyloid proteins (plaques) outside the neurons and an accumulation of abnormal tau proteins inside the neurons (neurofibrillary tangles) that damage the cortical areas of the brain. As a result, the synapses, which normally connect the neurons, decline; as the neurons are deprived of nutrients, they malfunction and eventually die. As the number of beta-amyloid and tau proteins increases, brain damage increases, initially to the part of the brain where memories are stored; therefore, memory loss is seen in all persons with AD, specifically the ability to remember new information.

❖ CLINICAL JUDGMENT TO PROMOTE HEALTHY AGING: AD

◆ Recognizing and Analyzing Cues

AD is described in three stages based on declines in cognitive function: early, middle, and late or mild,

moderate, or severe (AA, 2020; NIA, 2019). In the early stage, biological/neurological changes are underway, but the person functions independently. They may be working, driving, and maintaining a usual lifestyle but having mild memory problems such as forgetting certain words or the location of everyday objects. These cues may be recognizable to close family and friends and can be tested.

The middle stage (moderate dementia) may last many years but becomes increasingly recognizable: impaired thinking, difficulty finding words (anomia), and changes in judgment and behavior. Memory loss extends to personal history, leaving the person frustrated and sometimes angry. As this stage progresses, the person will have difficulty with bowel and bladder habits and sleeping. Although able to participate in personal care, assistance is eventually required.

When the late stage is reached, around-the-clock care is needed. Changes in physical abilities occur, such as difficulty walking. The ability to communicate needs is ultimately difficult or impossible. Those suffering from AD are particularly vulnerable to infection (AA, 2020). During the COVID-19 outbreak, those with late-stage AD, especially when living in group settings such as nursing homes, were among the first to contract the virus. A more in-depth discussion is available at www.alz.org. Details describing the recognizable cues suggestive of AD and their associated analyses can be found in Chapter 8, Table 8.2.

Diagnosis of AD requires that there has been a decline in the person's cognitive functioning from a previous level, that it developed slowly, that the changes are "greater than expected for the person's age and educational background," and that these changes can be documented with standardized neuropsychological testing (NIA, 2019) (Box 23.7).

◆ Nursing Actions

Like PD, AD is neurodegenerative in nature and impossible to cure. Pharmacological therapy is limited to medications with the potential to slow the cognitive decline. They are not always effective, but when they are, they can help sufferers continue to function to the best of

---

BOX 23.7 "I Just Can't Seem to Remember ..."

Mr. Phillipe had been coming to see me regularly in the clinic. One day when we had a little extra time, he looked at me and said, "You know a lot of people come up and talk to me like I should know them. I am polite and smile but more and more I don't know who they are. Sometimes I think I am losing my mind."

their ability longer and therefore maximize their quality of life and that of their loved ones. Cholinesterase inhibitors such as Aricept are for those with early- or middle-stage AD, and N-methyl-D-aspartate (NMDA) antagonists such as Namenda are for middle- to late-stage AD. The effectiveness of the medications and the side effects vary from person to person. They have not been found to extend the life of a person with AD.

Depression and other mental health issues are common in persons with AD. Too often the cues remain unrecognized and untreated. Nursing actions include close monitoring for these cues and assuring that they are treated appropriately and promptly should they be recognized (see Chapter 25).

Nursing actions when caring for people with neurological disorders in the acute care setting begin with becoming familiar with the person's baseline abilities and then enacting strategies to prevent loss of function during episodes of future acute illness. Because of the usually slow progression and disability that accompanies these disorders, individuals experience a change in activities and social participation. Because the changes are neurodegenerative in nature, eventually older adults experience changes in roles and may avoid social situations because of the accompanying cues.

Everyone, especially those with strong family histories of neurodegenerative disorders, would like to find ways to prevent them. Unfortunately, this is not possible, but promoting healthy aging is (Box 23.8). Nurses work with the individual and those who are either already providing care or will be doing so. Early comprehensive health, safety and fall risk, and gait assessments are important to help the caregivers and nursing staff provide the highest-quality and most empowering care possible. These should be repeated

periodically to monitor changes and make modifications to the hypotheses, actions, and, at times, expected outcomes as needed.

In the skilled nursing setting, periodic reassessments are done through the RAI process (see Chapter 8); however, it is just as important in the outpatient setting. This information guides the actions related to both meeting day-to-day needs and end-of-life planning and care. Legal preparation is needed for when the point of cognitive incapacity nears (see Chapters 7 and 28).

The recognition of cues indicating possible pain should be ongoing (see Chapter 18). A person with AD may not be able to understand or express pain but nonetheless experiences it as anyone else would under the same circumstances. Too often pain in persons with AD is unrecognized. Gerontological nurses should recognize this and use alternative means to analyze the cues of potential pain or discomfort (see Chapter 18).

Nowhere in the care of older adults is a skilled and caring multidisciplinary team more essential than in the care of persons with neurodegenerative disorders. It includes a nurse and neurologist; a physiatrist; speech, occupational, and physical therapists; an ophthalmologist; a rehabilitation specialist; a psychologist; a movement disorders specialist; and eventually, the hospice team. Ideally, care actions are led by a physician and a nurse practitioner working as a primary care team. It may also include a spiritual advisor or indigenous healer. It always includes the person's significant other(s), who will be involved in day-to-day life at some point in time.

Persons with neurodegenerative disorders watch their own decline over time, challenging self-esteem. The nurse can direct the person and care partners to formal programs in stress management or group support and urge them to attempt to maintain former relationships for as long as possible (see Chapter 26).

◆ Evaluating Outcomes

The key outcomes in the care of those with neurodegenerative disorders are (1) prompt recognition and analysis of potential cues, (2) prompt treatment of all reversible conditions (e.g., infections) at any time, (3) appropriate use of available nonpharmacological and pharmacological interventions, and (4) coordination between all care providers, including family members or partners. Striving for optimal outcomes means that the nurse makes sure the person gets good care, preserves self-care abilities for as long as possible, complications and injury are prevented, and support and guidance in dealing with progressive loss are provided (see Chapter 28). (Box 23.9).

BOX 23.8   Tips for Best Practice

Promoting Healthy Aging and the Risk of Neurocognitive Disorders

- Maintain blood pressure within normal limits
- Keep lipids at healthy levels
- Aspirin 81 mg daily as indicated
- Maintain healthy body weight
- Have a regular sleep/wake schedule
- Avoid excess alcohol
- Control diabetes
- Maintain optimal control of heart failure
- Stop smoking or never start
- Exercise
- Maintain mental health and stimulation

Components of an Annual Medical Examination for the Person With Neurological Disorders

- Review of current medications
- Assessment of mental health (evidence of psychosis, depression, anxiety, impulse control disorders)
- Cognitive status
- Evidence of autonomic dysfunction: orthostatic hypotension, constipation, urinary or fecal incontinence or urinary retention, erectile dysfunction
- Sleep quality
- History of falls
- Outcome of rehabilitation if used
- Safety issues relative to the stage of the disease
- Safe use and effectiveness of current medications
- Psychosocial and support needs

COMMUNICATION AND PERSONS WITH NEUROLOGICAL DISORDERS

The most common type of impaired verbal communication arising from neurological and cerebrovascular disturbances is aphasia. It affects the production or comprehension of speech, or the ability to read or write, or all of them (Box 23.10).

Aphasia may occur suddenly such as following a stroke, or slowly from advancing AD or PD. Depending on the type and severity of the aphasia, there may be little or no speech, speech that is fragmented or broken, or speech that is fluent but empty in content. When a stroke affects the dominant half of the brain, some disruption will occur in the "word factories," which are specific to the Broca's and Wernicke's areas in the cerebral cortex. Aphasia can be so severe as to make communication

BOX 23.10   **Communication Impairments Associated with Neurological Disorders**

Anomia: Word-finding difficulties. Either in spontaneous speech, such as a conversation or when asked to name an object.
Aphasia: Impaired ability to use and understand spoken or written words.
Verbal apraxia: A disruption in the brain's transmission of signals to the muscles required to plan and sequence the voluntary muscle movements needed to produce speech. Apraxia frequently occurs with aphasia.

impossible or very mild and barely recognizable. The type of aphasia corresponds with the part of the brain that is damaged.

Fluent (Wernicke's) Aphasia

Fluent aphasia is most often caused by damage to a part of the brain adjacent to the primary auditory cortex. The person speaks easily with many long runs of words, but the content does not make sense. They often have anomia, substituting an incorrect word or phrase without realizing it. The speech sounds like what is sometimes referred to as "jabberwocky," with unrelated words strung together or syllables repeated. The person cannot understand what is spoken to them and may be unaware of their speech difficulties and cannot understand why others do not understand.

Nonfluent (Broca's) Aphasia

Nonfluent aphasia typically involves damage to the Broca's area. The person usually understands others and may be able to read but speaks very slowly, with effort, and uses minimal number of words. The person often struggles to articulate a word and seems to have lost the ability to voluntarily control the movements required to create speech. Difficulties are experienced in communicating both orally and in writing.

Global Aphasia

Global aphasia is the result of large lesions in the left hemisphere of the brain and affects most or all aspects of language. Persons with global aphasia cannot understand words or speak intelligibly. They may use meaningless syllables repetitiously.

Anomic Aphasia

Anomic aphasia is associated with lesions of the dominant temporoparietal regions of the brain, although no single location has been identified. Persons with anomic aphasia understand and speak readily but may have severe word-finding difficulty. They may be unable to remember crucial content words. This is a frequent form of aphasia characterized by the inability to name objects. They struggle to provide the correct noun and often become frustrated at their inability to do so.

Enhancing Communication

Treatment of communication disorders because of a neurological impairment depends on the cause, type, and severity of the symptoms with a goal of maximizing the effectiveness of the ability to express and understand language and meaning. A speech-language pathologist is the expert in this field and provides advice and instructions for the nurses, significant others, and affected persons.

If a person has retained at least some cognitive function, alternative or augmentative communication devices are frequently used, especially following a stroke or another traumatic brain injury. Communication tools exist for every imaginable type of language disability (e.g., an alphabet or picture board so that the individual can point to letters to spell out messages or point to pictures of common objects and situations). Speech-therapy software that displays a word or picture speaks the word using prerecorded human speech.

Communication with the older adult experiencing aphasia can be frustrating for affected persons and all others involved in their lives as they struggle to understand each other. It is important to remember that in most cases of aphasia, especially in PD, the person retains normal intellectual ability. Therefore, communication must always occur at an adult level but with special modifications as directed by a speech-language pathologist. Sensitivity and patience are essential to promote effective communication outcomes.

A nurse may encounter persons with communication difficulties across the continuum of care and illness. It is most helpful if both formal and informal caregivers remain consistent so that they can come to know and recognize the cues indicating the needs of the person and how these needs are communicated. It is exhausting for the person to have to try continually to communicate needs and desires to an array of different people.

For further discussion, see Chapter 25.

KEY CONCEPTS

- There are a number of things that an individual can do to reduce their risk of cerebrovascular disease.
- Ischemic strokes are the result of temporary loss of oxygen to the brain with resultant tissue damage.
- Hemorrhagic strokes are less common than ischemic strokes but much more deadly and result from a rupture in a blood vessel in the brain.
- For the best possible outcomes, immediate treatment is required for a person suffering a stroke; essential nursing actions include teaching all persons early cues and how to activate the emergency response system.
- Correct diagnosis of the type of stroke is necessary before treatment can begin.
- Parkinson's disease and Alzheimer's disease are neurodegenerative, i.e., progressive and incurable.
- Parkinson's disease is a disorder that affects voluntary control of movement.

- The initial cues of Parkinson's disease may be mistaken for other common disorders commonly seen in older adults.
- An early cue of Alzheimer's disease is always loss of recent memory.
- Neurological disorders ultimately affect one's ability to speak in a way that is understandable to others.
- Maximizing outcomes for persons with neurological disorders requires a team approach that includes professionals, the patient, and significant others.

ACTIVITIES AND DISCUSSION QUESTIONS

1. What would you say to a person who tells you, "I thought I had a 'mini-stroke' the other day"?
2. You are teaching a class in the community about the signs of a stroke and what to do in response to them. What is the most important message you want to give?
3. Consider the things you can do in your life to reduce your risk of a stroke. Write them on a piece of paper and then share them with a friend or family member. When you do so, discuss which strategies you can commit to doing to reduce your risk (e.g., stop smoking, eat more vegetables, etc.).
4. Suggest strategies to optimize communication with persons who have communication difficulties as a result of a neurological problem.

REFERENCES

Alzheimer's Association: *Facts and figures,* 2020. https://www.alz.org/alzheimers-dementia/facts-figures.

Boss, B., & Huether, S. E. (2019). Disorders of the central and peripheral nervous system and the neuromuscular junction. In S. E. McCance, & S. E. Huether (Eds.), *Pathophysiology: The biological basis for disease in adults and children* (8th ed.). St Louis: Elsevier.

Centers for Disease Control and Prevention (CDC). (2020a). *Stroke Facts.* https://www.cdc.gov/stroke/facts.htm.

Centers for Disease Control and Prevention (CDC). (2020b). *Types of stroke.* https://www.cdc.gov/stroke/types_of_stroke.htm#transient.

Gao, Q., Leung, A., Yanung, A., et al. (2014). Effects of Tai Chi on balance and fall prevention in Parkinson's disease: A randomized clinical trial. *Clin Rehabil, 11*(28), 748–753.

Li, F., Harmer, P., Liu, Y., et al. (2014). A randomized controlled trial of patient-reported outcomes with tai chi exercise in Parkinson's disease. *Mov Disord, 29*(4), 539–545.

Meara, J. (2017). Parkinsonism and other movement disorders. In H. M. Fillit, K. Rockwood, & J. Young (Eds.), *Brocklehurst's textbook of geriatric medicine and gerontology* (ed. 8, pp. 510–518). Philadelphia: Elsevier.

National Institute of Aging (NIA). (2017). *Parkinson's disease.* https://www.nia.nih.gov/health/parkinsons-disease.

NHLBI. (n.d.). *Stroke.* https://www.nhlbi.nih.gov/health-topics/stroke.

National Institute of Aging (NIA). (2019). *Alzheimer's disease fact sheet.* https://www.nia.nih.gov/health/alzheimers-disease-fact-sheet#symptoms.

National Institute of Neurological Disorders and Stroke (NINDS): *Brain basics: Preventing stroke,* 2019. https://www.ninds.nih.gov/Disorders/Patient-Caregiver-Education/Preventing-Stroke#Do You Know Your Stroke Risk?

Parkinson's Foundation (PF). (2020). *Statistics.* https://www.parkinson.org/Understanding-Parkinsons/Statistics.

Powers, W. J., Rabinstein, A. A., Ackerson, T., et al. (2018). On behalf of the American Heart Association Stroke Council: 2018 guideline for the early management of patients with acute ischemic stroke: a guideline for healthcare professionals from the American Heart Association. *Stroke, 49,* e46–e110. https://www.acc.org/latest-in-cardiology/ten-points-to-remember/2018/01/29/12/45/2018-guidelines-for-the-early-management-of-stroke.

Whitney, C. M. (2004). Managing the square: How older adults with Parkinson's disease sustain quality in their lives. *J Gerontol Nurs, 30*(1), 28–35.

24

Clinical Judgment to Promote Mental Health

Theris A. Touhy

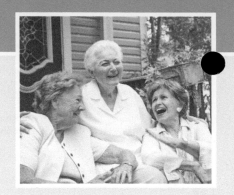

THE LIVED EXPERIENCE

I feel the older I get, the more I'm learning to handle life. Being on this quest for a long time, it's all about finding yourself.

Ringo Starr

MENTAL HEALTH

Mental health is not different in late life, but the level of challenge may be greater. Developmental transitions, life events, physical illness, cognitive impairment, and situations calling for psychic energy may interfere with mental health in older adults. These factors, though not unique to older adults, often influence adaptation. However, anyone who has lived for 80 or more years has been exposed to many stressors and crises and has developed tremendous resistance. Most older adults face life's challenges with equanimity, good humor, and courage. It is our task to discover the strengths and adaptive mechanisms that will assist them to cope with the challenges.

Older adults often experience multiple, simultaneous stressors (Box 24.1). Some older adults are in a chronic state of grief because new losses occur before prior ones are fully resolved; stress then becomes a constant state of being. The ability to tolerate stress varies between individuals and is influenced by current and ongoing stressors, by health, and also by coping ability. For example, if an individual has lost a significant person in the previous year, the grief may be manageable. If they have lost a significant person and developed painful, chronic health problems, the consequences may be quite different and can cause stress overload. In older adults, stress may appear as a cognitive impairment or behavior change that will be alleviated as the stress is reduced to the parameters of the individual's adaptability. Regardless of whether stress is physical or emotional, older adults will require more time to recover or return to prestress levels than younger people.

Any stressors that occur in the lives of older adults may actually be experienced as a crisis if the event occurs abruptly, is unanticipated, or requires skills or resources the individual does not possess. Through a lifetime of coping with stress, some individuals have developed

Abrupt internal and external body changes and illnesses

Other-oriented concerns: children, grandchildren, spouse, or partner

Loss of significant people

Functional impairment

Sensory impairments

Memory impairment (or fear of)

Loss of ability to drive (particularly men)

Acute discomfort and pain

Breach in significant relationships

Retirement (lost social roles, income)

Ageist attitudes

Fires, thefts

Injuries, falls

Major unexpected drain on economic resources (house repair, illness)

Abrupt changes in living arrangements to a new location (home, apartment, room, or institution)

Identity theft and fear of scams

a tremendous stress tolerance, whereas others will be thrown into crisis by changes in their lives with which they feel unable to cope. It is important to remember that there is great individual variability in the definition of a stressor. For some, the loss of a pet canary is a major stressor; others accept the loss of a good friend with grief but without personal disorganization. Some factors that influence a person's ability to manage stress are presented in Box 24.2.

Resilience is a factor that may explain the ability of some individuals to withstand stress. Resilience is defined as "flourishing despite adversity" (Hildon et al., 2009, p. 36). The process of resilience is characterized by successfully adapting to difficult and challenging life experiences, especially those that are highly stressful or traumatic. Resilient people "bend rather than break" during stressful conditions and are able to return to

BOX 24.2 **Factors Influencing Ability to Manage Stress**

- Health and fitness
- A sense of control over events
- Awareness of self and others
- Patience and tolerance
- Resilience
- Hardiness
- Resourcefulness
- Social support
- A strong sense of self

adequate (and sometimes better) functioning after stress ("bouncing back"). Characteristics associated with resilience include positive interpersonal relationships; a willingness to extend oneself to others; optimistic or positive affect; keeping things in perspective; setting goals and taking steps to achieve these goals; high self-esteem and self-efficacy; determination; a sense of purpose in life; creativity; humor; and a sense of curiosity. Older adults may demonstrate greater resilience and the ability to maintain a positive emotional state under stress than younger individuals (Clapp, 2016). Social support from the community, family, and professionals; access to care; and availability of resources can facilitate resilience.

MENTAL HEALTH DISORDERS

Mental, neurological, and substance (MNS) use disorders are prevalent in all regions of the world and are major contributors to morbidity and premature mortality. In the United States, including older adults with dementia, nearly 20% of people older than 55 years of age experience mental health disorders that are not part of normal aging (American Psychological Association, 2020a; World Health Organization, 2017). The most prevalent mental health problems in late life are anxiety, severe cognitive impairment, and mood disorders. Alcohol abuse and dependence are also growing concerns among older adults. Mental health disorders are associated with increased use of health care resources and overall costs of care. *Healthy People 2020* includes mental health and mental health disorders as a topic area (Box 24.3).

 BOX 24.3 **Healthy People 2020**

Mental Health and Mental Disorders (Older Adults)

- Reduce the suicide rate.
- Reduce the proportion of persons who experience major depressive episodes.
- Increase the proportion of primary care facilities that provide mental health treatment onsite or by paid referral.
- Increase the proportion of adults with mental disorders who receive treatment.
- Increase the proportion of persons with co-occurring substance abuse and mental disorders who receive treatment for both disorders.
- Increase depression screening by primary care providers.
- Increase the proportion of homeless adults with mental health problems who receive mental health services.

From US Department of Health and Human Services, Office of Disease Prevention and Health Promotion. (2012). *Healthy People 2020.* http://www.healthypeople.gov/2020.

The prevalence of mental health disorders may be even higher than reported statistics because these disorders are not always reported and not well researched, especially among non-White populations. Predictions are that the number of older adults with mental health disorders will soon overwhelm the mental health system. Many individuals in the baby boomer generation have experienced mental health consequences from military conflict, and the 20th century drug culture will also add to the burden of psychiatric illnesses in the future. The baby boomer generation is also more aware of mental health concerns and more comfortable seeking treatment, which will add to the challenges facing the mental health care system.

The focus of this chapter is on the differing presentation of mental health disturbances that may occur in older adults and the nursing interventions important in maintaining the mental health and self-esteem of older adults at the optimum of their capacity. Readers should refer to a comprehensive psychiatric–mental health text for more in-depth discussion of mental health disorders. A discussion of cognitive impairment and the behavioral symptoms that may accompany this disorder is found in Chapter 25.

FACTORS INFLUENCING MENTAL HEALTH CARE

Attitudes and Beliefs

Older adults with evidence of mental health disorders, regardless of race or ethnicity, are less likely than younger people to receive needed mental health care from mental health specialists. Some of the reasons for this include reluctance on the part of older adults to seek help because of pride of independence, stoic acceptance of difficulty, unawareness of resources, lack of geriatric mental health professionals and services, and lack of adequate insurance coverage for mental health problems. Stigma about having a mental health disorder, particularly for older adults, discourages many from seeking treatment. Agism also affects identification and treatment of mental health disorders in older adults. Similar to other conditions, cues of mental health problems may be looked at as a normal consequence of aging or blamed on dementia by both older adults and health care professionals. In older adults, the presence of comorbid medical conditions complicates the recognition and diagnosis of mental health disorders. Also, the myth that older adults do not respond well to treatment is still prevalent.

Other factors present barriers to appropriate diagnosis and treatment, including the lack of knowledge on

---

BOX 24.4 Resources for Best Practice

- **American Academy of Nursing:** Geropsychiatric Nursing Collaborative: https://www.aannet.org/initiatives/early-initiatives/geropsychiatric-nursing-collaborative.
- **American Society of Consultant Pharmacists STAMP Out Prescription Drug Misuse and Abuse Toolkit:** https://www.ascp.com/page/STAMPOut: Resource for health professionals to educate older adults and senior services providers about prescription drug misuse and abuse
- **Evidence-Based Practice Guideline: Secondary Prevention of Late-Life Suicide:** https://www.ncbi.nlm.nih.gov/pubmed/30208188.
- **Friendship Line (managed by the Institute on Aging), National Suicide Prevention Lifeline:** Available 24 hours per day, 7 days a week. Friendship Line: 1-800-971-0016; National Suicide Prevention Lifeline: 1-800-273-8255
- **Hartford Institute for Geriatric Nursing:** Geriatric nursing protocol: Depression in Older Adults; Impact of Event Scale-Revised (IES-R) (PTSD); Nursing standard of practice protocol: Substance misuse and alcohol use disorders
- **National Alliance on Mental Illness: Help for individuals and their families who are experiencing mental health disorders.** https://www.nami.org/
- **National Center for PTSD.** https://www.ptsd.va.gov/.
- **Online treatment navigator for alcohol use disorder:** Step by step guide for finding professionally led treatment: https://alcoholtreatment.niaaa.nih.gov/

---

the part of health care professionals about mental health in late life, inadequate numbers of geropsychiatrists, geropsychologists, and geropsychiatric nurses, and limited availability of psychiatric care, specifically geropsychiatric services. Increased attention to the preparation of mental health professionals specializing in geriatric care is important to improve mental health care delivery to older adults. An initiative to prepare advanced practice registered nurses (APRNs) in the specialty is the Geropsychiatric Nursing Initiative (GPNI), which provides guidelines and learning materials to improve the knowledge and skills of nurses in mental health care of older adults (Box 24.4).

Culture and Mental Health

Mental health disorders are found in all societies, but the frequency of different types of disorders varies, as do the social connotations. The standards that define "normal" behavior for any culture are determined by that culture itself. What may be defined as mental illness in one culture may be viewed as normal behavior in another. Different cultures and communities also exhibit and explain symptoms of mental distress in various ways

BOX 24.5 Cultural Variations in Expressing Mental Distress

- **Ataque de nervios (attack of nerves):** A syndrome among individuals of Latin descent, characterized by symptoms of intense emotional upset, including acute anxiety, anger, grief; screaming and shouting uncontrollably; attacks of crying, trembling, heat in the chest rising into the head; verbal and physical aggression. May include seizure-like or fainting episodes, suicidal gestures. Attacks frequently occur as a result of a stressful event relating to the family (such as death of a relative, conflict with spouse/children, witnessing an accident involving a family member). Symptoms are similar to acute anxiety, panic disorder. Related conditions are "blacking out" in southern United States and "falling out" in West Indies.
- **Susto (fright):** A cultural expression for distress and misfortune prevalent among some Latinos in the United States and among people in Mexico, Central America, and South America. Illness is attributed to a frightening event that causes the soul to leave the body and results in unhappiness, sickness, and difficulty functioning in social roles. Symptoms include appetite and sleep disturbances, feelings of sadness, low self-worth, lack of motivation. Symptoms are similar to PTSD, depression, and anxiety
- **Khyâl cap (wind attacks):** A syndrome found among Cambodians in the United States and in Cambodia. Symptoms include dizziness, palpitations, shortness of breath, and cold extremities. Concern that khyâl (a wind-like substance) may rise in the body, along with blood, and cause serious effects such as entering the lungs to cause shortness of breath/asphyxia or entering the brain to cause dizziness, tinnitus, and a fatal syncope. Attacks frequently brought about by worrisome thoughts. Symptoms include those of panic attacks, generalized anxiety disorder, and PTSD.

(Box 24.5). Cultural beliefs also influence who makes health care decisions, help-seeking behavior, preferences for type of treatment, and provider characteristics. Mental and behavioral health is a critical and frequently unaddressed matter in racial and ethnic minority communities. Cultural variation in beliefs about the causes of mental illness and the effects of treatment, past discrimination, and the lack of mental health treatments that are congruent with preferences, values, and beliefs contribute to disparities. Blacks, Latinos, American Indians/Alaska Natives, and Asian Americans are particularly at risk of mental health disorders. Minority individuals may experience symptoms that are underdiagnosed, undiagnosed, or misdiagnosed for cultural, linguistic, or historical reasons (American Psychological Association, 2020b).

Disparities are found in many groups. Although not well researched, sexual minority individuals, particularly older gay men, demonstrate higher rates of mental disorders, substance abuse, suicidal ideation, and deliberate self-harm than heterosexual populations (Hoy-Ellis et al., 2016). Sexual minority stress (gay-related stigma, discrimination or prejudice, concealment of sexual preferences, excessive human immunodeficiency virus [HIV] bereavements) and aging-related stress are thought to contribute to the unique mental health challenges of these individuals (Chapter 26). Research is also needed on the effect of other stressors such as war, terrorism, displacement, and immigration on mental health.

The Diagnostic and Statistical Manual of Mental Disorders (DSM-5) (American Psychiatric Association, 2013) has an increased emphasis on culture and mental health, including the range of psychopathology across the globe, not just illnesses common in the United States, western Europe, and Canada. Another significant change in the DSM-5 is the developmental approach and examination of disorders across the life span. This is particularly relevant for older adults because symptoms of mental distress may present differently from the presentation in younger individuals.

An increased understanding of the importance of cultural perspectives for individuals across the life span will facilitate more accurate assessment of mental health disorders, wellness, and illness and lead to fewer misdiagnoses. Enhancing the cultural proficiency of health care professionals will assist in structuring more culturally appropriate services, thus improving treatment outcomes and decreasing disparities. Box 24.6 presents best-practice tips for culture assessment. Research on all aspects of culture and mental health is critical. Chapter 3 discusses culture in more depth.

Availability of Mental Health Care

Dedicated financing for older adult mental health is limited even though about 20% of all Medicare beneficiaries experience some mental disorder each year. Medicare spends five times more on beneficiaries with severe mental illness and substance abuse disorders than on similar beneficiaries without these diagnoses. More than half of dual-eligible persons (those with both Medicare and Medicaid) have mental or cognitive impairments. The 2008 mental health parity legislations ended Medicare's discriminatory practice of imposing a 50% coinsurance requirement for outpatient mental health services. In 2014, coinsurance was reduced to 20%, bringing payments for mental health care in line with those required for all other Medicare Part B services (Center for Medicare Advocacy, 2020).

The Centers for Medicare and Medicaid Services (CMS) health risk assessment and annual wellness

---

BOX 24.6 Tips for Best Practice
Cultural Interview Questions

- "Sometimes people have different ways of describing their problem to their family, friends, or others in the community. How would you describe your problem to them?"
- "What troubles you most about your problem?"
- "Why do you think this is happening to you?"
- "What do you think are the causes of your problem?"
- "What do others in your family, friends, or others in your community think are the causes of your problem?"
- "Are there aspects of your background or identity that are causing other concerns or difficulties for you?"
- "Sometimes people have various ways of dealing with problems like your problem. What have you done to cope with your problems?"
- "Often people look for help from many different sources, including different kinds of doctors, helpers, or healers. In the past what kinds of treatment, help, advice, or healing have you sought for your problem? What have others advised?"
- "What do you think would be helpful?"
- "Do you have any concerns about the therapist-patient relationship?"

Adapted from American Psychiatric Association. (2013). *Diagnostic and statistical manual of mental disorders* (5th ed).Washington, DC: American Psychiatric Association.

---

visit for Medicare beneficiaries includes screening for depression, questions on alcohol consumption, and detection of cognitive impairment. Medicare also covers a yearly depression screening at no cost to beneficiaries. However, coverage for follow-up care for such problems remains limited (Jeste et al., 2018). Concerns remain about the 190-day lifetime limit for care in inpatient psychiatric facilities and the high out-of-pocket costs of prescription drugs. More comprehensive and integrated mental health care is needed, especially in light of the aging of the baby boomer generation.

Settings of Care

Older adults receive psychiatric services across a wide range of settings, including acute and long-term inpatient psychiatric units, primary care, and community and institutional settings. The majority of older adults treated for mental health services receive care from primary care providers. Less than 3% receive treatment from mental health professionals (American Psychological Association, 2020a). It is critical to integrate mental health and substance abuse with other health services including primary care, specialty care, home health care, and residential community–based care. Primary care providers must routinely screen for mental health problems in older adults and develop working relationships with mental health practitioners in their area to improve

access and communication. Successful models include mental health professionals in primary care offices; care managers; community-based, multidisciplinary geriatric mental health treatment teams; and use of advance practice nurses (SAMHSA-HRSA Center for Integrated Health Solutions, 2018).

In acute care settings, nurses will encounter older adults with mental health disorders in emergency departments or in general medical–surgical units. Admissions for medical problems are often exacerbated by depression, anxiety, cognitive impairment, substance abuse, or chronic mental illness, and these conditions are often unrecognized by primary care providers. Nurses who can identify mental health problems early and seek consultation and treatment will enhance timely recovery. Advanced practice psychiatric nursing consultation is an important and effective service in acute care settings.

Long-term care facilities and, increasingly, residential care/assisted living facilities (RC/ALFs), although not licensed as psychiatric facilities, provide the majority of care given to older adults with psychiatric conditions. Excluding dementia, individuals with behavioral illness account for close to 50% of all nursing facility residents. It is often difficult to find placement for an older adult with a mental health problem in these types of facilities, and few are structured to provide best practice care to individuals with mental illness. Additionally, patients with mental health diagnoses had lower access to high-quality facilities as measured by the overall quality of care and by facility staffing (Temkin-Greener et al., 2018).

The following are some of the obstacles to mental health care in nursing facilities and RC/ALFs: (1) shortage of trained personnel; (2) limited availability and access for psychiatric services; (3) lack of staff training related to mental health and mental illness; and (4) inadequate Medicaid and Medicare reimbursement for mental health services. An insufficient number of trained personnel affects the quality of mental health care in nursing homes and often causes great stress for staff.

New models of mental health care and services are needed for nursing homes and RC/ALFs to address the growing needs of older adults in these settings. Psychiatric services in nursing facilities, when they are available, are commonly provided by psychiatric consultants who are not full-time staff members, and their services are inadequate to meet the needs of residents and staff. Training and education of front-line staff who provide basic care to residents are essential. There is an urgent need for well-designed controlled studies to examine mental health concerns in both nursing facilities and RC/ALFs and the effectiveness of mental health services in improving clinical outcomes. Chapter 6 discusses long-term care in more depth.

MENTAL HEALTH DISORDERS

Anxiety Disorders

Anxiety disorders are not considered part of the normal aging process, but the changes and challenges that older adults often face may contribute to the development of anxiety symptoms and disorders or reactivate prior anxiety disorders. Increasing frailty, medical illness, losses, pain, lack of social support, traumatic events, medications, poor self-rated health, the presence of another psychiatric illness, and an early-onset anxiety disorder are all risk factors for late-life anxiety disorders. Older adults who experience anxiety have more visits to primary care providers with an increased average length of visit. Anxiety symptoms and disorders are associated with many negative consequences including increased hospitalizations, decreased physical activity and functional status, sleep disturbances, increased health service use, substance abuse, decreased life satisfaction, and increased mortality (Brenes et al., 2014).

Late-life anxiety is often comorbid with major depressive disorder, cognitive decline and dementia, and substance abuse. Almost half of older adults diagnosed with major depression also meet the criteria for anxiety. Current evidence suggests that anxiety is even more common than depression in community-dwelling older adults and may precede depressive disorders. There is some evidence to suggest anxiety may be predictive of cognitive decline, but anxiety also develops in response to cognitive decline (Fung et al., 2018). Symptoms of anxiety may occur in 75% of individuals diagnosed with dementia (Clifford et al., 2015). Further investigation is needed on all aspects of anxiety in older adults. Older adults who experience anxiety have more visits to primary care providers with an increased average length of visit.

❖ USING CLINICAL JUDGMENT TO PROMOTE HEALTHY AGING: ANXIETY

◆ Recognizing and Analyzing Cues to Anxiety

Data suggest that approximately 70% of all primary care visits are driven by psychological factors (e.g., panic, generalized anxiety, stress, somatization) (American Psychological Association, 2020a). This means that nurses often encounter anxious older adults and can identify anxiety-related symptoms and initiate actions that will lead to appropriate treatment and management. General issues in the psychosocial assessment of older adults involve distinguishing between normal, idiosyncratic, and diverse characteristics of the individual and pathological conditions. To recognize and analyze

cues to anxiety and other mental health concerns, it is important to have an understanding of past and present history, behavior patterns, personality, coping ability, the degree of social support, and the effect of life events. The cornerstones of assessment are listening carefully to the individual's life story, appreciating the individual's strengths, and coming to know the individual in their own uniqueness (Chapter 5).

The general and pervasive nature of anxiety may make diagnosis difficult in older adults. In addition, older adults tend to deny the psychological symptoms, attribute anxiety-related symptoms to physical illness, and have coexistent medical conditions that mimic symptoms of anxiety. Cues to anxiety most often present in physical complaint such as difficulty sleeping, stomach complaints, and general malaise. In addition, stigma associated with mental disorders is a factor for older adults. Avoiding previously enjoyed activities and increasing social isolation are major signs of both anxiety and depression. Often, health care providers may attribute these symptoms to "getting older," as a result of age-related stereotypes.

Some of the medical disorders that cause anxiety include cardiac arrhythmias, mitral valve prolapse, delirium, dementia, chronic obstructive pulmonary disease (COPD), heart failure, hyperthyroidism, hypoglycemia, postural hypotension, pulmonary edema, and pulmonary embolism. The presence of cognitive impairment may also make diagnosis complicated. Anxiety is also a common side effect of many drugs (Box 24.7). A review of medications, including over-the-counter (OTC) and herbal or home remedies, is essential with elimination of those that cause anxiety if possible (Chapter 9).

It is important to investigate all possible causes of anxiety, such as medical conditions and depression. Diagnostic and laboratory tests may be ordered as

---

BOX 24.7 Medications That May Cause Anxiety Symptoms

- Anticholinergics
- Digitalis
- Theophylline
- Antihypertensives
- Beta-blockers
- Beta-adrenergic stimulators
- Corticosteroids
- Over-the-counter medications such as appetite suppressants and cough and cold preparations
- Caffeine
- Nicotine
- Withdrawal from alcohol, sedatives, and hypnotics

indicated to rule out medical problems and cognitive evaluation conducted if impairment is suspected. When comorbid conditions are present, they must be treated. Several assessment/screening tools have been developed specifically for use with older adults: Geriatric Anxiety Inventory (GAI), Adult Manifest Anxiety Scale-Elder (AMAS-E), Geriatric Anxiety Scale (GAS), and Worry Scale (WS) (Balsamo et al., 2018). If such instruments are used, they should be weighed carefully with other data—complaints, physical examination, history, and interview data.

When assessing anxiety reactions in individuals residing in nursing facilities, look for daily disturbances, such as with staff or caregiver changes, room changes, or events over which the individual feels a lack of control or influence. By themselves, these circumstances seldom provoke an anxiety reaction, but they may be "the straw that breaks the camel's back," particularly in frail older adults. Nurses must be alert to the signs of anxiety in frail older adults or those with dementia because symptoms are subtle and the individual may be unable to tell us how they are feeling. Carefully observing behavior and searching for possible reasons for changes in behavior or patterns are important (Chapter 25).

◆ Nursing Actions: Anxiety

Although further research is needed to provide evidence to guide treatment, existing studies suggest that anxiety disorders in older adults can be treated effectively. Treatment choices depend on the symptoms, the specific anxiety diagnosis, comorbid medical conditions, and any current medication regimen. Creighton and colleagues (2018) found that pharmacotherapy was typically the first line of treatment, even though there is growing evidence that nonpharmacological interventions such as cognitive-behavioral therapy (CBT) and alternative medications are the recommended treatments. If the individual has more than one anxiety disorder or suffers from comorbid depression, substance abuse, or medical problems, treatment may be complicated. Suggested interventions for anxiety in older adults are presented in Box 24.8.

◆ Pharmacological Treatment

Pharmacotherapy is a treatment option for many patients with anxiety disorders, either in combination with CBT or as stand-alone treatment. However, research on the effectiveness of medication in treating anxiety in older adults is limited. Age-related changes in pharmacodynamics and issues of polypharmacy make prescribing and monitoring in older adults a complex undertaking. Antidepressants in the form of selective serotonin reuptake inhibitors (SSRIs) are usually the

---

BOX 24.8   Tips for Best Practice

Nursing Actions for Anxiety in Older Adults

- Establish a therapeutic relationship and come to know the person.
- Listen attentively to what is said and unsaid; pay attention to nonverbal behavior; use a nonjudgmental approach.
- Support the person's strengths and have faith in their ability to cope, drawing on past successes.
- Encourage expression of needs, concerns, and questions.
- Screen for depression.
- Evaluate medications for anxiety side effects; adjust as needed.
- Manage physical conditions.
- Accept the person's defenses; do not confront, argue, or debate.
- Help the person identify precipitants of anxiety and their reactions.
- Teach the person about anxiety, symptoms, and their effects on the body.
- If irrational thoughts are present, offer accurate information while encouraging the expression of the meaning of events contributing to anxiety; reassure the person of their safety and your presence in supporting the person.
- Intervene when possible to remove the source of anxiety.
- Encourage positive self-talk, such as "I can do this one step at a time" and "Right now I need to breathe deeply."
- Teach distraction or diversion tactics; progressive relaxation exercises; deep breathing.
- Encourage participation in physical activity, adapted to the person's capabilities.
- Encourage the use of community resources such as friends, family, churches, socialization groups, self-help and support groups, and mental health counseling.

From Flood, M., & Buckwalter, K. (2009). Recommendations for the mental health care of older adults: Part 1—An overview of depression and anxiety. *J Gerontol Nurs, 35*(2):26–34.

---

first-line treatment. Within this class of drugs, those with sedating rather than stimulating properties are preferred. Careful monitoring of response and side effects is important.

Second-line treatment may include short-acting benzodiazepines (alprazolam, lorazepam, mirtazapine). Treatment with benzodiazepines should be used for short-term therapy only (less than 3 months) and relief of immediate symptoms, but they must be used carefully in older adults. Use of these medications may be appropriate for only a few select indications, including severe generalized anxiety disorder (GAD) unresponsive to other therapies. However, benzodiazepine use continues to increase with age. Nearly one-third of users are 65–80 years old. Additionally, only a small proportion of individuals who received prescriptions for benzodiazepines were referred to or received psychotherapy or antidepressant therapy. Older adults are not receiving treatments that are both more appropriate and safer (Maust et al., 2016).

Benzodiazepines in older adults can cause cognitive impairment, falls, and other serious side effects. Fall risk is significantly increased with use of benzodiazepines, particularly among older adults with osteoporosis, sensory loss, Parkinson's disease, arthritis, polypharmacy, orthostasis, those who use the restroom frequently at night, and those with a history of falls (Markota et al., 2016). Use of older drugs, such as diazepam or chlordiazepoxide, should be avoided because of their long half-lives and the increased risk of accumulation and toxicity in older people. Nonbenzodiazepine anxiolytic agents (buspirone) may also be used, but not on an as-needed basis (prn). Buspirone has fewer side effects, but it requires a longer period of administration (up to 4 weeks) for effectiveness. See Chapters 9, 13, 15, and 25 for discussions on the use of benzodiazepines in older adults.

◆ Nonpharmacological Treatment

Psychotherapeutic approaches include CBT, exposure therapy, mindfulness-based stress reduction (MBSR), and interpersonal therapy. Increasing evidence supports the effectiveness of psychotherapy in treating anxiety in older adults, often in combination with pharmacotherapy. CBT is designed to modify thought patterns, improve skills, and alter the environmental states that contribute to anxiety. CBT may involve relaxation training and cognitive restructuring (replacing anxiety-producing thoughts with more realistic, less catastrophic ones) and education about signs and symptoms of anxiety. Telephone-delivered and Internet-based CBT are increasingly available and preliminary evaluation has shown improved patient outcomes, increased access to care, low cost, and ease of use (Kruse et al., 2017).

MBSR is a new technique that introduces the concept of mindfulness through the practice of techniques such as yoga, mindful breathing, and other forms of meditation (Clifford et al., 2015). Exposure therapy, also used in treatment of posttraumatic stress disorder (PTSD), involves controlled exposure to events/situations that cause anxiety until anxiety lessens and the body and mind are trained to view the situation with less distress.

Complementary and alternative therapies include biofeedback, progressive relaxation, acupuncture, yoga, massage therapy, art therapy, music therapy, dance therapy, meditation, prayer, and spiritual counseling. A systematic review of relaxation interventions for anxiety and depression with older adults found that yoga, music, and combined relaxation training was most effective for symptoms of anxiety (Klainin-Yobas et al., 2015). The therapeutic relationship between the patient and the health care provider is the foundation for any intervention. Support from family, referral to community resources and support groups, and provision of educational materials are other important interventions.

Posttraumatic Stress Disorder

Although originally considered an anxiety disorder, the DSM-5 removed PTSD from the classification of anxiety disorders and included it in a new chapter, "Trauma- and Stressor-Related Disorders." PTSD was once considered a psychological condition of combat veterans who were "shocked" by and unable to face their experience on the battlefield. Individuals with PTSD were labeled as weak, faced rejection from their military peers and society in general, and were removed from combat zones or discharged from the military. Today we know that PTSD is a psychobiological mental disorder associated with changes in brain function and structure and can affect survivors of combat experience but also terrorist attacks, natural disasters, mass trauma events, serious accidents, assault or abuse, and even sudden and major emotional losses (National Institute of Mental Health, 2019).

Prevalence

Most of the research on PTSD has been conducted with male veterans of military combat. The lifetime prevalence rate of PTSD for Vietnam veterans is estimated to be 30.9% of men and 26.9% of women; Gulf War veterans, 12.1%; and veterans of Operation Enduring Freedom/Operation Iraqi Freedom, 13.8% (Gradus, 2017). Prevalence rates of PTSD among older adults needs further study, but a study by Reynolds and colleagues (2016) reported PTSD rates for older adults (65 years and older) to be 2.6%, which is a lower prevalence rate than other age categories.

In addition to military combat, older adults in our care now have also experienced the Great Depression, the Holocaust, the Great Recession of 2008–2012, and racism—events that may also precipitate PTSD. Although they may have managed to keep symptoms under control, an individual who becomes cognitively impaired may no longer be able to control thoughts, flashbacks, or images. This can be the cause of great distress that may be exhibited by aggressive or hostile behavior. Older adults who are survivors of the Holocaust may experience PTSD symptoms when they are placed in group settings in institutions (Box 24.9). Older women with a history of rape or abuse as a child may also experience symptoms of PTSD when institutionalized, particularly during the provision of intimate bodily care activities, such as bathing.

Symptoms

The DSM-5 includes four major symptom clusters for diagnosis of PTSD: (1) reexperiencing; (2) avoidance;

BOX 24.9   Clinical Example of PTSD

Jack's Story

An 80-year-old WWII veteran resident with dementia was admitted to a large Veterans Administration (VA) nursing home. Jack's wife told the staff that he had been a high school principal who was very successful in his position. He had recurring frightening dreams throughout his life related to his war experiences and he would always turn off the radio or TV when there were programs about WWII. Now, because of his dementia, he was unable to control his thoughts and feelings. While in the nursing home, he would become very agitated and attempt to hit other residents around him when placed in the large day room. The staff recognized this as a PTSD reaction from his years as a prisoner of war. They always placed him in a smaller day room near the nursing station away from other residents, where he remained calm and pleasant. The aggression stopped without the need for medication.

PTSD, Posttraumatic stress disorder.

(3) persistent negative alterations in cognition and mood; and (4) alterations in arousal and receptivity (including irritable or aggressive behavior and reckless or self-destructive behavior) (American Psychiatric Association, 2013). Individuals often reexperience and relive the traumatic event in episodes of fear and experience symptoms such as helplessness, flashbacks (reliving the trauma over and over, including physical symptoms like a racing heart or sweating), frightening thoughts, bad dreams, avoidance of thoughts or situations that remind them of the traumatic event, poor concentration, irritability, increased startle reactions, and numbing of emotional responsiveness. Symptoms may be present within a short time period following the trauma, but a person may have a delayed response from a year to several years.

❖ USING CLINICAL JUDGMENT TO PROMOTE HEALTHY AGING: PTSD

◆ Recognizing and Analyzing Cues: PTSD

The care of individuals with PTSD involves awareness that certain events may trigger inappropriate reactions, and the pattern of these reactions should be identified when possible. Assessment of trauma and related symptoms should be routine in older adults because they may not report traumatic experiences or may minimize their importance. Similar to other mental health concerns, cues to PTSD symptoms include physical concerns, pain, sleep difficulties, or cognitive problems rather than emotional problems. PTSD often co-occurs with physical illness, substance use disorders, and chronic

pain. Reports of physical issues should be followed with questions about changes in mood and activities. Depression is present in half of individuals with PTSD, making it very important to assess routinely for depression and suicidal ideation. Cognitive screening for delirium/dementia is important. The Impact of Event Scale-Revised (IES-R) is a screening instrument for PTSD that may also be used (Christianson & Marren, 2013) (Box 24.4).

◆ Nursing Actions: PTSD

Effective coping with traumatic events seems to be associated with secure and supportive relationships; the ability to freely express or fully suppress the experience; favorable circumstances immediately following the trauma; productive and active lifestyles; strong faith, religion, and hope; a sense of humor; biological integrity; and resilience. As gene research and brain imaging technologies continue to improve, scientists are more likely to be able to pinpoint when and where in the brain PTSD begins. Other research is attempting to identify which factors determine whether someone with PTSD will respond well to one type of intervention or another, aiming to develop more personalized, effective treatments (National Institute of Mental Health, 2019).

The understanding of how to treat PTSD among older adults is still developing. Current treatment recommendations for older adults include CBT and prolonged exposure therapy (PE). A new study, the Warrior Wellness Study (Hall et al., 2018), examines the effects of exercise with older veterans with PTSD. Other therapies shown to improve PTSD symptoms include cognitive processing therapy, eye movement desensitization and reprocessing, and narrative exposure therapy. Cognitive therapy aims to isolate dysfunctional thoughts and assumptions about the trauma that seem to cause distress. Individuals are encouraged to challenge the truth of the beliefs and to substitute them with more balanced thoughts.

Exposure therapy involves recalling distressing memories of the trauma/event via controlled exposure to reminders of the event. Exposure can be done by imagining the trauma, reading descriptions of the event, or visiting the site of the trauma until distress associated with the memory lessens and the body and mind are retrained to view the situation as less dangerous than it was perceived to be.

Evidence-based psychospiritual interventions may also be effective in the treatment of veterans with PTSD and may be more acceptable among those who have a fear of mental illness–related stigma. Individuals able to find meaning and purpose in their traumatic experiences are less likely to develop chronic PTSD. Providers should inquire about the spiritual component of PTSD and help the individual to find meaning in their life (Chapter 5). Pharmacological therapy is also used, and sertraline and paroxetine have received approval by the US Food and Drug Administration (FDA) to treat PTSD. Careful monitoring of these medications is necessary in older adults (Chapter 9).

Therapies should be individualized to meet the specific concerns and needs of each unique patient and may include individual, group, and family therapy. Internet-based therapy, self-help therapy, and telephone-assisted therapy are other creative formats to make interventions more widely available, particularly for improving response to mass trauma events. Further research is necessary to understand the various presentations of PTSD in late life and validate and improve the effectiveness of available treatment approaches (Department of Veterans Affairs, 2019). Other resources for management of PTSD can be found in Box 24.4.

SCHIZOPHRENIA

Prevalence

Older adults are the fastest-growing segment of the total population of individuals living with schizophrenia, and the numbers are expected to grow in the coming decades with the increased longevity of the population. Onset of schizophrenia after the age of 45 years is identified as late-onset, and after the age of 60 years the onset of schizophrenia is considered to be rare (American Psychiatric Association, 2013).

Symptoms

The main symptoms associated with schizophrenia can be categorized into positive symptoms of delusions, hallucinations, disorganized speech, disorganized behavior; negative symptoms of flat or blunted affect, anhedonia, avolition; and cognitive symptoms of poor executive functioning and limited attention span (American Psychiatric Association, 2013). But by the age of 65 years, individuals living with schizophrenia experience fewer delusions and hallucinations but still experience some degree of impairment. Symptoms of cognitive impairment usually do not improve as the person ages. Mushkin and colleagues (2018) interviewed 20 aging adults living with schizophrenia to develop an understanding of living with schizophrenia and the person's well-being. Interestingly, the findings revealed that the participants viewed old age as "a window of opportunity" and "a chance to live a normal life" (Mushkin et al., 2018, p. 980).

Consequences

Individuals with severe persistent mental illnesses (SPMI) such as schizophrenia form a disenfranchised group whose access to medical care has been limited, leading to greater functional declines, morbidity, and mortality. Individuals with schizophrenia generally have a life expectancy 10–20 years shorter than the general population (World Health Organization, 2020). This reduction in years has been attributed to cardiovascular disease related to antipsychotics, poor diet, limited exercise, and smoking (Gates et al., 2015). Continued research is needed specifically to examine the effects of living with schizophrenia as an older adult across the globe.

Schizophrenia is a costly disease both in terms of personal challenges and with regard to medical care costs. The living situations for older adults who have schizophrenia can be challenging, with the majority living in nursing facilities, assisted living, boarding houses, or on the streets. Actions to improve independent functioning, irrespective of age and in conjunction with community services, would decrease the expenses associated with institutionalization. The management of older adults with schizophrenia is expected to become a serious burden for our health care system, requiring the development of integrated models of care across the continuum.

Nursing Actions: Schizophrenia

Treatment for schizophrenia includes both pharmacological and nonpharmacological approaches. First-generation antipsychotics (e.g., haloperidol) have been effective in managing the positive symptoms of schizophrenia but are problematic in older adults and carry a high risk of disabling and persistent side effects, such as tardive dyskinesia (TD). The abnormal involuntary movement scale (AIMS) is useful for evaluating early symptoms of TD (Chapter 9). The second-generation, atypical antipsychotic medications (e.g., risperidone, olanzapine, quetiapine), given in low doses, are associated with a lower risk of extrapyramidal symptoms (EPS) and TD. Another adverse effect of antipsychotics is the potential for weight gain and diabetes. The use of weight-neutral medications is recommended, and dietary education, waist circumference, and weight should be routinely included in assessment of individuals with schizophrenia (Hjorthøj et al., 2017). Federal guidelines for the use of antipsychotic medications in nursing facilities provide the indications for use of these medications in schizophrenia.

Other important interventions include a combination of support, education, physical activity, and CBT. A positive approach on the part of health care professionals, patients, and their families, combined with interventions to enhance quality of life, is important.

Families of older adults with schizophrenia experience the burden of caring for a family member with a chronic disability and dealing with their own personal aging. Community-based support services that include assistance with housing, medical care, recreation services, and services that help the family plan for the future of their relative are necessary. There are relatively few services in the community for older adults with schizophrenia. The National Alliance on Mental Illness (NAMI) (Box 24.4) is an important resource for clients and their families.

PSYCHOTIC SYMPTOMS IN OLDER ADULTS

The onset of true psychiatric disorders is low among older adults, but psychotic manifestations may occur as a secondary syndrome in a variety of disorders, the most common being neurocognitive disorders and Parkinson's disease (Chapters 23 and 25).

Paranoid Symptoms

New-onset paranoid symptoms are common among older adults and can present in a number of conditions in late life. Paranoid symptoms can signify an acute change in mental status as a result of a medical illness or delirium or they can be caused by an underlying affective or primary psychotic mental disorder. Paranoia is also an early symptom of Alzheimer's disease, appearing approximately 20 months before diagnosis. Medications, vision and hearing loss, social isolation, alcoholism, depression, the presence of negative life events, financial strain, and PTSD can also be precipitating factors of paranoid symptoms.

Delusions

Delusions are fixed beliefs that guide a person's interpretation of events and help make sense out of disorder, even though they are inconsistent with reality. The delusions may be comforting or threatening, but they always form a structure for understanding situations that might otherwise seem unmanageable. A delusional disorder is one in which conceivable ideas, without foundation in fact, persist for more than 1 month.

Common delusions of older adults are of being poisoned, personal objects being stolen, of children taking their assets, of being held prisoner, or of being deceived by a spouse, partner, or lover. In older adults, delusions often incorporate significant persons rather than the global grandiose or persecutory delusions. Fear and a lack of trust originating from a basis in reality may become magnified, especially if the person is isolated from others and does not receive reality feedback. It is always important to determine whether what "appears" to be

BOX 24.10   Clinical Examples of Delusions

Maggie's Story
Maggie persistently held onto the delusion that her son was a very important attorney and was coming to force the administration to discharge her from the nursing home. Her son, a factory worker, had been dead for 10 years. The events of her day, her hopes, and her status were all organized around this belief. It is clear that without her delusion she would have felt forlorn, lost, and abandoned.

Herman's Story
Herman was an 88-year-old man in a nursing home who insisted that he must go and visit his mother. His thoughts seemed clear in other respects (often the case with people who are delusional), and one of the authors (P. Ebersole) suspected that he had some unresolved conflicts about his dead mother or felt the need for comforting and caring. P.E. did not argue with Herman about his dead mother because arguing is never a useful approach to persons with delusions. Rather, she used the best techniques she could think of to assure Herman that she was interested in him as a person and recognized that he must feel very lonely sometimes. Herman continued to say that he must go and visit his mother. When P.E. could delay his leaving no longer, she walked with him to the nurses' station and found that his 104-year-old mother did indeed live in another wing of the institution and that he visited her every day.

delusional ideation is, in fact, based in reality. Box 24.10 presents some clinical examples.

Hallucinations

Hallucinations are best described as sensory perceptions that occur in the absence of external stimuli and may be spurred by the internal stimulation of any of the five senses. Although not attributable to environmental stimuli, hallucinations may occur as a combined result of environmental factors. Hallucinations arising from psychotic disorders are less common among older adults, and those that are generated are thought to begin in situations in which the person is feeling alone, abandoned, isolated, or alienated. To compensate for insecurity, a hallucinatory experience is stimulated, often an imaginary companion. Imagined companions may fill the immense void and provide some security, but they may also become accusatory and disturbing.

The character and stages of hallucinatory experiences in later life have not been adequately defined. Many hallucinations are in response to physical disorders, such as dementia, Parkinson's disease, sensory disorders, and medications. Older adults with hearing and vision deficits may also hear voices or see people and objects that

BOX 24.11 Clinical Example: Is It Hallucinations?

One older woman in a nursing home who had Alzheimer's disease and was experiencing agnosia would look in the mirror and talk to "the nice lady I see in there." "Do you want to eat or go out for a walk with me?" she would ask. It was comforting to her, and therefore she did not need medication for her "hallucination," as some would have labeled her behavior. As is the case with many disease symptoms, frail elders do not typically manifest the cardinal signs we have been taught to associate with certain physical and mental disorders. Diagnostic criteria, and often evidence-based practice guidelines, have been developed as a result of observation and research with younger people and may not always fit the older person. Until knowledge and research on the unique aspects of aging increase, nurses and other health care professionals are urged to individualize their assessment and treatment of older people using available guidelines specific to older people.

are not actually present (illusions). Some have explained this as the brain's attempt to create stimulation in the absence of adequate sensory input. If the hallucinations are not disturbing to the person, they do not necessitate treatment (Box 24.11)

❖ USING CLINICAL JUDGMENT TO PROMOTE HEALTHY AGING: PSYCHOTIC SYMPTOMS

Recognizing and Analyzing Cues: Psychotic Symptoms

The dilemma is often one of determining whether paranoia, delusions, and hallucinations are the result of medical illnesses, medications, dementia, psychoses, sensory deprivation or overload. Depending on the precipitating factors, treatment will vary. Treatment must be based on a comprehensive evaluation and determination of the nature of the psychotic behavior (primary or secondary psychosis). Treating the underlying cause of a secondary psychosis caused by medical illnesses, dementia, substance abuse, or delirium is a priority.

Determining adequacy of vision and hearing is also important because these impairments may predispose the older adult to paranoia or suspiciousness. Psychotic symptoms and/or paranoid ideation also present with depression, and therefore depression screening should also be conducted. Identification of suicide potential is also indicated because individuals experiencing paranoid symptoms are at significant risk of harm to self. It is never safe to conclude that someone is delusional

or paranoid or experiencing hallucinations unless there has been a thorough investigation of their claims, evaluation of physical and cognitive status, and identification of factors in the environment that may contribute to the behaviors.

◆ Nursing Actions: Psychotic symptoms

Frightening hallucinations or delusions, such as feeling that one is being poisoned, usually arise in response to anxiety-provoking situations and are best managed by reducing situational stress; being available to the person; providing a safe, nonjudgmental environment; and attending to the fears more than the content of the delusion or hallucination. Direct confrontation is likely to increase anxiety and agitation and the sense of vulnerability; it also may disrupt the relationship. A more useful approach is to establish a trusting relationship that is nondemanding and not too intense.

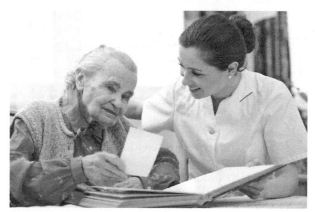

Demonstrating respect and a willingness to listen is the foundation for a caring nurse-patient relationship. (© iStock.com /AlexRaths.)

It is important to identify the individual's strengths and build on them. Demonstrating respect and a willingness to listen to concerns and fears are important. It is important that the nurse be trustworthy, give clear information, and present clear choices. Do not pretend to agree with paranoid beliefs or delusions, but rather ask what is troubling the person and provide reassurance of safety. It is important to try to understand the person's level of distress and how they are experiencing what is troubling. Other suggestions are to avoid television, which can be confusing, especially if the person awakens and finds it on or has a hearing or vision impairment. In addition, reduce clutter in the person's room and eliminate shadows that can appear threatening. Provide glasses and hearing aids to maximize sensory input and to decrease misinterpretations.

If symptoms are interfering with function and inter-personal and environmental strategies are not effective, antipsychotic drugs may be used. The newer atypical antipsychotics (risperidone, olanzapine) are preferred but must be used judiciously, with careful attention to side effects and monitoring of response. None of the antipsychotic medications is approved for use in treatment of behavioral responses in individuals with neuro-cognitive disorders. Atypical antipsychotic medications include a black box warning related to an increased risk of death when prescribed for older adults with dementia-related psychosis. Chapter 25 discusses behavior and psychological symptoms in dementia and nonpharmacological interventions.

BIPOLAR DISORDER

The DSM-5 defines bipolar disorder (BD) as a recurrent mood disorder that includes periods of mania and/or hypomania and major depression (bipolar I) or major depression and hypomanic episodes (bipolar II) (American Psychiatric Association, 2013). The length of the phases of depression and mania varies, lasting from days to weeks. BD is a lifelong disease that usually begins in adolescence. It is approximately one-third less common in older adults with lifetime prevalence rates of 0.5% to 1%. With the aging of the population, it is predicted that there will be a drastic increase of older adults with BD in the coming decades. BDs often stabilize in late life, but individuals tend to have longer periods of depression. Mania is a more frequent cause of hospitalization than depression, but depression may account for more disability. Similar to other psychiatric disorders in older adults, cues present differently than in younger adults. Comorbidities often mask the presence of the disorder and it is frequently misdiagnosed, underdiagnosed, and undertreated (Forester et al., 2015).

Recognizing and Analyzing Cues: BD

Diagnosis includes a thorough physical examination and laboratory and radiological testing to exclude physical causes of the symptoms and identify comorbidities. A medication review should be conducted because symptoms can be a side effect of medications. It is important to obtain an accurate history from the individual and the family, and this should include identification of symptoms associated with depression, mania, hypomania, and a family history of BD. Episodes of mania combined with depressed features and a family history of BD are highly indicative of the diagnosis (Box 24.12).

BOX 24.12   Focus on Genetics

Research on the genetic basis for mental health disorders such as depression, schizophrenia, and bipolar disorder is being conducted by the National Institute of Mental Health Center for Collaborative Genetic Studies on Mental Disorders (https://www.nimhgenetics .org/). The latest genome-wide study identified shared genetic risk factors between schizophrenia and bipolar disorder, bipolar disorder and depression, and schizophrenia and depression, the first evidence of overlap between these disorders. Continuous research on gene discovery for mental health disorders is ongoing.

Nursing Actions: BD

Pharmacotherapy

Lithium, the most commonly used substance for individuals with BDs, has neurological effects that make it difficult for older adults to tolerate. Lithium also has a long half-life (more than 36 hours), and dosing needs to be adjusted based on renal function. Medications that can affect urine production (diuretics) can alter lithium levels. Lithium levels, blood urea nitrogen (BUN) levels, and creatinine plasma levels need to be monitored closely. Anticonvulsant medications such as valproic acid, divalproex sodium, and lamotrigine are more commonly used in BD treatment, although the use of lamotrigine calls for monitoring for Stevens-Johnson syndrome. Medication levels and liver function tests must be monitored. Many of the anticonvulsant medications have an FDA warning that their use may increase suicide risk, therefore careful monitoring for changes in mood and behavior and signs of suicidal ideation is important.

Antidepressants such as fluoxetine, paroxetine, and venlafaxine can be used to treat depression in BD disorder in combination with other medications. Because these medications can trigger mania, careful assessment is important. Atypical antipsychotic drugs are also sometimes used, but with the same safety warnings discussed earlier, and are not to be used if neurocognitive disorders are suspected. Olanzapine, aripiprazole, and quetiapine are all approved for the treatment of BD and may relieve symptoms of severe mania and psychosis (Chapter 9).

Psychosocial Approaches

Patient and family education and support are essential, and the family must understand that the individual is not able to control mania and irritating behaviors because of a chemical imbalance in the brain. Treatment with medication and intensive psychotherapy; CBT; interpersonal and rhythm therapy (improving relationships with others and managing regular daily routines); and family-focused therapy have been reported to be effective in improving recovery rates.

Psychoeducation is an important component of all psychosocial interventions, and nurses can assist patients in learning about BD and its treatment. Psychoeducation should include developing an acceptance of the disorder, becoming aware of factors influencing symptoms and signs of relapse, learning how to communicate with others, and establishing regular sleep and activity habits. It is important to teach an individual to keep a log to monitor mood changes, activity levels, stressors, and amount of sleep. Medication regimens can be complicated, and many individuals struggle to adhere to them. An important nursing action is educating patients and families about the benefits and risks of prescribed medications, the importance of monitoring therapeutic effects, side effects, and the value of medication management systems.

DEPRESSION

Depression is not a normal part of aging, and studies show that most older adults are satisfied with their lives (National Institute on Aging, 2017). To understand depression, the nurse must understand the influence of late-life stressors and changes and the beliefs older adults, society, and health professionals may have about depression and its treatment.

Prevalence

Depression is a significant public issue and remains underdiagnosed and undertreated in the older adult population. The prevalence of depression among older adults ranges from 1% to 5%, but rates are at least two times higher in primary care and medical settings with 6% to 9% meeting the criteria for major depression (Bruce & Sirey, 2018; Centers for Disease Control and Prevention, 2017). Furthermore, depression is the leading cause of disability globally and a major factor in the burden of disease worldwide (World Health Organization, 2018). The prevalence of depressive disorders in older adults is expected to more than double by 2050 (Jeste et al., 2018).

Estimates are that 17% of older adults have symptoms of depression that do not meet the criteria for MDD; these symptoms are referred to as subsyndromal depression, dysthymic depression, and mild depression (Bruce & Sirey, 2018). The DSM-5 utilizes the term *persistent* depressive disorder to describe symptoms that are long-standing (lasting 2 years or longer) but do not meet the criteria for MDD. Recognition and treatment

are important because persistent depressive disorder has a negative impact on physical and social functioning and quality of life for many older adults and is associated with an increased risk of a subsequent major depression. There is limited research about older adults with mild depressive disorders.

Prevalence rates of depression in older adults probably underestimate the extent of the problem. The stigma associated with depression may be more prevalent in older adults, and they may not acknowledge depressive symptoms or seek treatment. Perceived stigma may be less of a concern for the future older adult population who are more aware of mental health concerns and more likely to seek treatment. Many older adults, particularly those who have survived the Great Depression, both world wars, the Holocaust, and other tragedies, may see depression as shameful, evidence of a flawed character, self-centered, a spiritual weakness, and sin or retribution.

Health professionals often expect older adults to be depressed and may not take appropriate action to assess for and treat depression. The differing presentation of depression in older adults and the increased prevalence of medical problems that may cause depressive symptoms also contribute to inadequate recognition and treatment. Even if depression is identified, most older adults with significant depression do not receive guideline-consistent, if any, depression treatment (Bruce & Sirey, 2018). All health care professionals must receive adequate education about depression in older adults in order to provide safe, effective care.

Consequences

Depression is a common and serious medical condition second only to heart disease in causing disability and harm to an individual's health and quality of life. Depression and depressive symptomatology are associated with negative consequences such as delayed recovery from illness and surgery, excess use of health services, cognitive impairment, exacerbation of coexisting medical illnesses, malnutrition, decreased quality of life, and increased suicide and non–suicide-related deaths. It is highly likely that nurses will encounter a large number of older adults with depressive symptoms in all settings. Recognizing depression and enhancing access to appropriate mental health care are important nursing roles to improve outcomes for older adults.

Etiology

The causes of depression in older adults are complex and must be examined in a biopsychosocial framework. Factors of health, gender, developmental needs, socioeconomics, environment, personality, losses, and

BOX 24.13 Medical Conditions and Depression

Cancers
Cardiovascular disorders
Endocrine disorders, such as thyroid problems and diabetes
Metabolic and nutritional disorders, such as vitamin B_{12} deficiency, malnutrition, diabetes
Neurological disorders, such as Alzheimer's disease, stroke, and Parkinson's disease
Viral infections, such as herpes zoster and hepatitis
Vision and hearing impairment

BOX 24.15 Risk Factors for Depression

- Chronic medical illnesses, disability, functional decline
- Alzheimer's disease and other dementias
- Bereavement
- Caregiving
- Female (2:1 risk)
- Socioeconomic deprivation
- Family history of depression
- Previous episode of depression
- Admission to long-term care or other change in environment
- Medications
- Alcohol or substance abuse
- Living alone
- Widowhood

functional decline are all significant to the development of depression in later life. Biological causes, such as neurotransmitter imbalances, have a strong association with many depressive disorders in late life. This may be a factor in the high incidence of depression in individuals with neurological conditions such as stroke, Parkinson's disease, and neurocognitive disorders.

Serious symptoms of depression occur in 30% to 50% of individuals with Alzheimer's disease, and depression is also a risk factor for dementia, particularly early-onset, recurrent, severe depression (Ryu, 2017). Among individuals with Alzheimer's disease, depression is the earliest observable symptom in at least one-third of cases (Jeste et al., 2018). Depression in individuals with Alzheimer's disease may be caused by an awareness of progressive decline, but research suggests that there may also be a biological connection between depression and Alzheimer's disease.

Medical disorders and medications can also result in depressive symptoms (Boxes 24.13 and 24.14). Other important factors influencing the development of depression are alcohol abuse, loss of a spouse or partner,

BOX 24.14 Medications and Depression

Antihypertensives
Angiotensin-converting enzyme (ACE) inhibitors
Methyldopa
Reserpine
Guanethidine
Antiarrhythmics
Anticholesteremic drugs
Antibiotics
Analgesics
Corticosteroids
Digoxin
L-Dopa

loss of social supports, lower income level, caregiver stress (particularly caring for a person with dementia), and gender. Some common risk factors for depression are presented in Box 24.15.

❖ USING CLINICAL JUDGMENT TO PROMOTE HEALTHY AGING: DEPRESSION

◆ Recognizing and Analyzing Cues: Depression

Making the diagnosis of depression in older adults can be challenging. Older adults who are depressed report more somatic complaints such as insomnia, loss of appetite, weight loss, memory loss, and chronic pain. It is often difficult to distinguish somatic complaints from the physical symptoms associated with chronic illness. Both symptoms must be evaluated. Decreased energy and motivation, lack of ability to experience pleasure, increased dependency, poor grooming and difficulty completing activities of daily living (ADLs), withdrawal from people or activities enjoyed in the past, decreased sexual interest, and a preoccupation with death or "giving up" are also signs of depression in older adults. Feelings of guilt and worthlessness, seen in younger depressed individuals, are less frequently seen in older adults.

Individuals often present with complaints of memory problems and a cognitive impairment of recent onset that mimics dementia but subsides upon remission of depression (previously called pseudodementia). It is important to note that a large percentage of these patients progress into irreversible dementia within 2 to 3 years, therefore recognition and treatment of depression are important. It is essential to differentiate between dementia and depression, and older adults with memory impairment should be evaluated for depression. Symptoms such as agitation, physically aggressive behavior, and repetitive verbalizations in persons with dementia may be indicators of depression (Cipriani et al., 2015) (Chapter 25).

Comprehensive evaluation involves a systematic and thorough evaluation using a depression screening instrument, interview, psychiatric and medical history, physical (with focused neurological examination), functional assessment, cognitive assessment, laboratory tests, medication review, determination of iatrogenic or medical causes, and family interview as indicated. A medication review including use of depressogenic medications, alcohol and substance abuse, and related comorbid physical conditions that may contribute to or complicate treatment of depression must also be included (Box 24.16).

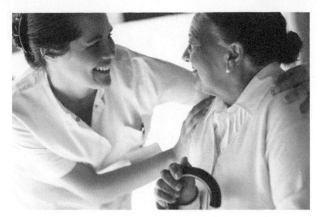

Creating hopeful environments in which meaningful activities and supportive relationships can be enjoyed is an important nursing role in the treatment of depression. (© iStock.com/Yuri.)

BOX 24.16 Tips for Best Practice

Depression

- Utilize a depression screening tool (GDS or Cornell if cognitive impairment).
- Assess for suicide: ask a direct question, "Have you thought of killing or harming yourself?"
- Investigate somatic complaints and look for underlying acute or chronic stressful events.
- Investigate sleep patterns, changes in appetite or weight, socialization pattern, level of physical activity, and substance abuse (past and present).
- Ask direct questions about psychosocial factors that may influence depression: elder abuse, poor environmental conditions, and changes in the patient role after death or disability of a spouse/partner.
- Obtain psychiatric and medical histories.
- Perform a physical exam including a focused neurological exam.
- Evaluate and treat chronic illnesses to improve outcomes and prevent exacerbations.
- Complete a functional assessment, paying close attention to changes in activities of daily living (ADL) function.
- Perform a cognitive assessment; depressed patients may show little effort during examination, answer "I don't know," and have inconsistent memory loss and performance during exam.
- Conduct a medication review (assessment for medications that may cause depressive symptoms).
- Assess for psychotic symptoms (delusions, hallucinations) and symptoms of bipolar disorder.
- Perform laboratory tests as appropriate to rule out other causes of symptoms (e.g., thyroid-stimulating hormone [TSH], T4, serum B12, vitamin D, folate, complete blood count, urinalysis).
- Utilize family/significant others in obtaining key information to correlate patient's symptoms with others' observations; always assess and interview patient first.

Screening all older adults for depression should be incorporated into routine health assessments across the continuum of care—in hospitals, primary care, long-term care, home care, and community-based settings. The Geriatric Depression Scale (GDS) was developed specifically for screening older adults and has been tested extensively in a number of settings. The Cornell Scale for Depression in Dementia (CSDD) is recommended for the assessment of depression in older adults with dementia (Chapter 8).

◆ Nursing Actions: Depression

The goals of depression treatment in older adults are to decrease symptoms, reduce relapse and recurrence, enhance function and quality of life, and reduce mortality and health care costs. Interventions are individualized and are based on history, severity of symptoms, concomitant illnesses, and level of disability. There are a wide range of treatments for depression, and outcomes for older adults are generally similar to those observed for younger populations. However, this may not be true for older adults who are frail with multiple medical comorbidities. Guidelines suggest that effective treatment for major depression is a combination of pharmacological therapy and psychotherapy or counseling with psychotherapy alone recommended as a first-line treatment in mild major depression. Psychotherapy is comparable to effective antidepressants (Kok & Reynolds, 2017).

◆ Nonpharmacological Approaches

Evidence-based nonpharmacological treatment options are needed for the treatment of depression, especially in primary care. CBT meets the highest level of evidence with a small but beneficial effect after meta-analysis. However, there are other promising options

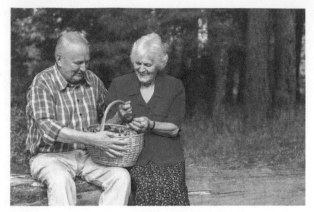

Older adults enjoying an activity together. (© iStock.com/Fred -Froese.)

for treatment, particularly in community settings, that could be delivered by nurses. Types of nonpharmacological treatment that have been found to be helpful in depression include family and social support, education, grief management, exercise, humor, spirituality, CBT, brief psychodynamic therapy, interpersonal therapy, reminiscence and life review therapy (Chapter 5), problem-solving therapy, and complementary therapy (e.g., tai chi) (Holvast et al., 2017). Exercise has been associated with a significant reduction in depressive symptoms (Seo & Chao, 2018) (Chapter 13). The development of effective, simplified, and accessible psychotherapeutic approaches, including Internet-based programs, geared toward older adults is important.

Despite evidence-based guidelines calling for combined pharmacological and psychotherapeutic treatment and the fact that older adults often prefer psychotherapy to psychiatric medications, psychological interventions are often not offered as an alternative. Reasons for this include time, reimbursement constraints, and a limited well-trained geriatric mental health workforce.

◆ Integrated care

The majority of older adults prefer to be treated for depression by primary care providers rather than mental health specialists. New models of care providing both primary and behavioral care in the same setting are designed to promote collaboration between primary care providers and mental health specialists in treating older adults. There is evidence that integrated care improves access, quality, and outcomes of depression treatment. The most effective models involve systematic depression screening, a depression care manager to work directly with the patients over time (often nurses), and the use of evidence-based depression treatment (Bruce & Sirey, 2018; Gilbody et al., 2017).

◆ Pharmacological Approaches

Antidepressants may effectively treat depression in older adults but have a high risk of adverse effects because of multiple medical comorbidities and drug–drug interactions from polypharmacy. Two-thirds of older adults who use antidepressants receive drugs that are either contraindicated or have the potential for moderate to major interactions (Holvast et al., 2017; Kok & Reynolds, 2017). Choice of medication depends on comorbidities, drug side effects, and the type of effect desired. People with agitated depression and sleep disturbances may benefit from medications with a more sedating effect, whereas those who are not eating may do better taking medications that have an appetite-stimulating effect.

The most commonly prescribed antidepressants are the SSRIs. These agents work selectively on neurotransmitters in the brain to alleviate depression. The SSRIs are generally well tolerated in older adults, but anticholinergic and sedative effects may be associated with physical and cognitive impairment. For those who do not respond to an adequate trial of SSRIs, there is another group of antidepressants that combines the inhibition of both serotonin and norepinephrine reuptake inhibitors (SNRIs) (e.g., venlafaxine [Effexor]). These may also be preferred by those who are engaged in or who anticipate sexual activity because they are less likely to have sexual side effects.

One of the atypical antidepressants, such as bupropion (Wellbutrin) or trazodone, may be used. In the context of reducing polypharmacy, Wellbutrin also reduces nicotine dependency, and trazodone is sedating—for a person who has difficulty getting to or staying asleep. Since the development of the SSRIs and SNRIs, the older monoamine oxidase (MAO) inhibitors and tricyclic antidepressants are no longer indicated because of their high side effect profile, including risk of falls.

All antidepressant medications must be closely monitored for side effects and therapeutic response. There are more than 20 antidepressants approved by the FDA for the treatment of depression in older adults, and several may have to be evaluated to determine the medication most effective for the individual. Similar to other medications for older adults, doses should be lower at first (50% of the target dose) and titrated as indicated until adequate treatment effect is ensured. If the patient has responded to treatment, it is not clear how long the medication should be continued, but if there is a lifetime history of depression, recommendations are that pharmacotherapy should be maintained for at least 2 years to prevent recurrence (Kok & Reynolds, 2017) (Chapter 9).

◆ Other Treatments

Electroconvulsive therapy (ECT) is the most effective treatment for older adults with major depression with efficacy ranging from 60% to 80%. ECT is also indicated for patients at risk of severe harm because of psychotic depression, suicidal ideation, severe malnutrition, or a medical condition that worsens because they refuse medication (Kok & Reynolds, 2017). ECT results in a more immediate response in symptoms and is also a useful alternative for frail older adults with multiple comorbid conditions who are unable to tolerate antidepressant treatment. ECT is much improved, but older adults will need a careful explanation of the treatment because they may have many misconceptions.

Rapid transcranial magnetic stimulation (rTMS) is a treatment approved in 2008 by the FDA to treat MDD in adults for whom medication was not effective or tolerated. The treatment consists of administering brief magnetic pulses to the brain by passing high currents through an electromagnetic coil adjacent to the patient's scalp. The targeted magnetic pulses stimulate the circuits in the brain that are underactive in patients with depression with the goal of restoring normal function and mood. For most patients, treatment is administered in 30- to 40-minute sessions over a period of 4 to 6 weeks. The effectiveness of the treatment is still being evaluated in older adults. TMS is contraindicated for persons who have seizures, stroke, brain injury/trauma/surgery, pacemakers, or intracranial magnetic devices. Box 24.17 presents suggestions for families and professionals caring for older adults with depression.

SUICIDE

Suicide is the 10th leading cause of death in the United States. In 2017, the highest suicide rate was among adults between 45 and 54 years of age. The second highest rate occurred in those 85 years or older. Among racial/ethnic populations, Whites had the highest suicide rate (accounting for 69.6% of suicide deaths), followed by American Indian/Alaska Natives (American Foundation for Suicide Prevention, 2020). Women in all countries have much lower suicide rates, possibly because of greater flexibility in coping skills based on multiple roles that women fill throughout their lives. Despite these alarming statistics, there is little research on suicide ideation and behavior among older adults.

In most cases, depression and other mental health problems, including anxiety, contribute significantly to suicide risk. Common precipitants of suicide in older adults include physical or mental illness, death of a spouse or partner, substance abuse, chronic pain, limited social support, living alone, financial strain, and a history of suicide attempts. One of the major

---

BOX 24.17   Tips for Best Practice

Family and Professional Support for Depression

- Provide relief from discomfort of physical illness.
- Enhance physical function (i.e., regular exercise and/or activity; physical, occupational, recreational therapies).
- Develop a daily activity schedule that includes pleasant activities, opportunities for socialization and social support
- Provide opportunities for decision-making and the exercise of control.
- Focus on spiritual renewal and rediscovery of meanings.
- Reactivate latent interests, or develop new ones.
- Validate depressed feelings as aiding recovery; do not try to bolster the person's mood or deny his or her despair.
- Help the person become aware of the presence of depression, the nature of the symptoms, and the availability of effective treatments.
- Emphasize depression as a medical, not mental, illness that must be treated like any other disorder.
- Provide easy-to-use educational materials to older adults and family members
- Demonstrate faith in the person's strengths.
- Praise any and all efforts at recovery, no matter how small.
- Assist in expressing and dealing with anger.
- Do not stifle the grief process; grief cannot be hurried.

---

differences in suicidal behavior in the old and the young is the lethality of method. Eight out of 10 suicides for men older than 65 years of age were with firearms and firearms account for 51% of all suicides (American Foundation for Suicide Prevention, 2020) (Chapter 16).

Many older adults who commit suicide reached out for help before they took their own life. Three-fourths of older adults who commit suicide had seen their physician within 1 month before death; 40% had visited within 1 week of the suicide, and 20% had visited the physician on the day of the suicide (American Psychological Association, 2018). Depression is frequently missed, and older adults with suicide ideation or with other mental health concerns often present with somatic complaints. The statistics suggest that opportunities for assessment of suicidal risk are present, but the need for intervention is not seen as urgent or even recognized. Consequently, it is very important for providers in all settings to inquire about recent life events, implement depression screening, evaluate for anxiety disorders, assess for suicidal thoughts and ideas based on depression assessment, and recognize warning signs and risk factors for suicide.

❖ USING CLINICAL JUDGMENT TO PROMOTE HEALTHY AGING: SUICIDAL RISK

◆ Recognizing and Analyzing Cues: Suicidal Risk

Older adults with suicidal intent are encountered in many settings. It is our professional obligation to prevent, whenever possible, an impulsive destruction of life that may be a response to a crisis or a disintegrative reaction. The lethality potential of an older adult must always be assessed when elements of depression, disease, and spousal loss are evident. Any direct, indirect, or enigmatic references to the ending of life must be taken seriously and discussed.

In the nursing home setting, the Minimum Data Set (MDS) (Chapter 8) includes screening for suicide risk and mandates that long-term care facilities have effective protocols for managing suicide risk. "Suicide prevention cannot be limited to hospital, primary care, and clinic settings, but rather must reach into communities and culture" (Butcher & Ingram, 2018, p. 29). Every older adult should be screened for suicidal ideation at each primary care visit. If the older adult has personal, medical, or situational risk factors, screening should take place every 6 months or more frequently if indicated.

Recognition and analysis of cues to potential suicide should include: (1) identification of risk factors, medical problems, medications, functional status, nutritional status, personal and family psychiatric history, alcohol or substance drug use, and complete physical and neurological exam; (2) evaluation of cognitive function; (3) psychological strengths, coping skills, spirituality, sexuality, suicidal ideation, past attempts at suicide; and (4) quantity and quality of social support, financial status, legal history, and potential for elder abuse (Butcher & Ingram, 2018). Evaluating gun safety and risk of injury is important in older adults. Older adults have the highest rates of gun ownership in the United States, and gun ownership is a significant risk factor for suicide in this age group. Chapter 16 provides a protocol for gun safety assessment. Other resources can be found in Box 24.4.

The most important consideration for a nurse is to establish a trusting and respectful relationship with the person. Because many older adults have grown up in an era when suicide bore stigma and even criminal implications, they may not discuss their feelings in this area. It is also important to remember that in older adults, typical behavioral clues such as putting personal affairs in order, giving away possessions, and making wills and funeral plans are indications of maturity and good judgment in late life and cannot be construed as indicative of suicidal intent. Even statements such as "I won't be around long" or "I'm ready to die" may be only a realistic appraisal of the situation in old age.

If there is suspicion that the older adult is suicidal, use direct and straightforward questions such as the following:
- Have you ever thought about killing yourself?
- How often have you had these thoughts?
- How would you kill yourself if you decided to do it?

⚡ SAFETY ALERT

Always ask direct questions of the patient and family about suicide risks and suicide ideation.

◆ Nursing Actions: Suicidal Risk

It is important to have a suicide protocol in place that clearly defines how the nurse will intervene if a positive response is obtained from any of the questions. The person should never be left alone for any period of time until help arrives to assist and care for him or her. Patients at high risk should be hospitalized, especially if they have current psychological stressors and/or access to lethal means. Patients at lower risk may be treated as outpatients provided they have adequate social support and no access to lethal means. Other crisis interventions include partial hospitalization, day treatment, antidepressant medications, communicating risk to family, care management, counseling, support groups, assistance with financial stress, increased social involvement, and increased activity with faith community (Butcher & Ingram, 2018).

Suicide is a taboo topic for most of us, and there is a lingering fear that the introduction of the topic will be suggestive to the patient and may incite suicidal action. Precisely the opposite is true. By introducing the topic, we demonstrate interest in the individual and open the door to honest human interaction and connection on the deep levels of psychological need. It is the nature of our concern and our ability to connect with the alienation and desperation of the individual that will make a difference.

SUBSTANCE USE DISORDERS

Substance abuse among older adults is one of the fastest-growing health problems in the United States. The baby boomer generation has had more exposure to alcohol and illegal drugs in their youth and has a more lenient attitude about substance abuse. Additionally, psychoactive drugs became more readily available for dealing with anxiety, pain, and stress. Although alcohol remains the most frequent reason for admission to substance abuse treatment, this proportion is declining. Cocaine- and

BOX 24.18 Healthy People 2020

Substance Abuse Objectives for Adults

- Increase the proportion of persons who need alcohol and/or illicit drug treatment and received specialty treatment for abuse or dependence in the past year.
- Increase the proportion of persons who are referred for follow-up care for alcohol problems, drug problems after diagnosis, or treatment for one of these conditions in a hospital emergency department.
- Increase the number of Level I and Level II trauma centers and primary care settings that implement evidence-based alcohol Screening and Brief Intervention (SBI).
- Reduce the proportion of adults who drank excessively in the previous 30 days.
- Reduce average alcohol consumption.
- Reduce the past-year nonmedical use of prescription drugs (pain relievers, tranquilizers, stimulants, sedatives, any psychotherapeutic drug).
- Decrease the number of deaths attributable to alcohol.

From US Department of Health and Human Services, Office of Disease Prevention and Health Promotion. (2012). *Healthy People 2020*. http://www.healthypeople.gov/2020.

heroin-related admissions are on the rise in the older adults and the incidence of opioid abuse and misuse is also increasing (Jeste et al., 2018). Despite these increases, substance abuse in older adults remains an underrecognized and undertreated public health concern. "Screening and prevention of unhealthy substance abuse is critical to address the potential enormous public health impact of increasing substance use by older adults" (Han & Moore, 2018, p. 117) (Box 24.18).

Alcohol Use Disorder

Prevalence and Characteristics

Alcoholism is the third most prevalent psychiatric disorder (after dementia and anxiety) among older men. Alcohol remains the most commonly used substance among older adults and is expected to increase considerably. The most severe alcohol abuse is seen in people aged 60 to 80 years, but not in those older than 80 years. Two-thirds of older adults with alcohol abuse are early-onset drinkers (alcohol use began at 30 or 40 years of age), and one-third are late-onset drinkers (use began after 60 years of age). Late-onset drinking may be related to situational events such as illness, retirement, or death of a spouse and includes a higher number of women (Campbell et al., 2014). Alcohol-related problems in older adults often go unrecognized, although the residual effects of alcohol abuse complicate the presentation and treatment of many chronic disorders.

Gender Issues

Although men (particularly older widowers) are four times more likely to abuse alcohol than women, the prevalence in women may be underestimated. The number and impact of older female drinkers are expected to increase over the next 20 years as the disparity between men's and women's drinking decreases. Women of all ages are significantly more vulnerable to the effects of alcohol misuse, including faster progression to dependence and earlier onset of adverse consequences. Even low-risk drinking levels (no more than one standard drink per day) can be hazardous for older women. Older women also experience unique barriers to detection of and treatment for alcohol problems.

Physiology

Older adults, especially females, develop higher blood alcohol levels because of age-related changes (increased body fat, decreased lean body mass, and total body water content) that alter absorption and distribution of alcohol. Decreases in hepatic metabolism and kidney function also slow alcohol metabolism and elimination. A decrease in the gastric enzyme alcohol dehydrogenase results in slower metabolism of alcohol and higher blood levels for a longer time.

Consequences

The health consequences of long-term alcohol use disorder include cirrhosis of the liver, cancer, immune system disorders, cardiomyopathy, cerebral atrophy, dementia, and suicide. Other effects of alcohol in older adults include urinary incontinence, which results from rapid bladder filling and diminished neuromuscular control of the bladder; gait disturbances from alcohol-induced cerebellar degeneration and peripheral neuropathy; depression; functional decline; increased risk for injury; and sleep disturbances and insomnia. Alcohol misuse has also been implicated as a major factor in morbidity and mortality as a result of trauma, including falls, drownings, fires, motor vehicle crashes, homicide, and suicide.

Alcohol use also exacerbates conditions such as osteoporosis, diabetes, hypertension, and ulcers. Many drugs that older adults use for chronic illnesses cause adverse effects when combined with alcohol (Box 24.19). All older adults should be given precise instructions regarding the interaction of alcohol with their medications.

Alcohol Guidelines for Older Adults

The possible health benefits of alcohol in moderation have been reported in the literature (reduced risk of coronary artery disease, ischemic stroke, Alzheimer's disease, and vascular dementia). As a result, older adults

---

BOX 24.19 Medications Interacting With Alcohol

Analgesics

Antibiotics

Antidepressants

Antipsychotics

Benzodiazepines

H2-receptor antagonists

Nonsteroidal anti-inflammatory drugs (NSAIDs)

Herbal medications (echinacea, valerian)

Acetaminophen taken on a regular basis, when combined with alcohol, may lead to liver failure

Alcohol diminishes the effects of oral hypoglycemics, anticoagulants, and anticonvulsants

---

may not perceive alcohol use as potentially harmful. Because of the increased risk of adverse effects from alcohol use, the National Institute of Alcohol Abuse and Alcoholism defines "at-risk drinking" for men and women aged 65 years and older as more than one drink per day (Box 24.20). Health professionals must share information with older adults about safe drinking limits and the deleterious effects of alcohol intake.

BOX 24.20 National Institute on Alcohol Abuse and Alcoholism Guidelines for Alcohol Use in Older Adults

Definition of a Standard Drink

- One 12-ounce can or bottle of regular beer, ale, or wine cooler
- One 8- or 9-ounce can or bottle of malt liquor
- One 5-ounce glass of red or white wine
- One 1.5 ounce shot glass of distilled spirit (gin, rum, tequila, vodka, whiskey, etc.). Label on bottle will say 80 proof or less

From National Institute on Alcohol Abuse and Alcoholism. *What is a standard drink?* https://www.niaaa.nih.gov/what-standard-drink.

❖ USING CLINICAL JUDGMENT TO PROMOTE HEALTHY AGING: ALCOHOL USE DISORDER

◆ Recognizing and Analyzing Cues: Alcohol Use Disorder

Alcohol and other substance use–related problems among older adults are too frequently undetected by health care professionals. The challenges associated with recognizing and analyzing cues of alcohol use problems include poor symptom recognition, lack of provider training, inadequate knowledge of screening instruments, lack of time, skepticism about benefits, fear of patient reactions, and the belief that patients will not be candid about substance use (DiBartolo et al., 2017). Alcohol-related problems may be overlooked in older adults because they do not drastically disrupt their lives or are not clearly linked to physical disorders. Health care providers may also be pessimistic about the ability of older adults to change long-standing problems.

The US Preventive Services Task Force (2018) recommends that adults 18 years and older in primary care should be screened by clinicians for alcohol misuse. Screening should be a part of health visits for people older than the age of 60 years in primary, acute, and long-term care settings (Sorrell, 2017). Although alcohol is the drug most often used among older adults, assessment should include all substances used (recreational drugs, prescription, nicotine, and OTC medications) (Han & Moore, 2018).

The Hartford Institute of Geriatric Nursing recommends that the Short Michigan Alcoholism Screening Test–Geriatric Version be used with older adults because it is more age appropriate than other instruments (Table 24.1). A single question can also be used for alcohol screening: "How many times in the past year have you had 5 or more drinks in a day (if a man), or 4 or more drinks (if you are a woman older than 65 years of age)?" If the individual acknowledges drinking that much, follow-up assessment is indicated.

Depression is often comorbid with alcohol abuse, and both alcohol and depression screenings should be offered routinely at health fairs and other sites where older adults may seek health information. A medication review should be conducted and screening should be done both before prescribing any new medications that may interact with alcohol and as needed after life-changing events. Alcohol abuse should be suspected in an older adult who presents with a history of falling, unexplained bruises, or medical problems associated with alcohol abuse problems.

Alcoholism is a disease of denial and not easy to diagnose, particularly in older adults with psychosocial and functional decline from other conditions that may mask decline caused by alcohol. Early signs such as weight loss, irritability, insomnia, and falls may not be recognized as indicators of possible alcohol problems and may be attributed to "just getting older." Box 24.21 presents signs and symptoms that may indicate the presence of alcohol problems in older adults.

Alcohol users often reject or deny the diagnosis or they may take offense at the suggestion of it. Feelings of shame or disgrace may make older adults reluctant to disclose a drinking problem. Families of older adults with substance use disorders, particularly their adult children, may be ashamed of the problem and choose

TABLE 24.1 Short Michigan Alcoholism Screening Test—Geriatric Version (S-MAST-G)ᵃ

	Yes (1)	No (0)
1. When talking with others, do you ever underestimate how much you drink?		
2. After a few drinks, have you sometimes not eaten, or been able to skip a meal, because you didn't feel hungry?		
3. Does having a few drinks help decrease your shakiness or tremors?		
4. Does alcohol sometimes make it hard for you to remember parts of the day or night?		
5. Do you usually take a drink to relax or to calm your nerves?		
6. Do you drink alcohol to take your mind off your problems?		
7. Have you ever increased your drinking after experiencing a loss in your life?		
8. Has a doctor or nurse ever said they were worried or concerned about your drinking?		
9. Have you ever made rules to manage your drinking?		
10. When you feel lonely, does having a drink help?		
TOTAL S-MAST-G SCORE* (1–10)		

ᵃScoring: 2 or more "Yes" responses indicate an alcohol problem.
From the Regents of the University of Michigan. (1991). *Short Michigan alcohol screening test—geriatric version (S-MAST-G)*. Ann Arbor, MI, University of Michigan Alcohol Research Center.

BOX 24.21 Recognizing and Analyzing Cues to Potential Alcohol Problems in Older Adults

Anxiety
Irritability (feeling worried or "crabby")
Blackouts
Dizziness
Indigestion
Heartburn
Sadness or depression
Chronic pain
Excessive mood swings
New problems making decisions
Lack of interest in usual activities
Falls
Bruises, burns, or other injuries
Family conflict, abuse
Headaches
Incontinence
Memory loss
Poor hygiene
Poor nutrition
Insomnia
Sleep apnea
Social isolation
Out of touch with family or friends
Unusual response to medications
Frequent physical complaints and physician visits
Financial problems

not to address it. Health care providers may feel helpless over alcoholism or uncomfortable with direct questioning or may approach the person in a judgmental manner. A caring and supportive approach that provides a safe and open atmosphere is the foundation for the therapeutic relationship. It is always important to search for the pain beneath the behavior.

◆ Nursing Actions: Alcohol Use Disorder

Alcohol problems affect physical, mental, spiritual, and emotional health. Actions must address quality of life in all of these spheres and be adapted to meet the unique needs of the older adult. Abstinence from alcohol is seen as the desired goal, but a focus on education, alcohol reduction, and reducing harm is also appropriate. Increasing the awareness of older adults about the risks and benefits of alcohol consumption in the context of their own situation is an important goal. Treatment and intervention strategies include cognitive-behavioral approaches, individual and group counseling, medical and psychiatric approaches, referral to Alcoholics Anonymous, family therapy, case management and community and home care services, and formalized substance abuse treatment. Treatment outcomes for older adults have been shown to be equal to or better than those for younger people (Campbell et al., 2014). Providing education about alcohol use to older adults and their families and referring to community resources are important nursing roles and essential to best practices.

Unless the person is in immediate danger, a stepped-care intervention approach beginning with brief interventions followed by more intensive therapies, if necessary, should be used. The US Preventive Services Task Force (2018) recommends brief counseling interventions to reduce alcohol use by adults. Brief intervention is a time-limited, patient-centered strategy focused on changing behavior and assessing patient readiness to change. Sessions can range from one meeting of 10 to 30 minutes to four or five short sessions. The goals of brief intervention are (1) to reduce or stop alcohol consumption and (2) to facilitate entry into formalized treatment if needed. Research results indicate that this type of intervention, with counseling by nurses in primary care settings, is effective for reducing alcohol consumption, and older adults may be more likely to accept treatment given by their primary care provider.

Long-term self-help treatment programs for older adults show high rates of success, especially when social outlets are emphasized and cohort supports are available. A significant concern is the lack of programs designed specifically for older adults, particularly older women, whose concerns are very different from those of a younger population who abuse drugs or alcohol. Health status, availability of transportation, and mobility impairments may further limit access to treatment. Development of treatment sites in senior centers and ALFs and telemedicine programs would increase accessibility.

Pharmacological treatment has not played a major role in the long-term treatment of alcohol-dependent older adults, but two medications, naltrexone (Revia) and acamprosate (Campral), are approved for treatment and have been used effectively with older adults. Disulfiram (Antabuse) is seldom used in older adults because of concerns about cardiovascular adverse effects (Campbell et al., 2014). Additional resources are presented in Box 24.4.

Acute Alcohol Withdrawal

When there is significant physical dependence, withdrawal from alcohol can become a life-threatening emergency. Detoxification should be done in an inpatient setting because of the potential medical complications and because withdrawal symptoms in older adults can be prolonged. Older adults who drink are at risk of experiencing acute alcohol withdrawal if admitted to the hospital for treatment of acute illnesses or emergencies. All patients admitted to acute care settings should be screened for alcohol use and assessed for signs and symptoms of alcohol-related problems. Older adults with a long history of consuming excess alcohol, previous episodes of acute withdrawal, and/or a history of prior detoxification are at increased risk of acute alcohol withdrawal.

OTHER SUBSTANCE ABUSE CONCERNS

Cannabis Use

The same physiologic changes with aging that increase the effect of alcohol in older adults also increase the effect of other drugs including benzodiazepines, opioids, and cannabis. With changes in attitudes toward cannabis, its legalization for recreational use in several states, and its increasing use for medicinal purposes, there has been a sharp increase in cannabis use among older adults. Health care providers need to be aware that their older patients may be using cannabis. A majority of older adults use cannabis medically or recreationally without problems, but there has been limited research of its effects on older adults. It is important to better understand both the benefits and risks of cannabis use so that health care professionals can educate and advise patients. Co-use of alcohol and the interaction of cannabis with other drugs and prescription medications needs further study (Choi et al., 2019; Han & Palamore, 2020; Wallace, 2019).

Prescription Drug Misuse

A more common concern seen among older adults is the misuse and abuse of prescription psychoactive medications. Dependence on sedative, hypnotic, or anxiolytic drugs, often prescribed for anxiety or insomnia and taken for many years with resulting dependence, is especially problematic for older women, who are more likely than men to receive prescriptions for these drugs (Markota et al., 2016). There have been dramatic increases in emergency department visits involving prescription misuse by adults 50 years and older with pain relievers and medications for insomnia and anxiety most often involved (Han & Moore, 2018).

Some of the reasons for the abuse of psychoactive prescription medications may be inappropriate prescribing and ineffective monitoring of response and follow-up. In many instances, older adults are given prescriptions for benzodiazepines or sedatives because of complaints of insomnia or nervousness, without adequate assessment for depression, anxiety, or other conditions that may be causing the symptoms. Older adults may not be informed of the side effects of these medications, including interactions with alcohol, dependence, and withdrawal symptoms. More importantly, conditions such as anxiety and depression may not be recognized and treated appropriately. STAMP Out Prescription Drug Misuse and Abuse Toolkit is an excellent resource for health care professionals to use in education about prescription drug misuse and abuse in older adults (Box 24.4).

KEY CONCEPTS

- The prevalence of mental health disorders is expected to increase significantly with the aging of the baby boomers.
- Older adults present with different cues of mental health problems. Recognizing and analyzing cues and identification of evaluation of nursing actions to promote mental health are essential.
- Mental health disorders are underreported and underdiagnosed among older adults. Somatic complaints are often the presenting symptoms of mental health disorders, making recognition of cues difficult and different than in younger adults.
- The incidence of psychotic disorders with late-life onset is low among older adults, but psychotic manifestations can occur as secondary symptoms in a variety of disorders, the most common being Alzheimer's disease.
- Psychotic symptoms in Alzheimer's disease necessitate different analysis and treatment than do long-standing psychotic disorders.
- Anxiety disorders are common in late life, and reestablishing feelings of adequacy and control is the heart of crisis resolution and stress management.
- Depression remains underdiagnosed and undertreated in the older population and is considered a significant public health issue. Depression in older adults can be effectively treated. Unfortunately, it is often neglected or assumed to be a condition of aging that one must "learn to live with." Screening and identification of depression is an important nursing action.
- Suicide is a significant problem among older men, particularly widowers. Many persons considering suicide are seen by the health care professional with physical complaints shortly before they commit suicide. Identification of depression and suicidal intent is important in primary care visits.
- Substance abuse, particularly alcohol, and misuse of prescription drugs are often underrecognized and undertreated problems of older adults, particularly older women. Screening and appropriate identification of concerns and intervention are important in all settings.
- Treatment outcomes for substance abuse for older adults are equal to or better than those for younger people.

ACTIVITIES AND DISCUSSION QUESTIONS

1. Discuss the three most common mental health disturbances that older adults are likely to experience and describe appropriate assessment and treatment.
2. What is likely to be different in the appearance of depression in a person who is 70 years old compared with its appearance in a person who is 20 years old?
3. Describe a time when you were depressed and discuss the feelings you experienced. What did you do about it?
4. Ask classmates who are from a different race or cultural group how they view depression.
5. What behaviors are indicative of suicidal intent in an older adult?
6. With a partner, assess for suicidal intent using the questions posed in the text.
7. What type of teaching would you provide to an older adult related to the use of alcohol and medications?

NEXT-GENERATION NCLEX® EXAMINATION-STYLE QUESTIONS

Mrs. Andrews, a 68-year-old female, is admitted to the medical/surgical unit with acute cystitis. She has a history of type 2 diabetes, hypertension, osteoporosis, and coronary artery disease. She has a 60-pack-year history of smoking and states she usually has a glass of wine at night to help her sleep. Admission laboratory work from the morning reveals a WBC count of 12.5×10^9/L, hemoglobin of 10.5 g/dL and hematocrit of 32%, MCV 105/dL, platelet count of 150×10^9/L, BUN 27 mg/dL creatinine 1.8 mg/dL, sodium 145 mmol/L, GGT 100 U/L, ALT 110 U/L, AST 96, and albumin 3.0 g/dL. While making hourly rounds, the nurse notes Mrs. Andrews is awake and restless at midnight. The nurse checks her vital signs and records a blood pressure of 150/88 mmHg, heart rate of 115 beats per minutes, respirations of 18 breaths per minute, and a temperature of 99.1°F. Mrs. Andrews states she has an upset stomach and can't get comfortable because of the noise "from her neighbor's constant partying."

Which interventions should the nurse include to best address the client's needs? Select all that apply.

1. Reduce environmental stimuli
2. Keep TV on to reorient the client
3. Request order for nutritional assessment
4. Monitor body temperature
5. Assess response to commands
6. Ensure consistent caregivers
7. Put all side rails up for safety
8. Ensure fluid balance is maintained

REFERENCES

American Foundation for Suicide Prevention. (2020). *Suicide statistics.* https://afsp.org/about-suicide/suicide-statistics/.
American Psychiatric Association. (2013). *Diagnostic and statistical manual of mental disorders* (ed. 5). Arlington: American Psychiatric Publishing.

American Psychological Association. (2020a). *Growing mental and behavioral concerns facing older adults*. https://www.apa.org/advocacy/health/older-americans-mental-behavioral-health.

American Psychological Association. (2020b). *Disparities in mental health status and mental health care*. https://www.apa.org/advocacy/health-disparities/health-care-reform.

Balsamo, M., Cataldi, F., Carlucci, L., & Fairfield, B. (2018). Assessment of anxiety in older adults: a review of self-report measures. *Clinical Intervention Aging, 13*, 573–593.

Butcher, H., & Ingram, T. (2018). Evidence-based practice guideline. Secondary prevention of late-life suicide. *Journal of Gerontology Nursing, 44*(11), 20–32.

Brenes, G. A., Danhauer, S. C., Lyles, M. F., & Miller, M. E. (2014). Telephone-delivered psychotherapy for rural-dwelling older adults with generalized anxiety disorder: study protocol of a randomized controlled trial. *BMC Psychiatry, 14*, 34.

Bruce, M. L., & Sirey, J. A. (2018). Integrated care for depression in older primary care patients. *Canadian Journal of Psychiatry, 63*(7), 439–446.

Campbell, J., Resnick, B., & Warshaw, G. (2014). Alcoholism. In R. Ham, P. Sloane, & G. Warshaw (Eds.), *Primary care geriatrics* (ed. 6, pp. 365–371). Philadelphia, PA: Elsevier.

Center for Medicare Advocacy: *Medical coverage of mental health and substance abuse services*. https://www.medicareadvocacy.org/medicare-info/medicare-coverage-of-mental-health-services/.

Centers for Disease Control and Prevention. (2017). *Depression is not a normal part of growing older*. https://www.cdc.gov/aging/mentalhealth/depression.htm.

Choi, N. G., DiNitto, D., & Arndt, S. (2019). Potential harms of marijuana use among older adults. *Public Policy & Aging Report, 29*(3), 88–94.

Christianson, S., & Marren, J. (2013). *Impact of Event Scale-Revised (IES-R)*. New York, NY: Hartford Institute for Geriatric Nursing.

Cipriani, G., Lucetti, C., Carlesi, C., Danti, S., & Nuti, A. (2015). Depression and dementia: a review. *European Geriatrics Medicine, 6*(5), 479–486.

Clapp, J. (2016). The diagnosis and treatment of post-traumatic stress disorder in older adults. *Annals Longterm Care, 24*(2), 12–16.

Clifford, K. M., Duncan, N. A., Heinrich, K., & Shaw, J. (2015). Update on managing generalized anxiety disorder in older adults. *Journal Gerontology Nursing, 41*(4), 10–20.

Creighton, A. S., Davison, T. E., & Kissane, D. W. (2018). The prevalence, reporting, and treatment of anxiety among older adults in nursing homes and other residential aged care facilities. *Journal of Affective Disorder, 227*, 416–423.

DiBartolo, M. C., & Jarosinski, J. M. (2017). Alcohol use disorder in older adults: challenges in assessment and treatment. *Issues in Mental Health Nursing, 38*(1), 25–32.

Department of Veterans Affairs. (2019). *PTSD treatment basics*. https://www.ptsd.va.gov/understand_tx/tx_basics.asp.

Forester, B., Aijilore, O., Spino, C., & Lehmann, S. (2015). Clinical characteristics of patients with late life bipolar disorder in the community: data from the NNDC registry. *The American Journal of Geriatric Psychiatry, 23*(9), 977–984.

Fung, A. W. T., Lee, J. S. W., Lee, A. T. C., & Lam, L. C. W. (2018). Anxiety symptoms predicted decline in episodic memory in cognitively health older adults: a 3-year prospective study. *International Journal Geriatrics Psychiatry, 33*(5), 748–754.

Gates, J., Killackey, E., Phillips, L., & Álvarez-Jiménez, M. (2015). Mental health starts with physical health: current status and future directions of non-pharmacological interventions to improve physical health in first-episode psychosis. *Lancet Psychiatry, 2*, 726–742.

Gilbody, S., Lewis, H., Adamson, J., et al. (2017). Effect of collaborative care vs. usual care on depressive symptoms in older adults with subthreshold depression: the CASPER randomized clinical trial. *JAMA, 317*(7), 728–737.

Gradus, J. L. (2017). *Epidemiology of PTSD. U.S. Department of Veterans Affairs*. https://www.ptsd.va.gov/professional/treat/essentials/epidemiology.asp.

Hall, K. S., Morey, M. C., Beckham, J. C., et al. (2018). The Warrior Wellness study: a randomized controlled exercise trial for older veterans with PTSD. *Translational Journal of American Collage Sports Medicine, 3*(6), 43–51.

Han, B. H., & Moore, A. A. (2018). Prevention and screening of unhealthy substance use by older adults. *Clinics in Geriatrics Medicine, 34*(1), 117–129.

Han, B., & Palamore, J. (2020). Trends in cannabis use among older adults in the United States, 2015-2018. *JAMA International Medicine*. doi.org/10.1001/jamainternmed.2019.7517. Published online February 24, 2020.

Hildon, Z., Montgomery, S., Blane, D., et al. (2009). Examining resilience of quality of life in the face of health-related and psychosocial adversity at older ages: What is "right" about the way we age?. *Gerontologist, 50*, 36–47.

Holvast, F., Massoudi, B., Oude Voshaar, R. C., & Verhaak, P. F. (2017). Non-pharmacological treatment for depressed older patients in primary care: a systematic review and meta-analysis. *PLOS One, 12*(9), e0184666.

Hoy-Ellis, C. P., Ator, M., Kerr, C., & Milford, J. (2016). Innovative approaches address aging and mental health needs in LGBTQ communities. *Journal American Society Aging, 40*(2), 56–62.

Hjorthøj, C., Stürup, A. E., McGrath, J. J., & Nordentoft, M. (2017). Life expectancy and years of potential life lost in schizophrenia: a systematic review and meta-analysis. *Lancet Psychiatry, 4*(4), 295–301.

Jeste, D. V., Peschin, S., Buckwalter, K., et al. (2018). Promoting wellness in older adults with mental illnesses and substance use disorders: call to action to all stakeholders. *American Journal of Geriatrics Psychiatry, 26*(6), 617–630.

Klainin-Yobas, P., Oo, W. N., Suzanne Yew, P. Y., & Lau, Y. (2015). Effects of relaxation interventions on depression and anxiety among older adults: a systematic review. *Aging Mental Health, 19*(12), 1043–1055.

Kok, R. M., & Reynolds, C. F, III. (2017). Management of depression in older adults a review. *JAMA, 317*(20), 2114–2122.

Kruse, C. S., Krowski, N., Rodriguez, B., Tran, L., Vela, J., & Brooks, M. (2017). Telehealth and patient satisfaction: systematic review and narrative analysis. *BMJ Open, 7*(8), e016242.

Markota, M., Rummans, T. A., Bostwick, J. M., & Lapid, M. I. (2016). Benzodiazepine use in older adults: dangers, management, and alternative therapies. *Mayo Clinic Proceeding, 91*(11), 1632–1639.

Maust, D. T., Kales, H. C., Wiechers, I. R., Blow, F. C., & Olfson, M. (2016). No end in sight: benzodiazepine use among older adults in the United States. *Journal of the American Geriatric Society, 64*(12), 2546–2553.

Mushkin, P., Band-Winterstein, T., & Avieli, H. (2018). Like every normal person?!" The paradoxical effect of aging with schizophrenia. *Quality Health Research, 28*(6), 977–986.

National Institute of Mental Health: *Post-traumatic stress disorder*. (2019). https://www.nimh.nih.gov/health/topics/post-traumatic-stress-disorder-ptsd/index.shtml.

National Institute on Aging: *Depression and older adults*. (2017). https://www.nia.nih.gov/health/depression-and-older-adults.

Reynolds, K., Pietrzak, R. H., Mackenzie, C. S., Chou, K. L., & Sareen, J. (2016). Post-traumatic stress disorder across the adult life span: findings from a nationally representative survey. *American Journal Geriatric Psychiatry, 24*(1), 81–93.

Ryu, S. H, Jung, H. Y., Lee, K. J., et al. (2017). Incidence and course of description in patients with Alzheimer's disease. *Psychiatry Investig, 14*(3), 271–280.

Seo, J. Y., & Chao, Y. Y. (2018). Effects of exercise intervention on depressive symptoms among community-dwelling older adults in the United States: a systematic review. *Journal of the Gerontology Nursing, 44*(3), 31–38.

SAMHSA-HRSA Center for Integrated Health Solutions: *Behavioral health in primary care.* (2018). https://www .integration.samhsa.gov/integrated-care-models/behavioral -health-in-primary-care.

Sorrell, J. M. (2017). Substance use disorders in long-term care settings: a crisis of care for older adults. *Journal of Psychosocial Nursing Mental Health Service, 55*(1), 24–27.

Temkin-Greener, H., Campbell, L., Cai, X., Hasselberg, M. J., & Li, Y. (2018). Are post-acute patients with behavioral health disorders admitted to lower-quality nursing homes? *American Journal of Geriatric Psychiatry, 26*(6), 643–654.

US Preventive Services Task Force: *Unhealthy alcohol use in adolescents and adults: screening and behavioral counseling interventions.* (2018). https://www.uspreventiveservicestaskforce.org/Page/Document/ UpdateSummaryDraft/unhealthy-alcohol-use-in-adolescents-and -adults-screening-and-behavioral-counseling-interventions.

Wallace R. (2019). The 2017 cannabis report of the national academy of medicine: a summary of findings and directions for research addressing cannabis use among older persons. *Public Policy & Aging Report, 29*(3), 85–87.

World Health Organization: *Mental health of older adults.* (2017). http://www.who.int/news-room/fact-sheets/detail /mental-health-of-older-adults.

World Health Organization: Mental health. *Key publications.* (2018). http://www.who.int/mental_health/publications/en/.

World Health Organization: *Mental health: WHO guidelines management of physical health conditions in adults with severe mental disorders.* (2020). https://www.who.int/mental_health/evidence /guidelines_physical_health_and_severe_mental_disorders/en/.

25

Clinical Judgment in Care of Individuals With Neurocognitive Disorders

Theris A. Touhy

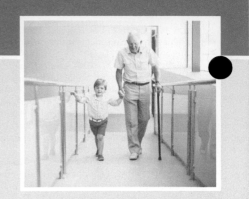

http://evolve.elsevier.com/Touhy/gerontological/

LEARNING OBJECTIVES

Upon completion of this chapter, the reader will be able to:

- Identify the characteristics of delirium and differentiate between delirium and mild and major neurocognitive disorders (dementia) and depression.
- Recognize and analyze cues to delirium and implement nursing actions for prevention, early identification, and treatment.
- Describe nursing models of care for individuals with mild and major neurocognitive disorders.
- Discuss common concerns in care of individuals with major neurocognitive disorders (communication, behavior, personal care, safety, nutrition) and nursing actions.
- Utilize clinical judgment to identify and evaluate nursing actions to provide supportive relationships and environments for individuals with dementia.

THE LIVED EXPERIENCE

The Alzheimer's patient asks nothing more than a hand to hold, a heart to care, and a mind to think for them when they cannot; someone to protect them as they travel through the dangerous twists and turns of the labyrinth. These thoughts must be put on paper now. Tomorrow they may be gone, as fleeting as the bloom of night jasmine beside my front door.

Diana Friel McGowin, who was diagnosed with Alzheimer's disease when she was 45 years old (McGowin, 1993, p. viii)

This chapter focuses on care of older adults with mild and major neurocognitive disorders (dementia) and delirium with an emphasis on nursing actions. The term *dementia* has been replaced with mild and major neurocognitive disorders (NCDs) in the DSM-5 (American Psychiatric Association, 2013), but the terms *dementia* and *cognitive impairment* will also be used in this chapter. Chapter 23 provides information about neurocognitive disorders including classification, etiology, disease-specific information, and pharmacological treatment. Cognitive function in aging is discussed in Chapter 5 and cognitive screening instruments in Chapter 8.

NEUROCOGNITIVE DISORDER: DELIRIUM

Although delirium is common in older adults, it often goes unrecognized, which increases the risk of functional decline, mortality, and health care costs (Inouye et al., 2014). Recognition and analysis of cues to delirium are very important because cues are often subtle and easily missed. Nurses play a key role in early identification and implementation of interventions aimed at reducing delirium and associated risks. Depression, delirium, and the mild and major NCDs (dementia) are called the *three Ds* of cognitive impairment because they occur frequently in older adults. An estimated 50% of individuals over the age of 65 years admitted to hospital settings have either delirium and/dementia (Gilmore-Bykovskyi et al., 2020). These important geriatric syndromes are not a normal consequence of aging, even though the incidence and prevalence are highest in older adults.

Because cognitive and behavioral changes characterize all three Ds, it can be difficult to diagnose delirium, delirium superimposed on dementia, or depression (Chapter 23). In the presence of depression, it is difficult to determine the true contribution of cognitive impairment; thus, depression should be treated and the individual should undergo reevaluation of cognitive status once stable. It is also important to note that an individual should not be newly diagnosed with dementia while in the hospital because it is very likely that the person has delirium superimposed on dementia that may be mild but interpreted as more advanced.

Differences Between Delirium, Dementia (Mild and Major NCD), and Depression

Delirium is characterized by an acute or subacute onset, with symptoms developing over a short period of time (usually hours to days). Symptoms tend to fluctuate over the course of the day, often worsening at night. People often experience reduced ability to focus, sustain, or shift attention, which leads to cognitive or perceptual disturbances. Perceptual disturbances are often accompanied by delusional (paranoid) thoughts and behavior and hallucinations. Often the hallucinations are related to seeing deceased family members, for example the person may report talking with their mother.

In contrast, major and mild NCDs typically have a gradual onset and a slow, steady pattern of decline without alterations in consciousness. These disorders represent serious pathological alterations and require assessment and interventions. However, a change in cognitive function in older adults is often seen as normal and therefore is not investigated. Any change in mental status in older adults requires a comprehensive geriatric assessment with a strong focus on cognitive function (Chapters 5, 8, and 23). Knowledge about cognitive function in aging and appropriate assessment and evaluation are keys to differentiating these three syndromes. Table 25.1 presents the clinical features and the differences in cognitive and behavioral characteristics in delirium, mild and major NCDs, and depression. The accepted criteria for a diagnosis of delirium are presented in the DSM-5 (American Psychiatric Association, 2013).

Etiology

Regardless of the etiology, the goal of delirium care is prevention and early identification. It is important to note that the development of delirium is a result of complex interactions among multiple causes. Delirium results from the interaction of predisposing factors (e.g., vulnerability on the part of the individual because of predisposing conditions, such as underlying cognitive impairment, functional impairment, depression, acute illness, sensory impairment) and precipitating factors/insults (e.g., medications, procedures, restraints, iatrogenic events, sleep deprivation, bladder catheterization, pain, and environmental factors). For example, an older adult with preexisting dementia may experience delirium after receiving just a single dose of sleep medication. Although a single factor, such as an infection, can trigger an episode of delirium, several coexisting factors are also likely to be present. A highly vulnerable older individual requires a lesser amount of precipitating factors to develop delirium (Inouye, 2018).

The exact pathophysiological mechanisms involved in the development and progression of delirium remain uncertain. One single cause or mechanism is not likely, but rather emerging evidence supports the theory of complex interaction of biological factors leading to the disruption of neuronal networks (Inouye, 2018). The causes of delirium are potentially reversible; therefore, early identification of clues, evaluation, and diagnosis are critical. Delirium is given many labels: acute confusional state, acute brain syndrome, confusion, reversible dementia, metabolic encephalopathy, and toxic psychosis.

Incidence and Prevalence

Delirium is a prevalent and serious neuropsychiatric syndrome that commonly occurs in older adults across the continuum of care. It is associated with short- and long-term consequences that can negatively influence health outcomes. Among medical inpatients, delirium is present on admission to the hospital in 10% to 31% of older adults. During hospitalization, 11% to 42% of older adults develop delirium. Up to 80% of patients in the intensive care unit (ICU) develop delirium. Patients undergoing coronary artery bypass surgery have the highest rates of delirium, followed by those experiencing trauma-related admissions. Joint replacement surgery had the lowest rates (Institute for Healthcare Improvement, 2019). In subacute settings, delirium is highly prevalent and persistent and still present on discharge and up to 3 months after discharge (Forsberg, 2017; Miu et al., 2016).

Delirium Superimposed on Dementia (DSD)

Older adults with mild and major NCDs are three to five times more likely to develop delirium; however, delirium is less likely to be recognized and treated as compared to delirium that occurs in those without mild

TABLE 25.1 **Differentiating Delirium, Depression, and Dementia (Mild or Moderate NCD)**

Characteristic	Delirium	Depression	Dementia
Onset	Sudden, abrupt	Recent, may relate to life change; can be chronic	Insidious, slow, over years and often unrecognized until deficits obvious In vascular dementia will see stair step pattern so may see sudden change in cognitive function but should always be evaluated
Course over 24 hours	Fluctuating, often worse at night	Fairly stable, may be worse in the morning	Fairly stable, may see changes with stress; some individuals have more symptoms toward nighttime (sundowning); may see sudden change when microvascular infarct occurs in vascular dementia
Consciousness	Reduced	Clear	Clear
Alertness	Increased, decreased, or variable	Normal	Generally normal
Psychomotor activity	Increased, decreased, or mixedSometimes increased, other times decreased	Variable, agitation or retardation	Normal, may have apraxia or agnosia
Duration	Hours to weeks	Variable and may be chronic	Years
Attention	Disordered, fluctuates	Most often no impairment; however, can have difficulty concentrating	Generally normal but may have trouble focusing
Orientation	Usually impaired, fluctuates	Usually normal; may answer "I don't know" to questions or may not try to answer	Often impaired; may make up answers or answer close to the right thing or may confabulate but try to answer
Speech	Often incoherent, slow, or rapid; may call out repeatedly or repeat the same phrase	May be slow	Difficulty finding word, perseveration
Affect	Variable but may look disturbed, frightened	Flat	Slowed response, may be labile

NCD, Neurocognitive disorder.
From Sendelbach S., Guthrie P. (2009). Acute Confusion/Delirium: Identification, Assessment, Treatment, and Prevention. *J Gerontol Nurs*, 35(11):11–18. doi:10.3928/00989134-20090930-01.

and major NCD. The prevalence of DSD in community and hospital populations ranges from 22% to 89%. An incidence of 40% in the community has been reported (Moon & Park, 2018). The presence of delirium can accelerate the trajectory of cognitive decline in older adults with preexisting NCD. DSD is associated with high mortality and morbidity among hospitalized older adults. Changes in the mental status of older adults with dementia are often attributed to underlying dementia, or "sundowning," and therefore not identified or even considered as a possible reason for changes in cognitive function. Despite its prevalence, DSD has not been well investigated and there is a need for more research on this topic as well as development of protocols for evaluation and treatment (Morandi et al., 2017).

Recognition of Delirium

Delirium, one of the most significant geriatric syndromes, is considered a medical emergency. Interestingly, as previously stated, despite a high incidence and prevalence of delirium, it is underrecognized. A comprehensive review of the literature suggests "nurses are missing key symptoms of delirium and appear to be doing superficial mental status assessments" (Steis & Fick, 2008, p. 47). Delirium in the ICU may be difficult to identify because of sedation and hypoactive disorders. Other factors contributing to the lack of recognition of delirium among health care professionals include inadequate education about delirium, limited use of formal assessment methods, a view that delirium is not as essential to the patient's well-being in light of more serious medical problems, and ageist attitudes. Failure to recognize delirium, to identify the underlying causes, and to implement timely interventions contributes to the negative sequelae associated with the condition. In a study of interventions nurses use to assess, prevent, and treat delirium in the acute care setting, cognitive changes in older adults are often labeled as confusion, frequently accepted as part of normal aging, and rarely questioned. Confusion in a child or younger adult would be recognized as a medical emergency, but confusion in older adults may be accepted as a natural occurrence (Dahlke & Phinney, 2008).

Clearly, attitudes about care of older adults and education about delirium assessment, prevention, and treatment are essential to improve care outcomes. Several recent studies investigating the effect of educational interventions on nurses' knowledge and practice of delirium care reported positive findings (Birge & Aydin, 2017).

Precipitating Factors for Delirium

There are many predisposing and precipitating factors for delirium (Box 25.1). The risk of delirium increases with the number of risk factors present. The more vulnerable the individual, the greater the risk. Identification of high-risk patients, risk factors, early and appropriate evaluation, and continued surveillance is the cornerstone of delirium prevention. Among the most predictive risk factors are immobility, functional deficits, use of restraints or indwelling catheters, medications, acute illness, infections, alcohol or drug abuse, sensory impairments, malnutrition, dehydration, respiratory insufficiency, surgery, and cognitive impairment.

Unrelieved or inadequately treated pain significantly increases the risk of delirium. Invasive equipment, such as nasogastric tubes, intravenous (IV) lines, catheters, and restraints, also contributes to delirium by interfering with the normal feedback mechanisms of the body. Medications can contribute to delirium and all medications, particularly those with anticholinergic effects and any new medications, should be considered suspect. Certain high-risk medications should be avoided, if possible; however, it is equally important to start medications when needed. For example, uncontrolled pain can lead to delirium, therefore starting an analgesic may be the best treatment. A mnemonic representing causes of delirium can be found in Box 25.2.

BOX 25.1   Precipitating Factors for Delirium

- Age greater than 65 years
- Cognitive impairment
- Severe illness or comorbidity burden
- Hearing or vision impairment
- Current hip fracture
- Presence of infection
- Inadequately controlled pain
- Polypharmacy and use of psychotropic medications (benzodiazepines, anticholinergics, antihistamines, antipsychotics)
- Depression
- Alcohol use
- Sleep deprivation or disturbance
- Renal insufficiency
- Aortic procedures
- Anemia
- Hypoxia or hypercarbia
- Poor nutrition
- Dehydration
- Electrolyte abnormalities
- Poor functional status
- Immobilization or limited mobility
- Risk of urinary retention or constipation
- Use of invasive equipment, restraints

From American Geriatrics Society. (2014). *Clinical practice guidelines for postoperative delirium in older adults.* https://geriatricscareonline.org /ProductAbstract/american-geriatrics-society-clinical-practice-guideline-for -postoperative-delirium-in-older-adults/CL018.

BOX 25.2   What Causes Delirium?[a]

D	Dementia
E	Electrolytes
L	Lungs, liver, heart, kidney, brain
I	Infection
Rx	Polypharmacy, psychotropics
I	Injury, pain, stress
U	Unfamiliar environment
M	Metabolic

[a]There is usually more than one cause.

Clinical Subtypes of Delirium

Delirium is categorized according to the level of alertness and psychomotor activity. The clinical subtypes are hyperactive, hypoactive, and mixed. Box 25.3 presents the characteristics of each of hyperactive and hypoactive delirium. Because of the increased severity of illness and the use of psychoactive medications, hypoactive delirium may be more prevalent in the ICU. Although the negative consequences of hyperactive delirium are serious, the hypoactive subtype may be more often missed and is associated with a worse prognosis because of the development of complications such as aspiration, pulmonary embolism, pressure injuries, and pneumonia.

BOX 25.3   Clinical Subtypes of Delirium

Hypoactive Delirium
- "Quiet or pleasantly confused"
- Reduced activity
- Lack of facial expression
- Passive demeanor
- Lethargy
- Inactivity
- Withdrawn and sluggish state
- Limited, slow, and wavering vocalizations

Hyperactive Delirium
- Excessive alertness
- Easy distractibility
- Increased psychomotor activity
- Hallucinations, delusions
- Agitation and aggressive actions
- Fast or loud speech
- Wandering, nonpurposeful repetitive movement
- Verbal behaviors (yelling, calling out)
- Removing tubes
- Attempting to get out of bed
- Unpredictable fluctuations between hypoactivity and hyperactivity

BOX 25.4   Resources for Best Practice

Delirium and Dementia

Advance Directive for Dementia: www.dementia-directive.org

Dementia Live: Simulation experience to immerse participants into life with dementia. https://ageucate.com/.

Hartford Institute for Geriatric Nursing: Delirium: Nursing Standard of Practice Protocol: Prevention, early recognition, and treatment; Assessment and management of delirium in older adults with dementia; Confusion Assessment Method (CAM), CAM ICU. https://consultgeri.org/try-this/general-assessment.

Hartford Institute for Geriatric Nursing: Dementia Series. https://consultgeri.org/try-this/dementia.

Hospital Elder Life Program (HELP): Program materials, Family-HELP program, The Family Confusion Assessment Method (FAM-CAM). https://www.hospitalelderlifeprogram.org/.

ICU Delirium and Cognitive Impairment Study Group: Patient and Family Report: Memories from the ICU. https://www.icudelirium .org/patients-and-families/overview.

Nursing Home Toolkit: Promoting Positive Behavioral Health: http://www.nursinghometoolkit.com/.

Society of Critical Care Medicine: Clinical practice guidelines for the management of pain, agitation, and delirium in adult patients in the ICU. https://www.sccm.org/Research/Guidelines/Guidelines /Guidelines-for-the-Prevention-and-Management-of-Pa.

WeCare Advisor: http://www.programforpositiveaging.org /wecareadvisor/.

ICU, Intensive care unit.

Consequences of Delirium

Delirium is a terrifying experience for the individual and their family and significant others and people often think the individual is "going crazy." Delirium is associated with increased length of hospital stay and hospital readmissions, increased services after discharge, and increased morbidity, mortality, and institutionalization, independent of age, coexisting illnesses, or illness severity (Flaherty et al., 2017). Posttraumatic stress disorder (PTSD) symptoms (nightmares, flashbacks, memories, and dreams individuals were unable to comprehend), although often not recognized, may occur in adults with delirium (Battle et al., 2017) (Chapter 28). Resources on delirium including video descriptions of delirium by patients can be found in Box 25.4.

Although the majority of hospital inpatients recover fully from delirium, a substantial minority will never recover or recover only partially. The more severe the delirium and the longer it lasts, the worse the outcome. Each episode of delirium increases the vulnerability of the brain, which further enhances the risk of dementia (Inouye, 2018). The persistence of delirium after discharge may interfere with the ability to manage chronic conditions and contribute to poor outcomes (Hain et al., 2012). Further research is needed to determine the reasons for the long-term poor outcomes, whether characteristics of the delirium itself (subtype or duration) influence prognosis, and how the long-term effects might be decreased.

⚡ SAFETY ALERT

Older adults with risk factors for delirium should be screened for delirium upon admission to the hospital, when transitioning from one area of care to another, and before discharge to other care settings or home. If experiencing symptoms, conduct a comprehensive geriatric assessment with a particular focus on cognitive status and potential reversible causes of delirium.

❖ USING CLINICAL JUDGMENT TO PROMOTE HEALTHY AGING: DELIRIUM

◆ Recognizing and Analyzing Cues: Delirium

Prevention of delirium is the first step in caring for vulnerable older adults who are at risk of delirium. An awareness and identification of the risk factors for delirium and a formal evaluation for delirium are the first-line interventions for prevention. Delirium has been called a critical vital sign of cognitive health and assessment should be given the same attention as other vital signs (Fick, 2018). Nurses play a pivotal role in the identification of delirium, and early intervention increases the chance for positive outcomes.

Evaluation of delirium begins with a thorough history and identification of key diagnostic features. Several instruments can be used to assess the presence and severity of delirium. To detect changes, it is very important to determine a person's baseline cognitive status. If the person cannot tell you this, family members or other caregivers can be asked to provide this information. Family members and other caregivers know the person well and will notice subtle changes in behavior. They can provide information about whether or not these behaviors are normal for this person and, if not, when they first appeared.

If the patient is alone, the responsible party or the institution transferring the patient can provide this information by phone. Determining baseline cognitive function is essential. Do not assume the person's current mental status represents their usual state and do not attribute altered mental status to age alone or assume that dementia is present. All older adults, regardless of their current cognitive function, should be evaluated with valid and reliable instruments to identify possible delirium when admitted to the hospital. Several delirium-specific instruments are available, such as the Confusion Assessment Method (CAM) (Inouye et al., 1990) and the NEECHAM (Neelon and Champagne) Confusion Scale (Neelon et al., 1996).

The ADAPT (Actions for Delirium Assessment Prevention and Treatment Program) at Hartford Hospital screens all patients 65 years of age and older in the emergency department with a Single Question in Delirium (SQID) screening technique that has also been noted as effective in identifying delirium. These patients are asked whether they have been more confused lately. If a family member or someone else is with them, that individual is asked the same question about the patient. If the answer is "yes", the patient gets an intentional test—counting backward from 20 to 1 (attentional deficit is the key element of delirium) (Cheney, 2019). If the patient answers yes to the SQID and is unable to perform the counting test, the ADAPT program, a coordinated approach to assessment, prevention, and treatment of delirium is instituted (Institute for Healthcare Improvement, 2019).

The CAM-ICU is another instrument specifically designed to identify delirium in an intensive care population and has been validated for use in critically ill, nonverbal patients who are on mechanical ventilation (Ely et al., 2001; Rigney, 2006). Many acute care settings have made the CAM a part of the electronic medical record.

The Confusion Assessment Method-Family Assessment Method (CAM-FAM) (Steis et al., 2012) can be used to identify symptoms based on reports from family members and closely correlates with the CAM in identification of delirium (Flanagan & Spencer, 2015) (Box 25.4). Chapter 8 provides more information regarding assessment of cognitive status.

Once an individual is identified as having delirium, re-evaluation should be conducted every shift. Documenting specific objective indicators of alterations in mental status rather than using the global, nonspecific term *confusion* will lead to more appropriate prevention, detection, and management of delirium and its negative consequences. Findings from a validated instrument are combined with nursing observation and evaluation, chart review, and physiological findings such as laboratory studies. Delirium often has a fluctuating course and can be difficult to recognize, therefore monitoring must be ongoing and include multiple data sources.

◆ Nursing Actions: Delirium

Because the etiology of delirium is multifactorial, multicomponent actions that address more than one risk factor are more likely to be effective. There is strong evidence that multicomponent interventions can prevent delirium in both medical and surgical settings and less robust evidence that they reduce the severity of delirium. Early engagement of the interdisciplinary team in assessment of risk factors as soon as the patient is admitted is key to a successful delirium prevention program (Oberai et al., 2018). Continued research is needed to evaluate what type of approach has the most beneficial effect in different clinical settings. A person-centered approach to care, rather than a disease-focused approach, can yield the best outcomes (Box 25.5).

BOX 25.5 Clinical Exemplar: Delirium

Mr. M., an 81-year-old male, was admitted to an acute care facility 2 days ago because of a change in his behavior. The admitting diagnoses were dehydration and acute kidney injury. Suddenly one day he became agitated and yelled loudly. The nurse caring for him was busy with an unstable patient in the next bed, therefore her first response was to medicate Mr. M. with an antianxiety medication. The clinical practice specialist just happened to be present and recalled the risks for delirium and that nonpharmacological approaches were best. She quickly suggested to the nurse: "Let's move him out of this room to a quieter area." This simple change in environment was effective in reducing Mr. M.'s agitation and for the next few days before discharge, he remained calm. This exemplar demonstrates the importance of working together to reduce the use of pharmacological interventions in individuals with delirium.

From Candice Hickman, MSN, RN, Clinical Practice Specialist.

A well-researched program of delirium prevention in the acute care setting, the Hospital Elder Life Program (HELP) (Hshieh et al., 2015; Inouye et al., 1999), focuses on managing six risk factors for delirium: cognitive impairment, sleep deprivation, immobility, visual impairments, hearing impairments, and dehydration. An interprofessional team of geriatric specialists, including nurses, takes a multifaceted approach to maintain cognitive and physical function for high-risk older adults, maximize independence at discharge, assist with transitions, and prevent unnecessary readmissions. Trained volunteers are also utilized in the HELP program. The program is used in more than 200 hospitals in the United States and internationally. The Family-HELP program (Box 25.4), an adaptation and extension of the original HELP program, trains family caregivers in selected protocols (e.g., orientation, therapeutic activities, vision, and hearing). Initial research demonstrates that active engagement of family caregivers in preventive interventions for delirium is feasible and supports a culture of family-oriented care.

Most of the interventions in the HELP program can be considered quite simple and part of good nursing care. Interventions include the following: offering herbal tea or warm milk instead of sleeping medications; keeping the ward quiet at night by using vibrating beepers instead of paging systems; removing catheters and other devices that hamper movement as soon as possible; encouraging mobilization; assessing and managing pain; and correcting hearing and vision deficits. Fall risk–reduction interventions—such as bed and chair alarms, low beds, reclining chairs, volunteers to sit with restless patients, and keeping routines as normal as possible with consistent caregivers—are other examples of interventions. Box 25.6 presents tips for prevention of delirium.

◆ **Pharmacological Approaches**

Pharmacological interventions to treat the symptoms of delirium may be necessary for patients who are in danger of harming themselves or others, or if nonpharmacological interventions are not effective. However, pharmacological interventions should be viewed as one approach in a multicomponent program of prevention and treatment but should not replace thoughtful and careful evaluation and management of the underlying causes of delirium. Research on the pharmacological management of delirium is limited, but with increased understanding of the neuropathogenesis of delirium, drug therapy may become more important.

Antipsychotic drugs are routinely used to treat delirium even though the US Food and Drug Administration has not approved their use for treating the condition. A systematic review and meta-analysis evaluating the effectiveness of antipsychotics for the prevention or treatment of delirium concluded that current evidence does not support the use of these medications and does not reduce the duration of delirium or improve other outcomes (Singu et al., 2020). Limited use of antipsychotic drugs may be considered if patients have hyperactive delirium that puts them or others at risk of injury or harm and all other nonpharmacological approaches have failed. If used, these medications should be given at the lowest possible dose for the shortest possible duration (Singu et al., 2020).

Caring for patients with delirium can be a challenging experience because the individual has difficulty communicating and may demonstrate disturbing behaviors, such as pulling out IV lines or attempting to get out of bed, disrupt medical treatment, and compromise their own safety or that of others. It is essential that nurses realize any such behavior is an attempt to communicate

---

BOX 25.6   Tips for Best Practice

Prevention of Delirium

- Sensory enhancement (ensuring glasses, hearing aids, listening amplifiers)
- Mobility enhancement (ambulating at least twice a day if possible)
- Bedside presence of a family member whenever possible
- Cognitive orientation and therapeutic activities (tailored to the individual)
- Pain management
- Cognitive stimulation (if possible, tailored to individual's interests and mental status)
- Simple communication standards and approaches to prevent escalation of behaviors
- Nutritional and fluid repletion enhancement
- Sleep enhancement (sleep hygiene, nonpharmacological sleep protocol)
- Medication review and appropriate medication management
- Adequate oxygenation
- Prevention of constipation
- Minimize the use of invasive medical devices, restraints, or immobilizing devices
- Pay attention to environmental noise, light, temperature
- Normalize the environment (provide familiar items, routines, clocks, calendars)
- Minimize the number of room changes and interfacility transfers

Adapted from American College of Surgeons NSQIP and American Geriatrics Society. (2016). *Optimal perioperative management of the geriatric patient.* https://www.facs.org/~/media/files/quality%20programs/geriatric /acs%20nsqip%20geriatric%202016%20guidelines.ashx; and American Geriatrics Society. (2014). *Clinical Practice Guidelines for Postoperative Delirium in Older Adults.* http://www.sciencedirect.com/science/article/pii /S1072751514017931.

BOX 25.7   Tips for Best Practice

Communicating With a Person Experiencing Delirium

- Know the person's past patterns.
- Look at nonverbal signs, such as tone of voice, facial expressions, and gestures.
- Speak slowly.
- Be calm and patient.
- Face the person and keep eye contact; get to the level of the person rather than standing over him or her.
- Explain all actions.
- Smile.
- Use simple, familiar words.
- Repeat as needed and allow adequate time for response.
- Repeated reorientation.
- Tell the person what you want them to do rather than what you do not want them to do.
- Give one-step directions; use gestures and demonstration to augment words.
- Reassure person's safety.
- Keep caregivers consistent.
- Assume that communication and behavior are meaningful and an attempt to tell us something or express needs.
- Do not assume that the person is unable to understand or has dementia.

something and express needs therefore it is important to implement strategies to address these unmet needs. Older adults experiencing delirium feel frightened and may have a sense of having lost control of their lives. The calmer and more reassuring the nurse is, the safer the patient will feel. Box 25.7 presents some communication strategies that are helpful in caring for individuals experiencing delirium.

CARE OF INDIVIDUALS WITH NEUROCOGNITIVE DISORDERS

Nurses provide direct care for people with neurocognitive disorders (NCDs) in the community, hospitals, and long-term care facilities. They also work with families and staff, teaching best practice approaches to care and providing education and support. With the rising incidence of NCDs, nurses will play an even greater role in the design and implementation of evidence-based practice and provision of education, counseling, and supportive services to individuals with NCDs and their caregivers. The overriding goals in caring for older adults with NCDs are to maintain function and prevent excess disability, to structure the

environment and relationships to maintain stability, to compensate for the losses associated with the disease, and to create a therapeutic milieu that nurtures the personhood of the individual and maintains well-being and quality of life.

Nutrition, activities of daily living (ADLs), maintenance of health and function, safety, communication, behavioral changes, caregiver needs and support, and quality of life are the major care concerns for patients, families, and staff caring for individuals with dementia. Five common care concerns for individuals with a diagnosis of a major NCD and nursing actions are discussed in the remainder of this chapter: communication, behavior concerns, ADL care, wandering, and nutrition. Caregiving for persons with NCDs is discussed in Chapter 26 and other care concerns such as falls and incontinence are discussed in earlier chapters of this book.

Person-Centered Care

Irreversible NCDs have no cure and although new medications offer hope for improved function, the most important treatment for the disease is competent and compassionate person-centered care. Person-centered care is one of the six major aims in the redesign of the US health care system and considers

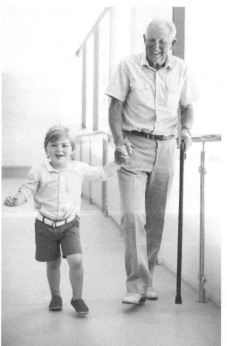

Maintaining Function and Preventing Unnecessary Decline Are Important. (© iStock.com/Squaredpixels.)

"what matters most" to individuals. Person-centered care looks beyond the disease and the tasks we must perform to the person within and our relationship with them. The focus is not on what we need to do to the person but on the person themselves and how to enhance their well-being and quality of life. "The person with dementia is not an object, not a vegetable, not an empty body, not a child, but an adult, who, given support, might exercise choices and respond to a respectful approach" (Woods, 1999, p. 35).

Person-centered care fosters abilities, supports limitations, ensures safety, enhances quality of life, prevents excess disability, and offers hope. Special skills and attitudes are required to nurse the person with dementia, and caring is paramount. It is not an area of nursing that "just anyone can do" (Splete, 2008, p. 11). The overarching principles of person-centered dementia care and resources are presented in Box 25.8.

Nutrition, activities of daily living (ADLs), maintenance of health and function, safety, communication, behavioral changes, caregiver needs and support, and quality of life are the major care concerns for patients, families, and staff caring for individuals with dementia. Five common care concerns for individuals with a diagnosis of a major NCD and nursing interventions are discussed in the remainder

of this chapter: communication, behavior concerns, ADL care, wandering, and nutrition.

Differing Needs in Younger-Onset Dementia and Mild NCD

Although the focus of this chapter is on care concerns of individuals with major NCDs, it is important to note that the concerns of individuals and their caregivers living with younger-onset dementia (onset before 65 years of age), mild NCD, and early stages of major NCD are quite different. To date, the preponderance of research and intervention programs has been directed toward individuals and their families living with major NCDs and has focused on preparing caregivers to cope with issues such as behavior problems, incontinence, ADL care, and nursing home placement. Many of these issues are not relevant to those with younger-onset dementia and mild NCD, therefore they will not be of interest to them and can even be frightening and misleading.

A significant number of individuals are diagnosed with dementia earlier in their lives, even as young as in their 30s and 40s (Chapter 23). According to the Alzheimer's Association (2018), up to 5% of Americans living with Alzheimer's disease belong to that group. Therefore, the current language guidelines suggest using the term *younger-onset dementia* instead of the previously used *early-onset dementia*, because it could be confused with early stages of symptoms of dementia at any age.

The individual may have dependent children at home and still be employed. They may be forced to retire and experience a loss of income, work roles, and related benefits during prime working years. Most dementia services are designed for older adults and do not meet the specific needs of younger individuals. Because the individual is younger, they are likely to be in better health than older adults and meeting the safety needs of someone who is still physically able can be challenging (Greenwood & Smith, 2016; Sakamoto et al. 2017).

Areas of concern for caregivers of persons with mild NCD and early-stage major NCD center less on personal care needs and more on communication, behavior, and relationships. Interventions that help both the person and their caregiver to deal with changing roles, stress, frustration, loss, communication difficulties, and the couple relationship are particularly needed. Continued research and development of programs of support and services for individuals with mild NCD, younger-onset stage dementia, and early stage major NCD and their caregivers are a priority, as is continued evaluation of the effectiveness of interventions in practice. Research must include the voices of those experiencing the health challenge of living with an NCD.

BOX 25.8 Person-Centered Nursing Interventions in Care of Individuals With NCDs

- Get to know the person
- Build and nurture authentic caring relationships
- Recognize and accept the person's reality
- Obtain input from the individual and engage in shared decision making to the extent possible
- Maximize abilities to make choices
- Structure daily living to maximize remaining abilities and support limitations
- Identify characteristics of the social and physical environment that may cause distress for the person or exacerbate behavior and psychological symptoms
- Provide meaningful activities and relationships to enhance quality of life
- Ensure safety
- Monitor general health and impact of the NCD on management of other medical conditions.
- Collaborate with caregivers in the areas of problem-solving, resource access; long-range planning, emotional support, and respite
- Support advance care planning and advance directives.

Adapted from Fazio, S., Pace, D., Maslow, K., et al. (2018). Alzheimer's Association dementia care practice recommendations. *Gerontologist, 58*, S1–S9.

COMMUNICATION

The experience of losing cognitive and expressive abilities is both frightening and frustrating. Early in the disease, word finding is difficult (anomia) and remembering the exact facts of a conversation is challenging (Box 25.9). As the disease progresses, memory, speech, and communication also decline. NCD affects both receptive and expressive communication components and alters the way people speak. Automatic language skills (e.g., hello) are retained for the longest time. The person may wander from the topic of conversation and bring up seemingly unrelated topics. The person may fail to pick up on humor or sarcasm or abstract ideas in conversation. Nonverbal and behavioral responses become especially important as a way of communication as verbal skills become more limited. As the disease progresses, verbal output may become less frequent although the grammar and sounds of the language being spoken remain relatively intact. Even in the later stages of NCD, the individual may understand more than you realize and still needs opportunities for interaction and caring communication, both verbal and nonverbal.

Communication is essential to person-centered care. No group of patients is more in need of supportive relationships with skilled, caring health care providers. People with cognitive and communication impairments "depend on their relationship with and trust of others to provide emotional support, solve problems, and coordinate complex activities" (Buckwalter et al., 1995, p. 15). Communication with individuals experiencing NCDs requires special skills and patience. Caregivers experience frustration and anxiety when their attempts to communicate with the person who has cognitive limitations are unsuccessful, often resulting in short interactions that are mostly task-oriented. Communication may be seen as a low priority because of heavy workloads and lack of awareness of the importance of communication.

BOX 25.9 Patient's Descriptions of Communication Difficulties

"I forget words. Sometimes it doesn't mean much and other times it means a great deal. I have learned ways to avoid making mistakes like shaking hands when I don't remember the person's name, joking, looking at their faces for a reaction."

(Hain et al., 2014, p. 85)

"There are a range of things you want to say over and over because I think it was a word that was important to say and I'll forget . . . I hope that what I am saying makes sense."

(Hain et al., 2010, p. 165)

When individuals cannot communicate their needs, behavioral problems may occur (Machiels et al., 2017).

To communicate effectively with a person experiencing a NCD, it is essential to believe that the person is trying to communicate something that is important. It is critical that nurses recognize various ways a person with dementia may communicate by getting to know the person. The best thing we can do is to discover what the person is trying to communicate and intervene according to needs. However jumbled it may seem, the person is attempting to tell us something. It is our responsibility as professionals to understand and know how to respond. The person with NCD cannot change their communication; we must change ours.

Nurses can overcome barriers to communication by taking a person-centered approach. Such framework encourages coming to know the person by taking time to find out the individual's story. In some cases, people are unable to disclose a lifetime of memories but taking the time to find out what their background is and making time to be present can contribute to effective communication. A communication intervention in long-term care demonstrated the value of tailored communication plans based on the abilities of the residents with dementia. The plans included how to communicate with the individual, how the resident communicates with others, and an "about me" section that gives information about the person (where they were born, work, family, interests). The results suggest that the communication intervention had positive effects on residents' quality of living (QOL) and care providers' mood and burden (McGilton et al., 2017).

Evidence-Based Communication Strategies

Classic research conducted by Ruth Tappen of Florida Atlantic University (Boca Raton, FL) and colleagues (Tappen et al., 1997, 1999) provided insight into communication strategies that were helpful in creating and maintaining a therapeutic relationship with people with moderate to major NCDs. Findings of this study were compared with recommendations in the literature and specific communication strategies were developed. More than 80% of the participants' responses in communication with a clinical nurse specialist were relevant in the context of the conversation. The research challenged some of the commonly held beliefs about communication with persons with NCDs, for example, avoiding the use of open-ended questions and keeping communication focused only on simple topics, task-oriented topics, and questions that can be answered with yes or no responses.

Findings of this study provided suggestions for specific communication strategies effective in various nursing

BOX 25.10 Tips for Best Practice

Four Useful Strategies for Communicating With Individuals Experiencing Cognitive Impairment

Simplification Strategies

Simplification strategies are useful with ADLs:

- Give one-step directions.
- Speak slowly and clearly.
- Allow time for response.
- Reduce distractions.
- One-to-one conversations; avoid multiple caregivers interacting at the same time.
- Give clues and cues as to what you want the person to do. Use gestures or pantomime to demonstrate what it is you want the person to do, e.g., put the chair in front of the person, point to it, pat the seat, and say, "Sit here."

Facilitation Strategies

Facilitation strategies are useful in encouraging expression of thoughts and feelings:

- Establish commonalities.
- Share self.
- Allow the person to choose subjects to discuss.
- Speak as if to an equal.
- Use broad openings, such as "How are you today?"
- Employ appropriate use of humor.
- Follow the person's lead.

Comprehension Strategies

Comprehension strategies are useful in assisting with understanding of communication:

- Identify time confusion (in what time frame is the person operating at the moment?).

- Find the theme (what connection is there between apparently disparate topics?). Recognize an important theme, such as fear, loss, or happiness.
- Recognize the hidden meanings (what did the person mean to say?).

Supportive Strategies

Supportive strategies are useful in encouraging continued communication and supporting personhood:

- Introduce yourself, and explain why you are there. Reach out to shake hands, and note the response to touch.
- If the person does not want to talk, go away and return later. Do not push or force.
- Sit closely and face the person at eye level.
- Limit corrections.
- Use multiple ways of communicating (gestures, touch).
- Search for meaning in all communication.
- Know the person's past life history, and daily life experiences and events.
- Recognize feelings, and respond.
- Treat the person with respect and dignity.
- Show interest through body posture, facial expression, nodding, and eye contact. Assume a pleasant, relaxed attitude.
- Attend to vision and hearing losses.
- Do not try to bring the person to the present or use reality orientation. Go to where the person is and enjoy the conversation.
- When leaving, thank the person for their time and attention and information.
- Remember that the quality, not the content or quantity, of the interaction is basic to therapeutic communication.

ADLs, Activities of daily living.

situations and hope for nurses to establish meaningful relationships that nurture the personhood of people with NCDs (Box 25.10). Communication strategies differ depending on the purpose of communication (e.g., performing ADLs, encouraging expression of feelings). Approaches to communication must be adapted not only to the person's ability to understand but also to the purpose of the interaction. What is appropriate for assessment may be a barrier to conversation that is designed to facilitate expression of concerns and feelings.

In the past, structured programs of reality orientation (RO) (orienting the person to the day, date, time, year, weather, upcoming holidays) were often used in long-term care facilities and chronic psychiatric units as a way to stimulate interaction and enhance memory. This intervention is still often noted as being of benefit to persons with NCDs. However, structured RO may place unrealistic expectations on persons with major NCDs

and may be distressing if the individual cannot remember these things. Families and professional caregivers can often be heard asking people with NCDs to name relatives, state their birth year, and remember other current facts. One can imagine how upsetting and demoralizing this might be to a person unable to remember.

This does not imply that we should not orient the person to daily activities, time of day, and other important events, but it should be offered without the expectation that the person will remember. Caregivers can provide orienting information as part of general conversation (e.g., "It's quite warm for December 10, but it will be a beautiful day for our lunch date"). Rather than structured RO, a better approach is to go where the person is in their own world rather than trying to bring the person's world into yours. For example, if the individual insists that they need to leave the house to meet the school bus, it is more helpful to ask the individual to talk about the times they did this activity rather than informing the person that their children are grown and do not ride the school bus.

Validation therapy, developed by Naomi Feil in the 1980s, involves following the person's lead and responding to feelings expressed rather than interrupting to supply factual data. Communication techniques include using nonthreatening words to establish understanding; rephrasing the person's words; maintaining eye contact and a gentle tone of voice; responding in general terms when meaning is unclear; and using touch if appropriate (Scales et al., 2018). "Although the evidence base for validation therapy is underdeveloped, the concept of honoring the feelings of the person living with dementia has face validity as part of person-centered dementia care" (Scales et al., 2018, p. S95). Helping families and caregivers understand validation therapy can assist in enhancing quality time with their loved ones.

BEHAVIOR CONCERNS AND NURSING MODELS OF CARE

Estimates are that behavioral and psychological symptoms of dementia (BPSD) occur in as many as 75% of individuals of individuals with NCD (at least one symptom) and become more common as the disease progresses. Compared with those who do not have BPSD symptoms, these individuals are institutionalized earlier and have poorer ability to complete ADLs, greater cognitive decline, lower quality of life, and increased risk of death. In addition, their caregivers report worse quality of life than caregivers of patients without BPSD symptoms (Watt et al., 2019).

Symptoms often co-occur, increasing their impact even more. BPSDs occur in clusters or syndromes identified as psychosis (delusions and hallucinations), agitation, aggression, depression, anxiety, apathy, disinhibition (socially and sexually inappropriate behaviors), motor disturbances, night-time behaviors, and appetite and eating problems. The most common symptoms are apathy, depression, and anxiety. Lifelong psychiatric disorders (Chapter 28) and their management may also affect the development of these symptoms (Kales et al., 2015).

BPSDs appear to be a consequence of multiple, but sometimes modifiable, interacting factors. These factors are both external and internal and result in part from heightened vulnerability to the environment as cognitive function declines. Neurodegeneration associated with dementia also plays a role in BPSDs (Molony et al., 2018; Scales et al., 2018). The quality of the interaction between the caregiver and the person living with dementia also influences behavioral symptoms (Kales et al., 2015). A recent scoping review of the evidence on determinants of BPSDs reported the following causes as common across

several behavioral symptoms: neurodegeneration, type of dementia, severity of cognitive impairments, declining functional abilities, caregiver burden, poor communication, and boredom (Kolanowski et al., 2017).

BPSD should be viewed as a form of communication that is meaningful (rather than a problem), an expression of unmet needs, and/or a reflection of lower tolerance for stressors in the physical and psychosocial environment. They are the individual's best attempt to communicate a variety of unmet needs. BPSDs symptoms cause a great deal of distress to the person and the caregivers, contribute to increased financial cost, caregiver burden, and nursing stress, poor quality of life for the person with dementia and their caregiver, significant declines in function, risk for physical abuse, and often precipitate institutionalization (Austrom et al., 2018; Kolanowski et al., 2017). Clinically significant BPSDs, if untreated, are associated with faster disease progression than in the absence of such symptoms.

Several nursing models of care are helpful in recognizing and understanding the behavior of individuals with NCDs and can be used to guide practice and to assist families and staff in providing care from a more person-centered framework. The *Progressively Lowered Stress Threshold* (PLST) model and the *Need-Driven Dementia-Compromised Behavior* (NDDB) model focus on the close interplay between person, context, and environment. These models propose that behavior is used to communicate or express, in the best way the person has available, unmet needs (physiological, psychosocial, disturbing environment, uncomfortable social surroundings) and/or difficulty managing stress as the disease progresses.

The Progressively Lowered Stress Threshold Model

The PLST model (Hall, 1994; Hall & Buckwalter, 1987) was one of the first models used to plan and evaluate care for people with NCDs in every setting. The model suggests that environmental antecedents produce stress, which is met by a coping response that is compromised by the impact of dementia (Scales et al., 2018). Symptoms such as agitation are a result of a progressive loss of the person's ability to cope with demands and stimuli when the person's stress threshold is exceeded. An example is the person who becomes agitated in response to excess noise in the environment (loudspeaker, loud talk).

Using this model, care is structured to decrease the stressors and provide a safe and predictable environment. Positive outcomes from use of the model include improved sleep; decreased sedative and tranquilizer use; increased food intake and weight; increased socialization; decreased episodes of aggressive, agitated, and disruptive behaviors; increased caregiver satisfaction with

BOX 25.11 Principles of Care Derived From PLST Model

1. Maximize functional abilities by supporting all losses in a prosthetic manner.
2. Establish a caring relationship and provide the person with unconditional positive regard.
3. Use patient behaviors indicating anxiety and avoidance to determine appropriate limits of activity and stimuli.
4. Teach caregivers to try to find causes of behavior and to observe and evaluate verbal and nonverbal responses.
5. Identify triggers related to discomfort or stress reactions (factors in the environment, caregiver communication).
6. Modify the environment to support losses and promote safe function.
7. Evaluate care routines and responses on a 24-hour basis and adjust plan of care accordingly.
8. Provide as much control as possible; encourage self-care, offer choices, explain all actions, do not push or force the person to do something.
9. Keep the environment stable and predictable.
10. Provide ongoing education, support, care, and problem solving for caregivers.

PLST, Progressively Lowered Stress Threshold.
Adapted from Hall, G. R., & Buckwalter, K. C. (1987). Progressively Lowered Stress Threshold: A conceptual model for care of adults with Alzheimer's disease. *Arch Psychiatr Nurs, 1*,399–406.

care; and increased functional level (DeYoung et al., 2003; Hall & Buckwalter, 1987). Box 25.11 presents the principles of care derived from the PLST model.

Need-Driven Dementia-Compromised Behavior Model

The NDDB model (Algase et al., 2003; Kolanowski, 1999; Richards et al., 2000) is a framework for the study and understanding of behavioral symptoms. All behaviors have meaning and are a form of communication, particularly as verbal communication becomes more limited. The NDDB model proposes that the behavior of persons with NCDs carries a message of need that can be addressed appropriately if the person's history and habits, physiological status, and physical and social environment are carefully evaluated. Rather than behavior being viewed as disruptive, it is viewed as having meaning and expressing needs. Behavior reflects the interaction of background factors (cognitive changes as a result of dementia, gender, ethnicity, culture, education, personality, responses to stress) and proximal factors (physiological needs such as hunger or pain, mood, physical environment [e.g., light, noise, temperature]) with the social environment (e.g., staff stability and mix, presence of others).

Optimal care is provided by manipulating the proximal factors that precipitate behavior and by maximizing strengths and minimizing the limitations of the background factors. For instance, sleep disruptions are common in people with dementia. If the person is not getting adequate sleep at night, agitated or aggressive behavior during the day may signal the need for more rest. Interventions to modify proximal factors interfering with sleep, such as noise, frequent awakenings during the night, and daytime boredom, can help meet the need for rest and sleep and decrease agitation or aggression.

❖ USING CLINICAL JUDGMENT TO PROMOTE HEALTHY AGING: BPSD

◆ Recognizing and Analyzing Cues: BPSD

Cues to recognizing potential causes of BPSDs vary widely and the behaviors have many potential causes. Analysis must be done in the context of the individual's history and situation and consideration of the multiple things that could be happening. The focus must be on understanding that behavioral expressions communicate distress and the response is to investigate the possible sources of distress and intervene appropriately.

There are many possible reasons for BPSDs. After ruling out medical problems (e.g., pneumonia, dehydration, impaction, infection/sepsis, fractures, pain, or depression) as a cause of the behavior, continued evaluation is important to identify why distressing symptoms are occurring. Conditions such as constipation or urinary tract infections can cause great distress for individuals with cognitive impairment and may lead to marked changes in behavior. In a study of community-dwelling older adults with dementia, 36% had undetected illness associated with BPSDs, making adequate assessment and treatment essential. Side effects of drugs or drug–drug interactions can also contribute to the development of symptoms (Kales et al., 2015).

Pain and discomfort are associated with aggressive behaviors in individuals with dementia. After careful evaluation of other possible causes of pain or discomfort, treatment with a trial of analgesics should be considered. Treatment of pain is challenging, especially in today's opioid epidemic where providers are often afraid to prescribe these medications. In some circumstances the person is not receiving enough medicine to control the pain and may therefore act out as a result of an inability to express symptoms verbally. It is essential for nurses to discover nonpharmacological approaches to pain and to advocate appropriate pharmacological interventions.

Understanding what triggers behavior is essential for development of interventions that address the

---

BOX 25.12   Stressors Triggering BPSDs (PLST Model)

Fatigue

Change of environment, routine, or caregiver

Misleading stimuli or inappropriate stimulus levels

Internal or external demands to perform beyond abilities

Physical stressors such as pain, discomfort, acute illness, and depression

---

BOX 25.13   Framework for Asking Questions About the Meaning of Behavior

What?

What is being sought? What is happening? Does the behavior have a physical or emotional component or both? What are the person's responses? What would be done if the person was 20 years old instead of 80? What is the behavior saying? What is the emotion being expressed?

Where?

Where is the behavior occurring? What are the environmental triggers?

When?

When does the behavior most frequently occur: after activities of daily living (ADLs), family visits, mealtimes?

Who?

Who is involved? Other residents, caregivers, family?

Why?

What happened before? Poor communication? Tasks too complicated? Physical or medical problem? Person being rushed or forced to do something? Has this happened before and why?

What Now?

Approaches and interventions (physical, psychosocial)

Changes needed and by whom?

Who else might know something about the person or the behavior or approaches?

Communicate to all and include in plan of care.

---

individual's unmet need. Fear, discomfort, unfamiliar surroundings and people, illness, fatigue, depression, need for autonomy and control, caregiver approaches, communication strategies, and environmental stressors are frequent precipitants of behavioral symptoms. "For the individual with late-stage dementia, a good deal of their discomfort comes from nonphysiological sources, for example, from difficulty sorting out and negotiating everyday life activities" (Kovach, 1999, p. 412).

The need for socialization and support and stimulation to address boredom can also contribute to changes in behavior. "Lack of meaningful activity is cited by people living with dementia and family members as one of the most persistent and critical unmet needs. The provision of individualized meaningful activities may help prevent or alleviate BPSDs by enhancing quality of life through engagement, enhanced social interaction, and opportunities for self-expression and self-determination" (Scales et al., 2018, p. S96). Box 25.12 presents precipitating factors for BPSDs.

Putting yourself in the place of the person with a NCD and trying to see the world from their eyes will help you understand their behavior. Questions of what, where, why, when, who, and what now are important components of the assessment of behavior. Box 25.13 presents a framework for asking questions about the possible meanings and messages behind observed behavior. Except in late-stage NCD, when verbal communication may be problematic, the perspective of the individual should be elicited to determine what they can describe about the situation. It is also important to understand what aspect of the behavior is most problematic or distressing for the individuals and the caregiver and design individually tailored interventions (Molony et al., 2018).

Use of a behavioral log or diary over a 2- to 3-day period to track when the behavior occurs, the circumstances, and the response to interventions is recommended and required in nursing facilities. The Behave-AD, the Cohen-Mansfield Agitation Inventory, and the Neuropsychiatric Inventory for Nursing Homes are examples of reliable instruments that can be used in assessment. The WeCare Advisor (WCA) (Box 25.4) is a web-based application designed to enable family caregivers to assess, manage, and track BPSDs using nonpharmacological approaches. Further testing of the tool is ongoing but use of the WCA seems to be associated with a significant decrease in caregiver stress (Kales et al., 2018; Kales et al., 2017). Box 25.14 presents examples of some common behaviors and possible strategies.

◆ Nursing Actions: BPSD

◆ Pharmacological Approaches

All evidence-based guidelines endorse an approach that begins with comprehensive evaluation of the behavior and possible causes followed by the use of nonpharmacological interventions as a first line of treatment except in emergency situations when BPSDs could lead to imminent danger or compromise safety (American Geriatrics Society, 2019). Medications, including antipsychotics, may be necessary and appropriate for the

BOX 25.14 Examples of Behavior and Environmental Modification Strategies for BPSDs

Behavior	Strategy
Hearing voices	Evaluate hearing or adjust amplification of hearing aids.
	Assess quality and severity of symptoms.
	Determine whether they present an actual threat to safety or function.
	Assess noise around patient's room (e.g., staff talking in hallway).
Aggression	Determine and modify underlying causes of aggression (e.g., pain, caregiver interaction, being forced to do something).
	Teach caregiver not to confront individual, use distraction, observe facial expression and body posture, leave individual alone if safe, return later for the task (e.g., bathing).
	Create a calmer, more soothing environment.
Repetitive questioning	Respond with a calm, reassuring voice.
	Use calm touch for reassurance.
	Place warm water bottle covered with soft fleece cover on the lap or abdomen.
	Inform individual of events only as they occur.
	Structure daily routines.
	Involve person in meaningful activities.

BPSDs, Behavioral and psychological symptoms of dementia.
Adapted from Kales, H., Gitlin, L., Lyketsos, C., et al. (2014). Management of neuropsychiatric symptoms of dementia in clinical settings: recommendations from a multidisciplinary expert panel. *J Am Geriatr Soc, 62,*762–769.

palliation of patient distress when nonpharmacological interventions fail (Kerns et al., 2018). Strict federal regulations monitor the use of psychotropic medications in SNFs. Prevalence rates of antipsychotic use has significantly declined in nursing homes as a result of several proactive measures (Chapter 6). Antipsychotic medication use in nursing facilities may be considered after all possible causes of behavior have been investigated and, if used, should be given at the lowest possible dosage for the shortest period of time, monitored closely for side effects, and subject to gradual dose reduction and review (CMS, 2013). Pharmacological approaches may be considered, in addition to nonpharmacological approaches, if there has been a comprehensive evaluation of reversible causes of behavior; the person presents a danger to self or others; nonpharmacological interventions have not been effective; and the risk/benefit profiles of the medications have been considered. There must be documentation of all care planning related to the individual's behaviors and use and effectiveness of nonpharmacological interventions.

⚡ SAFETY ALERT

Do not use antipsychotics as your first choice to treat behavioral and psychological symptoms of dementia (BPSDs). People with dementia often exhibit aggression, resistance to care, and other challenging or disruptive behaviors. In such instances, antipsychotic medications are often prescribed, but they provide limited benefit and can cause serious harm, including stroke and premature death. Use of these drugs should be limited to cases where nonpharmacological measures have failed and patients pose an imminent threat to themselves or others. Identifying and addressing causes of behavior change can make drug treatment unnecessary (American Geriatrics Society, 2015.)

The Centers for Medicare and Medicaid Services (CMS) has now expanded focus on reduction of other psychotropic medications such as antidepressant, anxiolytic, and hypnotic agents in nursing facilities. However, rates of antipsychotic use among individuals with dementia living in the community are rising. In the United States, 41.4% of adults aged 70 years and older take psychotropic medications (Basnet et al., 2020).

◆ Nonpharmacological Approaches

Nonpharmacological approaches are person-centered approaches that are informed by careful investigation of the possible causes and meaning of the individual's behavioral and psychological symptoms. Nonpharmacological approaches can be grouped into three categories: (1) those targeting the individual, (2) those targeting the caregiver, and (3) those targeting the environment (Kales et al., 2015). Approaches include the following: sensory practices (aromatherapy, massage, multisensory stimulation, bright-light therapy), psychosocial practices (validation therapy, reminiscence therapy, music therapy, animal-assisted therapy, meaningful activities), environmental design (e.g., special care units, homelike environment, gardens, safe walking areas), changes in mealtime and bathing environments, consistent staffing assignments and structured care protocols (bathing, mouth care), and support for caregivers (Scales et al., 2018).

There is a large amount of literature on nonpharmacological interventions and these approaches are recommended in the culture change movement (Chapter 6). In general, these interventions, despite a lack of rigorous testing, have shown promise for improving quality of life for persons with dementia at home and in residential care, have no harmful side effects, and require minimal to moderate investment (Scales et al., 2018). Nonpharmacological approaches that were found to be clinically efficacious for aggression and agitation compared with usual care are multidisciplinary care, massage and touch therapy, and music combined with massage and touch therapy. Exercise, outdoor activities, and modification of ADL also have been found effective for verbal aggression and physical agitation (Watt et al., 2019).

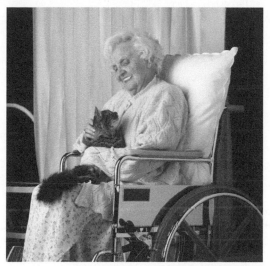

A nursing home resident enjoying pet therapy. (Courtesy Corbis.)

Continued attention to translating these interventions into real-world practice across settings in feasible and cost-effective ways is needed. Resnick and colleagues (2016) note that "despite regulatory requirements and availability of educational materials focused on nonpharmacological management of BPSDs, less than 2% of nursing homes consistently implement behavioral approaches" (p. 571). Identified barriers include lack of knowledge, skills, and hands-on experience with the many different approaches, belief that medication use is more effective, lack of belief in the effectiveness of non-pharmacological approaches, inadequate staffing, and lack of administrative support.

A toolkit approach that provides a variety of interventions may be useful in improving the use of nonpharmacological interventions in long-term care facilities. An online toolkit, *Promoting Positive Behavioral Health: A Nonpharmacological Toolkit for Senior Living Communities* (Kolanowski & Van Haitsma, 2013), provides many resources for nurses, other caregivers, and families including behavior assessment tools, clinical decision-making algorithms, and evidence-based approaches to ameliorate or prevent BPSDs (Box 25.4).

Clearly, the role of medications and nonpharmacological interventions to treat BPSDs needs further study. Our understanding of the comparative efficacy of pharmacological and nonpharmacological interventions for treating BPSDs has been limited by a lack of randomized controlled trials (Watt et al., 2019). Health care providers and family caregivers can benefit from training, better access, and practical assistance in implementing approaches for behavioral concerns. Behavioral health programs must be better integrated with primary medical care for individuals with dementia. Collaborative care management programs for the treatment of AD, often led by advanced practice nurses, have been shown to improve quality of care, decrease the incidence of BPSDs, and decrease caregiver stress (Callahan et al., 2006; Heintz et al., 2020; Reuben et al., 2014).

PROVIDING CARE FOR ACTIVITIES OF DAILY LIVING

The losses associated with dementia interfere with the person's communication patterns and ability to understand and express thoughts and feelings. Perceptual disturbances and misinterpretations of reality contribute to fear and misunderstanding. Often, bathing and the provision of other ADL care, such as dressing, grooming, and toileting, are the cause of much distress for both the person with dementia and the caregiver.

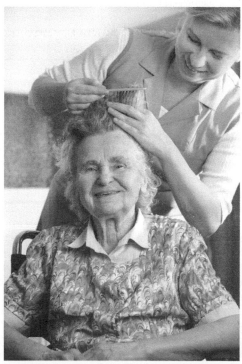

Activities of daily living care enhance self-esteem. (© iStock .com/AlexRaths.)

Bathing

Bathing is the ADL associated with the highest frequency of BPSD expressions of distress (Scales et al., 2018). Bathing is an essential aspect of everyday life that most people enjoy. However, bathing can be perceived as a personal attack by individuals with dementia who may respond by screaming or striking out. In institutional settings, a rigid focus on tasks or institutional care routines, such as a shower three mornings each week, can contribute to the distress and precipitate distressing behaviors. Being touched or bathed against a person's will violates the trust in caregiver relationships and can be considered a major affront (Rader & Barrick, 2000). The behaviors that may be exhibited are not deliberate attacks on caregivers by a violent person, but rather a way to express self in an uncertain situation. The message is: "Please find another way to keep me clean, because the way you are doing it now is intolerable" (Rader & Barrick, 2000, p. 49) (Box 25.15).

BOX 25.15 Understanding Behavior: Seeing Through the Eyes of the Person

You are asleep in the chair at home when suddenly you are awakened by a person you have never seen before trying to undress you. Then they put you naked into a hard, cold chair and wheels you down a hallway. Suddenly cold water hits you in the face and the person is touching your private areas. You don't understand why the person is trying to do this to you. You are embarrassed, frightened, cold, and angry. You hit and scream at this person and try to get away.

❖ USING CLINICAL JUDGMENT TO PROMOTE HEALTHY AGING: BATHING COMFORT

In research conducted in nursing homes, Rader and Barrick (2000) have provided comprehensive guidelines for bathing people with NCDs in ways that are pleasurable and decrease distress. Asking the question "What is the easiest, most comfortable, least frightening way for me to clean the person right now?" guides the choice of interventions. *Bathing Without a Battle* is an approach that can be used to create a better bathing experience for people with dementia. These techniques show positive results in reducing BPSD (Box 25.16). Another innovative approach being investigated in Sweden is caregiver singing and the use of background music during ADL care in nursing homes. Caregivers play and sing familiar songs during care routines. When compared with usual care practices, this approach enhanced the expression of positive moods and emotions, increased the mutuality of communication, and reduced aggression and resistive care behaviors (Hammar et al., 2011). The provision of

---

BOX 25.16 Tips for Best Practice
Techniques for Bathing Without a Battle

1. Rethink the bathing experience.
   - Make the experience comfortable and pleasurable.
   - Consider what makes the individual feel good.
   - Do not be in a hurry.
2. Approach techniques such as "let's get freshened up for the day" and avoiding bathing terminology (e.g., "it's time for your bath") can create a more positive environment. Tell person it is time to get freshened up and try not to ask, "do you want a bath?" because the answer may be no.
3. Have the room ready.
   - Keep the room warm and low-lit.
   - Handheld showerhead wets one area at a time.
   - Have a large towel or blanket to preserve dignity and keep person warm.
4. Begin bathing least sensitive area first.
   - Wash legs and feet first, followed by arms, trunk, perineum area, and face last.
5. Save washing hair until last or do separately.
6. Use distraction techniques.
   - Consider using music, calming sounds, or singing songs that the person likes.
   - Consider having the person hold a towel or something to provide distraction.
7. Consider a towel bath, under clothes bath, or sponge bath

From University of North Carolina Cecil G. Sheps Center for Health Services Research: *Bathing without a battle.* http://bathingwithoutabattle.unc.edu/.

---

oral care is another ADL that often precipitates anxiety and agitation for individuals with NCDs. Person-centered oral care protocols are discussed in Chapter 11.

WANDERING

Wandering associated with NCDs is one of the most difficult concerns encountered in home and institutional settings. Wandering is a complex behavior and is not well understood. Wandering is defined as "a syndrome of dementia-related locomotion behavior having a frequent, repetitive, temporally disordered and/or spatially disoriented nature that is manifested in lapping, random and/or pacing patterns, some of which is associated with eloping, eloping attempts or getting lost unless accompanied" (Algase et al., 2007, p. 696). Risk factors for wandering include visuospatial impairments, anxiety and depression, poor sleep patterns, unmet needs, and a more socially active and outgoing premorbid lifestyle. One in five persons with dementia wander and wandering frequency tends to increase as cognitive function decreases (Futrell et al., 2014).

Wandering presents safety concerns in all settings. Wandering behavior affects sleeping, eating, safety, and the caregiver's ability to provide care, and it also interferes with the privacy of others. The behavior can lead to falls, elopement (leaving the home or facility), injury, and death. The stimulus for wandering arises from many internal and external sources. Wandering can be considered a rhythm, intrinsically and extrinsically driven. Box 25.17 presents insight into the behavior of wandering from the perspective of individuals with an NCD.

❖ USING CLINICAL JUDGMENT TO PROMOTE HEALTHY AGING: WANDERING BEHAVIOR

It is important to recognize and analyze cues that may trigger wandering, such as acute illness, exacerbations of chronic illness, fatigue, medication effects, and constipation. Unmet needs or pain can increase wandering (Futrell et al., 2014). The need for social interaction or to relieve boredom may be a stimulus for wandering and research suggests that wandering is less likely to occur when the individual is involved in social interaction (Adekoya & Guse, 2019). Wandering behaviors can be predicted through careful observation and awareness of the person's patterns. For example, if a person with dementia starts wandering or trying to leave the home in the afternoon every day, meaningful activities such as music, exercise, and refreshments can be provided at this time.

Locked units and environmental modifications are also safety measures for individuals who wander. Wandering paths such as hallways with a continuous path or circular loop (including outside walking paths) and simple visual cues or artwork/objects to support therapeutic walking should be provided. Daily supervised walks and outside time in a safe area are important interventions. Although safety is a major concern, risks should not be the only focus. With a person-centered approach, the less wandering is seen as a problem, the more its benefits will be seen. Walking should be seen as exercise and an opportunity for socialization and care should be structured to support safety to maintain the positive benefits for some individuals (Adekoya & Guse, 2019). There are also several instruments to determine risk for wandering, and nurse researcher May Futrell and her colleagues (2010, 2014) developed an evidence-based protocol for wandering.

Wandering behavior may also result in people with NCDs going outside and getting lost. All people with dementia are considered capable of getting lost. Caregivers must prevent people with NCDs from leaving homes or care facilities unaccompanied, register the person in the Alzheimer's Association Safe Return program and Silver Alert if available, and have a plan of action in case the person does become lost. Protocols must be in place in care facilities that include identification of individuals who may wander; a wandering prevention program to ensure safety; and an elopement response plan (Futrell et al., 2014). There are a number of assistive technology devices and programs (e.g., electronic tagging and tracking devices) that can enhance the safety of persons who wander (Chapter 16).

NUTRITION

Older adults with NCDs are particularly at risk of weight loss and inadequate nutrition. Weight loss often becomes a considerable concern in later stages and about 90% of individuals with advanced dementia suffer from eating problems (Ijaopo & Ijaopo, 2019). Nutritional concerns are a major source of distress for people living with NCDs and their caregivers and are identified as a top research priority (Abelhamid et al., 2016). Some of the predisposing factors to nutritional inadequacy include lack of awareness of the need to eat, depression, loss of independence in self-feeding, agnosia, apraxia, vision impairments (deficient contrast sensitivity), wandering, pacing, and behavior disturbances. Weight loss increases the risk of infection, pressure injury development, poor wound healing, and hospitalization and is associated with higher mortality and morbidity. Nurses, as members of interprofessional teams, play a significant role in assessing nutrition in older adults with NCDs.

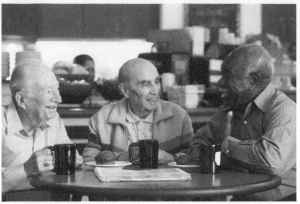

A pleasurable dining experience can enhance intake. (© iStock .com/monkeybusinessimages.)

❖ USING CLINICAL JUDGMENT TO PROMOTE HEALTHY AGING: NUTRITION

There has been little research on specific interventions to support food and fluid intake in individuals with NCDs and results of a systematic review found no definitive evidence on effectiveness, or lack of effectiveness, of specific interventions. Further research is needed and should include individuals with different NCDs, at different stages, and in different settings. However, Abdelhamid and colleagues (2016) suggest that individuals and their caregivers have to deal with eating problems despite a lack of evidence. Some promising interventions include: (1) establishing a routine so that the individual does not have to remember time and places for eating; (2) continue to serve foods and fluids that the person likes and has always eaten; (3) provide nutrient-dense foods (e.g., peanut butter, protein bars, yogurt); (4) pay attention to mealtime ambience; (5) allow as much time as needed to eat the foods that are preferred; (6) make food available 24 hours a day; and (7) allow the person to follow their accustomed eating schedule (e.g., late breakfast, early dinner).

Tube Feeding in End-Stage Dementia

Increasing evidence indicates that tube feeding in the end-stage of dementia does not prolong survival or improve quality of life. In fact, enteral feeding increases the risk of several complications, including aspiration and pressure injuries (Box 25.18). The proportion of nursing home residents with advanced dementia receiving feeding tubes has significantly decreased in recent years. The American Geriatrics Society (AGS) (2015) does not recommend feeding tubes for older adults with advanced dementia and suggests that careful hand feeding is at least as good as tube feeding for the outcomes

---

BOX 25.18   Myths and Facts About PEG Tubes in Advanced Dementia and End-of-Life Care

Myths

- PEGs prevent death from inadequate intake.
- PEGs reduce aspiration pneumonia.
- PEGs improve albumin levels and nutritional status.
- PEGs assist in healing pressure injuries.
- PEGs provide enhanced comfort for people at the end of life.
- Not feeding people is a form of euthanasia, and we cannot let people starve to death.

Facts

- PEGs do not improve quality of life.
- PEGs do not reduce risk of aspiration and increase the rate of pneumonia development. In one study, the use of feeding tubes was associated with an increased risk of pressure injuries among nursing home residents with advanced cognitive impairment (Teno et al., 2012).
- PEGs do not prolong survival in dementia.
- Nearly 50% of patients die within 6 months following PEG tube insertion.
- PEGs cause increased discomfort from both the tube presence and the use of restraints.
- PEGs are associated with infections, gastrointestinal symptoms, and abscesses.
- PEG tube feeding deprives people of the taste of food and contact with caregivers during feeding.
- PEGs are popular because they are convenient and labor beneficial.

PEG, Percutaneous endoscopic gastrostomy.
Data from Aparanji, K. & Dharmarajan, T. (2010). Pause before a PEG: a feeding tube may not be necessary in every candidate. *J Am Med Dir Assoc, 11,* 453–456; Teno, J., Gozalo, P., Mitchell, S., et al. (2012). Feeding tubes and the prevention or healing of pressure ulcers. *Arch Intern Med, 172*(9), 697–701; Vitale, C., Monteleoni, C., Burke, L., et al. (2009). Strategies for improving care for patients with advanced dementia and eating problems: optimizing care through physician and speech pathologist collaboration. *Ann Longterm Care, 17,* 32–39.

---

of death, aspiration pneumonia, functional status, and patient comfort.

Food and eating are closely tied to socialization, comfort, pleasure, love, and the meeting of basic biological needs. Feeding is often equated with caring, and not providing adequate nutrition may be viewed as cruel and inhumane. Decisions about feeding tube placement are challenging and require thoughtful discussion with patients and caregivers, who should be free to make decisions without duress and with careful consideration of the patient's advance directives, if available. Many considerations factor into decisions families and providers make about enteral feeding, including the individual's wishes in an advanced directive, cultural, religious and ethical beliefs, legal and financial concerns, and emotions.

Most feeding tube insertions occur during acute hospitalization and decisions to place a feeding tube are often taken without completely exhausting every means to maintain a normal oral intake. Research has shown that discussions surrounding the decision are often inadequate and health care surrogates claim they seldom have their informational needs completely met by health care providers (Ijaopo and Ijaopo, 2019; Teno et al., 2015). Discussion about advance directives and feeding support should begin early in the course of NCDs rather than waiting until a crisis develops. The best advice for individuals is to state preferences for the use of a feeding tube in a written advance directive. Individuals should be given information about the risks and benefits of enteral feeding in the end stages of NCDs (see Box 25.4 for reference to an advanced directive in dementia).

It is important that health care professionals provide the leadership to guide this complex decision-making process to promote true person-centered care (Gieniusz et al., 2018). Regardless of the decision, an important nursing role is to journey with the patient's loved ones, providing support and encouraging expression of feelings. Making these decisions is very difficult and loved ones "have to make peace with their decisions" (Teno et al., 2015). "Further research is required to establish whether tube feeding of individuals with advanced dementia provides more burdens than benefits or vice-versa and evaluate the impacts on quality of life and survival" (Ijaopo & Ijaopo, 2019).

NURSING ROLES IN THE CARE OF PERSONS WITH DEMENTIA

Caring for someone with an NCD, whether by family members or formal caregivers, requires special skills, knowledge of evidence-based practice, and a deep understanding of the person. A major focus of nursing education and continued education of practicing nurses should be on providing in-depth information on best practice care of individuals with NCDs. Current practice often does not reflect person-centered care and can cause great distress and poor outcomes for the individual and their caregivers. Rader and Tornquist (1995) reflected on the knowledge required and provide a view of caregiving roles that is quite useful and understandable for all caregivers. The authors have found that nurses and family caregivers can truly relate to the practical wisdom in these words.

- **Magician role:** To understand what the person is trying to communicate both verbally and nonverbally,

we must be a magician who can use our magical abilities to see the world through the eyes, the ears, and the feelings of the person. We know how to use tricks to turn an individual's behavior around or prevent it from occurring and causing distress.
- **Detective role:** The detective looks for clues and cues about what might be causing distress and how it might be changed. We have to investigate and know as much about the person as possible to be a good detective.
- **Carpenter role:** By having a wide variety of tools and selecting the right tools for the job, we build individualized plans of care for each person.
- **Jester role:** Many people with NCDs retain their sense of humor and respond well to the appropriate use of humor. This does not mean making fun of but rather sharing laughter and fun. "Those who love their work and do it well employ good doses of humor as part of the care of others, and for self-care" (Rader & Barrick, 2000, p. 42). The jester spreads joy, is creative, energizes, and lightens the burdens (Laurenhue, 2001; Rader & Barrick, 2000).

Fig. 25.1 presents a nursing situation that one nurse experienced in caring for individuals with NCDs who was being admitted to a nursing facility. Written from the perspective of the nurse and his knowledge of the patient, the story provides insight into important nursing responses, such as providing person-centered care, implementing therapeutic communication, and establishing meaningful relationships. It is a lovely example of expert gerontological nursing for individuals and a fitting way to end this chapter.

KEY CONCEPTS

- Cues to cognitive impairment are subtle, often missed, not adequately evaluated, and attributed to aging changes. Nurses must utilize clinical judgment in recognizing and analyzing cues of cognitive decline and inability to function in important aspects of life to design nursing actions to prevent unnecessary decline and promote cognitive health.
- Delirium results from the interaction of predisposing factors (e.g., vulnerability on the part of the individual attributable to predisposing conditions such as cognitive impairment, severe illness, sensory impairment) and precipitating factors/insults (e.g., medications, procedures, restraints).
- Delirium is characterized by fluctuating levels of consciousness, sometimes in a diurnal pattern, and frequent misperceptions and illusions. It is often unrecognized and is attributed to age or dementia. People with dementia are more susceptible to delirium. Knowledge of risk factors, preventive measures,

and treatment of underlying medical problems is essential to prevent serious consequences.

- Acute illness (e.g., UTIs, respiratory tract infections), medications, and pain are frequently the causes of delirium in older adults.

- It is essential to view all behavior as meaningful and an expression of needs. The focus must be on understanding that behavioral expressions communicate distress and the response is to investigate the possible source of distress and intervene appropriately.

- Fear, discomfort, unfamiliar surroundings and people, illness, fatigue, depression, need for autonomy and control, caregiver approaches and communication, and environmental stressors are frequent precipitants of behavioral symptoms.

- All evidence-based guidelines endorse an approach that begins with comprehensive assessment of BPSDs and possible causes followed by use of nonpharmacological interventions as a first-line treatment, except in emergency situations when symptoms could lead to imminent danger or compromise safety.

- Individuals with cognitive impairment respond best to calmness and patience, adaptations of communication techniques, and environments and relationships that enhance function, support limitations, ensure safety, and provide opportunities for a meaningful quality of life. Because cognitively impaired persons may be unable to express their feelings and needs in ways that are easily understood, the gerontological nurse must always try to understand the world from their perspective.

ACTIVITIES AND DISCUSSION QUESTIONS

1. What are the differences between delirium, dementia, and depression?
2. What are some of the risk factors for development of delirium?
3. Discuss communication strategies useful for a person experiencing delirium.
4. Why is it important to ensure that a person experiencing any change in mental status receives a thorough assessment and evaluation?
5. Brainstorm with fellow students how it would feel to be bathed by a total stranger.
6. The nursing assistants in a nursing home complain to you that Mr. G. hit them when they were trying to give him his required twice-weekly shower. How might you assist them in meeting Mr. G.'s need for bathing?
7. A family caregiver tells you that their loved one keeps trying to leave the house to find the children. What are some strategies you might share with the caregiver to deal with this situation?

NEXT-GENERATION NCLEX® EXAMINATION-STYLE QUESTIONS

Mrs. Landers is a newly admitted long-term care resident. She is 88 years old and has late dementia. In addition to Alzheimer's disease, her medical history includes hypertension, coronary artery disease, depression, and osteoporosis. The move to long-term care was planned when Mrs. Landers dementia was mild. She participated in the selection of the facility, along with her three children. She regularly wanders in and out of other resident's rooms, picking up objects and putting them down. The assistive personnel gently guide her out of the other residents' rooms without resistance when this happens and she smiles and repeats "yes" over and over. At 3 p.m. each day, she goes to the door and tries to leave; when assistive personnel or the nursing staff try to steer her to a diversional activity, she says, "no, no, no," pinches them, and resists redirection. Mrs. Landers eats finger foods as she wanders. She is incontinent of bowel and bladder. Her medications include memantine 10 mg twice daily, donepezil 10 mg at bedtime, fluoxetine 20 mg daily, aspirin 81 mg daily, ezetimibe 10 mg daily, valsartan/hydrochlorothiazide 160 mg/25 mg daily, and acetaminophen 500 mg every 4 hours as needed for pain. Her admission laboratory results reveal the following:

- Hemoglobin 11 mg/dL; hematocrit 34%
- WBC 8.2×10^9/L
- BUN/Creatinine 24 mg/dL and 1.4 mg/dL
- Na/Cl 144 mmol/L and 103 mmol/L
- Glucose 100 mg/dL
- Urine is amber and clear, pH 5.0, nitrite negative and leukocyte esterase trace, blood negative, WBC 1/hpf, and bacteria trace

Which actions will the nurse take to address the client's most pressing needs? Select all that apply.

1. Request the family schedule an appointment with the facility's contracted psychiatrist.
2. Put client on a toileting program to reduce incontinence.
3. Request dietary consult to ensure adequate intake to meet caloric needs.
4. Call the health care provider for antibiotic orders to treat a urinary tract infection.
5. Call the health care provider for as needed lorazepam to treat agitation.
6. Call the client's children to determine previous activities that took place around 3 p.m. daily.
7. Schedule meaningful activities for the client to promote cognitive stimulation.
8. Complete a behavioral diary over a 2–3-day period.

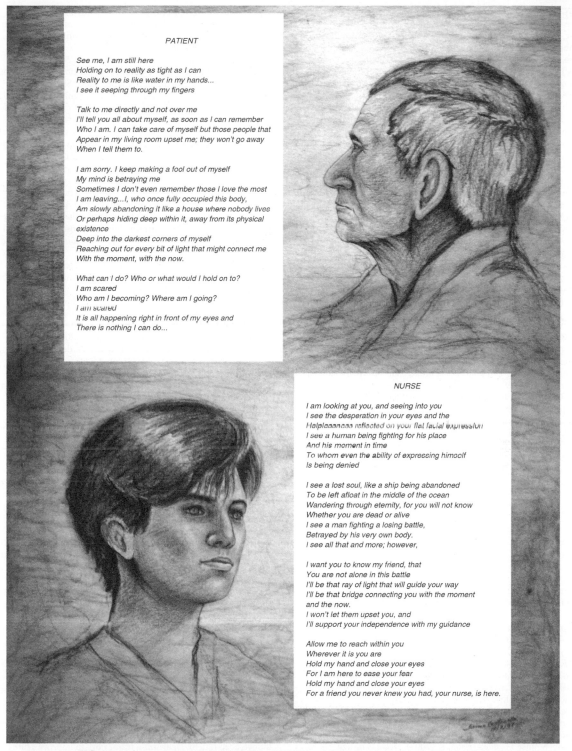

PATIENT

See me, I am still here
Holding on to reality as tight as I can
Reality to me is like water in my hands...
I see it seeping through my fingers

Talk to me directly and not over me
I'll tell you all about myself, as soon as I can remember
Who I am. I can take care of myself but those people that
Appear in my living room upset me; they won't go away
When I tell them to.

I am sorry. I keep making a fool out of myself
My mind is betraying me
Sometimes I don't even remember those I love the most
I am leaving...I, who once fully occupied this body,
Am slowly abandoning it like a house where nobody lives
Or perhaps hiding deep within it, away from its physical
existence
Deep into the darkest corners of myself
Reaching out for every bit of light that might connect me
With the moment, with the now.

What can I do? Who or what would I hold on to?
I am scared
Who am I becoming? Where am I going?
I am scared
It is all happening right in front of my eyes and
There is nothing I can do...

NURSE

I am looking at you, and seeing into you
I see the desperation in your eyes and the
Helplessness reflected on your flat facial expression
I see a human being fighting for his place
And his moment in time
To whom even the ability of expressing himself
Is being denied

I see a lost soul, like a ship being abandoned
To be left afloat in the middle of the ocean
Wandering through eternity, for you will not know
Whether you are dead or alive
I see a man fighting a losing battle,
Betrayed by his very own body.
I see all that and more; however,

I want you to know my friend, that
You are not alone in this battle
I'll be that ray of light that will guide your way
I'll be that bridge connecting you with the moment
and the now.
I won't let them upset you, and
I'll support your independence with my guidance

Allow me to reach within you
Wherever it is you are
Hold my hand and close your eyes
For I am here to ease your fear
Hold my hand and close your eyes
For a friend you never knew you had, your nurse, is here.

FIG. 25.1 Nurse and patient. (Copyright ©1998 by Jaime Castaneda, Lake Worth, FL.)

REFERENCES

Algase, D. L., Beel-Bates, C., & Beattie, E. R. A. (2003). Wandering in long-term care. *Annals Longterm Care, 11*, 33–39.

Algase, D. L., Moore, D. H., Vandeweerd, C., & Gavin-Dreschnack, D. J. (2007). Mapping the maze of terms and definitions in dementia-related wandering. *Aging & Mental Health, 11*, 686–698.

Abdelhamid, A., Bunn, D., Copley, M., et al. (2016). Effectiveness of interventions to directly support food and drink intake in people with dementia: systematic review and meta-analysis. *BMC Geriatrics, 16*, 26.

Adekoya, A., & Guse, L. (2019). Wandering behavior from the perspectives of older adults with mild to moderate dementia in long-term care. *Research Gerontology Nursing, 12*(5), 239–247.

Alzheimer's Association. (2018). *Younger/early onset Alzheimer's & Dementia.* https://www.alz.org/alzheimers_disease_early_onset .asp.

American Geriatrics Society. (2019). *Choosing wisely: ten things physicians and patients should question.* https://www.choosingwisely .org/societies/american-geriatrics-society/.

American Psychiatric Association. (2013). *Diagnostic and statistical manual of mental disorders*, 5th ed. *American Psychiatric Association.*

Austrom, M. G., Boustani, M., & LaMantia, M. A. (2018). Ongoing medical management to maximize health and well-being for persons living with dementia. *The Gerontologist, 58*(Suppl 1), S48–S57.

Basnet, P., Acton, G., & Requeijo, P. (2020). Psychotropic medication prescribing practice among resident with dementia in nursing homes: a person-centered care approach. *Journal Gerontologist Nursing, 46*(2), 9–15.

Battle, C. E., James, K., Bromfield, T., & Temblett, P. (2017). Predictors of post-traumatic stress disorder following critical illness: a mixed methods study. *Journal of Intensive Care Society, 18*(4), 289–293.

Birge, O., & Aydin, T. (2017). The effect of nonpharmacological training on delirium identification and intervention strategies of intensive care nurses. *Intensive & Critical Care Nursing: the official journal of the British Association of Critical Care Nurses, 41*, 33–42.

Buckwalter, K., Gerdner, L., Hall, G., et al. (1995). Shining through: The humor and individuality of persons with Alzheimer's disease. *Journal of Gerontological Nursing, 21*, 11–16.

Callahan, C. M., Boustani, M. A., Unverzagt, F. W., et al. (2006). Effectiveness of collaborative care for older adults with Alzheimer disease in primary care: a randomized controlled trial. *JAMA: the journal of the American Medical Association, 295*, 2148–2157.

Centers for Medicare and Medicaid Services (CMS): *Center for clinical standards and quality/survey and certification group,* (Memo), May 14, 2013. http://www.cms.gov/Medicare/Provider -Enrollment-and-Certification/SurveyCertificationGenInfo /Downloads/Survey-and-Cert-Letter-13-35.pdf.

Cheney, C. (2019). In-hospital delirium predictive of readmission, discharge to postacute facilities, ER visits. *Patient Safety and Quality Healthcare.* https://www.psqh.com/news/in-hospital -delirium-predictive-of-readmission-discharge-to-postacute -facilities-er-visits/. Accessed January 2021.

Dahlke, S., & Phinney, A. (2008). Caring for hospitalized older adults at risk for delirium: the silent, unspoken piece of nursing practice. *Journal of gerontological nursing, 34*, 41–47.

DeYoung, S., Just, G., & Harrison, R. (2003). Decreasing aggressive, agitated, or disruptive behavior: Participation in a behavior management unit. *Journal of gerontological nursing, 28*, 22–31.

Ely, E. W., Margolin, R., Francis, J., et al. (2001). Evaluation of delirium in critically ill patients: validation of the Confusion Assessment Method for the intensive care unit (CAM-ICU). *Critical Care Medicine, 29*, 1370–1379.

Fazio, S., Pace, D., Maslow, K., Zimmerman, S., & Kallmyer, B. (2018). Alzheimer's Association dementia care practice recommendations. *Gerontologist, 58*(Suppl 1), S1–S9.

Fick, D. M. (2018). The critical vital sign of cognitive health and delirium: whose responsibility is it? *Journal of gerontological nursing, 44*(8), 3–5.

Flaherty, J., Yue, J., Rudolph, J. (2017). Dissecting delirium. Phenotypes, screening, diagnosis, prevention, treatment, and program implementation. *Clinics in Geriatric Medicine, 33*(3), 393–413.

Flanagan, N. M., & Spencer, G. (2015). Informal caregivers and detection of delirium in postacute care: a correlational study of the confusion assessment method (CAM), confusion assessment method-family assessment method (CAM-FAM) and DSM-IV criteria. *International Journal of Older People Nursing, 11*(3), 176–183.

Forsberg, M. M. (2017). Delirium update for postacute care and long-term care settings: a narrative review. *The Journal of the American Osteopathic Association, 117*, 32–38.

Futrell, M., Melillo, K. D., Remington, R., & Butcher, H. K. (2014). Evidence-based practice guideline: wandering. *Journal of gerontological nursing, 40*(11), 16–23.

Futrell, M., Melillo, K. D., Remington, R., & Schoenfelder, D. P. (2010). Evidence-based practice guideline: wandering. *Journal of gerontological nursing, 36*, 6–16.

Gieniuz, M., Sinvani, L., Kozikowski, A, et al. (2018). Percutaneous feeding tubes in individuals with advanced dementia: are physicians "Choosing Wisely"? *JAGS, 66*, 64–69.

Gilmore-Bykovskyi, A. (2020). Gender differences in 30-day rehospitalizations among Medicare beneficiaries with Alzheimer's and dementia. *Innovation in Aging, 4* (Suppl_1), 697.

Greenwood, N., & Smith, R. (2016). The experiences of people with young-onset dementia: a meta-ethnographic review of the qualitative literature. *Maturitas, 92*, 102–109.

Hain, D. J., Tappen, R., Diaz, S., & Ouslander, J. G. (2012). Cognitive impairment and medication self-management errors in older adults discharged home from a community hospital. *Home Health Nurse, 30*(4), 246–254.

Hall, G. R. (1994). Caring for people with Alzheimer's disease using the conceptual model of progressively lowered stress threshold in the clinical setting. *The Nursing clinics of North America, 29*, 129–141.

Hall, G. R., & Buckwalter, K. C. (1987). Progressively lowered stress threshold: a conceptual model for care of adults with Alzheimer's disease. *Archives of psychiatric nursing, 1*, 399–406.

Hammar, L. M., Emami, A., Engström, G., & Götell, E. (2011). Communicating through caregiver singing during morning care situations in dementia care. *Scandinavian journal of caring sciences, 25*(1), 160–168.

Heintz, H., Monette, P., Epstein-Lubow, G., et al. (2020). Emerging collaborative care models for dementia care in the primary care setting: a narrative review. *American Journal of Geroatric Psychology, 28*(3), 320–330.

Hshieh, T. T., Yue, J., Oh, E., et al. (2015). Effectiveness of multicomponent nonpharmacological delirium interventions: a meta-analysis. *JAMA Internal Medicine, 175*(4), 512–520.

Ijaopo, E., & Ijaopo, R. (2019). Tube feeding in individuals with advanced dementia: a review of its burdens and perceived benefits. *Open Access.* https://doi.org/10.1155/2019/7272067.

Inouye, S. K. (2018). Delirium-a framework to improve acute care for older persons. *Journal of the American Geriatrics Society, 66*(3), 446–451.

Inouye, S. K., Bogardus, S. T. Jr., Charpentier, P. A., et al. (1999). A multicomponent intervention to prevent delirium in hospitalized older patients. *The New England journal of medicine, 340,* 669–676.

Inouye, S. K., van Dyck, C. H., Alessi, C. A., Balkin, S., Siegal, A. P., & Horwitz, R. I. (1990). Clarifying confusion: the confusion assessment method: a new method for detection of delirium. *Annals of Internal Medicine, 113,* 941–948.

Inouye, S. K., Westendorp, R. G., & Saczynski, J. S. (2014). Delirium in elderly people. *Lancet, 383,* 911–922.

Institute for Healthcare Improvement. (2019). Delirium prevention and treatment: how to improve care and avoid unnecessary costs. http://www.ihi.org/communities/blogs/delirium-prevention-and-treatment-how-to-improve-care-and-avoid-unnecessary-costs.

Kales, H. C., Gitlin, L. N., & Lyketsos, C. G. (2015). Assessment and management of behavioral and psychological symptoms of dementia. *BMJ, 350,* h369.

Kales, H. C., Gitlin, L. N., Stanislawski, B., et al. (2017). We Care Advisor™: the development of a caregiver-focused, web-based program to assess and manage behavioral and psychological symptoms of dementia. *Alzheimer Disease and Associated Disorders, 31*(3), 263–270.

Kales, H., Gitlin, L., Stanislawski, B, et al. (2018). Effect of the WeCareAdvisor on family caregiver outcomes in dementia: a randomized controlled trial. *BMC Geriatrics, 18,* 113.

Kerns, J. W., Winter, J. D., Winter, K. M., Kerns, C. C., & Etz, R. S. (2018). Caregiver perspectives about using antipsychotics and other medications for symptoms of dementia. *Gerontologist, 58*(2), e35–e45.

Kolanowski, A. M. (1999). An overview of the need-driven dementia-compromised behavior model. *Journal of gerontological nursing, 25,* 7–9.

Kolanowski, A., Boltz, M., Galik, E., et al. (2017). Determinants of behavioral and psychological symptoms of dementia: a scoping review of the evidence. *Nursing Outlook, 65,* 515–529.

Kolanowski, A., Van Haitsma, K. (2013). *Promoting positive behavioral health: a non-pharmacologic toolkit for senior living communities.* https://www.nursinghometoolkit.com/toolkitoverview.html.

Kovach, C. (1999). Assessment and treatment of discomfort for people with late-stage dementia. *Journal of Pain, Symptom Manage, 18*(6), 412–419.

Laurenhue, K. (2001). Each person's journey is unique. *Alzheimers Care Q, 2,* 79–83.

Machiels, M., Metzelthin, S. F., Hamers, J. P., & Zwakhalen, S. M. (2017). Interventions to improve communication between people with dementia and nursing staff during daily nursing care: a systematic review. *International Journal of Nursing Studies, 66,* 37–46.

McGilton, K. S., Rochon, E., Sidani, S., et al. (2017). Can we help care providers communicate more effectively with persons having dementia living in long-term care homes? *American Journal of Alzheimer's Disease and Other Dementias, 32*(1), 41–50.

McGowin, D. F. (1993). *Living in the labyrinth: A personal journey through the maze of Alzheimer's.* New York: Dell.

Miu, D. K., Chan, C. W., & Kok, C. (2016). Delirium among elderly patients admitted to a post-acute care facility and 3-months outcome. *Geriatric Gerontology International, 16*(5), 586–592.

Molony, S. L., Kolanowski, A., Van Haitsma, K., & Rooney, K. E. (2018). Person-centered assessment and care planning. *Gerontologist, 58*(Suppl 1), S32–S47.

Moon, K. J., & Park, H. (2018). Outcomes of patients with delirium in long-term care facilities: a prospective cohort study. *Journal Gerontology Nursing, 44*(9), 41–50.

Morandi, A., Davis, D., Bellelli, G., et al. (2017). The diagnosis of delirium superimposed on dementia: an emerging challenge. *Journal of the American Medical Directors Association, 18*(1), 12–18.

Neelon, V. J., Champagne, M. T., Carlson, J. R., & Funk, S. G. (1996). The NEECHAM confusion scale: construction, validation, and clinical testing. *Nursing Research, 45,* 324–330.

Oberai, T., Laver, K., Crotty, M., Killington, M., & Jaarsma, R. (2018). Effectiveness of multicomponent interventions on incidence of delirium in hospitalized older patients with hip fracture: a systematic review. *International psychogeriatrics /IPA, 30*(4), 481–492.

Rader, J., & Barrick, A. (2000). Ways that work: bathing without a battle. *Alzheimers Care Quarterly, 1*(4), 35–49.

Rader, J., & Tornquist, E. (1995). *Individualized Dementias Care.* New York, NY: Springer.

Resnick, B., Kolanowski, A., Van Haitsma, K., et al. (2016). Pilot testing of the EIT-4-BPSD intervention. *American journal of Alzheimer's disease and other dementias, 31*(7), 570–579.

Reuben, D. B., Ganz, D. A., Roth, C. P., et al. (2014). Effect of nurse practitioner comanagement on the care of geriatric conditions. *Journal of the American Geriatrics Society, 61*(8), 857–867.

Richards, K., Lambert, C., & Beck, C. (2000). Deriving interventions for challenging behaviors from the need-driven dementia-compromised behavior model. *Alzheimers Care Q, 1,* 62–72.

Rigney, T. S. (2006). Delirium in the hospitalized elder and recommendations for practice. *Geriatric nursing (New York, N. Y.), 27*(3), 151–157.

Sakamoto, M. L., Moore, S. L., & Johnson, S. T. (2017). "I'm still here": personhood and the early-onset dementia experience. *Journal of gerontological nursing, 43*(5), 12–17.

Singu, S., Koneru, M., Robinson, K., et al. (2020). Are antipsychotics helpful for preventing or treating delirium? *Jour Gerontol Nurs, 16*(1), 3–5.

Scales, K., Zimmerman, S., & Miller, S. J. (2018). Evidence-based nonpharmacological practices to address behavioral and psychological symptoms of dementia. *Gerontologist, 58,* S88–S102.

Splete, H. (2008). Nurses have special strategies for dementia. *Caring Ages, 9,* 11.

Steis, M. R., & Fick, D. M. (2008). Are nurses recognizing delirium? A systematic review. *Journal of gerontological nursing, 34,* 40–48.

Steis, M. R., Evans, L., Hirschman, K. B., et al. (2012). Screening for delirium using family caregivers: convergent validity of the Family Confusion Assessment Method and interviewer-rated Confusion Assessment Method. *Journal of the American Geriatrics Society, 60*(11), 2121–2126.

Tappen, R. M., Williams-Burgess, C., Edelstein, J., Touhy, T., & Fishman, S. (1997). Communicating with individuals with Alzheimer's disease: examination of recommended strategies. *Archives of psychiatric nursing, 11,* 249–256.

Tappen, R. M., Williams, C., Fishman, S., & Touhy, T. (1999). Persistence of self in advanced Alzheimer's disease. *Image J Nurs Sch, 31,* 121–125.

Teno, J. M., Freedman, V. A., Kasper, J. D., Gozalo, P., & Mor, V. (2015). Is care for the dying improving in the United States. *Journal of palliative medicine, 18*(8), 662–666.

Watt, J., Goodarzi, J., Veroniki, A., et al. (2019). Comparative efficacy of interventions for aggressive and agitated behaviors in dementia. *Annals of International Medical, 171,* 633–642.

Woods, B. (1999). Dementia challenges and assumptions about what it means to be a person. *Generations, 13,* 39.

26

Clinical Judgment to Promote Healthy Relationships, Roles, and Transitions

Theris A. Touhy

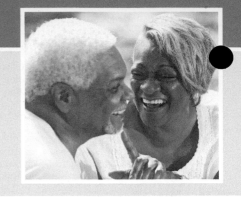

http://evolve.elsevier.com/Touhy/gerontological/

THE LIVED EXPERIENCE

It is so irritating when Madge tries to help me do things. After all, I have lived 85 years and have done very well. I think she wants to put me away somewhere. I wish she would just leave me alone. I'm sure I could manage if she just wouldn't interfere.

John, the father

I just can't stand watching as my father becomes weaker and is unable to do the things he always did so naturally and well. Yesterday he got lost on his way to the market. He was always my guide and protector. I knew I could count on him no matter what. It makes me feel sort of alone in the world.

Madge, the daughter

LATER LIFE TRANSITIONS

This chapter examines the various relationships, roles, and transitions that characteristically play a part in later life. The transitions of retirement, widowhood, and widowerhood and the concepts of family structure and function, as well as intimacy and sexuality, are examined. Nursing actions to support older adults in maintaining fulfilling roles and relationships and adapting to transitions are discussed. Transition to becoming a caregiver or recipient of care is discussed in Chapter 27.

Retirement

Issues of work and retirement for older adults are a cultural universal topic because every culture has mechanisms for retiring their older citizens. Although retirement patterns differ across the world, in industrialized nations and in many developing nations, the expectation is that older workers will cease full-time career job employment and be entitled to economic support. However, whether that support will be adequate, or even available, is a growing concern worldwide. In the United States and many European countries and in Australia, the problems are emerging as the generation born after World War II moves into retirement. Developing countries face similar issues with the growth of the older population combined with decreasing birth rates. Governments may not be able to afford retirement systems to replace the tradition of children caring for aging parents. Most countries are not ready to meet what is projected to be one of the defining challenges of the twenty-first century.

Retirement, as we formerly knew it, has changed. The transitions are blurring, and the numerous patterns and styles of retiring have produced more varied experiences in retirement. Retirement is no longer just a few years of rest from the rigors of work before death. It is a developmental stage that may occupy 30 or more years of a person's life and involve many stages. Some individuals will be retired longer than they worked. Retirees are living longer, and declining birth rates mean there will be fewer workers to support them. Countries are scaling down retirement benefits and raising the age when individuals can collect them. Individuals can expect to work longer before retirement, and many plan to continue to work after they retire. Some do so because of economic need, whereas others have a desire to remain involved and productive. However, only a quarter of retirees actually receive income from work (Employee Benefit Research Institute, 2019).

People are starting to retire later as they realize the obstacles financial challenges or obligations present to successful retirement and future independence (Plawecki & Plawecki, 2016). Sixty-nine percent of Baby Boomers either expect to or are already working past age 65 years. There may be financial reasons they want to keep working, or it might be that they want to stay mentally alert. The most frequently cited retirement fear across generations is outliving savings and investments (O'Brien, 2020; Transamerica Center for Retirement Studies, 2019). Retirement confidence continues to be closely related to having a retirement plan. The effect of the COVID-19 pandemic on retirement confidence may not be as optimistic.

Special Considerations in Retirement

The three-legged stool for retirement (Social Security, savings, and private pensions) has become one-legged for a sizable proportion of Americans because of limited personal retirement savings and decline in pension plans (Morley, 2017). Older adults with disabilities, those who had less access to education or held low-paying jobs with no benefits, and those not eligible for Social Security are at increased economic risk during retirement years. Older minority women, never-married women, and divorced women are more likely to be in poverty and are less likely to receive Social Security (Shelton, 2016).

Prior to the legalization of same-sex marriage in the United States, individuals were denied access to Social Security survivor benefits. After legalization of same-sex marriage, married same-sex couples now have access to Social Security survivor benefits, Medicaid spend-downs, bereavement leave, and tax exemptions upon inheritance of jointly owned real estate and personal property.

Inadequate coverage for women in retirement is common because their work histories have been sporadic and diverse. Women often retire earlier than anticipated because of family needs. Whereas most men have always worked outside the home, it is only within the past 30 years that this has been the expectation of women. Therefore large cohort differences exist. Traditionally, the variability of women's work histories, interrupted careers, the residuals of sexist pension policies, Social Security inequities, and low-paying jobs created hazards for adequacy of income in retirement. The scene is gradually changing in many respects, but the gender bias remains (Chapter 7).

Retirement Planning

Current research suggests that retirement has positive effects on life satisfaction and health, although this may vary depending on the individual's circumstances. Decisions to retire are often based on financial resources; attitudes toward work, family roles, and responsibilities; the nature of the job; access to health insurance; chronological age; health; and self-perceptions of ability to adjust to retirement. Retirement planning is advisable during early adulthood and essential in middle age. However, people differ in their focus on the past, present, and future and their realistic ability to "put away something" for future needs.

Retirement preparation programs are usually aimed at employees with high levels of education and occupational status, those with private pension coverage, and government employees. Thus, the people most in need of planning assistance may be those least likely to have any available, let alone the resources for an adequate retirement. Individuals who are retiring in poor health, minorities, women, those in lower socioeconomic levels, and those with the least education may experience greater concerns in retirement and may need specialized counseling and targeted education efforts.

❖ USING CLINICAL JUDGMENT TO PROMOTE HEALTHY AGING: RETIREMENT

Successful retirement adjustment depends on socialization needs, energy levels, health, adequate income, variety of interests, amount of self-esteem derived from work, presence of intimate relationships, social support, and general adaptability (Box 26.1). Nurses may have the opportunity to work with people in different phases of retirement or participate in retirement education and counseling programs.

Talking with individuals over the age of 50 years about retirement plans, providing anticipatory guidance about the transition to retirement, identifying those who

---

BOX 26.1   Predictors of Retirement Satisfaction

- Good health
- Functional abilities
- Adequate income
- Suitable living environment
- Strong social support system characterized by reciprocal relationships
- Decision to retire involved choice, autonomy, adequate preparation, higher-status job before retirement
- Retirement activities that offer an opportunity to feel useful, learn, grow, and enjoy oneself
- Positive outlook, sense of mastery, resilience, resourcefulness
- Good marital or partner relationship
- Sharing similar interests to spouse/significant other

Data from Hooyman, N., & Kiyak, H. (2011). *Social gerontology: A multidisciplinary perspective* (9th ed.). Boston: Allyn & Bacon.

---

may be at risk of lowered income and health concerns, and referring to appropriate resources for retirement planning and support are important nursing actions. Additionally, the period of preretirement and retirement may be an opportune time to enhance the focus on health promotion and illness and injury prevention (Chapter 2). It is important to build on the strengths of the individual's life experiences and coping skills and to provide appropriate counseling and support to assist individuals to continue to grow and develop in meaningful ways during the transition from the work role.

In ideal situations, retirement offers the opportunity to pursue interests that may have been neglected while fulfilling other obligations. However, for too many individuals, retirement presents challenges that affect both health and well-being, and nurses must be advocates for policies and conditions that allow all older adults to maintain quality of life in retirement.

Death of a Spouse or Life Partner

Losing a spouse or other life partner after a long, close, and satisfying relationship is the most difficult adjustment a person can face, aside from the loss of a child. This loss is a stage in the life course that can be anticipated but seldom is considered. Spousal bereavement in later life is a high probability for women, and although less common among men, it is still a significant event. Widowhood includes 6.4% of men and 19.5% of women aged 65 to 74 years; 14.7% of men and 42.9% of women aged 75 to 84 years; and 35.3% of men and 71.9% of women aged 85 years and older (Biddle et al., 2020).

Older women are substantially more likely to be widowed (and not remarried) than older men, and the majority of these older widowed women live alone. The number of widows has declined, especially for women whose spouses are now living longer. The decline in widowhood in recent decades also results from the rising share of divorced older adults who have not remarried.

Although a change in marital status is accepted as a normal life experience, the death of a spouse is a significant life event for older adults. With the loss of the intimate partner, several changes occur simultaneously in almost every domain of life and have a significant impact on well-being: physical, psychological, social, practical, and economic. Individuals who have been self-confident and resilient seem to fare best. Having frequent contact with family and friends is key to resilience in handling the loss. The transitional phase of grief, if handled appropriately, leads to the confirmation of a new identity, the end of one stage of life, and the beginning of another.

Gender differences on widowhood are found in the literature. Bereaved husbands may be more socially and emotionally vulnerable. Suicide risk is highest among men older than 80 years of age who have experienced the death of a spouse (Chapter 24). Widowers adapt more slowly than widows to the loss of a spouse and often remarry quickly. Loneliness and the need to be cared for are factors influencing widowers to pursue new partners. Having associations with family and friends, being members of a church community, and continuing to work or engage in activities can all be helpful in the adjustment period following the death of a wife. Common bereavement reactions of widowers are listed in Box 26.2 and should be discussed with male clients.

BOX 26.2   Common Widower Bereavement Reactions

- Search for the lost mate
- Neglect of self
- Inability to share grief
- Loss of social contacts
- Struggle to view women as other than wife
- Erosion of self-confidence and sexuality
- Protracted grief period

❖ USING CLINICAL JUDGMENT TO PROMOTE HEALTHY AGING: LOSS OF SPOUSE/LIFE PARTNER

Losing a spouse can have serious physical and mental health consequences. There is an elevated risk of morbidity and mortality, particularly in the early bereavement period. Physiological arousal, manifested as higher heart rate, higher systolic blood pressure, and elevation in morning cortisol level, can occur and persist for months after spousal loss. The risk seems likely to be the result of adverse physiological responses associated with acute grief. The likelihood of a heart attack or stroke doubles in the critical 30-day period after a partner's death (Biddle et al., 2020). The bereavement period is also associated with an elevated risk of multiple psychiatric disorders, particularly if the death was unexpected. However, the risks of effects of spousal bereavement and increasing age on health, particularly chronic issues, remain elevated even among those long past the event (10+ years), and ongoing surveillance and assessment are therefore indicated.

BOX 26.3   Patterns of Adjustment to Widowhood

Stage 1: Reactionary (First Few Weeks)
Early responses of disbelief, anger, indecision, detachment, and inability to communicate in a logical, sustained manner are common. Searching for the mate, visions, hallucinations, and depersonalization may be experienced.
Intervention: Support, validate, be available, listen to individual talk about mate, reduce expectations.

Stage 2: Withdrawal (First Few Months)
Depression, apathy, physiological vulnerability; movement and cognition are slowed; insomnia, unpredictable waves of grief, sighing, and anorexia occur.
Intervention: Protect individual against suicide, monitor health status, and involve in support groups.

Stage 3: Recuperation (Second 6 Months)
Periods of depression are interspersed with characteristic capability. Feelings of personal control begin to return.
Intervention: Support accustomed lifestyle patterns that sustain and assist individual to explore new possibilities.

Stage 4: Exploration (Second Year)
Individual begins new ventures, testing suitability of new roles; anniversaries, holidays, birthdays, and date of death may be especially difficult.
Intervention: Prepare individual for unexpected reactions during anniversaries. Encourage and support new trial roles.

Stage 5: Integration (Fifth Year)
Individual will feel fully integrated into new and satisfying roles if grief has been resolved in a healthy manner.
Intervention: Assist individual to recognize and share own pattern of growth through the trauma of loss.

◆ Nursing Actions: Loss of Spouse/Life Partner

Nurses will interact with bereaved older adults in many settings. This is an important time for nurses to assess the health status of the individual and provide actions to assist in coping. Knowing the stages of transition to a new role as a widow or widower will be useful in determining appropriate actions, although each individual is unique in this respect. Individuals respond to losses in ways that reflect the nature and meaning of the relationships and the unique characteristics of the bereaved. Patterns of adjustment are presented in Box 26.3. With adequate support, reintegration can be expected in 2 to 4 years. People with few familial or social supports may need professional help to get through the early months of grief in a way that will facilitate recovery. Additional information about dying, death, and grief can be found in Chapter 28.

RELATIONSHIPS IN LATER LIFE

Friendships

Friends are often a significant source of support in later life. The number of friends may decline, but the majority of older adults have at least one close friend with whom they maintain close contact, share confidences, and can turn to in an emergency. The social network may narrow as one ages, with intimate personal relationships being maintained and the more instrumental relationships discontinued. Research across the globe supports the value of friendship for older adults in promoting health and well-being.

Friendships are often sustaining in the face of overwhelming circumstances. Friends provide the critical elements of satisfactory living that families may not, providing commitment and affection without judgment. Personality characteristics between friends are compatible because the relationships are chosen and caring is shared without obligation. Trust, demonstrations of caring, and mutual problem solving are important aspects of the friendships.

Friends may share a lifelong perspective or may bring a totally new intergenerational viewpoint into a person's life. Late-life friendships often develop out of changing situations, such as relocation to retirement or assisted living communities, widowhood, and involvement in volunteer pursuits. As desires and pursuits change, some friendships evolve that the person never would have considered in their youth.

Considering the obvious importance of friendship, it seems to be a neglected area of exploration and a seldom considered resource for professionals working with older adults. Because close friendships have such influence on the sense of well-being of older adults, anything done to sustain them or assist in building new friendships and social networks will be helpful. Internet access and social media offer new opportunities to interact with friends or even to form new friendships. Generally, women tend to have more sustaining friendships than do men, and this factor contributes to resilience, a characteristic linked to successful aging (Chapter 24). It is important to ask older adults about their friendships and their importance and availability. Although friendships do provide much support, they are also a further source of grief in old age. The loss of friends through death occurs often, and nurses must appreciate the nature of this loss. Encouraging intergenerational friendships and linking older adults to resources for social participation and meaningful activities are important interventions.

FAMILIES

Changing Family Structure

The idea of family evokes strong impressions of whatever an individual believes the typical family should be. Because everyone comes from a family, these impressions have powerful symbolic meanings. However, in today's world, the definition of family is in a state of flux. As recently as 100 years ago, the norm was the extended family made up of parents, their grown children, and the children's children, often living together and sharing resources, strengths, and challenges. As cities grew and adult children moved in pursuit of work, parents did not always come along, and the nuclear family evolved. The norm in the United States became two parents and their two children (nuclear family), or at least that was the norm in what has been considered mainstream America. This pattern was not as common among ethnically diverse families where the extended family is often the norm. However, families are changing, and today the nuclear family is much less common.

Changing family patterns pose significant challenges for the future of long-term care because 80% to 90% of all long-term care services and supports are provided by spouses, adult children, and other informal caregivers. Baby Boomers are more likely to live alone than previous generations, and single-person households are increasing (Vespa & Schondelmyer, 2015). Other countries are also experiencing changes in family composition and even values as the numbers of older adults increase and the younger members of society become more mobile and move away from their home. In China, the extended family is disappearing, and in 2013 the country enacted a new law mandating that family members must attend to the spiritual needs of older family members and visit them frequently if they live apart. Nearly half of older adults in Japan live apart from their children (United Nations Economic and Social Commission for Asia and the Pacific, 2018).

A decrease in fertility rates has reduced family size, and American families are smaller today than ever before. The high divorce and remarriage rate results in households of blended families of children from previous marriages and the new marriage. The new modern family includes single-parent families, blended families, gay and lesbian families, domestic partnerships, and childless families. Older adults without families, either by choice or by circumstance, may create their own "families" through communal living with siblings, friends, or others. Indeed, it is not unusual for childless older adults residing in long-term care facilities to refer to the staff as their new "family."

Multigenerational Families

The US Census Bureau defines multigenerational families as those consisting of more than two generations living under the same roof. One in five Americans lives in a multigenerational household, about 19% of the population. In the United States, multigenerational families have grown by approximately 60% since 1990 (Generations United, 2021). Multigenerational families are more common among other cultures but it is growing among nearly all US racial groups and Hispanics, among all age groups, and among both men and women. In recent years, young adults have been the age group most likely to live in multigenerational households (previously, it had been older adults). The growth of multigenerational households in the United States accelerated during the economic downturn, and this growing trend is expected to continue. "Multigen" remodeling or new home building to accommodate intergenerational families is an increasing trend. Box 26.4 presents tips when planning to add an older adult to the household.

Family Relationships

Family members, however they are defined, form the nucleus of relationships for the majority of older adults and their support system if they become dependent. A long-standing myth in society is that families are alienated from their older family members and abandon their care to institutions. Nothing could be further from the truth. Family relationships remain strong in old age, and most older adults have frequent contact with their families. Most older adults possess a large intergenerational web of significant people, including sons, daughters, stepchildren, in-laws, nieces, nephews, grandchildren, and great-grandchildren, and partners and former partners of their offspring. Families provide the majority of care for older adults. Changes in family structure will have a significant impact on the availability of family members to provide care for older adults in the future.

BOX 26.4 Tips for Best Practice

Adding an Older Adult to the Household

Questions to Ask
- What are the needs of the new member and of the family?
- Where will space be allotted for the new member?
- How will the new member be included in existing family patterns?
- How will responsibilities be shared?
- What resources in the community will assist in the adjustment phase?
- Is the environment safe for the new member?
- How will family life change with the added member and how does the family feel about it?
- What are the differences in socialization and sleeping patterns?
- What are the older adult's needs and expectations?
- What are the older adult's skills and talents?

Modifications That May Need to Be Made
- Arrange semiprivate living quarters if possible.
- Regularly schedule visits to other relatives to give each family time for respite and privacy.
- Arrange adult day health programs and senior activities for the older adult to help keep contact with members of their own generation. Consider how the older adult will feel about giving up familiar surroundings and friends.

Potential Areas of Conflict
- Space: especially if someone has given up their space to the older relative

- Possessions: older adults may want to move possessions into the house; others may not find them attractive or may insist on replacing them with new things.
- Entertaining: times when old and young feel the need or desire to exclude the other from social events.
- Responsibilities and chores: the older adult may feel useless if they do nothing and may feel in the way if they do something.
- Expenses: increased cost of home maintenance, food, clothing, and recreation may not be shared appropriately.
- Vacations: whether to go together or alone; young persons may feel uneasy not taking the older adult out and may feel resentful if they must.
- Childrearing: disagreement over childrearing methods.
- Childcare: finding a balance between the amount of responsibility grandparents will assume for childcare if desired and family needs/ desires.

Ways to Decrease Areas of Conflict
- Respect privacy.
- Discuss space allocations.
- Discuss the older adult's furnishings before the move.
- Make it clear in advance when social events include everyone or exclude someone.
- Make clear decisions about household tasks; all should have responsibility geared to ability.
- Have the older adult pay a share of expenses if able.

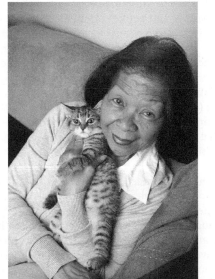

Pets are a part of the family and are particularly beneficial to older adults. They provide companionship, comfort, and caring. (© iStock.com/michellegibson.)

As families change, the roles of the members or expectations of one another may also change. Grandparents may assume parental roles for their grandchildren if their children are unable to care for them; or grandparents and older aunts and uncles may assume temporary caregiving roles while the children, nieces, and nephews work. Adult children of any age may provide limited or extensive caregiving to their own parents or aging relatives who may become ill or impaired. A spouse, sibling, or grandchild may also become a caregiver.

Close-knit families are more aware of the needs of their members and work to resolve problems and find ways to meet the needs of members, even if they are not always successful. Emotionally distant families are less available in times of need and have greater potential for conflict. If the family has never been close and supportive, it will not magically become so when members grow older. Resentments long buried may crop up and produce friction or psychological pain. Long-submerged conflicts and feelings may return if the needs of one family member exceed those of the others.

In getting to know older adults, gerontological nurses also get to know the family, learning of their special gifts and their life challenges. Nurses work with older adults within the unique culture of their family of origin, present family, and support networks, including friends.

Types of Families

Traditional Couples

The marital or partnered relationship in the United States is a critical source of support for older adults, and over half of noninstitutionalized older adults live with their spouse or partner. The proportion living with their spouse decreases with age, especially for women. Women older than 65 years of age are three times as likely as men of the same age to be widowed. Almost half of women 75 years and older live alone (Administration on Aging, Administration for Community Living, US Department of Health and Human Services, 2019). Men who survive their spouse into old age ordinarily have multiple opportunities to remarry if they wish. Even among the oldest, the majority of men are married. A woman is less likely to have an opportunity for remarriage in later life.

Often, older couples live together but do not marry because of economic and inheritance reasons. An increasing number of adults aged 50 years and older are in cohabitating relationships, and the rate of cohabitation has risen 75% since 2007. The rising number of cohabiters often coincides with rising divorce rates among this group. Most cohabiters aged 50 years and older have previously been married, including a majority who are divorced or widowed.

The needs, tasks, and expectations of couples in late life differ from those in earlier years. Some couples have been married more than 60 or 70 years. These years together may have been filled with love and companionship or abuse and resentment, or anything in between. However, in general, marital status (or the presence of a long-time partner) is positively related to health, life satisfaction, and well-being. For all couples, the normal physical and sociological circumstances in late life present challenges. Some of the issues that strain many of these relationships include (1) the deteriorating health of one or both partners; (2) limitations in income; (3) conflicts with children or other relatives; (4) incompatible sexual needs; and (5) mismatched needs for activity and socialization.

Divorce. In the past, divorce was considered a stigmatizing event. Today, however, it is so common that a person is inclined to forget the ostracizing effects of divorce from years ago. Older couples are becoming less likely to stay in an unsatisfactory marriage, and with the aging of the Baby Boomers, divorce rates will continue to rise. The divorce rate among people 50 years of age and older has doubled in the past 25 years. Among

adults 50 years and older who divorced in the past year, about a third had been in their prior marriage for at least 30 years. Research indicates that many late-life (gray) divorcees have grown unsatisfied with their marriages over the years and are seeking opportunities to pursue their own interests and independence for the remaining years of their lives. Health care professionals must avoid making assumptions and be alert to the possibility of marital dissatisfaction among older adults. Nurses should ask, "How would you describe your marriage?"

Long-term relationships are varied and complex, with many factors forming the glue that holds them together. Marital breakdown may be more devastating in older adults because it is often unanticipated and may occur concurrently with other significant losses. Nurses and other health care professionals must be concerned with supporting a client's decision to seek a divorce and with assisting him or her in seeking counseling in the transition. Divorce will initiate a grieving process similar to the death of a spouse, and a severe disruption in coping capacity may occur until the individual adjusts to a new life. The grief may be more difficult to cope with because no socially sanctioned patterns have been established. In addition, tax and fiscal policies favor married couples, and many divorced older women are at a serious economic disadvantage in retirement.

Other Types of Coupled Relationships

As the variations in families grow, so do the types of coupled relationships. Lesbian, gay, bisexual, transgender (LGBT) is the most commonly known term to describe sexual and gender orientation, but as we learn more, newer descriptions have evolved to be more inclusive. Lesbian, gay, bisexual, transgender, and/or queer, and intersex (LGBTQI) is the term now often seen when describing sexual and gender orientation. Gender and sexual minority is also a term seen in the literature (Zanetos & Skipper, 2020). Landry (2017) provides a comprehensive list and description of the various terms that nurses might find useful in delivering culturally sensitive care to LGBTQI individuals. This text will use the term *LGBT* because more data are available at present, but nurses need to be aware of the full range of sexual and gender orientation and coupled relationships among the growing number of older adults.

Although the number of individuals identifying as LGBT of any age has remained elusive given the reluctance many have about disclosing their status, an estimated 2.4 million Americans more than 60 years of age identify as LGBT, with projections that this figure will increase to 10 million by 2030 (Wardecker & Matsick, 2020). It is important to recognize that there are considerable differences in the experiences of younger LGBT individuals when compared with those who are older. Older

LGBT individuals did not have the benefit of antidiscrimination laws and support for same-sex partners and are more likely to have kept their relationships hidden than those who grew up in the modern-day gay liberation movement. Those older adults identifying as LGBT who came out to family members and faced the negative consequences of becoming estranged from their families of origin often created "families of choice" or chosen families. Chosen families are individuals who are chosen to play a significant role in the life of the individual even though they are not biologically or legally related. Families of choice usually include partners, friends, coworkers, neighbors, and ex-partners—individuals who provide the same supportive functions as would be expected from a person's family of origin (Orel & Coon, 2016).

Transgender and bisexual individuals are less likely to "be out." Some LGBT individuals may have developed social networks of friends, members of their family of origin, and the larger community, but many lack support. Because many LGBT couples may have no or fewer children, they will have fewer caregivers as they age (Chapter 27). Increasing numbers of same-sex couples are choosing to have families, and this will necessitate greater understanding of these "new" types of families, young and old. The majority of research has involved gay and lesbian couples and much less is known about bisexual and transgender relationships. Much more knowledge of cohort, cultural, and generational differences among age groups is needed to understand the dramatic changes in the lives of LGBT individuals in family lifestyles.

Coming to know LGBT individuals will assist nurses in providing more culturally competent, holistic care by addressing specific health issues faced by this vulnerable population (Zanetos & Skipper, 2020). "It is important for health care providers to not only understand the risk and stress associated with LGBT health disparities but also to learn more about how LGBT individuals live, socialize, and build relationships with others" (Wardecker & Matsick, 2020, p. 6). Nurse researchers are encouraged to consider study designs, methods, and procedures that support inclusion and visibility of LGBT older adults (Cloyes, 2016). Organizations that serve LGBT older adults in the community need to enhance outreach and support mechanisms to enable them to maintain independence and age safely and in good health. Box 26.5 includes resources for LGBT older adults.

Older Adults and Their Adult Children

In adulthood, relationships between the generations become increasingly important for most people. Older parents enjoy being told about the various activities and successes of their offspring, and these adult children begin to see aspects of themselves that have developed

---

> **BOX 26.5**   **Resources for Best Practice**
>
> **Lavender Health:** Site maintained by a team of nurses; educational resources and PowerPoint presentations on LGBT health issues and best practices for LGBT communities. https://lavenderhealth.org/.
>
> **Lesbian and Gay Aging Issues Network (LGAIN):** A constituent group of the American Society on Aging that works to raise awareness about the concerns of LGBT older adults and the unique barriers they encounter in gaining access to housing, health care, long-term care, and other needed services. https://www.asaging.org/lain.
>
> **Services and Advocacy for Gay, Lesbian, Bisexual, and Transgender Elders (SAGE):** https://sagenyc.org/nyc/.
>
> **National Center for Transgender Equality:** https://transequality.org/.

---

from their parents. At times, the relationships may become strained because the younger adults are more concerned with their own spouses, partners, and children. The parents are no longer central to their lives, although offspring may be central to the lives of their parents. The most difficult situations occur when the parents are openly critical or judgmental about the lives of their offspring. In the best of situations, adult children shift to the role of friend, companion, and confidant to the older adult, a concept known as filial maturity.

By and large, older adults and their children have relationships that are reciprocal in nature and characterized by affection and mutual support. These relationships are both the most important and potentially the most conflicted. Family resources are shared from birth and usually in some way until and after death. These resources may be tangible, such as money, belongings, and housing. Intangible resources may include advice, support, guidance, and day-to-day assistance with life. Older adults provide a family history perspective, models for growing old, assistance with grandchildren, a sense of continuity, and a philosophy of aging.

Most older adults see their children on a regular basis, and even children who do not live close to their older parents maintain close connections, so *"intimacy at a distance"* can therefore occur. Nine in 10 older adults living with others say they are in contact with their children at least weekly, and about 4 in 10 say they communicate with their children on a daily basis (Stepler, 2016).

Never-Married Older Adults

The number of adults who have never married is increasing in the United States. Older adults who have lived alone most of their lives often develop supportive networks with siblings, friends, and neighbors. Never-married older adults may demonstrate resilience to the challenges of aging as a result of their independence and may not feel lonely or isolated. Furthermore, they may have had longer lifetime employment and may enjoy greater financial security as they age. Single older adults will increase in the future because being single is increasingly more common in younger years.

Grandparents

The role of grandparenthood, and increasingly great-grandparenthood, is experienced by most older adults. The numbers of grandparents are at record highs and still growing at more than twice the overall population growth rate. Most Americans (83%) 65 years and older have grandchildren. Of these grandparents, two-thirds have at least four grandchildren. Four in 10 grandparents today are in the workforce. Seventy-two percent think being a grandparent is the single most important and satisfying thing in their life. Great-grandparenthood will become more common in the future in light of projections of healthier aging (Krogstad, 2015).

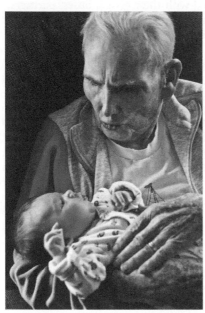

The author's grandson and his maternal great-grandfather. (Photo courtesy Ben Aronoff, Fogline Studios.)

As the term implies, the "grands" are a step beyond parents in their concerns, exposure, and responsibility. The majority of grandparents derive great emotional satisfaction from their grandchildren. Historically, the emphasis has been on the progressive aging of the grandparent as it affects the relationship with the grandchild, but little has been said about the effects of the growth and maturation of the grandchild on the relationship. Many young adults who have had close contact with their grandparents

> ### BOX 26.6   A Grandmother as Seen by an 8-Year-Old Child
>
> "A grandmother is a woman who has no children of her own. That is why she loves other people's children."
>
> "Grandmothers have nothing to do. They are just there: when they take us for a walk they go slowly, like caterpillars along beautiful leaves. They never say, 'Come on, faster, hurry up!'"
>
> "Everyone should try to have a grandmother, especially those who don't have a TV."

report that this relationship was very meaningful in their lives. Growing numbers of adult grandchildren are assisting in caregiving for their grandparents.

The age, vitality, and proximity of both grandchild and grandparent produce a kaleidoscope of possible activities and interactions as both progress through their aging processes. Grandparents are in frequent contact with their grandchildren, with 60% in contact on at least a weekly basis (Stepler, 2016). Geographic distance does not significantly affect the quality of the relationship between grandparents and their grandchildren. The Internet is increasingly being used by distant grandparents as a way of staying involved in their grandchildren's lives and forging close bonds (Chapter 5). Younger grandparents typically live closer to their grandchildren and are more involved in childcare and recreational activities (Box 26.6). Older grandparents with sufficient incomes may provide more financial assistance and other types of instrumental help. Grandparent-headed households are one of the fastest-growing US family groups, and this phenomenon is also taking place in other countries. This phenomenon is discussed in Chapter 27.

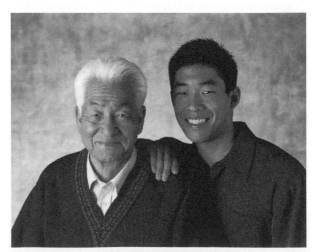

Grandparenting is an important role for older adults. (Copyright © Getty Images.)

Siblings

Late-life sibling relationships are poorly understood and have been neglected by researchers. As individuals age, they often have more contact with siblings than they did in the years when family and work demands were more pressing. About 80% of older adults have at least one sibling and they are often strong sources of support in the lives of never-married older adults, widowed persons, and those without children. For many older adults, these relationships become increasingly important because they have a long history of memories and are of the same generation and similar backgrounds.

Sibling relationships become particularly important when they are part of the support system, especially among single or widowed older adults living alone. The strongest of sibling bonds is thought to be the relationship between sisters. When blessed with survival, these relationships remain important into late old age. Service providers should inquire about sibling relationships of past and present significance. The loss of siblings has a profound effect in terms of awareness of one's own mortality, particularly when those of the same gender die. When an older adult reaches the age of the sibling who died, the reaction can be quite disruptive. Not only is grieving activated, but also rehearsal for one's own death may occur. In some cases in which an older sibling survives younger ones, there may be not only a deep grief but also pangs of guilt: "Why them and not me?" (Chapter 28).

Fictive Kin

Fictive kin are nonblood kin who serve as "genuine fake families," as originally expressed by Virginia Satir. These nonrelatives become surrogate family and take on some of the instrumental and affectional attributes of family. Fictive kin are important in the lives of many older adults, especially those with no close or satisfying family relationships and those living alone or in institutions. Fictive kin includes both friends and, often, paid caregivers. Primary care providers, such as nursing assistants, nurses, or case managers, often become fictive kin. Professionals who work with older adults need to recognize the instrumental and emotional support and the mutually satisfying relationships that occur between friends, neighbors, and other fictive kin who assist older adults who are dependent.

INTIMACY

Intimacy is the degree to which we express and have a need for closeness with another person. Although intimacy is often thought of in the context of sexual performance, it encompasses more than sexuality and includes five major relational components: commitment, affective intimacy, cognitive intimacy, physical intimacy, and interdependence (Youngkin, 2004). It is a warm, meaningful feeling of joy. Intimacy includes the need for close friendships; relationships with family, friends, and formal caregivers; spiritual connections; knowing that one matters in someone else's life; and the ability to form satisfying social relationships with others (Syme, 2015.) Intimacy needs change over time, but the need for intimacy and satisfying social relationships remains an important component of healthy aging.

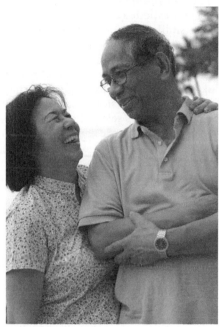

Older couples enjoy love and companionship. (© iStock.com /DanielBendjy.)

SEXUALITY

Sexuality is a central aspect of being human throughout life and encompasses sex, gender identities and roles, sexual orientation, eroticism, pleasure, intimacy, and reproduction. Sexuality is experienced and expressed in thoughts, fantasies, desires, beliefs, attitudes, values, behaviors, practices, roles, and relationships. Although sexuality can include all of these dimensions, not all of them are always experienced or expressed. Sexuality is influenced by the interaction of biological, psychological, social, economic, political, cultural, legal, historical, religious, and spiritual factors (World Health Organization, 2020). "Sexuality begins in utero as we are developing as human beings and ends with our death. Sexuality is the total expression of who we are as human beings. It is the most complex human attribute and encompasses our whole psycho-social development—our values, attitudes, physical appearance, beliefs, emotions, attractions, our likes/dislikes, our spiritual selves" (Clark, 2015). As a major aspect of intimacy, sexuality includes the physical act of intercourse and many other types of intimate activity. Enjoying and expressing one's sexuality leads to feelings of pleasure and well-being that are essential at any age to meet human needs for intimacy and belonging. Sexuality also allows a general affirmation of life (especially joy) and a continuing opportunity to search for new growth and experience.

Sexuality, similar to food and water, is a basic human need, yet it goes beyond the biological realm to include psychological, social, and moral dimensions (Fig. 26.1). The constant interaction among these spheres of sexuality works to produce harmony. The linkage of the four dimensions composes the holistic quality of an individual's sexuality. "Historically, sexuality has been perceived more narrowly in a biomedical context, with emphasis placed on the sexual response cycle, heteronormative behaviors (e.g., penile-vaginal intercourse), and heterosexist and ageist assumptions" (Syme, 2015, p. 36). A holistic view better reflects

 BOX 26.7 **Healthy People 2020**
Goals for Sexual Health

- Improve the health, safety, and well-being of lesbian, gay, bisexual, and transgender (LGBT) individuals.
- Promote healthy sexual behaviors, strengthen community capacity, and increase access to quality services to prevent sexually transmitted diseases (STDs) and their complications.
- Prevent human immunodeficiency virus (HIV) infection and its related illness and death.

Data from US Department of Health and Human Services, Office of Disease Prevention and Health Promotion: *Healthy People 2020*, 2012. http://www.healthypeople.gov/2020.

the philosophy of healthy aging for all individuals. *Healthy People 2020* includes goals for sexual health (Box 26.7).

The **social sphere of sexuality** is the sum of cultural factors that influence an individual's thoughts and actions related to interpersonal relationships, and sexuality related to ideas and learned behavior. Television, radio, literature, and the more traditional sources of family, school, and religious teachings combine to influence social sexuality.

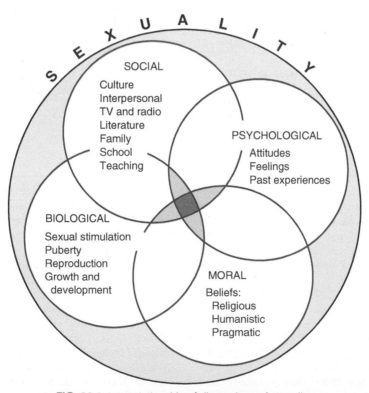

FIG. 26.1 Interrelationship of dimensions of sexuality.

The belief of that which constitutes masculine and feminine is deeply rooted in an individual's exposure to cultural factors (Chapter 3).

The psychological sphere of sexuality reflects a person's attitudes, feelings toward self and others and learning from experiences. Beginning with birth, the individual is bombarded with cues and signals of how a person should act and think about the use of "dirty words" or body parts. Conversation is self-censored in the presence of or in discussion with certain people. The moral aspect of sexuality, the "I should" or "I shouldn't," makes a difference that is based in religious and cultural beliefs or in a pragmatic or humanistic outlook.

The final sphere, **biological sexuality**, is reflected in physiological responses to sexual stimulation, reproduction, puberty, and growth and development. Because of the interrelatedness, these dimensions affect each other directly or indirectly whenever an aspect of sexuality is out of harmony.

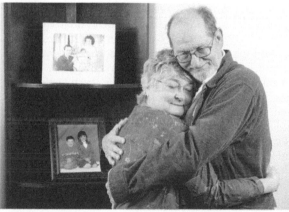

Love and affection are important to older adults. (From Sorrentino, S. A., & Gorek, B. (2006). *Mosby's textbook for long-term care assistants* (5th ed.). St Louis: Mosby.)

SEXUAL HEALTH

The World Health Organization defines sexual health as a state of physical, emotional, mental, and social well-being in relation to sexuality; it is not merely the absence of disease, dysfunction, or infirmity. Sexual health requires a positive and respectful approach to sexuality and sexual relationships, and the possibility of having pleasurable and safe sexual experiences, free of coercion, discrimination, and violence. For sexual health to be attained and maintained, the sexual rights of all persons must be respected, protected, and fulfilled (World Health Organization, 2020).

Sexual health is a realistic phenomenon that includes four components: personal and social behaviors in

agreement with individual gender identity; comfort with a range of sexual role behaviors and engagement in effective interpersonal relations with both sexes in a loving relationship or long-term commitment; response to erotic stimulation that produces positive and pleasurable sexual activity; and the ability to make mature judgments about sexual behavior that is culturally and socially acceptable. These interpretations address the multifaceted nature of the biological, psychosocial, cultural, and spiritual components of sexuality and imply that sexual behavior is the capacity to enhance self and others. Sexual health is individually defined and wholesome if it leads to intimacy (not necessarily coitus) and enriches the involved parties.

Factors Influencing Sexual Health

Expectations

Older adults are becoming increasingly open in their attitudes and beliefs about sexuality. However, a large number of cultural, biological, psychosocial, and environmental factors can influence the sexual behavior of older adults. Older adults may be confronted with barriers to the expression of their sexuality by reflected attitudes, health, culture, economics, opportunity, and historic trends. Factors affecting a person's attitudes on intimacy and sexuality include family dynamics and upbringing and cultural and religious beliefs (Chapter 3).

Older adults often internalize the broad cultural proscriptions of sexual behavior in later life that hinder the continuance of sexual expression. There remains a prevailing assumption that as we age, we become sexually undesirable, incapable of sex, or asexual. "It is erroneously believed that older adults (especially older women) are unattractive, that older sex is disgusting, risky, or 'wrong,' aging entails sexual dysfunction and sex, as a rule, should be discouraged in old age homes and other facilities" (Dhingra et al., 2016). Health care professionals are not immune to these stereotypes and may assume sexual issues are of lesser concern to older adults and neglect to address this important aspect of healthy aging. It is refreshing to see more movies with older actors that incorporate more positive views of older adults enjoying intimate and satisfying, sexual relationships (e.g., *Best Exotic Marigold Hotel* and *Our Souls at Night*).

Much sexual behavior stems from incorporating other people's reactions. Older adults do not feel old until they are faced with the fact that others around them consider them old. Similarly, older adults do not feel asexual until they are continually treated as such. An often quoted statement by Alex Comfort (1974) sums it up nicely: "In our experiences, old folks stop having sex for the same reasons they stop riding a bicycle—general infirmity, thinking it looks ridiculous, no bicycle."

Activity Levels

For all heterosexual, lesbian, gay, bisexual, transgender (LGBT) individuals, research supports that liberal and positive attitudes toward sexuality, greater sexual knowledge, satisfaction with a long-term relationship or a current intimate relationship, good social networks, psychological well-being, and a sense of self-worth are associated with greater sexual interest, activity, and satisfaction. Both early studies of sexual behavior in older adults and more recent ones indicate that older adults are continuing to enjoy active sex lives well into their 70s and 80s. More than half of men and almost a third of women over the age of 70 years reported that they were still sexually active, with a third of these men and women having sex at least twice a month, although sexual problems are relatively prevalent (Heidari, 2016).

Determinants of sexual activity and functioning include the interaction of each partner's sexual capacity, physical health, motivation, conduct, and attitudes, and the quality of the dyadic relationship. Having a sexual partner, frequent intercourse, good health, low level of stress, and an absence of financial worries enhanced a happy sexual relationship. Sexual activity is closely tied to overall health and individuals with better health are more likely to be sexually active. The most common reason for sexual inactivity among heterosexual couples is the male partner's health. Patterns of sexual activity in earlier years are a major predictor of sexual activity in later life and individuals with higher levels of sexual activity in middle age show less decline as they age. Regular sexual expression enhances psychological and physical well-being in older adulthood and may improve cognitive functioning (Schafer et al., 2018; Wright, 2019).

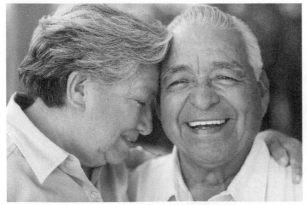

Sexuality is an important need in late life and affects pleasure, adaptation, and a general feeling of well-being. (© iStock.com /Aldo Murillo.)

Cohort and Cultural Influences

The era in which a person was born influences attitudes about sexuality. Women in their 80s today may have been strongly influenced by the prudish Victorian atmosphere of their youth and may have experienced difficult marital adjustments and serious sexual problems early in their marriages. Sexuality was not openly expressed or discussed, and this was a time when pleasurable sex was for men only; women engaged in sexual activity to satisfy their husbands and to make babies. These kinds of experiences shape beliefs and knowledge about sexual expression and comfort with sexuality, particularly for older women. It is important to come to know and understand older adults within their social and cultural background and not make judgments based on one's own belief system.

The next generation of older adults (Baby Boomers) has experienced other influences, including more liberal attitudes toward sexuality, the women's movement, a higher number of divorced adults, the human immunodeficiency virus (HIV) epidemic, and increased numbers of LGBT individuals, that will affect their views and attitudes as they age. The Baby Boomers and beyond, as they find themselves experiencing sexuality beyond the age they had assigned to their elders, may alter current perceptions. Most of what is known about sexuality in aging has been gained through research with well-educated, healthy, White older adults. Further research is needed among culturally, socially, and ethnically diverse older adults, those with chronic illness, and LGBT older adults.

Biological Changes

Acknowledgment and understanding of the age changes that influence sexual physiology, anatomy, and the stages of sexual response may partially explain alteration in sexual behavior to accommodate these changes and facilitate continued pleasurable sex. Characteristic physiological changes during the sexual response cycle do occur with aging, but these vary among individuals depending on general health factors. The changes occur abruptly in women starting with menopause but more gradually in men, a phenomenon called andropause. The "use it or lose it" phenomenon applies here: the more sexually active a person is, the fewer changes they are likely to experience in the pattern of sexual response. Changes in the appearance of the body (wrinkles, sagging skin) may also affect an older adult's security about their sexual attractiveness. Table 26.1 summarizes physical changes in the sexual response cycle. A major nursing role is to provide information about these changes and appropriate assessment and counseling within the context of an individual's needs.

TABLE 26.1 Physical Changes in Sexual Response in Old Age

Female	Male
Excitation Phase	
Diminished or delayed lubrication (1 to 3 minutes may be required for adequate amounts to appear)	Less intense and slower erection (but can be maintained longer without ejaculation)
Diminished flattening and separation of labia majora	Increased difficulty regaining an erection if lost
Disappearance of elevation of labia majora	Less vasocongestion of scrotal sac
Decreased vasocongestion of labia minora	Less pronounced elevation and congestion of testicles
Decreased elastic expansion of vagina (depth and breadth)	
Breasts not as engorged	
Sex flush absent	
Plateau Phase	
Slower and less prominent uterine elevation or tenting	Decreased muscle tension
Nipple erection and sexual flush less often	No color change at coronal edge of penis
Decreased capacity for vasocongestion	Slower penile erection pattern
Decreased areolar engorgement	Delayed or diminished erectile and testicular elevation
Labial color change less evident	
Less intense swelling or orgasmic platform	
Less sexual flush	
Decreased secretions of Bartholin's glands	
Orgasmic Phase	
Fewer number and less intense orgasmic contractions	Decreased or absent secretory activity (lubrication) by Cowper's gland before ejaculation
Rectal sphincter contraction with severe tension only	Fewer penile contractions
	Fewer rectal sphincter contractions
	Decreased force of ejaculation (approximately 50%) with decreased amount of semen (if ejaculation is long, seepage of semen occurs)
Resolution Phase	
Observably slower loss of nipple erection	Vasocongestion of nipples and scrotum slowly subsides
Vasocongestion of clitoris and orgasmic platform	Very rapid loss of erection and descent of testicles shortly after ejaculation
	Refractory time extended (time required before another erection ranges from several to 24 hours, occasionally longer)

SEXUAL RESPONSE

The most prevalent sexual problem in men is erectile dysfunction (ED). ED is defined as the inability to achieve a full erection or the inability to maintain an erection adequate for sexual intimacy. Although most men will experience periodic episodes of ED, these episodes tend to become more frequent with advancing age. Approximately 60% of men at 60 years old and 70% of men at 70 years old have ED (Mobley et al., 2017). When discussing ED with older men, it is important to also provide education about normal age-related changes. Older men require more physical penile stimulation and a longer time to achieve erection, and the duration of orgasm may be shorter and less intense.

An erection is governed by the interaction among the hormonal, vascular, and nervous systems. A problem in any of these systems can cause ED. Multiple causes can contribute to this problem in older men. Nearly one-third of ED is a complication of diabetes. Cardiovascular disease (CVD) and hypertension cause a narrowing and hardening of the arteries, leading to reduced blood flow to the corporal bodies, which is essential for achieving an erection. Recent studies have confirmed that ED also serves as a predictor of future CVD and individuals who present with ED and

CVD risk factors should be evaluated for silent CVD (Mobley et al., 2017). Alcohol abuse, smoking, medications, prostate cancer and treatment, obesity, anxiety, depression, and relationship discord are also causes of ED in older men (Marchese, 2017). The new nerve-saving microsurgical techniques used for prostatectomies often spare erectile function.

The use of phosphodiesterase inhibitors such as sildenafil (Viagra), vardenafil (Levitra), and tadalafil (Cialis) has revolutionized treatment for ED regardless of cause. Contraindications to the use of these medications include use of nitrate therapy, heart failure with low blood pressure, certain antihypertensive regimens, and other medications and cardiovascular conditions (Chapter 9). Before the availability of these medications, intracavernosal injections with the drugs papaverine and phentolamine, vasoactive agents that reduce resistance of arteriolar and cavernosal smooth muscle tissue of the penis, were used.

Penile implants of the semirigid, adjustable-malleable, or hinged and inflatable types are available when impotence does not respond to other treatments or is irreversible. The hinged and inflatable types, which are inserted in the testicular area, are the most popular. Another alternative is the vacuum pump device, which works by creating a vacuum that draws blood into the penis, causing an erection. Vacuum pumps are available in manual and battery-operated versions and may be covered by Medicare if deemed medically necessary.

Our understanding of the female response is still not well understood, and the definition and diagnostic criteria of sexual dysfunction are controversial and still under development. Difficulties reported by sexually active women related to becoming sexually aroused and achieving orgasm (Lee et al., 2016). Female sexual function can be influenced by factors such as culture, ethnicity, emotional state, age, and previous sexual experiences, and age-related changes in sexual response. Frequency of intimacy depends more on the age, health, and sexual function of the partner or the availability of a partner, rather than on their own sexual capacity.

Postmenopausal changes in the urinary or genital tract as a result of lower estrogen levels can make sexual activity less pleasurable. Dyspareunia, resulting from vaginal dryness and thinning of the vaginal tissue, occurs in one-third of women over the age of 65 years. In many instances, using water-soluble lubricants such as K-Y Jelly, Astroglide, Slip, and HR lubricating jelly during foreplay or intercourse can resolve the difficulty. Topical low-dose estrogen creams, rings, or pills that are introduced into the vagina may also help to plump

tissues and restore lubrication, with less absorption than oral hormones.

Women can experience arousal disorders resulting from drugs such as anticholinergics, antidepressants, and chemotherapeutic agents and from lack of lubrication from radiation, surgery, and stress. Unlike ED, studies of vascular insufficiency are less clear in women. Prolapse of the uterus, rectoceles, and cystoceles can be surgically repaired to facilitate continued sexual activity. Urinary incontinence (UI) is another condition that may affect sexual activity for both men and women. Appropriate assessment and treatment are important because many causes of UI are treatable (Chapter 12).

SEXUALITY AND LGBT INDIVIDUALS

Discrimination in health and social systems affects gay, lesbian, bisexual, and transgender individuals of all ages. Discrimination ranges from refusal of care, biases or incorrect assumptions, to overt derogatory statements (American Geriatrics Society, 2015). Older adults may be even more at risk of discrimination as a result of lifelong experiences with marginalization and oppression. They may have been shunned by family or friends, religious organizations, and the medical community; ridiculed or physically attacked; or labeled as sinners, perverts, or criminals. In the 1950s, same-sex behaviors were typically characterized as sodomy, were criminal, and the American Psychiatric Association classified homosexuality as a psychiatric disorder (Fredriksen-Goldsen, 2016). It was not until 1973 that homosexuality was removed from the *Diagnostic and Statistical Manual of Mental Disorders*. LGBT individuals may face dual discrimination because of their age and their sexual orientation or gender identity, and older women in lesbian relationships face the triple threat of being women, being old, and having a different sexual orientation (American Psychological Association, 2018).

As a result of lifelong discrimination and negative experiences with health care agencies and personnel, LGBT older adults are much less likely than their heterosexual peers to access needed health and social services or identify themselves as gay or lesbian to health care providers. As a result, they are at greater risk for poorer health than their heterosexual counterparts. Gay and bisexual adults 50 years of age and older are more likely to report higher prevalence of poor general health, disabling chronic conditions, high rates of substance abuse, and suicide (Franc et al., 2018). Transgender and bisexual older adults and individuals living with HIV are at greater risk for disparities and poorer health outcomes (Emlet, 2016). *Healthy People 2020* highlighted LGBT people for the first time as a health-disparate population and outlined goals to improve their health, safety, and well-being.

Health care providers may assume that their LGBT patients are heterosexual and neglect to obtain a sexual history, discuss sexuality, or be aware of their particular medical needs. Providers receive little education and training in the needs of this population and may lack sensitivity when caring for older LGBT individuals (Zanetos & Skipper, 2020). Health history forms need to be inclusive and not heterosexist. Using gender-neutral terms like partner or significant other is preferred over asking, "Are you married?" (Franc et al., 2018). This form of the question allows the nurse to look beyond the rigid category of family.

You can ask individuals if they consider themselves primarily heterosexual, homosexual, or bisexual. This question conveys recognition of sexual variety. If the patient identifies as transgender, it is important to ask how the patient wishes to be addressed. Use the name the person has asked you to call them and the pronouns they want you to use (National Center for Transgender Equality, 2016). Appropriate health-teaching materials, including those that depict same-sex couples, are important, as is not making assumptions about a person's sex based on their appearance.

Euphemisms are frequently used for a life partner (e.g., roommate, close friend). An older lesbian woman in a health care situation may refer to herself indirectly by saying "people like us." Nurses need to become more aware of these nuances and try to understand the fear of discovery that is apparent in older gay men and lesbian women. These older adults are of a generation in which they were, and may still be, closeted because of the homophobic experiences they had throughout their younger years.

Better support and care services for LGBT individuals by care providers should include working through homophobic attitudes and discomfort discussing sexuality, learning about special issues facing LGBT individuals, learning more about gender identity and the life experiences of individuals who identify as LGBT, and becoming aware of resources in the community specific to this population. "Health care professionals cannot change societal norms nor force the majority population to accept any race, religion, culture, or sexual orientation, but we are responsible for their health care collectively" (Landry, 2017, p. 344).

Facilities or agencies in the community need to be assessed from the perspective of the client, patient, or resident who may be gay, lesbian, bisexual, or transgender. It is important that service providers create programs that are inclusive and culturally appropriate for all individuals (Chapter 3). LGBT individuals look for indications of an inclusive and welcoming environment, which may include the display of nondiscrimination policies or a rainbow flag (Franc et al., 2018). Programs to increase awareness of the needs of LGBT older adults and reduce discrimination are necessary especially in light of the anticipated increase in older adults who identify as LGBT (Fredriksen-Goldsen, 2016).

INTIMACY AND CHRONIC ILLNESS

Chronic illnesses and their related treatments may bring many challenges to intimacy and sexual activity. Physical capacity for sexual activity may be affected by illness and psychological factors (anxiety, depression). Patients and their partners are given little or no information about the effect of illnesses on sexual activity or strategies to continue sexual activity within functional limitations. Individuals want and need information on sexual functioning, and health care professionals need to become more knowledgeable and more actively involved in sexual counseling (Byrne et al., 2017). Table 26.2 presents suggestions for individuals with chronic illness.

Timing of intercourse (mornings or when energy level is highest), oral or anal sex, masturbation, appropriate pain relief, and different sexual positions are all strategies that may assist in continued sexual activity. There is no consensus on what kind of position the individual should assume for sexual activity, but a lesser amount of energy is expended with the person on the bottom during use of the missionary position. Alternative positions may require less energy and may be more comfortable depending on the situation (Steinke, 2013; Steinke et al., 2013).

For individuals with cardiac conditions, manual stimulation (masturbation) may be an alternative that can be used to maintain sexual function if the practice is not objectionable to the patient. Studies show that masturbation is less taxing on the heart and makes less oxygen demand. Although self-stimulation is steeped in myth and fear, masturbation is a common and healthy practice in later life. Individuals without partners or those whose spouses are ill or incapacitated find that masturbation is helpful. As children, today's older population was discouraged from practicing this pleasurable activity with stories of the evils of fondling a person's own genitals. Masturbation provides an avenue for resolution of sexual tensions, keeps sexual desire alive, maintains lubrication and muscle tone of the vagina, provides mild physical exercise, and preserves sexual function in individuals who have no other outlet for sexual activity and gratification of their sexual need.

TABLE 26.2   Chronic Illness and Sexual Function: Effects and Interventions

Condition	Effects/Problems	Interventions
Arthritis	Pain, fatigue, limited motion Steroid therapy may decrease sexual interest or desire	Advise patient to perform sexual activity at time of day when less fatigued and most relaxed Suggest use of analgesics and other pain-relief methods before sexual activity Encourage use of relaxation techniques before sexual activity, such as a warm bath or shower, application of hot packs to affected joints Advise patient to maintain optimal health through a balance of good nutrition, proper rest, and activity Suggest that they experiment with different positions, use pillows for comfort and support Recommend use of a vibrator if massage ability is limited Suggest use of water-soluble jelly for vaginal lubrication
Cardiovascular disease	Most men have no change in physical effects on sexual function; one-fourth may not return to pre–heart attack function; one-fourth may not resume sexual activity Women do not experience sexual dysfunction after heart attack Fear of another heart attack or death during sex Shortness of breath	Encourage counseling on realistic restrictions that may be necessary **Post–myocardial infarction (MI):** Those able to engage in mild to moderate physical activity without symptoms can generally resume sexual activity; those with a complicated MI may need to resume sexual activity gradually over a longer period of time Avoid large meals several hours before sex Avoid anal sex Instruct patient and spouse on alternative positions to avoid strain and allow for unrestricted breathing Stop and rest if chest pain is experienced, take nitroglycerin if prescribed, and seek emergency treatment for sustained chest pain **Post-CABG or pacemaker or ICD insertion:** Avoid strain or direct pressure on device/incision Individuals with poorly controlled arrhythmias should not engage in sexual activity until the condition is well managed Instruct individual that ICD could fire with sex, although uncommon; a change in device setting may be needed
Cerebrovascular accident (stroke)	Depression May or may not have sexual activity changes Often erectile disorders occur Change in role and function of partners Decreased physical endurance, fatigue Mobility and sensory deficits Perceptual and visual deficits Communication deficits Cognitive and behavioral deficits Fear of relapse or sudden death	Encourage counseling Instruct patient to use alternative positions Suggest use of a vibrator if massage ability is limited Suggest use of pillows for positioning and support Suggest use of water-soluble jelly for lubrication Suggest alternate forms of sexual expression acceptable to the individuals

Continued

TABLE 26.2   Chronic Illness and Sexual Function: Effects and Interventions—cont'd

Condition	Effects/Problems	Interventions
Chronic obstructive pulmonary disease (COPD)	No direct impairment of sexual activity, although affected by coughing, exertional dyspnea, positions, and activity intolerance Medications may lead to erectile difficulties	Encourage patient to plan sexual activity when energy is highest Instruct patient to use alternative positions; use ample pillows for support and elevate the upper body, or use a sitting upright position; avoid any pressure on the chest Advise patient to plan sexual activity at time medications are most effective Suggest use of oxygen before, during, or after sex, depending on when it provides the most benefit Teach partner to observe for breathing difficulty and allow time for change of positions and time to catch breath when needed
Diabetes	Sexual desire and interest unaffected Neuropathy and/or vascular damage may interfere with erectile ability; about 50% to 75% of men have erectile disorders; a small portion have retrograde ejaculation Some men regain function if diagnosis of diabetes is well accepted, if diabetes is well controlled, or both Women have less sexual desire and vaginal lubrication Decrease in orgasms/absence of orgasm can occur; less frequent sexual activity; local genital infections	Recommend possible candidates for penile prosthesis Suggest use of alternative forms of sexual expression Recommend immediate treatment of genital infections
Cancers		
Breast	No direct physical affect; there is a strong psychological effect: loss of sexual desire, body-image change, depression/reaction of partner	Refer to support groups, sex therapists, counselors Encourage open expression of sexual concerns
Prostate	Incontinence can occur following surgery Erectile dysfunction Psychological effects Use of nerve-sparing surgery causes less dysfunction	Kegel exercises and routine toileting Use of phosphodiesterase inhibitors Provide information related to sexual functioning/continence
Most other cancers	Men and women may lose sexual desire temporarily Men may have erectile dysfunction; dry ejaculation; retrograde ejaculation Women may have vaginal dryness, dyspareunia Both men and women may experience anxiety, depression, pain, nausea from chemotherapy, radiation, hormone therapy, and nerve damage from pelvic surgery	New sexual positions may be helpful; explore alternative sexual activities

CABG, Coronary artery bypass graft; *ICD*, implantable cardioverter-defibrillator.
Data from Steinke, E. E. (2013). Sexuality and chronic illness, *J Gerontol Nurs 39*(11), 18–27.

INTIMACY AND SEXUALITY IN LONG-TERM CARE FACILITIES

Research is needed on sexuality in residential care facilities, but surveys suggest that a significant number of older adults living in these settings might choose to be sexually active if they had privacy and a sexual partner (Syme et al., 2017). Intimacy and sexuality among residents includes the opportunity to have not only intercourse but also other forms of intimate expressions, such as touching, hugging, kissing, hand holding, and masturbation. The sexual needs of older adults in long-term care facilities should receive the same attention as nutrition, hydration, and other well-accepted needs. Institutionalized older adults have the same rights as noninstitutionalized older adults to engage in or refrain from sexual activity

Attitudes about intimacy and sexuality among long-term care staff and, often, family members may reflect general societal attitudes that older adults do not have sexual needs or that sexual activity is inappropriate. Families may have difficulty understanding that their older relative may want to have a new relationship.

Nursing home staff generally have limited knowledge of late-life sexuality and may view residents' sexual acts as problems rather than as expressions of the need for love and intimacy. Reactions may include disapproval, discomfort, and embarrassment, and caregivers may explicitly or implicitly discourage or deny intimacy needs. LGBT older adults are particularly at risk for being discriminated against by both staff and other residents and may not receive care that is culturally safe and appropriate (Neville et al., 2014). Fears of being outed, disrespected, mistreated, and harmed are common and they often choose to stay in the closet (Steelman, 2018).

The majority of nursing facilities do not have policies addressing any aspect of resident sexuality and provide little training for staff. The evidence is clear that communication between older adults and health care professionals about sexual issues is currently poor (Syme et al., 2017). Privacy is a major issue in care facilities that can prevent fulfillment of intimacy and sexual needs. Suggestions for providing privacy and an atmosphere accepting of sexual activity include the availability of a private room, not interrupting when doors are closed and sexual activity is taking place, allowing residents to have sexually explicit materials in their rooms, and providing adaptive equipment, such as side rails or trapezes and double beds. In one facility where the author worked, the staff would assist one of the female residents to be freshly showered, perfumed, and in a lovely nightgown when she and her partner wanted to have sexual relations.

Nursing Actions: Enhancing Sexual Health in Long-Term Care

Staff, family, and resident education programs to promote awareness, provide education on sexuality and intimacy in later life, involve residents in discussions of sexuality, and discuss interventions to respond to residents' needs are important in long-term care settings. Staff education should include the opportunity to discuss personal feelings about sexuality, changes associated with aging, the impact of diseases and medications on sexual function, sexual expression among same-sex residents, and role-playing and skill training in sexual assessment and intervention.

The facility should clearly demonstrate its acceptance of sexuality and the rights and needs of residents of all sexual orientations to have their sexual needs accepted. Information about sexuality and sexual health in informational booklets, promotional flyers, and other documents produced for current and future residents would assist in normalizing the expression of sexuality in care environments.

Sexual expression policies need to be developed with input from staff, residents, and families, displayed prominently, and reviewed with staff members. Special attention is needed to ensure that LGBT identity is respected in long-term care facilities. Issues related to sexuality and sexual health should be discussed without anxiety or discomfort so that older adults receive optimal care and treatment (Bauer et al., 2016). The care facility should be a place where all older adults can be comfortable living (Neville et al., 2014).

INTIMACY, SEXUALITY, AND DEMENTIA

Intimacy and sexuality remain important in the lives of persons with dementia and their partners throughout the illness. Intimacy and sexuality may serve as a nonverbal form of communication and intimacy when other cognitive skills and functions have declined. A recent study reported that the majority of partnered older men and women who experience mild to moderate changes in cognition are sexually active, including 40% of partnered people age 80 to 91 years. One-quarter of men and 1 in 10 women in the dementia group reported masturbating. Most people, including men and women with lower cognition, regarded sexuality as an important part of life and reported having sex less often than they would like. Yet sexual behavior between life partners when one has dementia is not often addressed and individuals with dementia may be viewed as asexual.

Individuals with lower cognitive scores infrequently discuss sex with a physician, and physicians rarely counsel individuals with dementia, especially women, about sexual changes that may result from dementia or other medical conditions (Lindau et al., 2018). Nurses need to have an awareness of the sexual needs of the individual with dementia and their partner and be comfortable discussing this area with both. Communication can be encouraged by asking the question: "How has dementia affected your sexual relationship?"

As dementia progresses, particularly in individuals living in care facilities, intimacy and sexuality issues may present challenges, especially regarding cognitively impaired individuals who may lack sexual consent capacity or the ability to make their own sexual decisions (Jones & Moyle, 2018; Syme et al., 2017). Inappropriate sexual behavior (exposing oneself, masturbating in public, or making inappropriate sexual advances or sexual comments) may also occur in long-term care settings. These behaviors are most distressing to families, staff, and other residents. Sexual inappropriateness (sexual disinhibition) is one of the least understood aspects of dementia. Individuals with subtypes of dementia that include frontal lobe impairment (Pick's disease and alcoholic dementia) may exhibit more sexually inappropriate behavior.

These kinds of behavior may be triggered by unmet intimacy needs or may be symptoms of an underlying physical problem, such as a urinary tract or vaginal infection. The lack of privacy in care facilities may lead to sexually inappropriate behavior in public areas. Social cues such as explicit television shows may also precipitate behaviors. Bodily contact, such as in bathing residents, may be misinterpreted as a sexual act or romantic advance.

An interprofessional sexual assessment is helpful in determining the underlying need that the individual is expressing and how it might be addressed. Encouraging family and friends to touch, hug, kiss, and hold hands when visiting may help to meet touch and intimacy needs and decrease inappropriate sexual behavior. Also, allowing the person to stroke a pet or hold a stuffed animal may be helpful. Behavioral and nonpharmacological interventions are first-line treatment. Aggressive or violent behavior may require limit setting, working with the resident and family, providing for sexual expression in a nonharmful manner, and pharmacological treatment if indicated. Staff will need opportunities for discussion and assistance with interventions.

Sexuality among nursing home residents with dementia is a sensitive topic, and there are no national guidelines for determining sexual consent capacity among individuals with severe dementia. This topic is poorly understood and inadequately researched, and consensus about standard of care on this issue is limited (American Medical Directors Association, 2016). Determination of ability to consent for sexual activity for an individual with cognitive impairment involves concepts of voluntary participation, mental competence, and an understanding of the risks and benefits. The Hebrew Home in Riverdale, New York, initiated model sexual policies in 1995 with the most recent update in 2014. The National Institute on Aging and the Alzheimer's Association provide helpful resources on sexuality and dementia (Box 26.5).

HIV/AIDS AND OLDER ADULTS

An increasingly significant trend in the global HIV epidemic is the growing number of people aged 50 years and older who are living with HIV. This trend is occurring in both developed and developing countries. Although rates of HIV/AIDS have remained relatively stable and even declined a little in younger age groups, the number of older adults infected with the virus is growing. One in six new HIV diagnoses were among people age 50 and older (CDC, 2020). Women older than age 60 make up one of the fastest-growing risk groups, and most contracted the virus from sex with infected partners. Transgender women are also at disproportionate risk of HIV, but prevalence data on older transgender individuals are not available (Karpiak & Brennan-Ing, 2016). The incidence among older adults is expected to continue to increase as more individuals become infected later in life and those who were infected in early adulthood live longer as a result of advances in disease treatment.

The compromised immune system of an older adult makes him or her even more susceptible to HIV or AIDS than a younger adult. Older women who are sexually active are at high risk of HIV/AIDS (and other sexually transmitted infections) from an infected partner, resulting, in part, from normal age changes of the vaginal tissue—a thinner, drier, friable vaginal lining that makes viral entry more efficient. Studies show that sexually active older men and women do not routinely use condoms, thus increasing their risk of sexually transmitted diseases (STDs). Recently widowed or divorced individuals may not understand the need for practicing safe sex because they do not worry about an unwanted pregnancy and may not understand the risk of STDs. Older women are more likely than their younger counterparts to be in noncommitted relationships, and difficulty negotiating safe sexual relationships can contribute to increased HIV risk (Coleman, 2017).

Recognizing and Analyzing Cues: HIV

Physicians, nurse practitioners, and other health professionals need to increase their knowledge of HIV in older adults and become comfortable taking a complete sexual history and talking about sex with all older adults. Sexual health issues such as sexually transmitted infections, sexual functioning, and the sexual history of adult patients should be incorporated as a routine part of the medical history throughout life. The idea that older adults are not sexually active limits health care providers' objectivity to recognize HIV/AIDS as a possible diagnosis. Cues may be subtle, and AIDS in older adults has been called the "Great Imitator" because many of the symptoms, such as fatigue, weakness, weight loss, and anorexia, are common to other disease conditions and may be attributed to normal aging. Additionally, older adults may blame possible symptoms on aging or be reluctant to seek testing or share symptoms because of the stigma they associate with the disease.

Most US guidelines recommend HIV testing among high-risk groups regardless of age, but routine screening recommendations differ and some have a cut-off age of 65 years. The Joint Academy of HIV Medicine, the American Geriatrics Society, and the AIDS Community Research Initiative of America recommend routine opt-out screening, regardless of age. Late diagnosis of HIV can occur because health care providers may not always test older adults for HIV infection. Medicare covers annual screenings for HIV for those who are at increased risk and those who ask for the test. Also covered is annual screening for those who are at increased risk for STDs (Centers for Disease Control and Prevention [CDC], 2019).

Nursing Actions: HIV

Lack of awareness about HIV in older adults results in diagnosis late in the course of the disease, late start to treatment, possibly more damage to their immune system, and poorer prognoses than younger individuals (CDC, 2019). Women tend to be diagnosed with HIV later in their disease than men, and fewer women are getting HIV treatment (The Well Project, 2020). Older adults with HIV may also be at increased risk of geriatric syndromes that complicate their treatment and face higher rates of CVD, diabetes, hypertension, and cancer.

HIV and its treatment can also have profound effects on the brain. Although AIDS-related dementia, once relatively common among people with HIV, is now rare, researchers estimate that more than 50% of people with HIV have HIV-associated neurocognitive disorder (HAND), which may include deficits in attention, language, motor skills, memory, and other aspects of cognitive function that may significantly affect a person's quality of life. People who have HAND may also experience depression or psychological distress. Researchers are studying how HIV and its treatment affect the brain, including the effects on older adults living with HIV (National Institute of Neurological Disorders and Stroke, 2020).

Highly active antiretroviral therapy (HAART) can be more complicated if there are chronic illnesses, comorbidities, and polypharmacy. Long-term effects of HAART are also not well studied. However, there is no evidence that response to therapy is different in older adults than in younger individuals, and some data suggest that older individuals may be more adherent to HAART. Presently, guidelines for care of adults 60 to 80 years of age with HIV are somewhat limited because this population has not been studied in clinical or pharmacokinetic trials.

Misinformation about HIV is more common in older adults, and they may know less about the disease than younger individuals. Educational materials and programs aimed at older adults need to be developed, particularly for older women. Educational materials should include information about what HIV/AIDS is and how it is (and is not) transmitted, risk-reduction counseling, symptoms of which to be aware, and the treatments that are available. For older women, including opportunities to practice communication skills with sexual partners, may be helpful in sexual discussions with partners later. Small, peer-aged groups may be more successful for providing education than larger groups (Coleman, 2017). Brochures and prevention posters need to depict older adults and be designed for older learners. Jane Fowler of the National HIV Wisdom for Older Women's Program asks the question: "How often does a wrinkled face appear on a prevention poster?" Box 26.8 provides additional resources on sexual health.

BOX 26.8 Resources for Best Practice

Centers for Disease Control and Prevention (CDC): Guide to Taking a Sexual History. https://www.cdc.gov/std/treatment/sexualhistory.pdf.

Hartford Institute for Geriatric Nursing: Video illustrating use of PLISSIT model. https://consultgeri.org/try-this/general-assessment/issue-10.

Hebrew Home for the Aged at Riverdale: Policy and guidelines for sexual expression among individuals with dementa in long term care. https://www.basicknowledge101.com/pdf/health/sexualexpressionpolicy.pdf.

HIVAge.org: Resources, research, HIV and Aging Toolkit for Health Care Providers.

National Institute on Aging: Sexuality in later life, changes in intimacy and sexuality in Alzheimer's disease, HIV, AIDS and older adults. https://www.nia.nih.gov/health/sexuality-later-life.

National Resource Center for LGBT Aging (SAGE): Resources aimed at improving the quality of services and supports offered to lesbian, gay, bisexual and transgender (LGBT) older adults.

STDS IN OLDER ADULTS

There have been significant increases in the rate of other STDs in older adults. Older adults who are sexually active may be at risk of diseases such as syphilis, chlamydia infection, gonorrhea, genital herpes, hepatitis B, genital warts, and trichomoniasis. Risk factors are similar to those for AIDS and include the increasing number of divorced older adults, unsafe sexual practices (seniors have the lowest rate of condom use compared to other age groups), access to medications to aid in sexual function, and inadequate assessment and testing for STDs in this population. Older adults are more likely to receive a diagnosis of an STD when it is too late and then are unable to benefit from the available medications in the early stages. Many older adults are embarrassed to ask to be tested for STDs. Assessment of older adults needs to include screening for STDs and sex education for prevention.

❖ USING CLINICAL JUDGMENT TO PROMOTE HEALTHY AGING: SEXUAL HEALTH

◆ Nursing Actions: Promoting Sexual Health

Nurses have multiple roles in the area of sexuality and older adults. The nurse is a facilitator of a milieu that is conducive to the person asking questions and expressing their sexuality. The nurse is also an educator and provides information and guidance to those who need it. Some older adults remain or want to remain sexually active, whereas others do not see this as an important part of their lives. Nurses should open the door to discussions of sexual concerns in a nonjudgmental manner, helping those who want to continue to be sexually active, and making it clear that stopping sex is an acceptable option for others.

Sexuality and intimacy are crucial to healthy aging, and the way these are expressed among older adults is changing, particularly with the aging of the Baby Boomers and upcoming generations. When promoting healthy aging, nurses must consider increasingly open attitudes toward sexuality, dating and developing new relationships, the challenges of facilitating intimacy in residential settings, and the importance of promoting sexual health and safe sex practices. Being aware of one's own feelings about sexuality and attitudes toward intimacy and sexuality in older adults of all sexual preferences is important. Only after confronting one's own attitudes, values, and beliefs can the nurse provide support without being judgmental. Discussion and evaluation of sexual health of healthy older adults and those with dementia need to be included in nursing education programs (Jones & Moyle, 2018).

Validation of the normalcy of sexual activity and a discussion of the physiological changes that occur either with age or as a result of illness are important. Anticipation of problems in older individuals' sexual experiences can ward off anxiety, misconceptions, and an arbitrary cessation of sexual pleasure. Adaptations that will promote sexual function for individuals with chronic illness should be provided. Screening for HIV/AIDS and other STDs and education about safe sexual practices are also important.

In addition, the myth that adults do not engage in sexual activity must be put to rest. When questions about sexual issues are asked or when the older adult is examined, the nurse needs to be particularly cognizant of the era and culture in which the individual has lived to understand the factors affecting conduct. A medication review is essential because many medications affect sexual functioning. Often, medications are prescribed to both older men and women without attention to the sexual side effects. If medications that affect sexual function are necessary, adjustment of doses, use of alternative agents, and prescription of antidotes to reverse the sexual side effects are important (Chapter 9).

The PLISSIT Model (Annon, 1976) is a helpful guide for evaluation and intervention (Box 26.9).

- **Permission**: Obtain permission from the client to initiate sexual discussion. Allow the person to discuss concerns related to sexual issues and gather information about what might have changed in the person's life to affect sexual needs and response. Questions such as the following can be used: "What concerns or questions do you have about fulfilling your sexual needs?" or "In this era of HIV and other sexually transmitted infections, I ask all my patients about sexual practices and concerns. Are there any questions I can answer for you?"
- **Limited Information**: Provide the limited information to function sexually. Offer teaching about the normal age-associated changes that affect sexual performance or how illness may affect sexuality. Encourage the person to learn more about the concern from books and other sources.
- **Specific Suggestions**: Offer suggestions for dealing with problems such as lubricants for atrophic vaginitis; use of condoms to prevent sexually transmitted infections; proper use of ED medications; how to communicate sexual and other needs; ways to increase comfort with coitus or ways to be intimate without coital relations.
- **Intensive Therapy**: Refer as appropriate for complex problems that require specialist intervention.

Actions will be individualized based on coming to know the older adult and may center on the following categories: (1) education regarding age-associated change in sexual function; (2) compensation for age-associated changes and effects of chronic illness; (3) effective management of acute and chronic illness affecting sexual function; (4) provision of education on HIV and STDs and reduction of risk factors; (5) removal of barriers associated with fulfilling sexual needs; and (6) special interventions to promote sexual health in older adults with cognitive impairment.

BOX 26.9   PLISSIT Model

P: Permission from the client to initiate sexual discussion

LI: Providing the **Limited Information** needed to function sexually

SS: Giving **Specific Suggestions** for the individual to proceed with sexual relations

IT: Providing **Intensive Therapy** surrounding the issues of sexuality for the clients (may mean referral to specialist)

From Annon, J. (1976). The PLISSIT model: A proposed conceptual scheme for behavioral treatment of sexual problems. *J Sex Educ Ther, 2,* 1–15.

KEY CONCEPTS

- The ability to negotiate transitions successfully and to develop new and gratifying roles in later life depends on personal and environmental supports, timing, clarity of expectations, personality, and degree of change required.
- Retirement is no longer just a few years of rest from the rigors of work before death. It is a developmental stage that may occupy 30 or more years of a person's life and involve many stages. Some individuals will be retired longer than they worked.
- Preretirement planning and postretirement follow-up significantly affect positive adaptation to the transition.
- Older adults and their family members carry a long history. Current family dynamics must be understood within the context of family history.
- Loss of a spouse is the role change that has the greatest potential for life disruption and poor health outcomes. Nursing support can make a positive difference in the transition.
- Sexuality is love, sharing, trust, and warmth, as well as physical acts. Sexuality provides an individual with self-identity and affirmation of life.
- Generally speaking, medications, ill health, and lack of a partner affect sexual activity as one ages.
- Further research is needed to promote knowledge and understanding of the sexual health of older adults who identify as LGBT.
- Nursing actions for enhancing the sexual health of older adults in the community and long-term care

settings include education and counseling about sexual function and adaptations for age-related changes and chronic conditions; prevention of HIV/AIDS and STDs in sexually active individuals; and the maintenance of sexuality for health, well-being, and pleasure.

- AIDS awareness and the practice of safe sex among older adults is still lacking. Older adults and health professionals may not consider older adults at risk for AIDS or STDs even though the incidence of these diseases in the older population is rapidly increasing.

ACTIVITIES AND DISCUSSION QUESTIONS

1. Discuss your position in the family and how that has affected your relationship with siblings and parents.
2. Write a brief essay discussing the ways in which your grandparents have affected your life.
3. With a classmate, role play how you would conduct a review of systems in the area of sexual health with an older adult.
4. What would be the most important factors to consider when providing education about sexuality and sexual health?
5. What resources are available for older adults who identify as LGBT in your community?

NEXT-GENERATION NCLEX® EXAMINATION-STYLE QUESTIONS

Ms. Booth, 68 years old, comes to the senior health clinic to establish care and is accompanied by Ms. Singh, her partner of 20 years. Ms. Booth has a history of osteoarthritis in her hips and knees, coronary artery disease, chronic obstructive pulmonary disease with a 53-pack/year history of smoking, and Type 2 diabetes with mild peripheral neuropathy. Her medications include meloxicam 15 mg daily, aspirin 81 mg daily, valsartan/hydrochlorothiazide 160 mg/25 mg daily, nitroglycerin SL 0.5 mg every 5 minutes × 3 as needed for chest pain, fluticasone/salmeterol 250 µg/50 µg inhaled twice a day, glipizide/metformin 5 mg/500 mg twice a day, and pregabalin 50 mg three times per day. Vital signs include a blood pressure of 145/88 mmHg, pulse of 92 beats per minute, respiration rate of 18 breaths per minute, temperature 97.9°F, and oxygen saturation on room air of 96%.

The nurse asks Ms. Singh to leave the room during Ms. Booth's physical examination; however, Ms. Booth asks for her partner to stay, saying they have some sensitive questions to ask and want to ask them together. Both women appear uncomfortable. The nurse sits down, leans forward, smiles, and asks how they can help. Ms. Singh looks at Ms. Booth, then says they are afraid to have intercourse since Ms. Booth's chest pain began 6 months ago. The nurse nods, then discusses with them ways to adapt to Ms. Booth's chronic illnesses.

Which strategies should the nurse recommend to improve the clients sexual health? (Select all that apply).
1. Engage in sexual activity at a time of day when most relaxed and less fatigued.
2. Use analgesics or other pain-relief methods, such as hot packs to affected joints, prior to sexual activity.
3. Experiment with different positions to avoid strain and allow for unrestricted breathing.
4. Use vaginal lubrication containing glycerin.
5. Treat genital infections immediately.
6. If chest pain is experienced, take a nitroglycerin then resume activities.
7. Consider alternative forms of sexual expression acceptable to both individuals.
8. Wear oxygen during sexual activity.

REFERENCES

Administration on Aging, Administration on Community Living, US Department of Health and Human Services: *Profile of older Americans*, 2019. https://acl.gov/aging-and-disability-in-america/data-and-research/profile-older-americans.

American Geriatrics Society. (2015). American Geriatrics Society Care of Lesbian, Gay, Bisexual, and Transgender Older Adults Position Statement. *Journal of the American Geriatrics Society, 63,* 423–426.

American Medical Directors Association. (2016). *Capacity for sexual consent in dementia in long-term care.* https://paltc.org/amda-white-papers-and-resolution-position-statements/capacity-sexual-consent-dementia-long-term-care.

American Psychological Association. (2018). *Lesbian, gay, bisexual and transgender aging.* http://www.apa.org/pi/lgbt/resources/aging.aspx.

Annon, J. S. (1976). The PLISSIT model: a proposed conceptual scheme for behavioral treatment of sexual problems. *Journal of Sex & Education Therapy, 2,* 1–15.

Bauer, M., Haesler, E., & Fetherstonhaugh, D. (2016). Let's talk about sex: older people's views on the recognition of sexuality and sexual health in the health-care setting. *Health Expectation, 19*(6), 1237–1250.

Biddle, K., Jacobs, H., d'Oleire Uquillas, F., et al. (2020). Association of widowhood and β Amyloid with cognitive decline in cognitively unimpaired older adults. *JAMA Network Open, 3*(2), e200121. doi.org/10.1001/jamanetworkopen.2020.0121.

Byrne, M., Murphy, P., D'Eath, M., Doherty, S., & Jaarsma, T (2017). Association between sexual problems and relationship satisfaction among people with cardiovascular disease. *The Journal Sex Medicine, 14*(5), 666–674.

Centers for Disease Control and Prevention (CDC). (2019). *Sexually transmitted disease surveillance.* https://www.cdc.gov/std/stats/default.htm.

Centers for Disease Control and Prevention (2020). HIV and older Americans. https://www.cdc.gov/hiv/group/age/olderamericans/index.html.

Clark, T. (2015). *The circles of sexuality and aging American Society on Aging.* https://www.asaging.org/blog/circles-sexuality-and-aging.

Cloyes, K. G. (2016). The silence of our science: nursing research on LGBT older adult health. *Research Gerontology Nursing, 9*(2), 92–104.

Cohn, D., & Passel, J. F. (2018). *A record 64.6 million Americans live in multigenerational households.* Washington, DC: Pew Research Center. http://www.pewresearch.org/fact-tank/2018/04/05/a-record-64-million-americans-live-in-multigenerational-households/.

Coleman, C. L. (2017). Women 50 and older and HIV. Prevention and implications for health care providers. *Journal of Gerontology Nursing, 43*(12), 29–34.

Comfort, A. (1974). Sexuality in old age. *Journal of the American Geriatrics Society, 22,* 440–442.

Dhingra, I., De Sousa, A., & Sonavane, S. (2016). Sexuality in older adults: clinical and psychosocial dilemmas. *Journal of Geriatrics Mental Health, 3*(2), 131–139.

Emlet, C. (2016). Social, economic, and health disparities among LGBT older adults. *Generations, 40*(2), 16–22.

Employee Benefit Research Institute. (2019). *Confidence in retirement security rebounds to pre-financial crisis levels.* https://www.ebri.org/retirement/retirement-confidence-survey.

Franc, L., Moukoulou, L., Scott, L., & Zerwic, J. (2018). LGBT inclusivity in health assessment textbooks. *Journal of Professional Nursing, 34*(6), 483–487.

Fredriksen-Goldsen, K. I. (2016). The future of LGBT + aging: a blueprint for action in services, policies, and research. *Gen J West Gerontol Soc, 40*(2), 6–15.

Generations United (2021). Multigenerational households. https://www.gu.org/explore-our-topics/multigenerational-households/. Accessed February 2021.

Heidari, S. (2016). Sexuality and older people: a neglected issue. *Reproductive Health Matters, 24*(48), 1–5.

Jones, C., & Moyle, W. (2018). Are gerontological nurses ready for the expression of sexuality by individuals with dementia?. *Journal of Gerontological Nursing, 44*(5), 2–4.

Karpiak, S, & Brennan-Ing, M. (2016). Aging with HIV: the challenges of providing care and social supports. *Gen J Am Soc Aging, 40*(2), 23–25.

Krogstad, J. M. (2015). *5 facts about American grandparents.* Washington, DC: Pew Research Center. http://www.pewresearch.org/fact-tank/2015/09/13/5-facts-about-american-grandparents/.

Landry, J. (2017). Delivering culturally sensitive care to LGBTQI patients. *The Jour for Nurse Practitioners, 13*(5), 342–347.

Lee, DM, Nazroo, J, O'Connor, DB, Blake, M, & Pendleton, N (2016). Sexual health and well-being among older men and women in England: findings from the English Longitudinal Study of Ageing. *Archives of Sex Behavior, 45*(1), 133–144.

Lindau, ST, Dale, W, Feldmeth, G, et al. (2018). Sexuality and cognitive status: a U.S. nationally representative study of home-dwelling older adults. *Journal of the American Geriatrics Society, 66,* 1902–1910.

Marchese, K. (2017). An overview of erectile dysfunction in the elderly population. *Urologic Nursing, 37*(3), 157–170.

Mobley, DF, Khera, M, & Baum, N. (2017). Recent advances in the treatment of erectile dysfunction. *Postgrad Medicine Journal, 93,* 679–685.

Morley, J. (2017). Vicissitudes: retirement with a long post-retirement future. *Gener J Am Soc Aging, 41*(2), 101–107.

National Center for Transgender Equality. (2016). *Understanding transgender people: The basics.* https://transequality.org/issues/resources/understanding-transgender-people-the-basics.

National Institute of Neurological Disorders and Stroke. (2020). *Clinical trials*. https://www.ninds.nih.gov/Disorders/Clinical-Trials/Anakinra-Recombinant-Human-IL-1-Receptor-Antagonist-Neuroinflammation-HIV.

Neville, S. J., Adams, J., Bellamy, G., Boyd, M., & George, N. (2014). Perceptions towards lesbian, gay and bisexual people in residential care facilities: a qualitative study. *International Journal of Older People Nursing, 10*(1), 73–80.

O'Brien, S. (2020). Majority of workers expect their "retirement" to include a job, survey shows. https://www.cnbc.com/2020/09/03/many-workers-expect-their-retirement-to-include-a-job-survey-shows.html#:~:text=Among%20baby%20boomers%20still%20in,study%20from%20Voya%20Financial%20shows.&text=Overall%2C%2054%25%20of%20all%20workers,a%20job%20of%20some%20sort. Accessed February 2021.

Orel, N. A., & Coon, D. (2016). The challenges of change: how can we meet the care needs of the ever-evolving LGBT family? *General Journal American Society Aging, 40*(2), 41–45.

Plawecki, H. M., & Plawecki, L. H. (2016). Challenges of retirement. *Journal Gerontological Nursing, 42*(11), 3–5.

Schafer, M. H, Upenieks, L., & Iveniuk, J. (2018). Putting sex into context in later life: environmental disorder and sexual interest among partnered seniors. *Gerontologist, 58*(1), 181–190.

Shelton, A. (2016). *Social Security: a key retirement resource for woman*: AARP Public Policy Institute. https://www.aarp.org/work/social-security/info-2014/social-security-a-key-retirement-income-source-for-older-minorities-ppi.html.

Steelman, R. E. (2018). Person-centered care for LGBT older adults. *Journal of Gerontological Nursing, 44*(2), 3–5.

Steinke, E. E. (2013). Sexuality and chronic illness. *Journal of Gerontological Nursing, 39*(11), 18–29.

Steinke, E. E., Jaarsma, T., Barnason, S. A., et al. (2013). Sexual counseling for individuals with CVD and their partners: a consensus statement from the American Heart Association and the ESC Council on Cardiovascular Nursing and Allied Professions (CCNAP). *Circulation, 128*, 2075–2096.

Steple, R. (2016). *Smaller share of women ages 65 and older are living alone*. Washington, DC: Pew Research Center.

http://www.pewsocialtrends.org/2016/02/18/smaller-share-of-women-ages-65-and-older-are-living-alone/.

Syme, M. L., Yelland, E., Cornelison, L., Poey, J. L., Krajicek, R., & Doll, G. (2017). Content analysis of public opinion on sexual expression and dementia: implications for nursing home policy development. *Health Expectations, 20*, 705–713.

Transamerica Center for Retirement Studies (2019). What is retirement? Three generations prepare for older age. https://transamericacenter.org/docs/default-source/retirement-survey-of-workers/tcrs2019_sr_what_is_retirement_by_generation.pdf. Accessed February 2021.

United Nations Economic and Social Commission for Asia and the Pacific. (2018). *China has a law that mandates children to care for their elderly parents*. http://www.unescap.org/ageing-asia/did-you-know/364/china-has-law-mandates-children-care-their-elderly-parents.

Vespa, J., & Schondelmyer, E. (2015). A gray revolution in living arrangements. *United States Census Bureau Census Blogs*. https://www.census.gov/newsroom/blogs/random-samplings/2015/07/a-gray-revolution-in-living-arrangements.html.

Wardecker, B., & Matcisk, J. (2020). Families of choice and community connectedness: a brief guide to the social strengths of LGTTQ older adults. *Journal Gerontology Nursing, 46*(2), 5–8.

The Well Project. (2020). *Women and HIV*. http://www.thewellproject.org/hiv-information/women-and-hiv.

Wright, H., Jenks, R. A., & Demeyere, N. (2019). Frequent sexual activity predicts specific cognitive abilities in older adults. *The Journal of Gerontology. Series B, Psychological Science and Social Science, 74*(1), 47–51.

World Health Organization. (2020). *Defining sexual health*. http://www.who.int/reproductivehealth/topics/sexual_health/sh_definitions/en/.

Youngkin, E. Q. (2004). The myths and truths of mature intimacy: mature guidance for nurse practitioners. *Advance for nurse practitioners, 12*, 45–48.

Zanetos, J., & Skipper, A. (2020). The effects of health care policies: LGBTQ aging adults. *Journal Gerontology Nursing, 46*(3), 9–12.

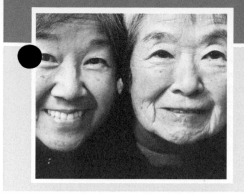

27

Clinical Judgment to Promote Caregiver Health

Theris A. Touhy

http://evolve.elsevier.com/Touhy/gerontological/

LEARNING OBJECTIVES

Upon completion of this chapter, the reader will be able to:
- Identify the range of caregiving situations and the potential challenges and opportunities of each.
- Differentiate between abuse and neglect.
- Define the nurse's role in the prevention of mistreatment of older adults.
- Utilize clinical judgment to identify and evaluate nursing actions to promote caregiver health.

THE LIVED EXPERIENCE

There are four kinds of people in the world: those who have been caregivers, those who are currently caregivers, those who will be caregivers, and those who will need caregivers.
Rosalyn Carter quoted in Alzheimer's Reading Room (2013)

CAREGIVING

Family caregiving has become a normative experience (similar to marriage, working, or retirement) for many of America's families and cuts across racial, ethnic, and social class distinctions. Gerontological nurses are most likely to encounter older adults with their family and friends in situations relating to caregiving of some kind. Informal caregivers (family members and other unpaid caregivers) provide the majority of care for older adults in the United States. Thirty-two percent of informal caregivers are caring for their parent and 36% are caring for their spouse.

Six in ten family caregivers across all race/ethnicity groups are employed. Since 2015 there has been an increase of 5 million employed caregivers. These caregivers often face great stressors in trying to manage jobs and families while caregiving (American Association of Retired Persons and National Alliance for Caregiving, 2020). Family caregives who are employed has increased by more than 5 million since 2015. Six in ten family caregivers are employed (AARP and National Alliance for Caregiving, 2020).

Caregivers are evenly split between men and women, although we know very little about the male caregiver experience (Accius, 2017). Family structures have chan-ged, as have family caregiving networks. It is important for nurses to understand the complexity of caregiving and the many forms it may take. Defining caregiving as a dyad of a caregiver and care recipient does not reflect today's patterns of caregiving (Epps et al., 2019). Informal care provided by caregivers is universally recognized as the foundation of the long-term care system. Informal caregivers basically provide free services to care recipients. It would cost an estimated $470 billion to replace the care that family caregivers provide, more than the amount of total Medicaid spending (Family Caregiver Alliance, 2019). Without family caregivers, the present level of long-term care could not be sustained. Box 27.1 presents some statistics on caregiving.

Caregiving in the LGBT community follows a different pattern. Nine percent of caregivers self-identify as LGBT and LGBT older adults largely care for each

BOX 27.1 Facts About Caregiving

- Approximately 34.2 million caregivers have provided care to an adult aged 50 years or older in the past 12 months in the United States.
- Family caregivers are children (41.3%), spouses (38.4%), and other family and friends (20.4%).
- The average duration of a caregiver's role is 4.6 years.
- Sixty-six percent of caregivers are female and their average age is 48 years.
- The number of male caregivers is smaller but increasing, and continued research is needed to address their unique needs. Among spousal caregivers 75 years and older, both sexes provide equal amounts of care.
- Between 12% and 18% of the total adult caregivers in the United States are estimated to be between the ages of 18 and 24 years.
- About 43.5 million adult family caregivers care for someone who has Alzheimer's disease or other dementia. They provide care an average of 1 to 4 years more than caregivers of individuals with other illnesses.
- Almost half of lesbian, gay, bisexual, and transgender (LGBT) older adults provide caregiving assistance to families or origin or families of choice.
- More than 2.7 million grandparents are providing primary care (custodial grandparents) for grandchildren in the United States and grandparent-headed households are one of the fastest-growing US family groups.
- Caregiving can have serious negative effects on mental and physical health. Approximately 40% to 70% of caregivers have clinically significant symptoms of depression.
- Caregiving can also present financial burdens, and women who are family caregivers are 2.5 times more likely than non-caregivers to live in poverty.

Data from Family Caregiver Alliance, National Center on Caregiving. (2019). *Caregiving statistics: demographics.* https://www.caregiver.org/caregiver-statistics-demographics.

other. However, LGBT baby boomers and millennials also take care of their aging parents at a disproportionate rate (National Resource Center on LGBT Aging, 2020). Spouses, partners, and friends provide almost 90% of the care received by older adults who identify as LGBT. The pattern reflects the importance of a "chosen family" in the lives of older adults who identify as LGBT. "These chosen families provide care to the LGBT older adult, but they often go unrecognized and are not provided with adequate information to care for patients or not acknowledged as caregivers in medical settings. Nurses need to give them the support, assistance, and information they need to provide proper care to their loved one" (Wardecker & Johnston, 2018, pp. 2–3). These patterns may change for future generations of older adults who identify as LGBT who have had the

benefits of marriage equality, greater social acceptance, and having children.

The concern over encountering anti-LGBT bias increases the demand for informal caregiving because older adults identifying as LGBT will go to great lengths to avoid entering senior housing and are often determined to age-in-place at all costs. They are also less likely to access supportive in-home services because of fear of discrimination and bias. In a number of areas across the country, LGBT community members have launched efforts to create senior housing and retirement communities specifically designed with their needs in mind. Many of these projects are still in development stages and are primarily designed for affluent individuals. Hopefully, as the community continues to advocate on behalf of LGBT seniors, a greater variety of housing options will ultimately be available. Local and national LGBT organizations can be another vital resource in locating community agencies that are sensitive and supportive (Chapter 26).

Caregiving is considered a major public health issue across the globe, and attention to the physical and mental health of caregivers is receiving increased attention. As a result of demographic changes, the demand for family caregivers of adults over the age of 65 years is increasing significantly but we do not have an eldercare system properly equipped to support them (Eldercare Workforce Alliance, 2018). Current trends suggest that the use of paid, formal care by older adults in the community has been decreasing, while their sole reliance on family caregivers has been increasing. The need for family caregivers will increase substantially, but the number of family caregivers who are available to provide care is also decreasing substantially.

The "caregiver support ratio" will start to drop when the first baby boomers begin to turn 80 years old in 2026 and by 2050, the ratio will fall to less than three potential caregivers for every person 80 years and older (Feinberg & Levine, 2015–2016). Additionally, there is a growing shortage of formal caregivers (nursing assistants, licensed practical nurses [LPNs] and registered nurses [RNs]) for long-term care services across the continuum (Chapters 1 and 6).

Some suggest that the conception of caregiving is different among the baby boomer generation. Although they recognize their responsibility to care for ill family members, they view themselves as partners in the organization of care and want to negotiate and set limits to the amount and kind of care they wish to undertake. This will require the existence of alternative resources to family care and policy and practice that no longer takes family caregiving for granted. Baby boomer caregivers and upcoming generations will expect more support and formal assistance from national and local agencies in a coordinated long-term care network (Chapter 6).

Impact of Caregiving

Although caregiving is a means to "give back" to a loved one and can be a source of joy in the giving, it is also stressful. "Caregiving is a very complex issue, and assuming a caregiving role is a time of transition that requires a restructuring of one's goals, behaviors, and responsibilities. It requires taking on something new, but it is also about loss—of what was and what could have been" (Lund, 2005, p. 152). Caregivers are considered to be "*the hidden patient*" (Schulz & Beach, 1999, p. 2216).

Family caregiving has been associated with increased levels of depression and anxiety, poorer self-reported physical health, compromised immune function, higher rates of insomnia, increased alcohol use, and increased mortality (Tang et al., 2018). Caregiver burden encompasses physical, psychological, emotional, relational, social, and financial problems due to caregiving (Pristavec, 2018). Unrelieved caregiver stress increases the potential for abuse and neglect, which is discussed later in this chapter. There are certain circumstances that are more likely to cause challenges with caregiving (Box 27.2).

Caregiving can be both rewarding and distressing, generating both feelings of benefit and burden for some caregivers and even with high burden, caregivers may experience high benefits. Caregivers experiencing benefits have better mental health and continue in the caregiving role longer than those experiencing burden (Pristavec, 2018). Positive benefits of caregiving may include enhanced self-esteem and well-being, personal growth and satisfaction, and finding or making meaning through caregiving.

Caregiving is more likely to be perceived as rewarding if the caregiver feels needed and useful, has a close and reciprocal relationship with the care recipient,

---

BOX 27.2 Circumstances Associated With Caregiver Stress

- Competing role responsibilities (e.g., work, home)
- Advanced age of the caregiver
- High-intensity caregiving need
- Insufficient resources
- Financial difficulty
- Poor self-reported health
- Living in the same household with the care recipient
- Dementia of the care recipient
- Length of time caregiving
- Prior relational conflicts between the caregiver and care recipient

---

BOX 27.3 Tips for Best Practice
Reducing Caregiver Stress

- Educate yourself about the disease or medical condition.
- Contact the appropriate disease-related organization to learn about resources and education and support groups to help you adapt to the challenges you encounter.
- Find a health care professional who understands the disease.
- Consult with other experts to help plan for the future (legal, financial).
- Tap your social resources for assistance.
- Take time for relaxation and exercise.
- Use community resources.
- Maintain your sense of humor.
- Explore religious beliefs and spiritual values.
- Participate in pleasant, nurturing activities such as reading a good book, taking a warm bath.
- Seek supportive counseling when you need it.
- Identify and acknowledge your feelings; you have a right to ALL of them.
- Set realistic goals.
- Attend to your own health care needs.

Data from https://www.mayoclinic.org/healthy-lifestyle/stress-management/in-depth/caregiver-stress/art-20044784.

---

believes their help is appreciated by the care recipient, and has an adequate support network (Monin et al., 2017). The positive benefits of caregiving have been given more attention in recent years, but further research is needed to help understand which factors influence how caregivers perceive the experience and how assistance programs can focus on increasing the perception of benefits (Pristavec, 2018) (Box 27.3).

Nurse researcher Patricia Archbold and colleagues (1990) studied caregiving as a role and examined how the relationships between the caregiver and care recipient (mutuality) and the preparation of the caregiver for the tasks and stresses of caregiving (preparedness) influence reactions to caregiving. Most caregivers are not prepared for the many responsibilities they face and receive no formal instruction in caregiving activities. Lack of preparedness can greatly increase the caregiver's stress.

Caregivers who report a high level of preparedness for the caregiving experience lower levels of caregiver strain after hospitalization of older adults and during cancer care and treatment (Zwicker, 2018). Several validated caregiver assessment instruments are available including the Preparedness for Caregiving Scale and the Modified Caregiver Strain Index (Fig. 27.1). Further research is needed to understand the complexities of the caregiving and care-receiving role and provide a theory

Directions: Here is a list of things that other caregivers have found to be difficult. Please put a checkmark in the columns that apply to you. We have included some examples that are common caregiver experiences to help you think about each item. Your situation may be slightly different, but the item could still apply.

	Yes, On a Regular Basis = 2	Yes, Sometimes = 1	No = 0
My sleep is disturbed (For example: the person I care for is in and out of bed or wanders around at night)	_____	_____	_____
Caregiving is inconvenient (For example: helping takes so much time or it's a long drive over to help)	_____	_____	_____
Caregiving is a physical strain (For example: lifting in or out of a chair; effort or concentration is required)	_____	_____	_____
Caregiving is confining (For example: helping restricts free time or I cannot go visiting)	_____	_____	_____
There have been family adjustments (For example: helping has disrupted my routine; there is no privacy)	_____	_____	_____
There have been changes in personal plans (For example: I had to turn down a job; I could not go on vacation)	_____	_____	_____
There have been other demands on my time (For example: other family members need me)	_____	_____	_____
There have been emotional adjustments (For example: severe arguments about caregiving)	_____	_____	_____
Some behavior is upsetting (For example: incontinence; the person cared for has trouble remembering things; or the person I care for accuses people of taking things)	_____	_____	_____
It is upsetting to find the person I care for has changed so much from his/her former self (For example: he/she is a different person than he/she used to be)	_____	_____	_____
There have been work adjustments (For example: I have to take time off for caregiving duties)	_____	_____	_____
Caregiving is a financial strain	_____	_____	_____
I feel completely overwhelmed (For example: I worry about the person I care for; I have concerns about how I will manage)	_____	_____	_____

[Sum responses for "Yes, on a regular basis" (2 pts each) and "yes, sometimes" (1 pt each)]

Total Score =

FIG. 27.1 Modified Caregiver Strain Index. (From Thornton, M., & Travis, S. S. (2003). Analysis of the reliability of the Modified Caregiver Strain Index. *J Gerontol B Psychol Sci Soc Sci, 58*(2), S129. Copyright The Gerontological Society of America. Reproduced by permission of the publisher.)

BOX 27.4   Resources for Best Practice

Administration for Community Living: National family caregiver support program: https://acl.gov/programs/support-caregivers/national-family-caregiver-support-program.

Alzheimer's Association: Respite Care Guide, Free online caregiver community. https://www.alz.org/help-support/caregiving/care-options/respite-care.

Caregiver Action Network: Caregiver Help Line, Caregiver Toolkit, Resources, education. https://www.caregiveraction.org/.

Caregiver Preparedness Scale: https://consultgeri.org/try-this/general-assessment/issue-28.pdf

Centers for Disease Control and Prevention: Violence Prevention. https://www.cdc.gov/violenceprevention/elderabuse/index.html.

Family Caregiver Alliance: Resources, education. https://www.caregiver.org/.

Hartford Institute for Geriatric Nursing: Family Caregiving Standard of Practice Protocol; Detection of Elder Mistreatment Nursing Standard of Practice Protocol; Modified Caregiver Strain Index.

National Alliance for Caregiving: International resources and best practices in caregiving. https://www.caregiving.org/.

National Center on Elder Abuse: https://ncea.acl.gov/.

National Respite Locator Service: Search for respite programs and providers. https://archrespite.org/respitelocator.

---

base for nursing actions. Other resources for caregivers are presented in Box 27.4.

Caregiving of Individuals With Dementia

Caregivers of individuals with dementia provide more intensive help than caregivers of individuals without dementia and experience greater financial, emotional, and physical challenges (Gaugler et al., 2017). Services for individuals with dementia used to be primarily institutional, such as in nursing homes, but now more than two-thirds to three-quarters of individuals with dementia live in the community (Lepore & Wiener, 2017). Factors that increase the stress of caregiving for an individual with dementia include grief over the multiple losses that occur, the physical demands and duration of caregiving (up to 20 years), communication difficulties, and a lack of resource availability.

Demands are intensified if the care recipient demonstrates behavioral disturbances and impairments in activities of daily living (ADLs) and instrumental activities of daily living (IADLs) (Gaugler et al., 2017) (Chapter 25). The effects of Alzheimer's disease and related dementias on marital relationships can be devastating for both partners and lead to loneliness, frustration, and estrangement. Enhancing communication between spousal caregivers and their loved one with dementia has been investigated by nurse researcher Dr. Christine

Williams (2015). The CARE (Communicating about Relationships and Emotions) intervention was found to improve communication for both spouses and promote spouses' engagement with one another.

Spousal Caregiving

Eighty percent of older adults who live with spouses with disabilities provide care for them. More wives than husbands provide care, but this is changing as the life expectancy for men increases. Caregiving spouses experience more mental and physical health problems from their caregiving, provide more intensive, time-consuming care than other family caregivers, and are less likely to receive assistance from other family members (Polenick & DePasquale, 2018). Older spouses often take on greater burdens than they can reasonably handle and get by with significantly less help in the home than other types of caregivers, yet their responsibilities increase over time (Park, 2017). Spousal caregivers who report a great deal of strain are almost two times more likely to die than caregivers reporting some strain (Perkins et al., 2013).

Older spouses caring for partners who are ill also face many role changes. Older women may need to learn to drive, manage money, or make decisions by themselves. Male caregivers may need to learn how to cook, shop, do laundry, and provide personal care to their wives. Spousal caregivers also deal with the added responsibilities of caregiving while at the same time dealing with the anticipated loss of their spouse. Nurses should be alert to situations in which health care personnel may be able to provide supports and resources that make it possible for an individual to assume new responsibilities without being totally overwhelmed. Adult day programs, respite care services, or periodic assistance from a home health aide or homemaker may make it possible for the couple to continue to live together and ease the strain of caregiving. It is important to pay attention to the physical and mental health needs of the caregiver and those of the care recipient.

Aging Parents Caring for Adult Children With Intellectual and Developmental Disabilities

Although we tend to think of caregivers as middle-aged adults caring for older adults, an unknown number of older adults are caring for their middle-aged children with intellectual and developmental disabilities (I/DD). In the past century, children with I/DD were typically in institutions and usually died before reaching adulthood. Today, about 75% of adults with I/DD now live with their parents or other family members and more than 25% live with parents aged 60 years and older (Baumbusch et al., 2017). For the first time in history, individuals with I/DD are outliving their parents and planning for their future is an area posing challenges for older adults and for service providers internationally.

With increased survival, adults with I/DD are also at risk of developing chronic illness and will need more care and services. For example, individuals with Down syndrome are more likely to develop dementia. Often, the burden of caring for a child with I/DD has been carried by parents for their entire adult life and will end only with the death of the parent or the adult child. Parental caregivers who are aging face changes in their financial resources and health that affect their continued caregiving ability.

A majority of these caregivers worry about how their child will receive care if they develop a debilitating illness or die. A recent study reported that aging parents were increasingly aware of their own aging process and the implications for their ability to continue providing care. They were fostering connections with both informal and formal sources of care that could supplement or replace their care activities. It was important to shift their care activities from providing physical support to a focus on social-economic support and communicating their intimate knowledge of their relative with I/DD to others who could provide care in the future. Engaging in conversations and planning for end-of-life care was a major challenge and depended to a certain extent on their relative's understanding of death and dying and their emotional readiness to live without their main care provider (Baumbusch et al., 2017).

In the United States, the Planned Lifetime Assistance Network (PLAN), available in some states through the National Alliance for the Mentally Ill, provides lifetime assistance to individuals with disabilities whose parents or other family members are deceased or can no longer provide for their care. The Alzheimer's Association and other aging organizations offer education and support programs for both parents and their developmentally disabled adult children in some communities. There is a continued need for the development of both in-home and community options for developmentally disabled adults who are aging. Additionally, there is a need for research exploring the experience of aging families caring for adult children with I/DD.

Grandparents Raising Grandchildren

Over the past decade grandparents have assumed the primary caregiving responsibility for their grandchildren at an unprecedented rate. Global figures indicate that grandparents represent the majority of all kinship carers and are the largest providers of formal childcare between birth and 12 years of age (McLaughlin et al., 2017). More than 2.7 million grandparents provide primary care (custodial grandparents) for grandchildren in the United States and grandparent-headed households are one of the fastest-growing US family groups. About 39% of grandparent caregivers are over the age of 60 years.

The reasons grandparents take a child into the home without their parents vary among countries, groups, and individuals. Many grandparents have become, by default, the primary caregivers of grandchildren because the parents are unable to provide the care needed as a result of child abuse, teen pregnancy, imprisonment, joblessness, military deployment, drug and alcohol addictions, illness, death, and other social problems. Drug addiction, especially to opioids, is behind much of the rise in the number of grandparents raising their grandchildren (Anderson, 2019). Research related to the effect of grandparent caregiving on health status is lacking, but existing literature suggests that there are economic, health, and social challenges inherent in this role.

As with other types of caregiving, there are both blessings and burdens and caregivers' experiences will be unique. For many grandparents, the challenges may include limited income and financial support through the welfare system, lack of informal support systems, loss of leisure activities in retirement, and shame or guilt related to their children's inability to parent (McLaughlin et al., 2017). Physical and mental stressors appear to be greater when grandparents are raising a chronically ill or special-needs child or a child with behavioral problems, or experiencing chronic illness themselves. The COVID-19 pandemic has presented many challenges for grandparents caring for grandchildren, particularly with school closures and the heightened risk of COVID-19 in older adults.

Often, crisis situations precipitate the decision of a grandparent to assume caring for a grandchild and time for preparation is not available. In many cases, grandparents assume care so that their grandchildren's care is not taken over by the public care system. However, many custodial grandparents are not licensed in the foster care system and are not eligible for the same services and financial support as licensed foster parents. About 25% of grandparent-headed households are in poverty and over half of grandmothers raising grandchildren live in poverty. Housing, food, and child care assistance are minimal for grandfamilies outside the system and only a small percentage get the help they need (Generations United, 2020).

The benefits for the children cared for by grandparents are better than for children in nonrelative care and include increased stability, greater safety, better behavioral and mental health outcomes, more positive feelings about placements, more likely to report they "always felt loved," more likely to live with or stay connected to siblings, and greater preservation of cultural identity and community connections (Generations United, 2020).

Nursing Actions: Supporting Grandparent Caregivers

Routine screening and monitoring of the psychological distress of primary care grandparents and offering support, advice, and referral to reduce stressors are important. Currently, evidence suggests that cognitive-behavioral interventions have the most empirical support for improving a grandparent caregiver's psychological well-being. Promising approaches that require further research to support their effectiveness include support groups, interdisciplinary case management, and psychoeducational interventions (McLaughlin et al., 2017). Another successful service is kinship navigator programs, which provide a single point of entry for connecting to housing, household resources, physical and mental health services, and financial and legal assistance (Generations United, 2020).

Some grandparent caregivers may be reluctant to seek assistance and often neglect their own health concerns. Delivering health promotional and financial assistance information within the nonjudgmental environment of grandparent support groups may be effective (Taylor et al., 2017). Resources to support grandparent caregivers should be available in communities and could be offered through health care institutions, schools, and churches. Nurses can be instrumental in developing and conducting programs for grandparent caregivers. The National Family Caregiver Support Program (NFCSP), under the Older Americans Act program, provides support services, education and training, counseling, and respite care and should be encouraged in all states. Nurses can refer the grandparents to their local area agency on aging to inquire about available resources (Box 27.4). Suggestions for nursing actions with older adults providing primary care to their grandchildren are presented in Box 27.5.

BOX 27.5   Tips for Best Practice
Nursing Actions With Grandparent Caregivers

- Early identification of at-risk grandparents
- Comprehensive evaluation of physical, psychosocial, and environmental factors affecting those in the caregiving role for grandchildren
- Anticipatory guidance and counseling about child growth and development and other child-raising issues
- Referral to resources for support, counseling, and financial assistance
- Advocacy for policies supportive of grandparents who have assumed a caregiving role

---

Long-Distance Caregiving

Because of the increasing mobility of today's global society, more children move away for education or employment and do not return home. When a parent needs help, it must be provided "long distance." This is perhaps one of the most difficult situations and it presents unique challenges. About 15% of all caregivers are long-distance caregivers and this is increasing. Issues that need to be considered in long-distance caregiving include identifying a local person who will be available quickly in emergency situations; identifying reliable individuals or services that will provide daily monitoring if necessary; identifying acceptable facilities for assisted living or nursing home care if that becomes necessary; determining which family member is most likely to be free to travel to the older adult if needed; and being sure that legalities regarding advance directives, a will, and power of attorney (for health care and financial) have been established.

A profession and industry has emerged to assist the geographically distant family member to ensure that an older relative will receive care. This profession is made up of geriatric care managers, some of whom are nurses or social workers. A care manager can be hired to do everything a family member would do if able, from being available in an emergency, to helping with estate planning, to making arrangements for a move to a nursing home. These services are available primarily to those who are able to pay for them because they are not covered by private insurance, Medicare, or any public agencies. Although these services are expensive, they may be far less expensive than alternative living arrangements or institutional placement.

Similar services may be available for persons with very low incomes through the local Area Agency on Aging "Community Care for the Elderly" programs. When incomes are too high to qualify for Medicaid and too low to pay for private care managers, the individual and their families must do the best they can. Long-distance care then depends on the goodness of neighbors, local friends, and apartment managers and frequent trips by the long-distance caregiver to the older adult.

❖ USING CLINICAL JUDGMENT TO PROMOTE HEALTHY AGING: CAREGIVING

◆ Recognizing and Analyzing Cues: Caregiver Health

Gathering information about the family is an important component of care for older adults. Often, nurses see families in times of crisis when an older family member needs care. When working with families, it is important for the nurse to be aware of their vision of what a "family" should be and what a "family" should do. Our values should not enter into evaluation of families and families should not be judged or labeled as dysfunctional (Feinberg & Levine, 2015–2016). It is necessary to identify the strengths within each family and to build on those strengths while recognizing the family's limitations in providing support and caregiving. Thus, the nurse's role is to teach, monitor, and strengthen the family system so as to maintain health and wellness of the entire family structure.

Gathering information about a caregiving situation helps identify the specific challenges, needs, strengths, and resources of the family caregiver, and the caregiver's ability to contribute to the needs of the care recipient (Feinberg & Levine, 2015–2016). A personalized plan of care for the family is developed and includes how the health care team can help the person providing care.

Family caregivers often perform tasks that nurses typically perform including injections, tube feedings, operating special equipment, managing multiple medications, catheter and colostomy care, and other complex care responsibilities: "the same tasks that make nursing students tremble the first time they have to perform them" (Kennedy, 2017).

Almost half of these family caregivers do these medical/nursing tasks without any preparation and few visits from home care providers (Reinhard et al., 2017). Only about a third of family caregivers reported that a doctor, nurse, or social worker asked them what was needed to care for their loved one, and even fewer said a health or social provider had asked what they needed to care for themselves (Feinberg & Levine, 2015–2016). Nurses play an important role in insuring that the family is included in plans of care for the older adult.

In response to these concerns, new laws in support of family caregivers have been enacted at both the state and federal levels. The Caregiver Advise, Record, and Enable or CARE Act is in effect in nearly three-quarters of the United States Provisions of the laws vary from state to state but the CARE Act generally institutes three basic reforms that require hospitals to (1) let patients identify a family caregiver when they're admitted; (2) notify the family caregiver in advance when the patient will be discharged; and (3) provide a simple instruction of the medical tasks they will be performing when their loved one returns home (Kennedy, 2017).

In 2018, the Recognize, Assist, Include, Support, and Engage (RAISE) Family Caregivers Act was signed into law (Govtrack, 2018). The law directs the US Secretary of Health and Human Services (HHS) to develop, maintain, and update an integrated national strategy to support family caregivers. The Lifespan Respite Care Act provides competitive grants to states in collaboration with a public or private nonprofit state respite coalition to enhance respite care and education of caregivers.

Nursing Actions: Caregiver Health

In designing actions to support caregiving, a partnership model, combining the nurse's professional expertise with the caregiver's knowledge of the family member, is recommended (Box 27.6). Given the range of caregiving situations and the uniqueness of each, interventions must be tailored to individual needs and build on the caregiver's existing strengths and resources. Actions include risk analysis, education about caregiving and stress, needed care skills, caregiver health and home safety, support groups, linkages to ongoing support, counseling, resource identification, relief/respite from daily care demands, and stress management.

BOX 27.6 Tips for Best Practice

Nursing Actions to Create and Sustain a Partnership With Caregivers

- Surveillance and ongoing monitoring
- Coaching: helping caregivers apply knowledge and develop skills
- Teaching: providing information and instruction
- Providing accurate and complete information about services; determine with the family referrals for services based on needs and preferences of caregiver and care recipient; mutually determine with the family services that are affordable, acceptable, and logistically feasible
- Fostering partnerships: fostering communication and collaboration between the caregiver and the care recipient and between them and the nurse
- Providing psychosocial support: attending to psychosocial well-being; help the caregiver and family identify effective coping strategies
- Coordinating: orchestrating the work of other health care team members and the activities of the caregiver

---

Education provided by nurses to help prepare the caregiver for the caregiving role, particularly at the time of discharge from the hospital or nursing home, can help to prevent role strain and lessen burden. Questions to be addressed with the caregiver include the following (Reinhard et al., 2017):

- What questions do you have regarding care today?
- What questions do you have about care at home?
- How are you doing and what are your needs?

With many caregivers trying to balance caregiving responsibilities while working, educational programs offered in the workplace can be beneficial for both the caregiver and the employer. When nurses work with families from a different culture that may have unfamiliar rituals and routines, the nurses need to be particularly careful to respect these differences. Service providers need to enhance cultural competence and design programs that are culturally acceptable (Chapter 3).

Linking caregivers to community resources, such as respite care, adult day programs, and financial support resources, is important. Respite care allows the caregiver to take a break from caregiving for various periods of time and can be one way family caregivers can take time for themselves and possibly avoid the need to relinquish their caregiving role (Roberts & Struckmeyer, 2018). Respite care may be provided in institutions, in the home, or in other community settings such as adult day service program (Chapter 6). However, respite care remains an important yet underutilized preventive resource despite it being the most commonly requested type or caregiver assistance (Rose et al., 2015).

Nurses should be aware of respite care resources in their communities and the local Area Agency on Aging can provide information on respite care and other caregiver services. Some government and nonprofit agencies offer free respite help but most respite services are paid privately by the family. For veterans, 30 days of respite care a year is available.

Respite care is covered through Medicare for individuals receiving hospice care but allows only 5 consecutive days of benefits. These interventions, when available, can alleviate much of the stress of caregiving but are utilized infrequently or very late in the course of caregiving in the United States. Many countries in Europe offer generous respite care services as part of the long-term care system. Chapter 6 discusses long-term care supports and services in more depth. *Healthy People 2020* objectives for long-term services and supports are presented in Box 27.7.

Tailored multicomponent programs designed to match a specific target population seem to have the most

positive outcomes on caregiver burden and stress—for example, groups designed to assist caregivers caring for individuals with early-stage dementia or those with Parkinson's disease. Programs that work collaboratively with care recipients and their families and are more intensive and modified to the caregiver's needs are also more successful. There are wide variations in caregiving experiences and the needs of an adult child caring for a parent with dementia may be quite different from those of a gay man or woman caring for a friend with cancer. Online training and support programs and telehealth tools seem to have great potential and need further research (Chi & Demiris, 2017; Egan et al., 2018).

Interventions with caregivers must always consider the great variability in family structures, resources, traditions, and history. The range of adaptations is enormous and the goal is always to restore the balance of the system to the greatest extent possible and support caregivers in their caring. Research suggests that differences exist in caregiving quality of life among individuals of different ages, male and female caregivers, and different racial and minority groups. Greater caregiving responsibilities are reported among females, racial and ethnic minorities, and low-income caregivers (Cook & Cohen, 2018). Resources for caregiving are presented in Box 27.4.

◆ Special Considerations for Caregivers of Individuals With Dementia

Therapeutic programs for both individuals and their caregivers should be individualized to meet the varied and changing needs over the course of the illness. The voice of the individual with Alzheimer's disease (AD) needs to be heard and they should be included in activities and support groups. Programs should be offered both in the community and in long-term care and assisted living facilities. Online psychoeducational programs for caregivers offer flexibility and can overcome the barriers of geographic distance and availability. The Alzheimer's Association is a valuable resource for both in-person and online support group formats (Box 27.4).

Access to a knowledgeable provider who can follow the individual and family throughout the course of the illness is essential and leads to improved outcomes and less distress. The current model of primary care does not adequately address the complexities of dementia care and most caregivers do not receive adequate support to help them with dementia-related problems throughout the course of the illness. Collaborative care management programs for the treatment of AD, often led by advanced practice nurses with expertise in dementia, have been shown to improve quality of care,

---

 BOX 27.7 Healthy People 2020

Long-Term Services and Supports

- Reduce the proportion of unpaid caregivers of older adults who report an unmet need for caregiver support services.
- Reduce the proportion of noninstitutionalized older adults with disabilities who have an unmet need for long-term services and supports.

Data from US Department of Health and Human Services, Office of Disease Prevention and Health Promotion. (2012). *Healthy People 2020*. http://www .healthypeople.gov/2020.

decrease the incidence of behavioral and psychological symptoms, and decrease caregiver stress. Care of individuals with neurocognitive disorders in discussed in Chapter 25.

Nursing actions with caregivers must always consider the great variability in family structures, resources, traditions, and history. The range of adaptations is enormous and the goal is always to restore the balance of the system to the greatest extent possible and support caregivers in their caring. The family can be visualized as a mobile structure with many parts and when one part is touched, each part shifts to regain the balance. The intrusion of professionals in a family system will temporarily unbalance the system and may provide an opportunity to restore the balance in a healthier manner, sometimes by adding an element or increasing the weight of one or decreasing the weight of another. Further research is needed to provide the foundation for nursing actions with family caregivers, particularly among racially and ethnically diverse families and nontraditional families.

ELDER MISTREATMENT

Elder mistreatment is a complex phenomenon that includes elder abuse and neglect. It is the infliction of actual harm, or a risk for harm, to vulnerable older persons through the action or behavior of others (American Psychological Association [APA], 2020). It is a universal problem and occurs in all educational, racial, cultural, religious, and socioeconomic groups, in any family configuration, and in every setting. It is one of the most unrecognized and underreported social problems today. Although there are no reliable statistics available related to the prevalence on a worldwide basis, the World Health Organization estimates that up to 15.7% of those older than 60 years of age have been or will be mistreated (World Health Organization [WHO], 2020).

In the United States, approximately 1 in 10 older adults has experienced some form of elder abuse. Estimates are that only 1 in 14 cases of abuse are reported to authorities (National Council on Aging, 2021). As the population of older adults continues to grow, so does the expectation that the prevalence of mistreatment will increase as well. The risk is further exacerbated with the shrinking pool of family caregivers (Chapter 26).

For mistreatment to occur, the perpetrator and a vulnerable older adult must have a trusting relationship of some kind. This may be as simple as a salesperson (financial exploitation) or as complex as a long-time caregiver such as a spouse or a child. Most often "elder mistreatment" occurs in the context of family caregiving. This may be a lifelong pattern that intensifies in the caregiving situation. The risk factors for a person to become

---

BOX 27.8   More Likely to Mistreat and Be Mistreated

More Likely to Abuse or Neglect
- Family member
- One with emotional or mental illnesses
- One who is abusing alcohol or other substances
- History of family violence
- Cultural acceptance of interpersonal violence
- Caregiver frustration
- Social isolation
- Impaired impulse control of caregiver

More Likely to Be Abused or Neglected
- Cognitive impairment, especially with aggressive features
- Dependent on abuser
- Physically or mentally frail
- Having abused the caregiver earlier in life
- Women either living alone or living in a household with family members
- Behavior that is considered aggressive, demanding, or unappreciative
- Living in an institutional setting
- Feeling deserving of abuse because of own inadequacies

Adapted from Sehgal, S. R., & Mosqueda, L. (2014). Mistreatment and neglect. In R. J. Ham, D. Sloane, & G. A. Warshaw, (Eds.). *Primary care geriatrics: A case-based approach* (6th ed., pp. 360–364). Philadelphia: Elsevier.

---

an abuser or to be abused are often interconnected (Box 27.8). Abusers can be men or women, of any age, race, or socioeconomic status. Individuals with dementia are especially vulnerable to mistreatment because the disease may prevent them from reporting abuse or recognizing it. They may also be vulnerable to strangers who take advantage of their cognitive impairment.

Mistreatment at the hands of formal caregivers occurs as well. When a number of different providers are giving care, monitoring becomes especially difficult. Situations of increased potential for formal caregiver abuse include those in which there is inadequate supervision of patient care, poor coordination of services, inadequate staff training, theft and fraud, drug and alcohol abuse by staff, tardiness and absenteeism, unprofessional and criminal conduct, and inadequate record keeping. Nurses should pay particular attention to the person who is alone with a formal caregiver for extended periods of time, with no support from others and no opportunities for respite for the caregiver.

Resident-to-resident elder mistreatment (inappropriate, disruptive, or hostile behavior among nursing home residents) is a sizable and growing problem. Among nursing home residents, reports are that 19.8% have experienced resident-to-resident mistreatment. Specific types of mistreatment include cursing, screaming, or yelling at another person; physical incidents such as hitting, kicking, or biting; and sexual incidents. These incidents are likely to cause emotional and/or physical harm and are stressful to staff. Further research is needed to develop actions for prevention and treatment. All residents have the right to be protected from abuse and mistreatment, and the facility is required to ensure the safety of all residents and investigate reports of abuse (Chapter 6).

Abuse

Abuse is intentional and may be physical, psychological, medical, financial, or sexual. Many states have reporting statutes that require certain persons, including nurses, who become aware of abuse, neglect, or exploitation to report it to the appropriate authorities. The designated authority can be found in each state's laws. Many factors interfere with the identification of those who are mistreated (Box 27.9). It is further complicated by varying cultural perspectives on abuse and expectations of care of older adults. Financial exploitation is common and often difficult to detect because there are no external signs of mistreatment. Changes in banking practices, access to a bank account by an unauthorized person, failure to pay medical or other bills, unexpected changes in a will, or the disappearance of personal items are all evidence of possible financial exploitation. Also "invisible, the most common form of abuse is verbal, emotional/psychological" (National Center on Elder Abuse [NCEA], 2021).

BOX 27.9 Factors Influencing Identification of Abuse of Older Adults

Cultural or societal tolerance of violence, especially against women
Shame and embarrassment
Fear of retaliation
Fear of institutionalization
Social isolation
Unacceptability of emotional expression, especially that of fear or distress

From World Health Organization. (2018). *Elder abuse.* http://www.who.int /mediacentre/factsheets/fs357/en/.

Impact of Elder Abuse

The abuse of older adults has effects that are more far-reaching than is usually discussed. Those subjected to even minimal abuse have been found to have a 300% higher risk for death than those who have never been abused (NCEA, 2021). In addition, older adults who have been victims of violence have more health problems than other older adults, including increased bone or joint problems, digestive problems, depression or anxiety, chronic pain, hypertension, and cardiovascular disease.

Neglect

Neglect is a form of mistreatment resulting from the failure of action by a caregiver or through a person's own behavior or choices. Neglect of self and neglect by caretakers are often difficult to define because they are intertwined with energy, lifestyle, and resources. Nurses are particularly challenged by issues of self-neglect when the ethical principle of beneficence (do good) counters that of autonomy (self-determination). In either case, the needs of the individual may not become known until there is a medical crisis when the person's unmet needs become visible to others.

Neglect by a Caregiver

Neglect by a caregiver requires a socially (formally or informally) recognized role and responsibility of a person to provide care to a vulnerable other. Neglect is most often passive mistreatment, such as an act of omission. It is not only the failure to provide the goods and services—such as food, medication, medical treatment, and personal care—necessary for the well-being of the care recipient, but also the failure or inability to recognize the responsibility to provide such goods and services. Neglect is active when care is withheld deliberately and for malicious reasons (NCOA, 2021). In some cases this level of neglect would be considered abuse as well. Neglect by caregivers occurs for many reasons (Box 27.10).

BOX 27.10 Possible Reasons for Neglect by Caregivers

Caregiver personal stress and exhaustion
Multiple role demands
Caregiver incompetence
Unawareness of importance of the neglected care
Financial burden of caregiving limiting resources available
Caregivers' own frailty and advanced age
Unawareness of community resources available for support and respite

---

Self-Neglect

Self-neglect is a behavior in which people fail to meet their own basic needs in the manner in which the average person would in similar circumstances. It generally manifests itself as a refusal to, or failure to, provide themselves with adequate safety, food, water, clothing, shelter, personal hygiene, or health care. It may be a result of diminished capacity, but it also may be the result of a long-standing lifestyle, homelessness, or alcoholism or other substance abuse. It is important for nurses to remember that there are many mentally competent people who understand the consequences of their decisions and make conscious and voluntary decisions to engage in acts that threaten their health or safety as a matter of personal choice. There are both ethical and legal questions as to how much health care professionals can and should intervene in these situations.

❖ USING CLINICAL JUDGMENT TO PROMOTE HEALTHY AGING: ELDER MISTREATMENT

◆ Recognizing and Analyzing Cues: Elder Mistreatment

When working with frail and vulnerable older adults, nurses must always be vigilant and sensitive to the signs and symptoms of mistreatment. Recognizing and analyzing cues to elder mistreatment includes the obvious indicators of physical abuse (e.g., unexplained bruises) and also more subtle signs. The range of signs and symptoms that may indicate mistreatment are presented in Box 27.11. For a person who is clearly competent and refuses assessment, this cannot be done. For a person with unmet needs or other signs of abuse or neglect, as well as questionable capacity, intervention is required.

A full and specialized evaluation includes the immediate determination of the person's safety. Further evaluation of possible mistreatment involves a number of very sensitive components and tools developed by experts in the field that may be very useful (Box 27.4). Because of the sensitive nature of such an assessment, specialized training is recommended for all nurses.

◆ Nursing Actions: Elder Mistreatment

In most states and US jurisdictions, licensed nurses are "mandatory reporters." This means that persons who have a reasonable belief that a vulnerable person either has been or is likely to be abused, neglected, or exploited are required to report this promptly to authorities identified by the jurisdiction where the person lives. Usually these reports are anonymous (Brent, 2019). If a nurse believes an older adult to be in immediate danger, the police are notified. How the nurse accomplishes this varies with the work setting.

In hospitals and nursing homes, suspicions of abuse are often reported first internally to the facility social worker. In a home care setting, the report is made to the nursing supervisor. It would be very unusual for the nurse not to approach this subject through their employer. However, a nurse who is a neighbor, friend, or privately paid caregiver may be under obligation to make the report directly. In the skilled nursing facility

---

BOX 27.11 Signs of Mistreatment

The first signs that further evaluation may be necessary are if the histories given by the (usually cognitively intact) older adult and the caregiver are inconsistent or the caregiver refuses to leave the individual alone with the nurse. Although it is always important to ask the older adult if they are a recipient of abuse/shame/suffering/family disharmony/moral cruelty, it cannot be assumed that this will be acknowledged. Although there is more than one category of abuse and abuse combined with neglect, the following specific signs would be included:

Physical Abuse
- Unexplained bruising or lacerations in unusual areas in various stages of healing
- Fractures inconsistent with functional ability

Sexual Abuse
- Bruises or scratches in the genital or breast area
- Fear or an unusual amount of anxiety related to either routine or necessary examination of the anogenital area
- Torn undergarments or presence of blood

Medical Abuse
- Caregiver repeatedly requesting procedures that are not recommended and not desired by the person receiving care

Medical Neglect
- Unusual delay between the beginning of a health problem and when help is sought
- Repeated missed appointments without reasonable explanations

Psychological Abuse
- Caregiver does all of the talking in a situation, even though the elderly person is capable
- Caregiver appears angry, frustrated, or indifferent while the elderly person appears hesitant or frightened
- Caregiver or the care recipient aggressive toward one another or the nurse

Neglect by Self or Caregiver
- Weight loss
- Uncharacteristically neglected grooming
- Evidence of malnutrition and dehydration
- Fecal/urine smell
- Inappropriate clothing to the situation or weather
- Insect infestation

---

or licensed assisted living facility, nurses have the additional resource of calling the state long-term care ombudsman for help.

If the abuse is triggered by the stress of caregiving, nurses can be very proactive and help all involved take action to lessen the stress. Interventions to assist caregivers are discussed in the first part of this chapter and Box 27.12 presents Tips for Best Practice to prevent mistreatment.

BOX 27.12   Tips for Best Practice

Prevention of Elder Mistreatment

- Make professionals aware of potentially abusive situations.
- Help families develop and nurture informal support systems.
- Link families with support groups.
- Teach families stress management techniques.
- Arrange comprehensive care resources.
- Provide counseling for troubled families.
- Encourage the use of respite care and day care.
- Obtain necessary home health care services.
- Inform families of resources for meals and transportation.
- Encourage caregivers to pursue their individual interests.

KEY CONCEPTS

- Family members and other unpaid caregivers provide 80% of care for older adults in the United States.
- Recognizing and analyzing cues to caregiver health may be different for the various types of caregiving roles (spousal, grandparent, LGBT individuals, individuals with dementia). Grandparents are increasingly assuming primary caregiving roles with grandchildren.
- Caregiving activities are one of the most major social issues of our time, as well as a significant global public health problem.
- Nursing actions with caregivers include risk evaluation, education about caregiving and stress, needed care skills, caregiver health and home safety, support groups, linkages to ongoing support, counseling, resource identification, relief/respite from daily care demands, and stress management.
- Elder mistreatment is an umbrella term that covers abuse, neglect, exploitation, and abandonment.
- Most abuse (90%) occurs in the home setting and is committed by adult children or spousal caregivers. Nursing actions can assist in mitigating the stress and burden of caregiving.

ACTIVITIES AND DISCUSSION QUESTIONS

1. What do you think your role will be when your parent or parents need help?
2. What would you find most difficult in regard to assisting your older parent/grandparent?
3. You are preparing an 81-year-old woman for discharge following a stroke. Her husband will be the caregiver. What teaching might you provide to prepare him for the caregiving role?

NEXT-GENERATION NCLEX® EXAMINATION-STYLE QUESTIONS

Ms. Carlyle, 73 years old, cares for her 105-year-old mother, Mrs. Stanton, who has end-stage Alzheimer's disease (AD). Ms. Carlyle has been her mother's caregiver for the past 15 years. In addition to AD, Mrs. Stanton has hypokalemia and constipation. She makes nonverbal vocalizations but no speech and has few voluntary movements of her extremities, except for banging her right wrist on her upper bedrails. She has been bedridden for the past 2 years and is incontinent of bowel and bladder. A percutaneous endoscopic gastrostomy tube was inserted 2 years ago, when dysphagia led to repeated episodes of pneumonia. She has tube feedings every four hours. Mrs. Stanton is 5'8" tall and weighs 125 pounds (BMI 19 kg/m²). Ms. Carlyle takes meticulous care of her mother and aside from perineal maceration and occasional yeast infections, there have been no pressure injuries.

The nurse conducts a home visit and completes a Modified Caregiver Strain Index. Ms. Carlyle scores 12 on the index, indicating her sleep is disturbed, it is physically stressful for her to provide care for her mother, and it is distressing to her to see her mother in this state. She has also had to make adjustments with family and her personal life in order to care for her mother. The nurse sits with Ms. Carlyle and discusses the situation and provides her with community resources to support her as a caregiver and educate her about self-care.

Which of the following indicate the caregiver has taken steps to reduce their stress? (Select all that apply).
1. "I joined an online Alzheimer's support group."
2. "I go for a short walk each afternoon while my mother sleeps."
3. "I arranged for respite care so that I can plan a weekend getaway."
4. "I spend time weeding my garden each day."
5. "My blood pressure is under control, so I cancelled my last two appointments."
6. "I withdrew money from my life insurance policy to care for Mom."
7. "I stopped going to my book club so that I wouldn't be away from Mom so long."
8. "I don't go to church anymore; it's too hard to go."

REFERENCES

Accius, J. (2017). *Breaking stereotypes: spotlight on male family caregivers.* AARP Public Policy Institute. https://www.aarp.org/ppi/info-2017/breaking-stereotypes-spotlight-on-male-family-caregivers.html.

American Psychological Association (APA): *Elder abuse and neglect: in search of solutions*, 2020. http://www.apa.org/pi/aging/resources/guides/elder-abuse.aspx?item=1.

American Association of Retired Persons and National Alliance for Caregiving (2020). Caregiving in the United States. https://doi.org/10.26419/ppi.00103.001.

Anderson, L. (2019). States with high opioid prescribing rates have higher rates of grandparents responsible for grandchildren. In United States Census Bureau, The Opioid Crisis, Grandparents raising grandchildren.

Archbold, P. G., Stewart, B. J., Greenlick, M. R., & Harvath, T. (1990). Mutuality and preparedness as predictors of caregiver role strain. *Res Nurs Health, 13*, 375–384.

Alzheimer's Reading Room: Quote of the day, 2013. http://www.alzheimersreadingroom.com/2009/11/quote-of-day-caregivers.html.

Baumbusch, J., Mayer, S., Phinney, A., & Baumbusch, S. (2017). Aging together: caring relations in families of adults with intellectual disabilities. *Gerontologist, 57*(2), 341–347.

Bonds, K., & Lyons, K. S. (2018). Formal service use by African American individuals with dementia and their caregivers: an integrative review. *J Gerontol Nurs, 44*(6), 33–39.

Brent, N. (2019). Nurses and mandatory reporting laws. *CPH and Associates*. https://www.cphins.com/nurses-and-mandatory-reporting-laws/.

Chi, N. C., & Demiris, D. (2017). The roles of telehealth tools in supporting family caregivers: current evidence, opportunities, and limitations. *J Gerontol Nurs, 43*(2), 3–4.

Cook, S., & Cohen, S. (2018). Sociodemographic disparities in adult child informal caregiving intensity in the United States. *J Gerontol Nurs, 44*(9), 15–20.

Egan, K. J., Pinto-Bruno, Á. C., Bighelli, I., et al. (2018). Online training and support programs designed to improve mental health and reduce burden among caregivers of people with dementia: a systematic review. *J Am Med Dir Assoc, 19*, 200–206.e1.

Eldercare Workforce Alliance (2018). *Advancing a well-trained workforce to care for us as we age*. http://eldercareworkforce.org/. Accessed February 2021.

Epps, F., Rose, K., & Lopez, R. (2019). Who's your family? African American caregivers of older adults with dementia. *Res Gerontol Nurs, 12*(1), 20–26.

Family Caregiver Alliance, National Center on Caregiving: *LGBT caregiving: frequently asked questions*, 2015. https://www.caregiver.org/print/32.

Family Caregiver Alliance (2019). Caregiver statistics: demographics. https://www.caregiver.org/caregiver-statistics-demographics. Accessed February 2021.

Feinberg, L. F., Levine, C. (2015–2016). Family caregiving: looking to the future. *Generations*, 39(4), 1119.

Gaugler, J., Jutkowitz, E., & Peterson, C. M. (2017). An overview of dementia caregiving in the United States. *Generations Fall* (ACL Suppl), 37–42.

Generations United: *State of grandfamilies: In loving arms: the protective role of grandparents and other relatives in raising children exposed to trauma*, 2020. https://www.gu.org/explore-our-topics/grandfamilies/state-of-grandfamilies-in-america-annual-reports/.

GovTrack. *HR 3759 (115th) RAISE Family Caregivers Act*, 2018. https://www.govtrack.us/congress/bills/115/hr3759.

Kennedy, MS. (2017). Family caregivers need our help–and now it's the law. *Am J Nurs, 117*(12), 7.

LePore, M., & Wiener, J. (2017). Improving services for people with Alzheimer's disease and related dementias and their caregivers. *Generations Fall*, (Suppl), 3–6.

Lund, M. (2005). Caregiver, take care. *Geriatr Nurs, 26*, 152–153.

McLaughlin, B., Ryder, D., & Taylor, M. F. (2017). Effectiveness of interventions for grandparent caregivers: a systematic review. *Marriage Fam Rev, 53*(6), 509–531.

Monin, J. K., Brown, S. L., Poulin, M. J., & Langa, K. M. (2017). Spouses' daily feelings of appreciation and self-reported well-being. *Health Psychol, 36*(12), 1135–1139.

National Center on Elder Abuse. Statistics and Data. https://ncea.acl.gov/What-We-Do/Research/Statistics-and-Data.aspx. Accessed February 2021.

National Council on Aging. Elder Abuse Facts. https://www.ncoa.org/public-policy-action/elder-justice/elder-abuse-facts/#:~:text=Approximately%201%20in%2010%20Americans,abuse%20are%20reported%20to%20authorities. Accessed February 2021.

National Resource Center on LGBT Aging. (2020). *Fact sheet: LGBT caregiving*. https://www.lgbtagingcenter.org/resources/resource.cfm?r=832.

Park, M. (2017). In sickness and in health: spousal caregivers and the correlates of caregiver outcomes. *Am J Geriatr Psychiatry, 25*(10), 1094–1096.

Perkins, M., Howard, V. J., Wadley, V. G., et al. (2013). Caregiving strain and all-cause mortality: evidence from the REGARDS study. *J Gerontol B Psychol Sci Soc Sci, 68*(4), 504–512.

Polenick, CA., & DePasquale, N. (2019). Predictors of secondary role strains among spousal caregivers of older adults with functional disability. *Gerontologist, 59*(3), 486–495.

Pristavec, T. (2018). The burden and benefits of caregiving: a latent class analysis. *Gerontologist*. doi.org/10.1093/geront/gny022.

Reinhard, S. C., Capezuti, E., Bricoli, B., & Choula, R. B. (2017). Feasibility of a family-centered hospital intervention. *J Gerontol Nurs, 43*(6), 9–16.

Roberts, E., & Struckmeyer, K. (2018). The impact of respite programming on caregiver resilience in dementia care: a qualitative examination of family caregiver perspectives. *Inquiry, 55*. doi.org/10.1177/0046958017751507.

Rose, M., Noelker, L., & Kagan, J. (2015). Improving policies for caregiver respite services. *The Gerontologist, 55*(2), 302–308.

Schulz, R., & Beach, S. R. (1999). Caregiving as a risk factor for mortality: the caregiver health effects study. *J Am Med Assoc, 282*(23), 2215–2219.

Tang, S. H., Chio, O., Chang, L. H., et al. (2018). Caregiver active participation in psychoeducational intervention improved caregiving skills and competency. *Geriatr Gerontol Int, 18*(5), 750–757.

Taylor, M. F., Marquis, R., Coall, D. A., Batten, R., & Werner, J. (2017). The physical health dilemmas facing custodial grandparent caregivers: policy considerations. *Cogent Med, 4*(1).

Wardecker, B., & Johnston, T. (2018). Seeing and supporting LGBT older adults' caregivers and families. *J Gerontol Nurs, 44*(11), 2–4.

Wettstein, G., & Zulkarnain, A. (2017). *How much long-term care do adult children provide?* Chestnut Hill, MA: Center for Retirement Research at Boston College.

Williams, C. L. (2015). Maintaining caring relationships in spouses affected by Alzheimer's disease. *Int J Human Caring, 19*(3), 12–18.

World Health Organization (WHO). (2020). *Elder abuse*. http://www.who.int/mediacentre/factsheets/fs357/en/.

Zwicker, D. (2018). Preparedness for caregiving scale. *Try This, 28*. https://consultgeri.org/try-this/general-assessment/issue-28.pdf.

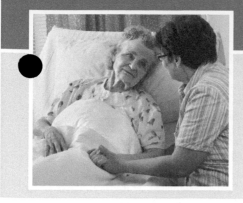

28

Loss, Death, and Palliative Care

Kathleen Jett

http://evolve.elsevier.com/Touhy/gerontological/

LEARNING OBJECTIVES

Upon completion of this chapter, the reader will be able to:
- Differentiate between loss and grief.
- Describe cues that suggest different types of grief.
- Explain the personal characteristics required of a nurse to be able to promote optimal outcomes for those who are grieving.
- Propose nursing actions when comfort is the desired outcome of care.
- Explain the role and responsibility of the nurse in assisting persons with advance care planning.
- Explain the difference between passive and active euthanasia.

THE LIVED EXPERIENCE

When we were in our sixties my friends and I met over cards, went on trips, and experienced all the joys of retirement. We didn't have much time to worry about aches and pains. In our seventies we had less time to play because we were busy visiting one another in the hospital or nursing home. In our eighties we met frequently again, but it was usually at our friends' funerals, leaving little time for cards or travel. Now that I am in my nineties hardly any of my friends are still alive; you know it gets kind of lonely, so you just have to make new younger friends!

Theresa, age 93

Life is like a pinwheel, a thing of beauty and change. Loss, like the wind, sets it in motion, beginning the life-changing process of grieving. Throughout a person's life the winds of loss will gently stir recurrent episodes of grief through sights, sounds, smells, anniversary dates, and other triggers. The arms of the pinwheel suggest movement by the bereaved, reaching out of the experience of grief by surrendering through resting or lowering a person's defenses toward life and reaching out to others and rejoining life through change. Each gust of wind may generate a resurgence of grief, but the pinwheel will never lose its beauty.

Loss, dying, and death are universal, incontestable events of the human experience. Some loss is associated with the normal changes with aging, such as the loss of flexibility in the joints (see Chapters 4 and 21). Some loss is related to the normal changes in everyday life and life transitions, such as moving and retirement. Other losses are those of loved ones through death. Some deaths are considered normative and expected, such as older parents and friends. Other deaths are considered non-normative and unexpected, such as the death of adult children or grandchildren.

Regardless of the type of loss, each one has the potential to trigger grief and a process we call bereavement or mourning. Grieving and mourning are usually used synonymously. However, grieving is an individual's emotional response to a loss and mourning is an active and evolving process that includes those behaviors used to incorporate the experience into a person's life after the loss. Mourning behaviors are strongly influenced by social and cultural norms that prescribe the appropriate ways of both reacting to the loss and coping with it (Gerdner et al., 2007). For example, in much of the world, widows are expected to wear black after the death of their husbands; but in India the traditional dress of a Hindu widow is a white saree. There is no single way to grieve or respond to loss; each person grieves in his or her own way.

Although there are also cultural expectations related to grief following death, there are no guidelines for behavior other types of loss actually. For example, an individual who moves to a nursing home (loses one's home) or who retires (loss of profession) may be very sad, irritable, and forgetful. The cues may lead to a hypothesis of dementia when the person is actually grieving. When the losses accumulate in quick succession, a state of bereavement overload may result. The griever may become temporarily incapacitated and require careful and skilled support and guidance from the nurse.

Gerontological nurses need to have basic knowledge of the morning rituals of those who receive their care and how to comfort and care for grievers, including one another. Additional knowledge and nursing actions are related to the care of a dying person and their survivors. Finally, nurses caring for the dying must be comfortable with their own mortality. In this chapter we hope to provide the basic information necessary to promote the outcomes of effective grieving, peaceful dying, and good and appropriate deaths.

GRIEF WORK

Researchers have tried for years to understand the grieving process (grief work), resulting in a number of models and theories to explain and predict the human response. Pioneer thanatologist (a person who studies the dying process) Elisabeth Kübler-Ross is best known for describing what became known as the stages of dying (1969). Other early theorists included Rando (1995), Corr and colleagues (2000), and Doka (2002). Each of these scholars described successful grieving as movement through predictable stages, phases, or tasks until one eventually was able to "let go" of that which was lost (Hall, 2011). The models have strongly influenced what caregivers and society in general have been taught about the grieving process.

Newer approaches have described grief work as more of a circular process in which a continued attachment to that which has been lost, at some level, is "normal" (Hall, 2011). Although the theories are intended to describe physical death and related grief, we propose that these same models can serve as a framework for understanding other types of meaningful losses in the lives of older adults.

A Loss Response Model

Jett's Loss Response Model (LRM) is influenced by the systems' work of nurse theorist Dr. Betty Newman (Alward, 2010) and the writings of nurse Barbara Giacquinta (1977), psychiatrist Avery Weisman (1979), and thanatological scholars Doka (2002) and Neimeyer and Sands (2011). It can be used to improve the understanding of grieving and to help nurses develop actions in the care and comfort of those who have experienced, or are experiencing, a loss of any kind.

According to the LRM, grievers are part of a greater system that is striving to achieve or maintain *equilibrium* (Fig. 28.1). However, the impact of the loss (or the anticipation of it) results in *disequilibrium* or instability within the system. The loss seems unreal and the system is in chaos; the grievers are emotionally and *functionally disrupted.* Many people will say, "I don't even know what I am feeling!" Common, simple activities, such as dressing, that normally take a few minutes may take much longer. Deciding which clothing to wear may seem too complex a task. Even as the tasks are accomplished, the person may complain of feeling distracted, restless, "at a loose end," and numb. Men who complained of numbness have been found to have higher cortisol levels (i.e., indicators of physiological stress) than women (Richardson et al., 2013).

As the system attempts to stabilize the grievers begin to make sense of the chaos and integrate the loss into their lives, they *search for meaning*, asking such questions of themselves and others: What did I do to have to leave my home? Could I have done more? Why did this happen to us (me)? How will we survive the loss? In reacting to the loss of a child or a grandchild, thoughts of "why wasn't it me?" are common. Searching for meaning is difficult and as it is done, *others are informed* of the loss.

Each time the story is repeated, *emotions are engaged* in ways that are consistent with the griever's culture and personality. The expression of emotions can be quite powerful: anger, frustration, or even relief. Nurses can and do listen to the stories about the loss over and over again. Each time the story is slightly different as the meaning is incorporated into the person's life. These discussions can be a dress rehearsal of sorts as the person prepares to tell outsiders of the loss (e.g., "I can't drive

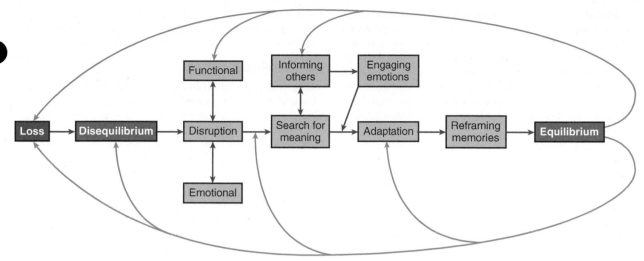

FIG. 28.1 The Loss Response Model and cyclical loss.

anymore"). Although acute grief may be **triggered** at each telling, the intensity lessens and the duration of the pain shortens.

As roles and circumstances in which persons find themselves change, adaptation is necessary. *Adaptation* is a process in which the system changes in order to survive. For example, when a person is no longer able to do a task because of loss of ability, someone else must step in to perform it; when the elder patriarch dies, it may be a cultural expectation that the eldest son assumes his father's roles and responsibilities.

Finally, if the system is to survive, it must redefine itself. This is accomplished not by forgetting or ignoring the loss but by *reframing memories*. In the case of a death, family portraits and reunions will still be possible, just different from before and new memories can and will be made. If celebrations had always been held at the home of the oldest parent (eliciting the sights, smells, and memories of childhood), a move to a nursing home will prevent this custom. New memories, rituals, and *adaptation* occurs when the celebrations are held at the home of another, such as that of a child. The system can return to a new but different steady state. The nurse serves as a role model who displays the behavioral qualities of responsiveness, authenticity, commitment, and competence—that is, caring.

The Loss Response Model is cyclical and especially applicable to those with multiple underlying chronic conditions and multiple losses as are common in later life. At any point in the movement toward stabilization new disturbances may lead to renewed instability. The grievers are finding ways to adapt to the functional disruption related to one loss when another occurs. A

home has been rearranged to make it safe for the person who has suffered a stroke (a loss in itself) when she falls and breaks her hip (loss of health), necessitating a nursing home stay (loss of home, independence, usual food, etc.), either short-term or permanent, because of the combined losses resulting in new losses as the cyclic continues.

Types of Grief

Grieving takes enormous amounts of physical and emotional energy. It is the hardest thing anyone can do and may be especially hard for older adults who must simultaneously face other challenges and losses discussed throughout this text. Emotions can be intense and this intensity may manifest as confusion, depression, or preoccupation with thoughts of the deceased or the loss. This reaction may be mistaken for other conditions, such as dementia, when it probably is a type of delirium, a temporary change in mental status due to psychological stress and requires that the nurse pay careful attention to cues and the need to develop caring nursing actions. The gerontological nurse is most likely to work with those who are experiencing anticipatory grief, acute grief, or chronic grief. A fourth type, disenfranchised grief, may be hidden, but when it occurs, it is nonetheless significant.

Anticipatory Grief

Anticipatory grief is the emotional response to a loss before it occurs, a dress rehearsal, so to speak. The nurse recognizes this grief as preparation for potential loss, such as losing belongings (e.g., selling of a home), moving (e.g., into a nursing home), or knowing that a body part or function is going to change (e.g., a mastectomy), or in anticipation of the loss of a spouse or oneself either through dementia or death. Behavioral cues that may signal anticipatory grief include preoccupation with the loss, unusually detailed planning, or a sudden change in attitude toward the thing or person to be lost (Coelho & Barbosa, 2017). High levels of preparation have been found to be associated with improved bereavement-related outcomes.

If the loss is certain but no one can say when it will occur or if it does not occur when or as expected, those awaiting the actual loss or death may become irritable, hostile, or impatient, not because they want the loss to occur, but in response to the emotional ups and downs of the waiting. Researchers Glaser and Strauss (1968) described this as an "interruption in the sentimental order" on nursing units. When this occurs, no one, including care staff, quite knows how to behave. It may be easier to cope with anticipated losses when they occur at an expected time or in an expected manner.

Anticipatory grief can result in the phenomenon of premature detachment from an individual who is dying or detachment of the dying person from the environment. Pattison (1977) called the premature withdrawal of others sociological death, and the premature withdrawal of the person, psychological death. In either case, the person who is dying is no longer involved in day-to-day activities of living and essentially suffers a premature death.

Acute Grief

Acute grief is a crisis. It has a definitive syndrome of somatic, psychological, and spiritual cues indicating distress that occur in waves lasting varying periods of time. It is always shaped by cultural heritage. Different cues may occur every time the loss is acknowledged, when others are informed, or even when condolences are offered. A preoccupation with the loss similar to daydreaming may occur, accompanied by a sense of unreality. Depending on the situation, feelings of relief, self-blame, or guilt may also be acute and manifest themselves as hostility or anger toward friends, depression, or withdrawal. The intense stress of acute grief may lead to significant declines in physical health and the cues suggestive of depression (Nakajima, 2018). A formerly conflicted relationship may be idealized and confusing to others.

During periods of acute grief, *functional disruption* is at its peak. Fortunately, it does not last forever. The system must find a way to adapt if it is to survive. Acute grief is most intense in the months immediately following the loss with the intensity of feelings lessening over time. A griever may cry in the first months any time the

loss is mentioned. Later, the person will still be grieving, but the tears are replaced by a surging sense of loss and sadness and still later by more fleeting reactions.

Shadow Grief

Grieving takes time, but over the months, the intense pain of the acute period of impact lessens as memories are reframed. But the old memories never go away completely. There are often moments of intermittent sadness referred to as shadow grief (Horacek, 1991). A cue is temporarily inhibited function but is considered a normal response. Although most often discussed in the context of perinatal death, a type of shadow grief can occur at any age and with any loss. It may be triggered by anniversary dates (birthdays, holidays, anniversaries) or by sensory stimuli, such as the smell of perfume, a color, or a sound (Carr et al., 2014) (Box 28.1).

Complicated Grief

Shadow grief is a type of chronic grief that is considered normal and restorative. Yet for others, such as survivors of major tragedies, war, rape, abuse, and other horrific events, the "shadows" may be debilitating and are now recognized as posttraumatic stress. This is a form of complicated grief regardless of the age of the person.

Complicated grief also comes in the form of acute grief that does not significantly lessen over the months and even years after the loss. Obstacles of one form or another interfere with the evolution toward the reestablishment of equilibrium of the system; stability is elusive. The memories resist being reframed. Issues of guilt, anger, and ambivalence toward the person who has died or the thing that has been lost will impede the grieving process until these issues are resolved. Reactions are exaggerated and memories are experienced as if they are fresh, over and over again.

Cues indicating possible complicated grief include excessive and irrational anger, outbursts in social settings, and insomnia that lingers for an extended time or surfaces months or years after the loss. Complicated grief may trigger a major depressive episode, exacerbations of chronic health problems, or even suicide

BOX 28.1   The Carved Birds

One day as I was browsing at an art show, I came across a booth of carved birds, a favorite design of my beloved mother. I turned to remark to her. Except she was not there: she had died 15 years earlier in my home. Sadness passed over me like a cloud and I wished she were there—I would buy her one as a special gift. Instead, I turned to my husband and shared reminiscences as I had done before. As the wind blows, so do the clouds pass.

(Nakajima, 2018). Families who have a loved one who has committed suicide have been found to be among those who have the greatest risk of complicated and chronic grief (Sveen & Walby, 2008). This type of grief necessitates the professional intervention of a grief counselor, a psychiatric nurse practitioner, or a psychologist who has skills at helping grieving elders and their loved ones.

Disenfranchised Grief

Disenfranchised grief is experienced by persons whose loss cannot be openly acknowledged or publicly mourned. The grief is socially disallowed or unsupported (Burns et al., 2018; Doka, 2002; Lathrop, 2017). The person does not have a socially recognized right to mourn and grieve. In other words, the relationship is not recognized; the loss is not sanctioned or the griever is not recognized and the grief cannot be made public. Disenfranchised grief has frequently been associated with domestic partnerships in which the family of the deceased does not acknowledge the partner or in secret relationships in which the involved party cannot tell others of the meaning or depth of the attachment. Disenfranchised grief can also occur in situations of family discord in which a member of the family is considered the "black sheep." Older adults can experience disenfranchised grief when persons close to them do not understand the full meaning of a loss, such as when others perceive the death of a loved one from Alzheimer's disease as a blessing and fail to support the griever or caregiver who has struggled for years with anticipatory grief and now must cope with the acute grief of the actual death (Paun & Farran, 2011).

Factors Affecting Coping With Loss

To cope effectively with loss is to have the ability to move from a state of chaos to one of stability; from disequilibrium to renewed equilibrium, if only for a moment. It is to find meaning in the loss and be able to find a way to reframe memories. Many factors affect the ability to cope with loss and grief (Box 28.2).

Psychiatrist Avery Weisman described those who are more likely to deal effectively with loss as "good copers"; that is, individuals or families who have successfully navigated through crises in the past (1979, pp. 42–43). They can acknowledge the loss and try to make sense of it. They can maintain composure when necessary, can generally use good judgment, and can remain optimistic and appropriately hopeful without denying the loss. Good copers seek guidance when it is needed.

On the contrary, those who cope less effectively have few, if any, of these abilities. They tend to be more rigid, pessimistic, and demanding. They are more likely to

---

> **BOX 28.2 Factors Influencing Grieving**
>
> **Physical**
> Number of concurrent medical conditions
> Use of sedatives (delays, but does not lessen grief)
> Nutritional state
> Exercise
> Mental health
>
> **Emotional**
> Unique nature and meaning of loss
> Coping strategies, personality, and maturity
> Previous experience with loss or death
> Sex-role conditioning
> Immediate circumstances surrounding loss
> Timeliness of the loss
> Perception of preventability (sudden versus expected)
> Number, type, and quality of secondary losses
>
> **Social**
> Individual support systems
> Sociocultural, ethnic, religious expectations, and rituals

Modified from Beare, P. G., & Myers, J. L. (1998). *Adult health nursing,* (3rd ed.). St Louis, MO: Mosby.

---

be dogmatic and expect perfection in themselves and others. Ineffective copers are more likely to live alone, socialize little, and have few close friends or have an ineffective support network. They may have a history of mental illness, or have guilt, anger, or ambivalence toward the person who has died or that which has been lost. The person is more likely to have unresolved past conflicts or be facing the loss at the same time as secondary life stressors. In some cases, the person will have fewer opportunities as a result of the loss. Those at special risk of significantly adverse effects of grief are older spouses and life partners of any kind. Intense grief may cause a temporary decrease in cognitive function that can be misinterpreted as dementia, isolating the griever. They are the persons most in need of the expert interventions of grief counselors and skilled, sensitive gerontological nurses.

❖ USING CLINICAL JUDGMENT TO PROMOTE HEALTHY AGING

Like good copers, good gerontological nurses must be flexible, practical, resourceful, and abundantly optimistic. The nurse fosters the griever's movement from disequilibrium to a new, albeit modified, steady state and positive outcome (Box 28.3).

BOX 28.3   Tips for Best Practice

Helping Grievers Move Through the Impact of Loss to the Reestablishment of Equilibrium

Functional Disruption
- Provide functional assistance

Searching for Meaning
- Provide reliable sources of information (e.g., websites).
- Inform appropriate providers of the person's need for information and make sure the person receives it.
- Engage in active listening.

Engaging Emotions
- "Give permission" to express emotions.
- Offer physical presence.
- Offer to locate usual sources of support during times of crisis (e.g., minister, tribal elder).
- Engage in active listening.

Informing Others
- Offer physical presence.
- Engage in active listening.

Adaptation
- Identify meaningful events influenced by the loss.
- Help find new ways of replacing that which has been lost.
- Offer discussions of how the loss has affected life.
- Engage in active listening.

Reframing Memories
- Offer to discuss mechanisms to develop new memories without denying connection with that or with whom has been lost.
- Encourage reminiscence.
- Facilitate opportunities for culturally based and desired bereavement rituals.
- Assure grievers that stability will return.
- Engage in active listening.

The actions of a nurse are not to prevent grief but to support those who are grieving. Although that which has been lost can never be replaced, the potential long-term detrimental outcomes can be lessened. Working with those who are grieving is part of the normal workday of gerontological nurses, who are professional grievers in their own way. It is one of the few areas in nursing where small actions can make a large difference in the quality of life for the person to whom we provide care.

◆ Recognizing and Analyzing Cues

The goal of grief assessment is to differentiate between those who are likely to cope effectively and those who are at risk of ineffective coping so that appropriate nursing

actions can be planned. The analysis of grief-related cues is based on knowledge of the unique mourning process and the subsequent grieving of the individual. Cues are obtained through observation of behavior of the individual and are analyzed within the context of the person's culture (Gire, 2014).

A thorough search for cues includes asking questions about recent significant life events, life or spiritual values, and relationship to that which has been lost. How many other stressful or demanding events or circumstances are occurring in the griever's life? Actions include getting to know the person and their family/significant others to understand their wishes and expectations. This information will help determine who is most at risk of complicated grieving. The more concurrent stressors in a person's life, the more they will need grief specialists. The nurse determines which stress management techniques have been used in the past and whether they were helpful (e.g., meditation) or potentially harmful (e.g., substance use or abuse). Was the griever's identity closely tied to that which is lost, such as a lifelong athlete who is faced with never walking again? If the loss is of a partner, how was the relationship? The loss of an abusive or controlling partner may liberate the survivor, who may feel guilty for not feeling the grief that is expected. For many older women who have been dependent financially on their spouses, death may leave them impoverished, significantly complicating their grief. Knowing more about the loss and the effect of the loss on the older adult's life will enable the nurse to construct and implement appropriate and caring responses.

◆ Nursing Actions

The first time a new nurse is confronted with cues indicating that a person is grieving may result in discomfort, fear, anxiety, and insecurity. The tendency is to be sympathetic rather than empathetic. Questions arise: What do I say? Should I be cheerful or serious? Should I talk about or even mention the dead person's name or the loss?

Nursing actions especially when older adults and their families are in crisis, include introducing themselves and explaining the nature of their roles (e.g., charge nurse, staff nurse, medication nurse) and the time they have available. Nurses gently establish rapport and learn the cultural, religious, and personal meaning of the loss or pending loss. If it is the time of impact (e.g., just after a new serious diagnosis, at the death of a family member, or upon becoming a new resident of a long-term care facility), the most that nursing actions may accomplish is to provide support and a safe environment and ensure that basic needs, such as meals, are met. A nurse can soften the despair by fostering *reasonable* hope, such as, "You will make it through this time, one moment at a time, and I will be here to help." Those with this nursing support are more likely to have good outcomes related to the loss (Clark, 2019).

Nurses make a significant contribution to the family in fostering even momentary stability by knowing which questions to ask at the time of death, such as the following: Which cultural or familial rituals are important right now? Is there anyone who should be called at this time (see informing others below)? Would a spiritual advisor be a support for you right now? Have prior funeral arrangements already been made; if not, who can help you with this? Had they made their wishes known for this time?

Nurses recognize *functional disruption* and offer support and direction. They may have to help the family decide what needs to be done immediately and find ways to do it—either the nurse offers to complete the task or the nurse finds a friend or family member who can step in so that the disruption does not have any deleterious effects (Box 28.4).

As grievers *search for meaning*, they may need help finding what they are looking for if this is possible. Sometimes it is information about a disease, a situation, or a person. Sometimes it is a spiritual search and help in finding a source of comfort such as a priest, rabbi, or medicine woman or a place of peace, such as the chapel or mosque. Often what is needed most is someone to listen to the "whys" and "hows"—questions that cannot be answered. Gerontological nursing actions include the provision of education about the consequences of both the loss and the death and dying process, preferably before the physical and psychological changes have begun.

Sometimes nurses offer to contact others for those who are grieving, thinking that this is something that will help. However, it is far more therapeutic for grievers to be the ones who inform others because it helps the

loss become part of their new reality. The nurse can offer to find a phone number or hold the griever's hand during the conversation or just "be there" when the news is being shared. In this way the nursing actions are supportive when the griever's emotions engage and move toward wellness and equilibrium.

As an older adult moves forward in adapting to the loss, such as a move from home to a nursing home, the nurse can talk with the person about what was most valued about living at home and what habits were comforting, and find ways to incorporate these in a new way into the new environment. If an older adult does not have access to a kitchen and always had a cup of tea before bed, this can become part of the nursing actions specific to the individual.

Memories are reframed so that they can accommodate for the loss without diminishing the value of that which has been lost, thus minimizing the risk of complicated grief (Maccallum & Bryant, 2011). Nurses can help memories to be reframes and help persons/systems move toward equilibrium through seemingly simple actions that can make a very big difference. The grandmother who had always hosted her eldest daughter's birthday party can still do that even as a resident in a long-term care facility. When a nurse has the information about this important ritual, they can act to help the person reserve a private space, send out invitations, and have the birthday party as always, just reframed in that it is catered by the facility in the new "home."

The nurse knows that at any point in the movement toward equilibrium a new loss can occur and the cycle begins again or moves back to an earlier point and movement forward starts afresh (Fig. 28.1).

Countercoping

Avery Weisman (1979) described the actions of health care professionals related to fostering positive outcomes to grieving as "countercoping." Although he was speaking of working with people with cancer, it is equally applicable to working with people who are grieving for loss of any kind and for families coping with pending or past loss. "Countercoping is like counterpoint in music, which blends melodies together into a basic harmony. The patient copes; the therapist [nurse] countercopes; together they work out a better fit" as the memories are reframed (Weisman, 1979, p. 109). Weisman suggests four very specific types of nursing actions or countercoping strategies: (1) clarification and control, (2) collaboration, (3) directed relief, and (4) cooling off.

Clarification and control. Nursing actions that help griever(s) cope with loss may be getting or receiving information, considering alternatives, and finding a way to make the grief manageable. A nurse helps persons

---

BOX 28.4 Functional Disruption: The Dirty Dishes

During a visit to the home of a woman who was in the last months of her life and getting progressively weaker so she could hardly stand, I noticed that there was a stack of dirty dishes in the sink. Her husband sat watching TV. Using the best therapeutic conversation I learned in nursing school I asked about the dishes. They both started crying. He said he did not know how to load the dishwasher—she had always done it and she did not know how to tell him that she could not do them. My "nursing intervention" that day was a lesson on using a dishwasher.

resume control by encouraging them to avoid acting on impulse. It may be necessary to say, "This is probably not a good time to make any major decisions."

Collaboration. A nurse collaborates by encouraging grievers to share stories as they inform others and repeat the stories as often as is necessary as they "talk it out." Acting as a collaborator is more directive than usual nursing activities; it may be acceptable to say, "Yes, this is a good time to talk."

Directed relief. Some temporary directed relief may be necessary, especially during the period of acute grief. Nursing actions to promote catharsis may be helpful. In many instances the nurse encourages the griever to cry or otherwise express feelings such as hurt or anger, if this is culturally acceptable to the griever. The nurse may have to say something like, "Expressing your feelings might help." Activity may also be recommended as a natural extension of feelings. For example, intense physical activity may give one person emotional relief and creative arts may help another. In some cultures, people may tear their clothes or cut their hair.

Cooling off. From time to time, grievers might need to be encouraged to avoid active grieving temporarily when things must be done or decisions must be made. Nurses ask about diversions that worked in the past during times of stress and encourage their use as needed. The nurse may need to suggest new tactics that may prove helpful. Although there is considerable cultural variation, cooling off also means encouraging the person to modulate emotional extremes at times and to think about ways to make sense of the loss, to build a new sense of self-esteem after the loss, and to help reestablish life patterns.

All nurses who participate in actions with grievers must have skills in therapeutic communication. Active listening is greatly preferable to giving advice. When listening, a nurse soon discovers that it is often not the actual loss that is of utmost concern, but rather the fear associated with the loss. If a nurse listens carefully to both the stated and the implied, what will be heard may be expressions such as the following: "How will I go on?" "What will I do now?" "What will become of me?" "What will happen to my loved ones, pets, etc.?" "I don't know what to do." "How could they do this to me?" "Will I be forgotten?" Because the nurse knows adaptation of some kind will ultimately occur, such comments may seem exaggerated or melodramatic, but to the person who is acutely grieving there seems to be no end to the pain be it physical or emotional. The person cannot yet look ahead and know that the despair will ever lessen. Like good copers, good gerontological nurses must be flexible, practical, resourceful, and abundantly optimistic.

DYING, DEATH, AND PALLIATIVE CARE

Many people have said that death is not the problem; it is the dying that takes the work. This is true for all involved: the person who is dying, the loved ones, and the professional caregivers, including nurses. Dying is both a challenging life experience and a private one. A major question arises when considering dying and death in late life today: When is a person with multiple chronic or repeated acute or progressive health problems considered to be "dying"? Both treatable chronic conditions and those associated with an irreversible terminal condition often occur at the same time, more so as we age. When these are combined with fatigue and frailty, care becomes even more complex (Capel, 2017).

How people deal with their own dying is often a reflection of the way they responded to earlier losses and stressors. Most people probably die as they have lived; that is, the way one faces dying is an expression of personality, circumstances, illness, and culture (National Cancer Institute [NCI], 2020). Although not all older adults have had fulfilling lives or have a sense of completion, transcendence, or self-actualization (see Chapter 26), they often consider their own deaths around the age of their parents as "normal." If dying occurs after a particularly prolonged or painful illness, it is sometimes rationalized as a relief, at least in part. At the same time, the deaths of persons subjected to catastrophic events, such as murder or as the result of terrorist acts are neither reliefs nor socially acceptable.

Although the cues attributed to terminal conditions may appear obvious, they can easily be confused with frailty and exacerbations of chronic diseases in later life. Anxiety, depression, restlessness, agitation, or withdrawal are behaviors that are frequently categorized as manifestations of worsened confusion or dementia but may also be the only way someone can express their feelings that death is near. Ensuring that the person remains comfortable, whether the condition is acute, near the end of life, or anywhere in between, are expected actions of the nurse and other members of the caring team.

The Family

Today's older adults are usually members of multigenerational and complex networks. Those considered "family" increasingly include friends, ex-spouses and partners, step-grandchildren, and fictive kin (those considered family as a result of affective bonds). Although children may be geographically distant filial ties continue to exist (see Chapter 26). When a family elder becomes seriously or terminally ill and cannot uphold their role or obligation, the family balance or dynamics are significantly altered (*functional disruption*). For example, new arrangements are needed when an older family member who has been providing childcare or meal preparation is no longer able to do so. This change may cause considerable familial and often financial distress, as will the need for elder-care when day-to-day help seems impossible because of the work demands and schedules of adult children. Part of the distress comes from the changing roles of the children. Although changes may not occur at the time of diagnosis, they will as frailty advances (see Chapter 27). Adult children begin to see their own mortality through the death of their parents as a new "family" is established.

The idea that family members can remain involved with the dying person may be a source of constant conflict as they anticipate and plan for life without the dying family member and as they provide or try to provide the high level of care that may be needed. This change requires enormous energy by family members who are already burdened with their own anticipatory grief, daily living, and, in many cases, raising their own children and possibly grandchildren. The physical, psychological, spiritual, and economic burden of parent care has the potential to spiral down to neglect, abuse, and worsening health (Capel, 2017).

Family members learn, sometimes early on, that reframing memories will be necessary to separate their own identities from that of the patient and learn to tolerate the reality that another family member will die while they live. The ability of the family to support, love, and provide intimacy may lead to exhaustion, impatience, anger, and a sense of futility if the dying is prolonged. Family members may be grieving differently from each other, hindering communication when it is needed the most. As the illness worsens, physical disability increases, and the patient's needs intensify, so may the family members' feelings of helplessness and frustration.

The family may feel extremely pressured to provide very personal care during the final days of a relative's life. They may feel caught between experiencing the present and remembering the person as they were, between pushing for more interventions with the potential to extend the dying and allowing a natural death to occur. Nurses often hear families lament that they "can't give up on them" at the same time they say, "I don't know how much longer I can do this."

Despite the family's grief and pain, they must give the person permission to die; let the loved one know that it is all right to let go and leave them and that while the person will be missed, the family will somehow eventually manage. This gesture is the last act of love and dignity that the family can offer. Occasionally, no family is available to say, "It's okay to let go." The task then falls to the nurse who has developed a meaningful relationship with the person through caring.

❖ USING CLINICAL JUDGMENT TO PROMOTE HEALTHY AGING WHILE DYING

The needs of the dying are like threads in a piece of cloth. Each thread is individual but necessary to the integrity and completeness of the fabric. If one thread is pulled, it affects the other threads, and the material's appearance, the thread placement, and the stability of the cloth. When one need is unmet, it will affect all others because they are interdependent and interwoven.

A good and appropriate death is one that a person would choose if choosing were possible. It is one in which a person's needs are met to the extent possible. The responsibility of the nurse is to provide safe conduct as the dying and their families navigate through unknown waters to a good and appropriate death (Boxes 28.5 and 28.6). There are several ways a nurse can intervene to promote healthy aging even while a person is dying; one of these is to apply Weisman's six Cs approach (1984).

BOX 28.5 Safe Conduct

The responsibility of a nurse is to provide what is referred to as "safe conduct," helping the dying and their families navigate through unknown waters to a good and appropriate death—that is, a death that the person would choose if choosing were possible. A good and appropriate death is one in which the person's needs are met for as long as possible and life is never without meaning.

BOX 28.6 A Good and Appropriate Death

- Care needed is received and it is timely and expert.
- One is able to control one's life and environment to the extent that is desired and possible and in a way that is culturally consistent with one's life.
- One is able to maintain composure when necessary and to the extent desired.
- One is able to initiate and maintain communication with significant others for as long as possible.
- Life continues as normal as possible while dying with the added tasks that may be needed to deal with and adjust to the inevitable death.
- One can maintain desirable hope at all times.
- One is able to reach a sense of closure in a way that is culturally consistent with one's practices and life patterns.

Recognizing Cues and Nursing Actions
The Six Cs Approach
Weisman (1984) identified six needs of many persons who are dying: care, control, composure, communication, continuity, and closure. Although some of these

needs are most applicable to those of northern European descent, they can provide a place to begin to think about caring for persons from all cultures.

Care. As an advocate, the gerontological nurse's actions assures that the best care is received; this includes expert management of the common problems of pain (see Chapter 18), nausea and vomiting, constipation (Chapter 12), bowel obstruction, diarrhea, fatigue, other symptoms, and the provision of support at all times (Capel, 2017). Nursing actions go beyond the physical to address psychological pain induced by depression, anxiety, fear, and unresolved emotional conflicts. When these needs are not met, the total pain experience is intensified and should be addressed in a manner that is acceptable to the person.

Dying calls for great amounts of energy for persons to cope with the emotional and physical assault of illness on the body. Two almost universal problems are a sense of breathlessness and fatigue. Caring means developing nursing actions that help the person conserve energy. Cues that will help formulate hypotheses include: How much can the individual do without becoming physically and emotionally taxed? Is there something in particular that causes more or less shortness of breath? Would having oxygen available provide comfort? Which everyday activities are most important for the person to do independently? How much energy is needed for the patient to be able to talk with visitors or staff without becoming exhausted? The nurse not only asks these questions of the person but also recognizes and analyses cues in persons who cannot make their needs known. Only when such issues are addressed can the person strive toward the outcomes of control and composure when needed.

Control. As people move toward physiological death and, in the case of dementia, loss of cognition, they are in the process of losing everything they have ever known or will ever know. The potential loss of identity, independence, and control over bodily functions can also lead to lost self-esteem. The person may begin to feel ashamed, humiliated, and a "burden." The nurse may recognize cues of distress related to loss of control, that is, the need to remain in a collaborative role relating to one's own living and dying and as an active participant in one's care to the extent desired and possible. Once nurses know the person's preferences and priorities, including cultural expectations, they can address these needs by taking every opportunity to design person-centered actions and in doing so bolster the person's self-esteem. Whenever possible, nursing actions, such as those related to grooming, eating, awakening, sleeping, visiting, and so forth can be done on the person's requested schedule rather than that of the nurse's or facility's. A nurse never

has the right to determine the activities of the individual, especially in relation to visitors and how time is spent.

Composure. Composure is the modulation of emotional extremes. Although Weisman describes this as a need for those who are dying, it is highly variable by culture: in some (e.g., Italian) it might be a time of great emotional expression; in others (e.g., German) it might be a time of stoicism. If the goal is one of composure, it is not to avoid the sadness but to have moments of relief.

Communication. When caring for those who are dying and their families there is a need for a great deal of different types of communication. A person may express a need for information as they *search for meaning*, make decisions, and *inform others* of the actual or pending loss. The style of communication that is acceptable varies by cultural expectations, personalities, and relationships (Chapter 3), the nurse has a responsibility to make sure that the person who is dying has an opportunity to communicate how, what, and to whom they choose. Expert communication between members of the care team (including families and patients) always leads to improved outcomes (Clark, 2019). The earlier the communication begins, the better a nurse can facilitate quality of life and healthy living while dying (Foley, 2019). Good communication means that the person and family feel that they have been heard.

In a classic study of terminal illness among the patient, family, and hospital staff, Glaser and Strauss (1963) identified four types of communication: *closed awareness, suspected awareness, mutual pretense,* and *open awareness.* Each of these influence the work on the nursing home or hospital unit and the care of the patient.

- *Closed awareness* is described as "keeping the secret." Hospital staff and the family and friends know that the patient is dying, but the patient does not know it or knows and keeps the secret. Generally, caregivers invent a fictitious future for the patient, in hopes that it will boost the patient's morale. Although this happens less today because of legislation related to patients' rights, it still occurs. In some cultures, such as in many Latino families, it may be expected.
- In *suspected awareness,* the person suspects they are dying, but because it is not discussed, it cannot be confirmed. Inquiries on the part of the person are indirect or avoided by others. Hints are bandied back and forth, and a contest ensues for control of the information.
- *Mutual pretense* is a situation of "let's pretend." Everyone knows the patient has a terminal illness, but no one talks about it—real feelings are kept hidden.
- *Open awareness* occurs when the patient, family, friends, nurses, and physicians openly acknowledge

the eventual death of the patient. The patient may ask, "Will I die?" and "How and when will I die?" The family grieves with the patient rather than for the patient. The nurse can encourage open awareness whenever possible while at the same time respecting the patient's wishes (Gire, 2014). In some cultures, talking about an anticipated death is deemed helpful. In others, one can be aware of the dying but talking about it openly may be taboo, such as in the traditional Haitian culture.

Depending on where the death occurs and the role of the nurse at the time, actions will differ. Nurses sometimes notify family members, a funeral home, or other care team members. Nurses always assure that cultural and religious expectations at the time of and following death are met. The nurse may be the one to prepare the body for the family's viewing prior to transport to the funeral home. Nurses always allow time for the family to ask questions, even if the same questions are asked over and over again.

Continuity. The need for continuity is a desire to preserve as normal a life as possible, for as long as possible; to maintain at least some level of equilibrium while dying. Too often a dying person can feel shut off from the rest of the world at a time when they are still capable of being involved and active in some way. Loneliness is the result of a loss of continuity with one's life. The nursing strategies to address this include asking about the person's life and those things most valued and working with the family and the patient or resident on a plan to remain engaged in as many of the activities and past roles as possible. A father who watches a certain ballgame with his son every Sunday can continue to do this regardless of the need to be in a hospital, in a nursing home, or an inpatient hospice unit. If the person is at home and is bedridden, it may make more sense to have the bed in a central area rather than in a distant room. Treating the person who is dying as an intelligent and competent adult at all times is a powerful expression of caring.

One approach people have taken to obtain continuity of their lives after death is in the establishment of legacies. Legacies can take many different forms and may range from memories that will live on in the minds of others to bequeathed fortunes. A grandmother who is likely to die before a favorite grandchild's wedding can create a legacy when she participates with planning, regardless of the age of the grandchild if this is important to them, thereby leaving an enduring and special legacy.

Closure. Finding closure is an opportunity for reconciliation and transcendence. Reminiscence is one way of putting one's life in order, in other words, to evaluate the pluses and minuses of one's life and find that it

had some value (Box 28.7). It is a means of resolving conflicts, giving up possessions, and making final good-byes. Learning to say "good-bye" today leaves open the possibility of many more "hellos." Pain and other symptoms that are not well controlled may interfere with this reconciliation, making appropriate nursing actions especially important.

If a person feels that physiological death is approaching, the nurse can look for cues when the person begins using "coded communication," such as saying goodbye instead of the usual goodnight, giving away cherished possessions as gifts, urgently contacting friends and relatives with whom the person has not communicated with for a long time, and having direct or symbolic premonitions that death is near.

For some, closure means coming to terms with their spiritual selves, with Jesus, God, Allah, or Buddha, for example. Pastoral support may be offered but should never be facilitated without the person's express permission. The nurse can foster transcendence by providing patients with the time and privacy for self-reflection as well as an opportunity to talk about whatever they need to talk about, especially about the meanings of their lives and the meanings of their deaths.

Care, control, composure, communication, continuity, and closure create the borders necessary to complete the fabric of needs of the dying. Their influence is omnipresent in the other needs. Without them, the cloth can fray and attempts to meet the needs will be limited.

DYING AND THE NURSE

Nurses are professional grievers experiencing the death of their patients and residents over and over again. Nursing assistants are often "invisible grievers" as they watch the slow death or decline of someone they have intimately cared for over the years (Mohlman et al., 2018). Some consider the death of a patient as a failure and that they have "lost" the person they cared for; yet, when it is a good death, it can be viewed as a professional success each time we share the special and very personal experience of providing safe conduct for those who are dying and gentle caring for their survivors. Nurses are instrumental in providing skillful care that is congruent with the values of the older adult (Foley, 2019). We can use the reminders of our own mortality as motivation to live the best we can with the time we have. Nurses can

seek support and give it to one another. As grievers, we too may need to tell the story of the dying, or the person, to those professionals around us, either in formal or in informal support groups; and we must listen to the stories of our colleagues over and over again until they also become part of the fabric of our colleagues' lives.

Caring for older adults requires knowledge of the grieving and dying processes as well as skills in providing symptom relief, i.e., palliative care (Table 28.1). However, it is also acknowledged that constantly working with the grieving or dying is an art. The development of the art calls for inner strength and personal

TABLE 28.1   Best Nursing Practice: Signs and Symptoms of Approaching Death

Physical	Rationale	Intervention
Coolness	Diminished peripheral circulation to increase circulation to vital organs	Socks, light cotton blankets or warm blankets if needed; do not use electric blanket
Increased sleeping	Conservation of energy	Respect need for increased rest; inquire as to patient's wishes regarding timing of companionship
Disorientation	Metabolic changes	Identify self by name before speaking to patient; speak normally, clearly, and truthfully
Fecal and/or urinary incontinence	Increased muscle relaxation	Change bedding as needed; use bed pads; avoid indwelling catheters
Noisy respirations	Poor circulation of body fluids, immobilization, and the inability to expectorate	Elevate the head with pillows, or raise the head of the bed, or both; gently turn the head to the side to drain
Restlessness	Metabolic changes and relative cerebral anoxia	Calm the patient by speech and action; reduce light; gently rub back, stroke arms, or read aloud; play soothing music; do not use restraints
Decreased intake of food and fluids	Body conservation of energy for function	Provide nutrition within limits expressed by patient or in advance directive; semisolid liquids easiest to swallow; protect mouth and lips from discomfort of dryness
Decreased urine output	Decreased fluid intake and decreased circulation to kidney	Explain to family that this is normal
Altered breathing pattern	Metabolic and oxygen changes	Elevate the head of bed; speak gently to patient
Emotional or Spiritual	**Presumed Rationale**	**Intervention**
Withdrawal	Prepares the patient for release and detachment and letting go	Continue communicating in a normal manner using a normal voice tone; identify self by name; give permission to let go
Vision-like experiences of dead friends or family; religious vision	Preparation for transition	Accept the reality of the experience for the person; reassure the person that the feeling is normal
Restlessness	Tension, fear, unfinished business	Listen to patient express their fears, sadness, and anger; facilitate completion of business if possible
Unusual communication	Signals readiness to let go	Say what needs to be said to the dying patient; kiss, hug, cry with him or her as appropriate

---

BOX 28.8 Nursing Skills Needed for Palliative Care

- Have ability to talk to patients and families about dying.
- Be knowledgeable about pain and symptom control.
- Have ability to provide comfort-oriented nursing interventions.
- Recognize physical changes that precede imminent death.
- Deal with own feelings.
- Deal with angry patients and families.
- Be knowledgeable and deal with the ethical issues in administering end-of-life palliative therapies.
- Be knowledgeable and inform patients about advance directives.
- Be knowledgeable of the legal issues in administering end-of-life palliative care.

Modified from White, K. R., Coyne, P. J., & Patel, U. B. (2001). Are nurses adequately prepared for end-of-life care? *J Nurs Scholarsh 33*,147–151.

---

coping skills (Box 28.8). The most important skills for nurses may be not only helping an older adult find meaning in their life as lived but also the nurse's ability to disengage emotionally after the death (Royal College of Nursing, 2016). The effective gerontological nurse has developed a personal philosophy of life and of death and of what each means. Although this can and does change over time, it will help when times are difficult. Emotional maturity allows the nurse to deal with disappointment and postponement of immediate needs or desires. Maturity means that the nurse can reach out for help when needed. Finally, to provide comfort to grieving persons, nurses must be comfortable with their own lives or at least be able to set aside their own sadness and grief while working with the sadness and grief of others.

Palliative Care

Gerontological nurses routinely care for older adults who have irreversible and progressive conditions, such as Alzheimer's disease and Parkinson's disease. Others have exhausted all treatment options for conditions such as cancer or heart disease. A nursing home resident may elect to remain at a care facility rather than return (ever) to a hospital, even if faced with an acute event such as a stroke or the more protracted end-stage heart disease. These elders are receiving a type of care called *palliative care*—with the goal of comfort rather than cure, the treatment of symptoms rather than disease, and the *quality* of life left rather than the *quantity* of life remaining (Aina & Kelsey, 2018). Nurses function in a variety of roles in the provision of palliative care: as a staff nurse giving direct care, as a coordinator implementing the plan of the interdisciplinary team, as

an executive officer responsible for clinical care, or as an advocate for humane care for persons who are dying and their families.

Nurses have also been involved in the establishment of programs such as the POLST (Physician Orders for Life-Sustaining Treatment) program. Originating in Oregon in the 1990s, the POLST program supports effective communication of patient desires and respect for these wishes in end-of-life care (https://polst.org). Master's degrees and national certifications in palliative care are now available from a number of organizations and schools.

Actions associated with palliative care can be provided anywhere by anyone sharing these goals and skills. It can even be provided at the same time a person is receiving curative care for something else, such as receiving treatment for a bladder infection while terminally ill with heart disease (Batchelor, 2010). Palliative care affirms life, regards dying as a normal process, and neither hastens nor postpones death (World Health Organization [WHO], 2020). Good end-of-life care should focus more on what we as nurses provide than what we forgo.

The scope and specialty of palliative care has grown considerably over the years; research has been conducted, professional organizations have been formed, and standardized curricula have been developed. With the support of the American Association of Colleges of Nursing and City of Hope Medical Center, a broad initiative (ANA-ELNEC) was organized in 1999, "Dedicated to Educating Nurses in Excellent Palliative Care" (https://www.aacnnursing.org/ELNEC). It is hoped that by training nurses and faculty, nursing as a profession can provide the highest level of palliative care. Whereas initially palliative care was the specialty of community-based organizations referred to as hospices, specialized units and staff are now seen in many long-term care and acute care facilities.

Hospice

The term *hospice* refers to a formalized structure from which a significant amount of the palliative care is delivered with a focus on pain and symptom control. It derives its meaning from the medieval concept of hospitality in which a community assisted a traveler at dangerous points along their journey. The dying are indeed travelers along the continuum of life within a community consisting of friends, family, and specially prepared people to care, that is, the hospice/palliative care team.

The concept of the contemporary hospice was made famous by Dr. Cicely Saunders, founder of Saint Christopher's Hospice in London in 1967. In 1974, Dr. Florence Wald (Dean of the College of Nursing at Yale), two pediatricians, and a chaplain brought the hospice concept to the United States when they established the Connecticut Hospice in Branford, Connecticut.

Both for-profit and not-for-profit hospice organizations are now in many locations in the United States and provide comprehensive and interdisciplinary care to persons assessed to be in the last 6 months of life. A hospice organization is expected to provide medical, nursing, nursing assistant, chaplain, social work, and volunteer support 24 hours per day if needed. Other services may include massage, music, art, and pet therapy. Hospices provide care not only to the dying but also to the dying person's families and friends through support before and after the death of loved ones.

The majority of hospice care occurs at home. The home becomes the primary center of care, provided by family members or friends who are taught basic nursing skills and how to administer the medications needed to ensure their loved one remains comfortable. A growing number of inpatient hospice facilities exist for those with symptoms that cannot be managed at home or those without caregivers, or to provide short periods of rest from caring (respite) for the caregivers. They are not usually intended for long-term stays. These may be associated with a community hospice program—freestanding or small units within other types of care facilities. Hospice nurses and others may also see patients who are residents in assisted living facilities and nursing homes. The nurses provide education and consultation regarding symptom management to facility staff and at times provide supplemental care. Special units in acute care hospitals may also provide palliative care services guided by traditional hospice principles. Pain control and the opportunity to die at home are the key principles that people associate with hospice services. Yet, hospice represents much more. The staff support and guide the family in personal care and ensures that the person will not die alone and that the family will not be abandoned. Bereavement services for the family extend for a period of time on an emergency and regular basis after the death of the patient. In contrast to palliative care, hospice services are limited to the time when a person's life expectancy is anticipated to be 6 months or less.

DECISION-MAKING AT THE END OF LIFE

Decision-making at the end of life has become a legal, ethical, medical, and personal concern. The lines between living and dying are blurred as a result of technology now available. This results in ambivalence concerning whether death is to be delayed and for how long and under what circumstances. Decisions need to be made if death is to be artificially delayed and is only acceptable when aggressive medical procedures (e.g., intubation) are no longer effective or if what is referred to as a "natural death" can occur without the use of death-delaying actions.

The issue of who has the authority to make end-of-life decisions and for whom has been the subject of research, debate, and, in the United States, federal legislation. An adult who has not been adjudicated to lack capacity (see Chapter 7) is recognized as the final decision-maker; however, this assumption is based on a very Euro-American or Western perspective. Persons who are from non-Western traditions place less emphasis on the individual and more on the needs of the family or community (see Chapter 3) (Mazanec & Tyler, 2003). Nurses have an obligation to know the legal requirements in their jurisdictions and then work with the older adult and the family to determine how the local laws can fit with their cultural patterns and needs related to end-of-life decisions.

Advance Directives

Whereas people have always had opinions about which medical care and procedures they would or would not want, their right to refuse medical treatment was not established in the United States until 1990 by the Patient Self-Determination Act (PSDA) and implemented in all states in 1991. Under the PSDA, the adult with capacity (Chapter 7) was recognized as the ultimate authority to accept or forego death-delaying treatment. Through the legislation related to the PSDA, adults were granted the legal authority to complete what are known as advance health care directives (AHCDs)—or statements about their wishes and directions to others before the need for a decision arises. These directives may be as vague as "no treatment if I am terminally ill" to as detailed as a breakdown of decisions about dialysis, antibiotics, tube feedings, cardiopulmonary resuscitation (CPR), and so on. The AHCD also provides a mechanism for an adult to appoint another adult (a proxy or surrogate) of their choosing to make decisions if they are no longer able to do so (see Chapter 7).

The common forms of advance directives are known as living wills, durable powers of attorney for health care (DPAHC), and medical powers of attorney (see Chapter 7) (Gittler, 2011). A living will is usually restricted to represent a person's wishes specific to a terminal illness. In contrast, a person appointed in a DPAHC can speak for the other in most or all matters of health care. In some states, advance directives are legally binding documents that nurses, physicians, and health care institutions are required to respect. Both the proxy and the health care surrogate are expected to use what is known as *substituted judgment,* that is, a decision the person would make if able to do so. This may include turning off a ventilator, turning off tube feedings, or stopping intravenous fluids and allowing natural deaths.

All agencies in the United States that receive Medicare and Medicaid funds are required to disseminate PSDA information to their patients and inquire as to the existence of advance directives. Hospitals and long-term care facilities are responsible for providing written information at the time of admission about the individual's rights under law both to refuse medical and surgical care and to provide this decision in writing and in advance. Health maintenance organizations (HMOs) are required to do the same at the time of member enrollment as are home health agencies as the patient comes under the care of the agency. Hospices are obliged to inform patients of their rights on the initial visit. Providers (physicians and nurse practitioners) are encouraged but are not under legal obligation to provide this same information to their patients, although a health care visit for the sole purpose of a discussion of advance planning is now covered (paid for) by Medicare.

Although the exact format and signature (e.g., notarization) requirements vary from state to state, the PSDA is a federal mandate and applies to persons in all jurisdictions. There are multiple sources of related information available on the Internet.

Nurses cannot provide legal information but do have a responsibility to serve as a resource person ready to answer basic questions people have about end-of-life decision-making. A nurse may be called upon to determine the cultural barriers to completing advance directives (Box 28.9). A nurse is often the person who asks about the presence of an existing advance directive such as a living will, ensures that it still reflects the person's wishes, advocates that the wishes are followed, and makes sure that existing or newly created advance directives are available in the appropriate locations in the medical record.

Euthanasia, Assisted Suicide, and Aid-in-Dying

The recognition of the right to refuse life-sustaining medical treatment renewed age-old questions over persons' rights to make their own decisions regarding the continuation of their natural lives. Some people, especially those who are suffering from a terminal illness, have ended their lives. Others have asked for assistance in accomplishing this in the most painless way possible. Many gerontological nurses are among those who have been asked (Box 28.10).

Euthanasia, physician-assisted suicide, and *physician aid-in-dying* are the phrases most commonly heard in discussions around this topic today. "…Euthanasia… occurs when someone other than the patient administers medication with the intention of hastening death" (ANA, 2019)." In both physician-assisted suicide and physician aid-in-dying, the patient is given the means to end their life (usually in the form of access to a lethal dose of medications) and instructions on the safe way to do this on their own, when and if they choose.

The potential for a person's ultimate control of their dying has risen to state and Supreme Court levels in the United States and to equivalent levels in other countries. In 1994 and again in 1997, voters in Oregon were the first to pass legislation legalizing a person's right to end their life in very specific circumstances. The voters in Washington State passed similar legislation in 2008 with identical restrictions. Vermont, Hawaii, Colorado, California, New Jersey, Maine, and the District of Columbia followed. Montana and California courts ruled that there was nothing in the state law prohibiting physician-assisted suicide, but no definitive laws have been passed (Death with Dignity, 2020).

Physician-assisted suicide is legal in Belgium, Canada, The Netherlands, Switzerland, Luxemburg, Australia (state of Victoria only), Sweden, and Colombia. Only The

---

BOX 28.9   Cultural Barriers to the Use of Advance Directives and Hospice

- Distrust of the health care system (especially in groups who have experienced violence or discrimination in the United States or their country of origin)
- Collectivism: Family rather than individual is "decision-maker"
- Preference for physician, as expert, to make the decision
- Taboo to talk about death or dying
- Influence of faith and spirituality: Illness as a test of faith
- Belief that life is a gift from God that must be protected
- Death as a part of the cycle of life and must not be disturbed
- Dying away from home may lead to a disturbance of the spirits
- Cannot die at home because the spirit will linger

From Coolen, P. R. (2012). Cultural relevance in end-of-life care. *EthnoMed,* May 1. https://ethnomed.org/clinical/end-of-life/cultural-relevance-in-end-of-life-care.

BOX 28.10   Can I Help You?

One day when checking on a woman with end-stage pulmonary disease, I asked, "Is there anything I can do for you?" She responded quickly asking if I knew how she could reach Dr. Kevorkian, a physician who had been known for assisting people commit suicide long before the physician-assisted suicide was even discussed. I knew that I had to be much more proactive in finding ways to make her more comfortable while she waited to die.

Kathleen Jett at 40

Netherlands, Colombia, Canada, Luxemburg, South Korea, and several other countries permit some type of active euthanasia. In most cases the person much be experiencing "unbearable suffering" to be eligible and in all cases very strict criteria must be met. The status of any one state or country is subject to change. The number of people who have chosen this route to end their suffering have been relatively few (My Death My Decision, 2018).

As the ethical questions surrounding end-of-life issues become increasingly complex, so do the questions regarding nurses' roles relative to these. Over the years, the American Nursing Association has developed several "Position Statements" that articulate professional expectations of American nurses and provide guidance related to the care they provide. The most recent, *The Nurse's Role When a Patient Requests Aid in Dying*, advises nurses to "remain objective when patients are exploring … end-of-life options" while reiterating that "euthanasia is … inconsistent with the core commitments of the nursing profession" (ANA, 2019). Individual statements include *The Ethical Responsibility to Manage Pain and the Suffering it Causes* (approved 2018), *Nurses Role and Responsibilities in Providing Care and Support at the End of Life* (approved 2016), and *Nursing Care and Do Not Resuscitate (DNR) and Allow Natural Death (AND) Decisions* (revised 2012). In all cases nurses are expected to strive to understand the desires of the patient, to explain the options available to the patient, and to provide the highest level of care needed to achieve comfort. It is recommended that the term "allow a natural death" instead of "do not resuscitate" be used because of vagueness of the latter term and the negative connotations that have been attributed to it (i.e., "doing nothing").

Palliative Sedation

Although the purpose of palliative nursing care is always to promote comfort and alleviate intractable suffering, there are times when this seems impossible. For some, refractory and unendurable symptoms cannot be controlled as death draws near. As far back as 1997, the US Supreme Court declared that although euthanasia was always illegal, pharmacological sedation for the relief of refractory symptoms (e.g., pain, nausea and vomiting, dyspnea) by whatever means necessary was acceptable even if death is a "side-effect" of the treatment, as long as the *intention* was not to hasten death. This has been referred to as *terminal sedation* but is more accurately *palliative sedation* (Cherny et al., 2020) (Box 28.11).

Palliative sedation is the controlled and carefully monitored use of medications to lower the patient's level of consciousness to the extent necessary to achieve

---

BOX 28.11 Providing Comfort in the Final Moments of a Natural Life: Palliative Sedation

A physician friend came to work one morning looking like he had not slept in days and was on the edge of tears. I knew that his dearest friend Mark, another physician, had been suffering greatly with end-stage cancer. I just sat quietly next to my friend until he was ready to tell me his story. Finally, sobbing he described sitting with his friend the last few days as his friend begged him to "do something, anything to stop the pain." I knew that they had not been able to make him comfortable. "I had to do something!" He began to give his friend sedatives slowly but steadily until at last he was able to quit trashing and crying but was still breathing. Whenever he began becoming uncomfortable, he received more medication. Several hours later Mark quietly died with his wife and best friend at his side.

---

comfort. The *intention* of palliative sedation is only for comfort and is considered neither euthanasia nor physician-assisted (or nurse-assisted) suicide. The ethical principles that support palliative sedation include the precepts of dignity, respect for autonomy, beneficence, fidelity, nonmaleficence, and the principle of double effect, which evaluates an action based on intended outcome of comfort and not the relief of suffering through death. Palliative sedation is also replete with controversy because of the "slippery slope" between it and euthanasia.

Nurses have had strong opinions related to all aspects of end-of-life care, yet the profession's opposition to nurse participation in euthanasia does not negate the obligation of the nurse to provide compassionate, ethically justified end-of-life care that includes actions that result in comfort, the alleviation of suffering, and the provision of adequate pain control. If a nurse is not able to do this, it is expected that an alternate person be assigned (ANA, 2019).

KEY CONCEPTS

- Loss occurs within a system consisting of the individual who has experienced the loss and their significant others. Loss includes the death of a member of the system.
- Grief is an emotional reaction and strongly influenced by the type of loss, the individual's ability to cope, and the system's ability to address ensuing chaos.
- Nursing actions that help persons who are dealing with loss are part of the daily work of the gerontological nurse.

- A dying older adult is a person with all the same needs as others for good and natural relationships with people.
- The desired outcome of palliative care is always comfort .
- Advance directives (including living wills) allow an individual control over life and death decisions by written communication and the appointment of a person (a proxy) to be an advocate when they are no longer able to dictate their wishes.
- Physician aid-in-dying and euthanasia are very different concepts as defined by both the World Health Organization and the American Nurses Association and any number of other organizations.
- The purpose of palliative sedation is only to reduce the person's level of awareness to the point of symptom relief. It is never for the purpose of hastening death, even if this occurs as a result of the sedation.

ACTIVITIES AND DISCUSSION QUESTIONS

1. Explore your response to being given a terminal diagnosis. What coping mechanisms work for you? With which awareness approach would you be comfortable?
2. Describe the priority nursing actions related to a dying person and their family when they are especially protective of one another.
3. Describe and strategize how you would bring up the topic of advance directives.
4. What advance directive related to end of life is legally recognized in your state?
5. Describe how you would introduce the topic of dying with a patient who is critically ill and not expected to live.

NEXT-GENERATION NCLEX® EXAMINATION-STYLE QUESTIONS

Mrs. Arroyo, 78 years old, is in a hospice for end-stage dementia. She lies in bed curled in the fetal position. She is on a pureed diet with nectar thick liquids. Over the last year, she has been treated for aspiration pneumonia four times. Her weight is steadily declining. Six months ago, she weighed 115 pounds (BMI 18.56 kg/m²) and yesterday she weighed 103.5 pounds (BMI 16.70 kg/m²). Her vital signs are 88/44 mmHg, heart rate of 60 beats per minute, respiration rate of 10 breaths per minute and irregular, and her temperature is 94.2°F. Her albumin level is 2.2 g/L. Over the last day, the nurse has

documented the presence of a stage 2 pressure injury measuring 5 mm × 2.5 mm × 2 mm on Mrs. Arroyo's coccyx; the wound base is pale. Her skin is cool to touch and purplish on hands and feet. She had one wet under pad in the last 24 hours. She is occasionally restlessness but is not responding to stimuli and is no longer eating or drinking. The nurse has called the family to come to the bedside, telling them death is approaching.

To facilitate a good death, which nursing actions should be implemented? (Select all that apply).
1. Offer small, spicy snacks to stimulate the client's appetite.
2. Provide a warm cotton blanket.
3. Start an IV of normal saline to prevent dehydration.
4. Identify self and speak softly when providing care.
5. Reduce environmental stimuli.
6. Encourage the family to talk to the client and give them permission to die.
7. Insert a foley catheter to control incontinence.
8. Use an electric blanket to keep the client warm.

REFERENCES

Aina, F., & Kelsey, B. (2018). Demystifying palliative and hospice care. *American Nurse Today*, January 3. https://www.americannursetoday .com/demystifying-palliative-hospice-care/.

Alward, P. D. (2010). Betty Newman's system model. In M. E. Parker, & M. C. Smith (Eds.), *Nursing theories and nursing practice* (3rd ed., pp. 182–201). Philadelphia: FA Davis.

American Nurses Association (ANA). (2019). *ANA advises objectivity in new medical aid in dying position*, June 26. https://www .nursingworld.org/news/news-releases/2019-news-releases /ana-advises-objectivity-in-new-medical-aid-in-dying-position/.

Batchelor, N. H. (2010). Palliative or hospice care? Understanding the similarities and differences. *Rehabil Nurs, 35*(2), 60–64.

Burns, V. F., Sussman, T., & Bourgeois-Guerin, V. (2018). Later-life homelessness as disenfranchised grief. *Can J Aging, 37*(2), 171–184.

Capel, M. M. (2017). Palliative medicine in older patients. In H. M. Fillit, K. Rockwood, & J. Young (Eds.), *Brocklehurst's textbook of geriatric medicine and gerontology* (8th ed., pp. 953–962). Philadelphia: Elsevier.

Carr, D., Sonnega, J., Nesse, R. M., et al. (2014). Do special occasions trigger psychological distress among older bereaved spouses? An empirical assessment of clinical wisdom. *J Gerontol B Psychol Sci Soc Sci, 69*(1), 113–122.

Cherny, N., Smith, T. J., & Savarese, D. M. F. (2020). *Palliative sedation*. https://www.uptodate.com/contents/palliative-sedation.

Clark, R. (2019). Letting go: the role of the nurse during death and dying. *JGN, 45*(9), 2–3.

Coelho, A., & Barbosa, A. (2017). Family anticipatory grief: An integrative literature review. *Am J Hosp Palliat Care, 34*(8), 774–785.

Corr, C. A., Nabe, C. M., & Corr, D. M. (2000). *Death and dying, life and living* (ed. 3). Stamford City, CT: Wadsworth.

Death with Dignity. *In your state*. June 23. https://www.deathwithdignity .org/take-action.

Doka, K. J. (2002). *Disenfranchised grief: New direction, challenges, and strategies for practice*. Champaign, IL: Research Press.

Foley, L. M. (2019). Improving end-of-life care for hospitalized older adults. *JGN, 45*(7), 2–4.

Gerdner, L. A., Yang, D, Cha, D, et al. (2007). The circle of life. *J Gerontol Nurs, 33*(5), 20–31.

Giacquinta, B. (1977). Helping families face the crisis of cancer. *Am J Nurs, 77*(10), 1585–1588.

Gire, J. (2014). How death imitates life: Cultural influences on conceptions of death and dying. *Online Readings in Psychology and Culture, 6*(2). https://scholarworks.gvsu.edu/cgi/viewcontent.cgi?article=1120&context=orpc.

Gittler, J. (2011). Advance care planning and surrogate health care decision making for older adults. *J Geriatr Nurs, 37*(5), 15–19.

Glaser, B. G., & Strauss, A. L. (1963). *Awareness of dying.* Chicago: Aldine.

Glaser, B. G., & Strauss, A. L. (1968). *Time for dying.* Chicago: Aldine.

Hall, C. (2011). Beyond Kübler-Ross: Recent developments in our understanding of grief and bereavement. *InPsych, 33*(6), 1–12.

Horacek, B. J. (1991). Toward a more viable model of grieving and consequences for older persons. *Death Stud, 15*, 459–472.

Kübler-Ross, E. (1969). *On death and dying.* New York: Macmillan.

Lathrop, D. (2017). Disenfranchised grief and physician burnout. *Ann Fam Med, 15*(4), 375–378.

Maccallum, F., & Bryant, R. A. (2011). Imagining the future in complicated grief. *Depress Anxiety, 28*(8), 658–665.

Mazanec, P., & Tyler, M. K. (2003). Cultural considerations in end-of-life care: How ethnicity, age and spirituality affect decisions when death is imminent. *Am J Nurs, 103*(3), 50–59.

My Death My Decision. (2018). *Assisted dying in other countries.* www.mydeath-mydecision.org.uk/info/assisted-dying-in-other-countries.

Mohlman, W., L., Dassel, K., & Supiano, K. P (2018). End-of-life education and discussions with assisted living certified nursing assistants. *JGN, 44*(6), 41–48.

Nakajima, S. (2018). Complicated grief: recent developments in diagnostic criteria and treatment. *Philos Trans R Soc London B Biol Sci, 373*, 1–10. https://www.ncbi.nlm.nih.gov/pmc/articles/PMC6053994/.

National Cancer Institute. (2020). *Grief, bereavement and coping with loss (PDQ) – Health professional version.* https://www.cancer.gov/about-cancer/advanced-cancer/caregivers/planning/bereavement-hp-pdq#_106.

Neimeyer, R. A., Sands, D. C., et al. (2011). Meaning reconstruction in bereavement: From principles to practice. In R. A. Neimeyer, D. L. Harris, & H. R. Winokuer, et al. (Eds.), *Grief and bereavement in contemporary society: Bridging research and practice.* New York: Routledge.

Pattison, E. M. (Ed.). (1977). *The experience of dying.* Englewood Cliffs, NJ: Prentice-Hall.

Paun, O., & Farran, C. J. (2011). Chronic grief management for dementia caregivers in transition. *JGN, 37*(12), 28–35.

Rando, T. A. (1995). Grief and mourning: Accommodating to loss. In H. Wass, & R. A. Neimyer (Eds.), *Dying—Facing the facts* (pp. 211–241). Philadelphia: Taylor & Francis.

Richardson, V. E., Bennett, K. M., Carr, D., et al. (2013). How does bereavement get under the skin? The effects of late-life spousal loss on cortisol levels. *J Gerontol B Psychol Sci Soc Sci, 70*(3), 341–347.

Royal College of Nursing: *Roles and responsibilities* (2016). https://rcni.com/hosted-content/rcn/fundamentals-of-end-of-life-care/roles-and-responsibilities.

Sveen, C. A., & Walby, F. A. (2008). Suicide survivors' mental health and grief reactions: A systematic review of controlled studies. *Suicide Life Threat Behav, 38*(1), 13–29.

Weisman, A. (1979). *Coping with cancer.* New York: McGraw-Hill.

Weisman, A. (1984). *The coping capacity: On the nature of being mortal.* New York: Human Sciences Press.

World Health Organization (WHO). (2020). WHO definition of palliative care. Available at http://www.who.int/cancer/palliative/definition/en.

Figure numbers followed by *b, f,* and *t* indicate boxes, figures, and tables, respectively.